Chronic
PAIN

Assessment, Diagnosis, and Management

Edited by

Michael S. Margoles, M.D., PH.D.

and

Richard Weiner, PH.D.

CRC Press
Boca Raton   London   New York   Washington, D.C.

Library of Congress Cataloging-in-Publication Data

Catalog information may be obtained from the Library of Congress

Table of Contents

Foreword

Anyone who has driven an automobile or watched the old comedies of the 1930s has felt the fear of the driver in the movie whose steering wheel becomes detached while the car is careening down a hill. It is not a feeling of excitement; it is a fearful feeling of loss of control. Happily, in the movies, the protagonist is always saved from disaster; however, the viewer is usually struck by the utter impossibility of a satisfactory ending to such a situation. The scenario does serve a purpose for modern-day clinicians. It serves as an analogy of what the chronic pain patient is perceiving.

All too often, chronic pain patients find themselves watching helplessly as their pain wrestles the steering wheel from their hands. Where once they felt themselves in control of their lives and the direction of their lives, now they have surrendered the direction of their lives to their pain. They have lost control — control of their immediate and ultimate destiny. Their pain tells them when they can sleep, when they will awaken, how long they can walk, how long they can sit, when they can work, and when they can have a satisfactory relationship with their loved ones. The pain may have started as a helpful warning signal of an organic problem that required medical attention, but it becomes a nagging impediment to all of the activities of daily living. Pain — chronic, debilitating pain — has taken the driver's seat.

Eighty percent of chronic pain patients develop depression secondary to their pain. Infrequently, depression is manifested as pain. Together, these two etiologies result in two problems — chronic pain followed by chronic pain and depression, or depression followed by depression and chronic pain — that affect as many as 85–90% of all chronic pain patients. While the degree of depression is as variable as the intensity of pain, the clinician is challenged with developing a measured, dual therapeutic approach to what has been called the chronic pain–depression complex.

The magnitude of the challenge that chronic pain has brought to Western medicine is evident when the extent of the public's turn to alternative care is considered. Americans are turning to alternative medical care in record numbers, and alternative medical care is now a $27 billion industry. We know that the public is very cautious with its health care dollar; therefore the public's commitment to alternative medical care is quite telling. And what does this tell us? It tells us that people's medical problems are not always satisfactorily resolved with traditional Western (allopathic) medicine, and chronic pain management is one of the major reasons for patients' feelings of dissatisfaction. Simply stated, if individuals with chronic pain complaints were being cared for adequately — even if they remained in some degree of pain but could foresee an eventual resolution to their disabling discomfort — they would have little need to seek out alternative medical care, including chiropractic, herbal medicine, homeopathy, biofeedback, acupuncture, acupressure, massage therapy, reflexology, and the like. It is the traditional medical approach itself that is driving patients to seek help elsewhere. Too many clinicians feel that if the "organic reason" for pain symptoms cannot be documented with the usual medical tools, such as MRIs and X-rays, then the pain cannot be "real," and clinicians do not feel their time is well spent if they are treating perceived "unreal" conditions. No wonder chronic pain patients feel abandoned.

To complicate matters further, almost all chronic pain patients do not "get well" in the sense that other patients with self-limited conditions recover. Rather, chronic pain patients "learn to cope," "resume work," and "manage their pain" with the help of competent medical and psychosocial assistance. But for many clinicians, this is not winning, and Americans love to win. Perhaps that is why medical disciplines such as pediatrics, orthopedic surgery, and cardiology are much more popular than geriatrics and pain management. A clinician perceives himself as a "winner" when he cures an infant of colic, surgically repairs a broken bone, or replaces a damaged heart valve. It is much more difficult to perceive oneself a "winner" when working with patients whose medical outcome is, at best, management of a problem or keeping a problem in check. This principle notwithstanding, thankfully, a few dedicated clinicians have chosen the less traveled path.

A salient characteristic of dedicated clinicians is their ability to learn as well as to teach. Dr. Michael Margoles epitomizes this characteristic. His daily practice is one of both teaching his patients as well as learning from them the nature of pain. Too many clinicians feel they understand pain as a symptom. Their knowledge and understanding of the problem, I suggest, fall short. Pain is a symptom, but it is also a medical condition in and of itself. Its nature, its manifestation, and its results are so complex that clinicians will practice a lifetime and still not fully understand it. This is why it is essential that clinicians assume roles as listeners as well as caregivers.

In this book, Dr. Margoles carefully focuses on what every chronic pain patient should know about his or her pain and the therapeutic approach to the management of that pain. What he teaches in this book is the lessons he only began to learn in medical school. He has woven into his teachings what he has learned, and continues to learn, from his patients. He is a listener who has gained significant insight into the modern pain phenomenon through his patients. While clearly his lessons are intended for people in pain and the families of individuals in pain, clinicians would do well to learn from these lessons also.

Chronic pain affects every aspect of life. It affects physical well-being, mood, nutrition, stamina, and feelings of self-worth and self-respect. Chronic pain affects not only the family member afflicted, but also affects the family unit itself. It must be carefully managed to minimize the trauma to the patient and to preserve the relationships within the family that make living a precious and rewarding endeavor. Chronic pain is the perfect affliction for the patient who wishes someone else, usually the physician, to attend to the cure without the patient's active involvement in the treatment plan, for surely chronic pain will continue in perpetuity for such an individual. But for the patient who wishes to learn, to understand, and to participate actively in the management of the problem, chronic pain can be conquered.

Robert B. Supernaw, Pharm.D.
Professor and Dean
University of the Pacific School of Pharmacy
Stockton, California

Prologue

Where there is no vision the people perish;
they are destroyed for lack of knowledge.

The Bible

Based on 21 years of experience with chronic pain patients, it is my opinion that most chronic pain and its victims are not being understood. This occurs with the medical profession, attorneys, insurance companies, government agencies, and more. The intent of this book is to supply answers that may help chronic intractable pain patients and, most importantly, may save lives.

This book is a compilation of works from authors in the field of pain management plus relevant contributions from patients. Each professional author selected to write in this book was asked to do so because he or she person has recognized expertise in the field of pain management.

Preface

Chronic pain is not a simple problem; there are no easy answers; this book does not have a simple message, but it does contain answers for those who are earnestly looking for them.

"Chronic pain has become America's most common, expensive, and debilitating disorder, yet many doctors and chronic pain sufferers know surprisingly little about the causes of pain and the wide variety of treatments that are available today" (Bresler and Turbo, 1979). This statement was made on the cover leaflet of a book written in 1979, and is still unfortunately true today.

The singular theme of this book, that runs from cover to cover, is conquering pain, and its related problems, through proper management. We are not marketing one idea of how to deal with pain, but rather relating numerous tools and concepts with which to attack chronic pain. Almost every specialty in the field of health care professionals has representation in the field of pain management.

Resolving chronic pain is not a simple problem. It is a serious, multifaceted illness. It can deeply affect you, your friends, your marriage, your family, and your job. Chronic pain is a problem of major proportion. Its diagnosis and treatment can frustrate patient and physician alike. In the United States, an estimated 35–40 million people suffer from chronic pain and more than 10 million of these are partially or totally disabled because of the pain. Many of these pain problems are resistant to the strongest of analgesics (pain-killing medication) and may only respond slowly to prolonged administration (two years or more) of appropriate management.

Some individuals may find some of the chapters too detailed and complex. In that case, skim through those chapters and read the areas you can understand. You will probably locate the information that is of interest to you. If you think a particular section may relate to you but you cannot understand the material, take it to a medical professional and ask him or her to explain it to you.

Currently, many medical doctors and therapists throughout the Western world believe that chronic pain is produced by something other than a physical abnormality. You may feel that something is really wrong with you, but your point of view is frequently cast aside for a model of chronic pain that is caused by "excessive psychological stress" (Bresler, 1979), "a supposed but unidentified and possibly nonexistent nociceptive (pain receiver) source" (Waddel, 1987), or a "dysthymic" (due to depression) pain disorder. You may be told, "There's nothing really wrong with you" or, worse, "The pain is all in your head" and "You'll just have to learn to live with it." Many chronic pain patients fail to respond to conventional treatment. They do not fit the usual acute patient model and they don't fit into the usual treatment plan. And so they may be labeled as having a purely emotional or "hysterical" problem.

The presence of pain may mean disease (i.e., myofascial pain syndrome, fibromyalgia, etc.), but it does not always mean tissue damage.

The authors of this book believe that all pain is real. And, it is what the patient says it is. If the pain is of a real nature, it is treated with physical approaches. If the pain is produced by the mind (psychogenic), it is treated with behavioral (psychological) methods (modalities). We believe that all chronic pain is a mixture of real (organic) and psychogenic (emotional) components.

Patients with chronic pain have frequently been rejected by the medical profession because of the complexity of their problems. A case history or narrative summary of one of the more complex patients, if properly prepared, will usually read like a condensed version of the *Merck Manual* (a medical reference book for the lay public), and that is a frightening reality to face.

Patients may see many doctors before seeing a pain therapist. They bounce from doctor to doctor with no one physician directing their course. After a routine quick exam and review of X-rays are found to be negative, they might be told: "It's all in your head," or "You should be feeling fine by now," or "You'll have to learn to live with it!" This type of thinking severely limits the physician's vision and the patient's hope of getting well.

If your doctor chooses to tell you "You're going to have to learn to live with it," what are you supposed to do? What are your options? Most people try another doctor. But what if that doctor tries the same treatment and you don't get better? Who do you go to then? Who will believe your pain is real?

One of the greatest problems facing chronic pain patients as they look for help is "selective perception." The most common example of this occurs after a patient relates his or her history and problem to a physician. He or she tells the doctor the pain is in the low back and the neck. At the finish of the whole evaluation, the doctor says "We need to do some studies, X-rays, MRI, and a scan on your low back pain problem." The patient tries to say, "But what about my neck pain?" The doctor says, "Take this ibuprofen and I will see you back in three weeks." We believe we have tried to remedy some of that problem in this book. What has been written in this book is aimed at the totality of your problems. While it won't get rid of the selective perception you may encounter in your physician's office, we hope it will address your concerns about multifocal (multiple areas) pain problems. If you are looking for a therapist with a "multifocal" emphasis, we suggest you contact the American Academy of Pain Management (13947 Mono Way, #A, Sonora, CA 95370, phone 209-533-9744).

At present, many therapies used in the treatment of chronic pain attempt to:

1. Apply some type of therapy externally (a balm, heat, ice)
2. Change the way you view your pain
   a. Psychotherapy
   b. Behavior modification
   c. Cognitive therapy
   d. Stress reduction
3. Work it out with physical therapy and exercises
4. Put over-the-counter or prescription medications into your system to relieve the pain, stress, or insomnia problem
5. Cut the pain out with surgery

All the above concepts are addressed in this book. It also addresses the balance or imbalance of your whole self and some of what is actually gone wrong inside of you (what is chemically out of balance inside). This will be covered in the numerous chapters relating to the use of diet, vitamins, minerals, and hormones that are crucial to getting the chronic pain patient to respond to the other therapies listed above. These commonly overlooked problems, if properly addressed, can spell a significant difference between chronic pain patients who get well and those who do not.

Many authorities in the medical field think of acute pain as having to do with something physically being wrong with you (broken bone, ruptured disc, etc.), but chronic pain is viewed as something psychologically wrong with you. In the chronic model many therapists say, "Just get a handle on your mind and/or your stress, and you can lick your pain problem." Before long, you and your family begin to think that there can't be anything really wrong, and your pain problem must be all in your head.

Some people lose faith because of the "it's all in your head model" of chronic pain, and suicide begins to look like a solution to their problems. But hold on! There are some real ways to understand what chronic pain really is, and this is what the authors of this book will relate.

With respect to acute pain, there is usually only one basis of thinking that is used to explain the pain problem. For example, in a ruptured disc problem, the basis of thinking is purely mechanical, with the ruptured disc pressing on a nerve root and causing the pain, numbness, and weakness problems.

However, in chronic pain there are usually a minimum of three concepts that explain the pain problem, and that is what makes it appear to be difficult. For example, concepts that might explain a person's chronic pain problem might be:

1. Pain in the muscles for low back and leg pain
2. Vitamin, mineral, and hormonal problems to account for decreased energy and stamina
3. Emotional problems that account for feelings of hopelessness and despair that accompany the chronic pain

All these concepts are explained and outlined in Chapter 2.

Expert opinions vary about the origin and timing of the events in persons afflicted by chronic pain. For example, some authorities believe psychological problems cause the pain, and others say the psychological problems are caused by the pain.

The purpose of this book is to promote understanding of the many problems and numerous needs of the chronic pain patient. We hope this book will serve as a valuable resource to chronic pain patients who are seeking solutions to their problems. These needs encompass many of the body's systems and frequently require more than one therapist to manage all the areas of involvement.

The emphasis of this material is to teach you an understanding of the many features (facets) of your chronic pain problem. The chapters do not run in a continuous fashion. Each section stands alone and may deal with an entirely different subject than the section before it.

Another goal is to either enhance your present treatment or to offer you ideas of what to look for in a program that treats chronic pain patients. It is not our intent to do away with the need for professional help in the treatment of your pain problem, but to offer you additional helpful advice from knowledgeable professionals who are familiar with the management of patients with chronic pain. The relationship that you have with your treating therapist is a special one, and we do not intend to interfere with that. You may want to discuss some of our ideas and concepts with your treating professional.

Much of what we have written is self-help techniques that may be useful in helping you control your pain and related disability.

"Every patient's situation is different, so there can be no universal cure-all for every kind of pain" (Bresler, 1979). The team approach is vital for the welfare of the patient and therapist.

Treatment of a chronic pain patient is somewhat like a progressive dinner. You get this treatment at this office or station, that treatment at that office or station, and so on. It is all part of the team effort to combine multiple specialists, of varying training and talents, to tackle a multifaceted problem. It is difficult to get definitive treatment from one source. However, for some patients, all the "courses" of the "dinner" aren't prepared yet. For those patients, the medical field has to evolve a bit more before definite treatment can be offered. Even if your pain problem has no definite treatment, your physician and you can agree to treat some of the pain symptoms while you are waiting for more definitive treatment to arrive in the pain management field. This will allow you to get on with your life.

While many of the authors present material that has gained acceptance for the treatment of chronic pain patients, some present material that is gaining acceptance.

Lastly, our hope is that this book will add to the many pieces of literature that are pushing the frontiers of chronic pain treatment forward. We hope this book will spell out more encouragement for those chronic pain patients who currently have none.

Michael S. Margoles, M.D., Ph.D.
Richard S. Weiner, Ph.D.

References

Bresler, D. and Turbo, R. (1979). *Free Yourself from Pain,* Simon and Schuster, New York.
Waddel, G. (1987). A new clinical model for the treatment of low-back pain, *Spine,* 12, 632.

The Editors

Michael S. Margoles, M.D., Ph.D., is an orthopedic surgeon and pain management specialist. He is in private practice in San Jose, California.

Dr. Margoles did his undergraduate work at San Jose State University and the University of California at Berkeley. He graduated from the University of California at Berkeley in 1965 with a degree in biochemistry. He obtained his M.D. degree from the University of California at Irvine in 1969. In 1974, he graduated, with honors, from the Orthopedic Institute of the Hospital for Joint Diseases and Medical Center, New York City.

In 1986, Dr. Margoles received an honorary Ph.D. for his work with chronic pain patients. Part of the honorary degree was based on his clinical use of colchicine in the treatment of some of his back and neck chronic pain patients who had disc disorders.

Dr. Margoles is board certified in orthopedic surgery and pain management. He is a member of the International Association for the Study of Pain and the American Pain Society, a Fellow of the American Academy of Neurological and Orthopedic Surgeons and the New York Academy of Sciences, and a charter member of the American Academy of Pain Management, the American Academy of Pain Medicine, and the National Chronic Pain Outreach Association.

Dr. Margoles has authored over 38 publications. He is a member of the editorial review boards of the *American Journal of Pain Management, Journal of Myofascial Medicine,* and *Journal of Neurological and Orthopedic Surgery.*

Richard S. Weiner, Ph.D., is executive director of the American Academy of Pain Management. He received a doctorate from the University of Delaware in urban affairs and public policy in 1981. He holds a master's degree in counseling and a bachelor of arts degree in psychology from the University of Delaware.

Dr. Weiner has been inducted into the John C. Liebeskind History of Pain Collection, UCLA Biomedical Library. He has served as a consultant in health care to the minister of health in several administrations. He has led and participated in numerous international medical exchange programs.

Dr. Weiner is the editor of *Pain Management: A Practical Guide for Clinicians* and *Innovations in Pain Management.* He has authored over 50 published articles on pain management and has lectured before multidisciplinary pain management professionals at many prestigious worldwide bodies. He has held various posts and chaired scientific committees regarding health care policy.

His important policy research interests include the relationship of pain to innovative treatment, coordinated multidisciplinary care, and measures of outcome.

Contributing Authors

Jay Bayer, D.O.

Beverly Breakey, R.N., C.M.T.

Geoffrey Brecher, D.C.

David A. Devine, Ph.D.

Lawrence A. Funt, D.D.S., M.S.D.

Joseph Lee, M.D.

Ronald J. Mackley, D.D.S., M.S.

Michael S. Margoles, M.D., Ph.D.

David D. Robinson, Ph.D.

Thomas Romano, M.D., Ph.D.

Harvey Rose, M.D.

Richard Weiner, Ph.D.

Dedication

This book is dedicated to all of our wonderful patients and to the patients who have not become aware that there is hope. We also wish to dedicate this work to our patients who have helped us realize what pain and suffering is all about. You have added greatly to our knowledge of the people we treat.

This book is dedicated to all those who suffer in silence, those who are waiting for hope, and those who have given up hope. Many have waited, and some have perished while waiting.

This book is dedicated to educating patients with chronic pain. It is dedicated to professionals who want to know more about chronic pain. This material has proved helpful in helping the authors and their patients attack the problem of chronic pain. The wheels of change move slowly, sometimes too slowly for some who wait or have waited.

Although this book offers much that is commonplace, it offers new dimensions of management for chronic pain that are just beginning to become commonplace in all the fields of health sciences represented in this book.

This book is dedicated to chronic pain patients who are looking for self-help that can be combined with the expertise of a qualified therapist or interdisciplinary team management program.

Because chronic pain is so complex, it takes years of research to discover what works and what does not. Studies in chronic pain are very difficult to conduct because it is a multifaceted problem.

This book is also dedicated to Janet G. Travell, M.D. (1901–1997) and David G. Simons, M.D. Their combined works, *Myofascial Pain and Dysfunction: The Trigger Point Manual,* Volumes 1 and 2, published in 1983 and 1992, represent the most significant breakthrough for the diagnosis and management of patients suffering chronic pain.

This work is also dedicated to those to who have fought with spouses, relatives, neighbors, employers, insurance companies, or government agencies, trying to get recognition for the disability caused by a pain problem. We hope you will find our work helpful.

This work is dedicated to the Lord with gratitude for all His inspiration.

Section I

Chronic Pain

1 I Am No Stranger to Pain

Michael S. Margoles, M.D., Ph.D.

JANUARY 30, 1991

I am now 48 years old and have been in pain for 35 years. When I was three years old, I accidentally opened the rear door of a moving car, fell to the curb, injured my head, and was in the hospital for a number of days with a concussion. When I was six, my mother hit the brakes too hard one day and I injured my head on the dashboard of our 1948 Buick; dashboards were not padded in those days. I grew up in the Midwest and enjoyed an active life of sports, including skating and football, among others. These were rugged sports and I frequently fell and/or was injured in skating and tobogganing. When I was eight, I was hospitalized at a university hospital for severe allergy problems. When I was ten, I was evaluated for thyroid abnormalities. The allergy testing resulted in some desensitization injections. The thyroid testing proved borderline and no treatment was undertaken. By the time I was 13, I was troubled with severe headaches at least once per week. My mother told me these were "sinus headaches." Sometimes they responded to aspirin and sometimes not. As I grew older, the frequency of the headaches increased. I played center on my high school football team, and by the time I got to college, I had so many aches and pains in my back that I decided not to participate in college football. During my years in college, the competition was rugged, the studies were demanding, and the stress was great. I frequently drank large amounts of caffeinated coffee to get more hours of study out of every day. By age 18, I was plagued by increasing episodes of irritable bowel syndrome which were marked by frequent indigestion and occasional attacks of diarrhea. Pizza seemed to be the food that most frequently gave me indigestion and milk was the food that most frequently gave me diarrhea. I went on from college to postgraduate studies at a very competitive university, carrying a tremendous load of course material that was extremely challenging. My knees began to ache during my postgraduate work. The problem increased over the years. My major course of studies was fiercely competitive and, struggling to achieve the highest grades possible, by the time I finished my postgraduate studies, I was plagued by three major headaches a week. The headaches were intensified by stress and aggravated by exposure to bright light. They frequently responded to two to three tablets of Excedrin®, but sometimes no amount of nonprescription medication controlled the headaches, and I had to recede to a dark room with a pillow over my head or merely sleep the headache off overnight.

My stomach problem progressed to a full-blown ulcer which was proven with a special study of the stomach called a GI series. Antacid medication helped, but was of limited value. Stress and tension made the problem worse. Pain had begun to occur in my right shoulder and felt as though it were a tendonitis problem. My knees were troublesome, especially if I sat with them bent for any length of time. I had to always take an aisle seat, whether I was in class or on a plane, to keep my knees extended and avoid the pain. Rarely could I attend a movie theater without the pain problem interfering with the joy of seeing the film.

The back pain problem waxed and waned, which left me with a sensation of stiffness and pain that gave me good days and bad. It got worse when I went on to further postgraduate training, this time in a somewhat hostile environment during an extremely stressful 5 years of further training. At that point, my sleep began to become markedly disturbed. There were nights that I could not get to sleep or sleep comfortably. If I slept more than 6 hours, my low back would begin to hurt. Nightmares became an intermittent, but progressive, problem. Shortly before my last stint of postgraduate training, I married the girl of my dreams. Through all my years of college and postgraduate training, I was a very compulsive person, did extra work on all my projects, received high grades, and worked diligently to earn the best possible results that I could achieve.

I started into practice in 1974. This was a very aggressive venture and I was employed by a large corporation. The hours were long and the work was hard and demanding. Frequently, I would be up all night long tending to the needs of people who needed my help, skill, and expertise. After almost 2 years of this work, my ulcer pains were worse, my headaches were disturbing, my knee pains were at times disabling, and the effects of stress began to take a tremendous toll on my nervous system. After nights of being up late and working long hours, my back would ache without letup. Pain would begin to radiate down my right leg at times and down my left leg at other times. Cramping in my calves became so severe that charley horses would awaken me in the middle of the night and I would scream due to the severity of the pain that locked up my lower leg. My body began to ache all over. Some days I felt better than others. Emotionally, I was reaching a breaking point. On occasion, I suffered from attacks of dizziness that were of a mild degree, but nonetheless distressing.

At numerous times over the past 20 years, I have consulted medical personnel for treatment of these conditions, but with no real significant relief. I experienced an emotional collapse in the spring of 1976 and had to quit working for almost 8 months. I had suffered depression due to burnout. The recovery from that depression was slow. During that period of time, my stress level went down and I obtained psychotherapy to help me with pacing and restructuring my life.

At the beginning of 1977, I opened a practice for myself with the idea in mind that I could control the stress in my life by going at a pace that I could tolerate. I still suffered from headaches, right shoulder pain, the ulcer pain problem, stress effects on the nervous system (including irritability, tiredness, and a low stress tolerance), the persistence of the knee pains, and pain which became problematic in my feet and which was accompanied by burning sensations and swelling from time to time.

I took a refresher course in 1977, spending a week at a conference. Following that conference, a stabbing pain began in the upper aspect of my left shoulder which felt as though a sword was being shoved into my upper back intermittently and with no association to work, stress, or other factors.

As I went into my own practice, I began to do consulting work for another office on a part-time basis. Most of my work related to the review of persons who have disability secondary to back or neck pain problems. What I saw, as I did my evaluations, intrigued me. I came to realize that numerous people with problems similar to mine were parading in front of me throughout the days that I worked there. I noted that these people, who were being treated by some of the best physicians in my area, were not obtaining relief of symptoms that were similar to mine.

I was intrigued by seeing these people for whom there were no answers in regard to their pain and suffering. I noted large numbers of the same types of patients in my own practice. I took these problem cases to an expert in myofascial pain syndrome in another city. He reviewed the cases and advised me to institute a program of myofascial pain syndrome therapy. I returned and began using this program with limited, but impressive, success. A year later, I went to see the same specialist with a series of more complex cases that had more resistant pain and suffering problems. He advised me to add a vitamin treatment program, both orally and by injection, to try to resolve the patient's problems. I proceeded to implement the recommended therapy in the people who were seeing me for those problems. When I began to use the recommended program, I saw results that were quite astonishing. I was so impressed at what the expert had recommended that I began to utilize this program in the management of my own pain, discomfort, and distress. Much to my amazement, my knee pain problems on both sides began to clear dramatically. Within 6 weeks of using that program, I literally threw away all the bottles of antacid that used to sit on my desk, at my bedside, and in my car. During that period of time, my middle back had become problematic by going out and becoming painful at least monthly. I consulted a chiropractor and found that the manipulation treatments provided good, but temporary, relief. Because I was encouraged by what the medical consultant had relayed to me, I began investigative work on my own.

Over the course of time, I sought out other consultants throughout the country and gained further knowledge in how to help people who came to me for relief of complex pain and disabling pain problems. Some had problems that were extremely severe and disabling. Some of the more severe cases could not be solved and could not be treated. Eventually the majority of people consulting me for help could be given hope of treatment available for their problem and also hope that active investigations were going on to further resolve what persistent problems they had.

I watched the people who came to me for help. I listened to their statements and comments about the therapy that was being offered to them and being utilized by them. I felt encouragement that what I was offering them was helping a great majority of people to resolve disabling pain problems and helping them cope with the parts of the problem that could not be resolved. I allowed some of my teaching to come from my patients about the type of pain they had and what therapies worked best for their suffering, pain, and distress.

I began to actively partake of these therapies myself. Over the course of the 15 years that I have been actively pursuing these methods of treatment, I have resolved all of my knee pain, 95% of my back pain, 98% of my headache pain, all of the pain in both my left and right shoulder (including the stabbing pain in the upper left shoulder), the dizziness problem, and the sleep and nightmare problem.

Since 1989, I had been on all the perpetuating factor treatments mentioned in Chapter 10 on myofascial pain syndrome, including the vitamin shots every other day.

In the summer of 1992, I consulted Bonnie Pruden, a trained myotherapist in my town. The purpose of the therapy was to increase the flexibility of my neck and back. The therapy was helpful.

My 40-year-old headaches are now gone unless I eat foods grown with organophosphate pesticides (most fruits and vegetables) or consume vitamin supplements that have any vitamin A in them. I have been off vitamin A supplements for about 4 years now. When my blood level for vitamin A was tested, I had a level of 101 (normal range = 60–97). Therefore I run a slightly elevated blood level on no supplements. Any supplements would put me into progressive vitamin A toxicity.

SEPTEMBER 1993

In September of 1993 my ex-wife left me. She was my bookkeeper, office manager, and head nurse. Because she did not have myofascial pain syndrome, she was more active in managing various aspects of the practice than I was. When she left, the weight of her responsibilities fell on me. I was also emotionally devastated by the fact that my wife of 26 years had left me. My overall activity level stepped up by an extra 40–50%. I also needed to stay up extra hours to accomplish all the work that she and I used to do as a team. Shortly after she left, I began to experience pain in both sides of my back, buttocks, and both of my legs that was severe and incapacitating. I tried a number of pain killers and found that none of the schedule three analgesics (Vicodin®, Lorcet® 10, and others) had much positive effect on my pain problem. I consulted a physician friend of mine who prescribed MS Contin® (time-release morphine) at 300 mg/day. The medication gave some help, but the side effects of constipation, difficulty urinating, and nausea were very bothersome. For a time I needed to use crutches to get around. It was embarrassing to see patients while I was on crutches and on the very pain medication I prescribed for a number of them.

My physician friend injected a number of myofascial trigger points in my back and buttock. Trigger point injections are extremely painful at times, but I toughed them out. When combined with the pain medication, they helped me slowly get up and get my business back up to speed.

I was determined to keep my very specialized practice going, if at all possible. I was then able to begin recruiting staff to take my ex-wife's place. It was difficult to do, and it was almost a year before I could find trustworthy people who could help me. By February of 1994 most of the severe pain flare-up had been brought under satisfactory control. I was down to taking two to three Lorcet® 10 tablets per day and doing pretty well. Pain was residual in the side of my left leg, just below the knee, and it was brought under good control by three injections in the side of the leg (tibialis anterior muscle).

1994

My ex-wife had asked a female family friend (of seven years) of the family to look in on me in her absence. With the passage of time, our family friend and I began dating and eventually were married in December of 1994.

Unfortunately, too much baggage was packed for the honeymoon. We spent the first night in town and then drove up the coast about 150 miles north to stay in a home we had rented for the week.

During the months before my marriage, I had been working tirelessly many hours per week. I was stressed and my body was run down before the honeymoon. Two days into the honeymoon, I got out of bed and began to experience severe pain in my right buttock and right leg. This was accompanied by an inability to urinate standing up. I thought for sure I had ruptured a disc in my back. However, since we were honeymooning in a fairly sparsely populated area, I decided to try myofascial trigger point injections to treat the pain problem.

At times the pain was unbearable, especially the dull knife-like pains that sizzled down my leg, into the outside of my lower leg. These pains made me clench my teeth very hard. The pain would respond only minimally to methadone or Dilaudid® tablets, which had been prescribed by the doctor in charge of my pain management.

I taught my bride how to administer injections to the myofascial trigger points in the muscles of my buttock. Each evening she would administer two to five myofascial trigger point injections. The first few injections were so painful that I almost decided to bear the pain and forget the myofascial trigger point injections. At one point, I tried a muscle stimulator, but that only caused more pain than I already had.

Then Dilaudid® injection was prescribed to be given before the myofascial trigger point injections. About 20 minutes before each myofascial trigger point injection, an injection of 2–2.5 mg of Dilaudid® was administered. This made the myofascial trigger point injections tolerable. Our honeymoon was somewhat compromised by the onset of my pain, but we managed to have a fairly memorable time during that week. The Dilaudid® injection 15–20 minutes before the myofascial trigger point injections made the trigger point injection pain more bearable, but by no means did it completely erase the pain effect.

By the end of the honeymoon, the sciatic pain on the right buttock and leg was coming under good control. I was able to urinate in a standing position. There was residual pain in my low back and left leg. This time all leg pain was abolished by injecting into the buttock and hip trigger points.

1996

From December of 1994 to 1996 a number of myofascial trigger point injections were necessary to keep peeling away the numerous layers of trigger points that were activated in 1993 and 1994. A number of therapists were helpful here.

In February of 1996 I went bowling with my daughter. We only bowled two games before I experienced severe pain in my buttocks. It flared up through the weekend.

I was left with a pain from my posterior lower ribs to posterior mid thigh every time I bent my head forward in the morning while trying to dress for work or administer the morning vitamin shot in my lower abdomen.

I now see the chiropractor once every 2–3 weeks and once per month I see a pain management doctor (an anesthesiologist who is the head of a local pain service) to have residual myofascial trigger points injected, for continuing improvement of my pain and overall functioning. As of 1996 I no longer needed premedication with Dilaudid® injectable before my myofascial trigger point injections.

Now, at 54 years of age, I no longer look like a severe arthritic when I get up from sitting in a theater, church, couch, etc., because my back pain has been significantly alleviated.

I know that I may have another attack of severe myofascial pain, but with each passing year, my response to attacks is better and my need for analgesic medication is less and less. I continue to take all the medications recommended for myofascial pain syndrome, which include calcium tablets, 0.25 mg of thyroid, B complex with C and E (Bronson), 1000 mg of time-release vitamin C, 300 mg of magnesium complex three times per day, B-complex injections every other day, 20-meq potassium tablets three times per day (prescription), and Mineral Insurance Formula (Bronson) three times per day.

I still can't "go all out," and I still have to pace myself during the day. Getting enough restful, uninterrupted sleep (usually 7–8 hours) is important. I have a number of active myofascial trigger points. At present they are a minimal problem to me. If I push too hard, they activate and cause problems of pain and restricted mobility.

The myofascial pain syndrome will be a lifelong disease. The results of proper management have paid off in relief of pain, ability to maintain gainful employment, and, currently, minimal crippling pain flare-ups.

I am no stranger to pain. I am Michael S. Margoles, M.D.

2 The Many Facets of Chronic Pain

Michael S. Margoles, M.D., Ph.D.
Lawrence A. Funt, D.D.S., M.S.D.

CONCEPTS

The major topics to be covered in this chapter are

- Concepts in chronic pain
- Evaluation of persons with chronic pain
- Formulating a working diagnosis
- Treatment of persons with chronic pain
- The Funt Orthopedic System

INTRODUCTION

This chapter is a five-part summary review of many of the problems and concepts relating to chronic pain and people who have chronic pain. Chronic pain is a complex problem. Frequently there are no simple answers.

Chronic pain is often referred to as "intractable." As used here, intractable pain means a pain state in which the cause of the pain cannot be removed or otherwise treated. In the generally accepted course of medical practice, no relief or cure of the cause of the pain is possible or none has been found after reasonable efforts to do so. "Reasonable efforts" include, but are not limited to, evaluation by the attending physician and one or more physicians specializing in the treatment of the area, system, or organ of the body perceived to be the source of pain.

The first part of this chapter deals with how to conceptualize or understand chronic pain. The second part addresses some of the components of how to properly evaluate a person with chronic pain. The third part addresses the concepts of formulating a diagnosis after the evaluation of the person has been performed. The fourth part addresses many treatments that are currently available to treat chronic pain. The final part presents one author's (Dr. Funt) system of dynamic application of all the components in the first four parts and represents concepts in how to diagnose and treat people with chronic pain. It is merely one good, sound system of approach. It provides a good "game plan" for diagnosis and treatment of people with chronic pain. There are other approaches available, and these will be detailed in other sections of the book.

Pain is arbitrarily designated as "chronic" if it has gone on for 6 months or more. Chronic pain is a problem with many concerns. It is not just a sprained back or an aching joint; it is that and more. It can cause chronic disability, depression, apathy, divorce, and suicide. It changes lives, frustrates attainment of life goals, and destroys families. To say the least, chronic pain is a frustrating problem for both the person and therapist.

The material in this section will briefly discuss some of the more prominent features of the problems which a person with chronic pain faces.

Onset and Origin

The onset and origin of a chronic pain problem are sometimes not a clear-cut cause-and-effect situation. Some of the pain problems begin slowly, without clear cause, and then progress slowly, worsening over time. Other cases may begin abruptly after an accident, fall, or other type of injury, but when the usual time for recovery has elapsed, the problem goes on to become chronic and disabling. In general, the greater the number of injuries that occurred before the pain problem began, the harder it is to resolve it.

Chronic pain may result from degeneration of a joint (arthrosis or arthritis) or degeneration of a nerve (neuropathy, myelopathy, etc.). For reasons as yet unknown, chronic pain tends to run in families and may affect a number of generations.

Chronic pain may be a complication of medical or surgical treatment. One example is scar tissue that forms in the low back after successful disc surgery. Another instance is the appearance of spine pain after radiation therapy for a tumor in the region of the spine.

One of the most frequent causes of chronic, nonmalignant pain is myofascial pain syndrome. Although this condition is common, and easy to diagnose, many people and professionals (doctors, dentists, chiropractors, etc.) are not aware of it.

Dynamic Process

Most chronic pain is a dynamic (changes over time) process. Its progression can change from hour to hour, day to day, week to week, or month to month. Many people use the expression "good days and bad." Without proper therapy to halt the downhill progression, the problem(s) continues on a ceaseless downhill course that borders on an advancing nightmare.

Economics

Economic disadvantages work against the chronic pain patient in five ways:

1. Failing health causes inability to provide an income.
2. Insurance premiums and other expenses become impossible to keep up with.
3. Payment for ongoing medical and surgical treatment becomes staggering. Some people may spend $15,000–$25,000 or more per year for treatment of their ongoing problem.
4. Some insurance companies eventually try to unload people with chronic pain because they are a continuing liability and a drain on insurance dollars. Insurance companies are often remiss in paying for medical problems which become chronic.

5.   Employers fear hiring people with back, neck, and other chronic pain, because of the risks of reinjury, the costs of escalated premiums, and time lost from work.

Emotional and Psychological

People frequently complain that the doctors they see regarding their severe and complex chronic pain problem tell them to either go home and live with or that it is all in their head. People treated this way feel hurt, angry, insulted, rejected, and misunderstood.

Any chronic problem is accompanied by emotional abnormalities of varying degree. However, some physicians who are not familiar with people who have chronic pain and related problems frequently mistake the resulting stress as a psychological problem. Too often, the person is labeled with a diagnosis of "functional overlay," "hysterical disorder," "conversion disorder," "dysthymic disorder," or some other primary psychiatric problem. What is even more alarming is that these psychiatric diagnoses are sometimes made by physicians who have had no formal psychiatric training!

In some cases the evaluating physician considers himself or herself a self-appointed "guardian." His or her disbelief and ignorance about people with chronic pain is used to "protect" the insurance companies from getting "ripped off" by discrediting people with ongoing chronic pain complaints. The person suffering with chronic pain gets no understanding or sympathy from this type of physician. The rejecting consultations from such a physician add to the confusion, dismay, and psychological distress. People then lose hope, become discouraged, and unfortunately become very angry at the professionals and at themselves.

Because of the pain and the associated disability, interpersonal problems of stress and distress may develop between the individual and his or her spouse, family, friends, relatives, fellow workers, and medical personnel. The ravages of a chronic pain problem may cause a family to fall apart. There may be accusations by friends and professionals that the person is faking it or emotionally triggering the pain. Even the person's spouse begins to question his or her standing and reliability. Finally, the person begins to think it's all in his or her head.

Grieving

There is a grieving process that accompanies chronic pain, and it relates to loss of previous lifestyle, loss of productivity, loss of self-esteem, sexual dysfunction, and being rejected and misunderstood by the medical community, family, spouse, friends, and co-workers. The person with chronic pain may go through a grieving process that lasts for the total duration of the pain problem, which can last 10 years or more. However, this usually maximizes within the first 2 years of the chronic pain problem. After that, the person may make peace with his or her pain part and accept the limitations that it has imposed.

Medications

There are a number of facets to the medication component of chronic pain. The chronic pain patient either depends on drugs, has a tolerance to them, cannot tolerate them, doesn't want any of them, or doctors have refused to prescribed them. There is much confusion and misunderstanding on both the part of the person and the physician in the proper use of medications in the treatment of chronic pain. Unfounded and unrealistic fears of addiction to narcotic pain relievers and sleeping medications are pervasive in the minds of both people and doctors.

Fortunately, some states have enacted legislation to encourage doctors to use narcotic pain medications when the doctor thinks they are needed as part of the treatment.

Long-term (greater than 6 weeks) use of medications such as nonsteroidal anti-inflammatory drugs (aspirin, Motrin®, Clinoril®, Advil®, Tolectin®, etc.) can cause ulcers, gastrointestinal bleeding, and liver and kidney problems.

Metabolic/Allergy/Hypersensitivity

Many people with chronic pain consume a diet that is too high in carbohydrates, a diet which has been found to antagonize pain problems. There are problems with respect to sensitivities and abnormal reactions (pain flare-ups) to various foods and chemicals used to process or protect foods. These can act to aggravate and "perpetuate" chronic pain.

The chronic stress of the pain problem causes depletion of vital nutrients. Blood testing often reveals vitamin, mineral, and other internal chemistry problems which relate to the chronic pain problem and act to perpetuate, aggravate, or initiate a chronic pain problem. Despite this readily available blood testing, many members of the medical profession are lacking when it comes to understanding the role of vital nutrients in the restoration and rehabilitation of chronic pain patients.

Hormonal

Decreased estrogen and thyroid levels in the blood antagonize the muscular component of the pain problem in myofascial pain syndrome (Travell and Simons, 1983; Sonkin, 1994). The same is true for decreased cortisone production (adrenal gland deficit) in the body (Sonkin, 1994).

Physical Problems

Physical impairment may be extensive in the person with chronic pain. Generally, the older the problem, and the less the specific therapy for it, the worse the physical impairment becomes.

Assistive aids are often necessary and helpful. These consist of wheelchairs, crutches, extension devices to assist in reaching and grasping, and raised toilet seats, among many others.

People with chronic pain who are untreated or improperly treated may have to curtail some or a great deal of their "up time" (activities) as the pain and dysfunction get worse. In extreme cases the "up time" is almost nonexistent or only minutes at a time. This lifestyle can extend from periods of days to years. This state of physical compromise makes seeking proper medical care nearly impossible. According to Pawlicki (1980), 45% of men and 59.5% of women in a recent survey said that there were days when the pain was so bad that they spent the whole day in bed. On the other hand, as the pain and dysfunction improve, the physical functioning improves spontaneously.

Mechanical

There are numerous mechanical factors that produce or aggravate chronic pain. Among these various items are poor posture, ruptured disc, pinched nerve, muscle spasms, excessive weight, abuse of muscles, and improper use of the neck or back.

Structural Problems

This relates to altered body structure that acts as a perpetuating factor to chronic pain. It usually has the greatest impact on myofascial pain syndrome. These problems relate to dental malocclusions, short arm, short pelvis on one side, short leg, and long second metatarsal (an important bone in the arch of the foot) accompanied by a short first metatarsal.

Physiological Abnormalities

These relate to the vital processes of the body such as muscle function, digesting food, etc. In the person with chronic pain there are a multitude of physiological functioning abnormalities of varying degree, and they may not be considered as relating to the chronic pain. These include decreased stress tolerance, irritable bowel, malabsorption of vital nutrients, failing memory, bumping into things, sleep problems, nerve malfunctions, allergies, accidental loss of urine, dry skin, easy bruising, catching more colds and flu, swelling of hands and feet, cold intolerance, failing health, and decreased energy.

Spiritual Issues

This sometimes includes loss of faith, feeling separated from God, and a sense of being punished by God. Frequently, people who have been plagued by severe ongoing pain have given up on God. A person who has spiritual or religious beliefs could benefit by seeking counsel from religious leadership for purposes of support and direction.

Rehabilitation Issues

Getting Well Is a Process and a Challenge

If rehabilitation is perceived in a positive manner, everyday life will be more fulfilling and more productive during the rehabilitation process, in spite of the presence of pain.

The person with chronic pain may state that movement and/or previous rehabilitation attempts cause pain, which frustrates the rehabilitation efforts.

The training that a person with chronic pain obtains must emphasize the nonmalignant nature of the pain and associated disability. The person must be made to see his or her pain as distressing but not dangerous.

After a proper assessment, the person with chronic pain must move into a position of understanding that there is no gain in physical functioning without the pain associated with moving the atrophied muscles toward rehabilitation. It is important for the person with chronic pain to learn what kind of pain is not destructive to tissues and what kind might signal the onset of more injury.

The person must understand that there are no easy answers and no magic overnight solutions!

The person must come to realize that rehabilitation and recovery are not a passive endeavor in which one sits and the doctor does all the work. Rehabilitation of the chronic pain person is an active endeavor where the burden of becoming rehabilitated falls heavily on the person experiencing the pain.

In some persons pain prevents gain. In some instances very active and pain-producing trigger points must be inactivated to promote physical rehabilitation. Sometimes adequate amounts of mild to strong pain-relieving medication must be used to promote physical rehabilitation. In some persons soft tissue pain is so great that physical rehabilitation is not possible.

There may be great struggle in getting well. Some of the people with severe chronic pain do not have the emotional stability, tenacity, and determination to adhere closely to programs aimed at getting them functioning productively again.

Slow Cure

Reducing the pain, increasing physical function, and, if necessary, changing one's attitude toward pain and disability is a lengthy process. Some of the milder cases may take 1–3 months to recover, but in some of the more severe cases, significant recovery may take a number of years.

EVALUATION AND ASSESSMENT OF THE PERSON WITH CHRONIC PAIN

Comprehensive Diagnostic and Evaluation Procedures

Multiple factors need to be considered in evaluation of the person with chronic pain, such as length of the illness, psychological reaction to it, family dynamics, work status, general health status, metabolic status, number of accidents or injuries, stress tolerance, motivation of the person, motivation of spouse, motivation of employer, and attitude of the insurance carrier, to mention only a few of the pertinent considerations.

The evaluation is accomplished by using multiple methods. This consists of history taking and physical examination and may also include X-rays, blood tests, occupational therapy evaluation, assessment of physical conditioning, physical therapy, electromyogram (nerve studies), computerized axial tomography (CAT) scan, magnetic resonance imaging (MRI) scan, diagnostic ultrasound, and others.

Evaluations are frequently accomplished by multiple specialists, drawing on expertise from orthopedic and neurological surgeons, physical therapists, neurologists, anesthesiologists, dietitians, practitioners in general and internal medicine, specially trained nursing personnel, counselors, and psychologists. Sometimes evaluation can be done by one specialist who has some expertise in all the above-mentioned areas.

History Taking

A detailed analysis with an emphasis on the mechanism of injury is crucial to the history taking in a person with pain. For instance, if the person was rear ended with his or her head turned to the left at the time of impact, then the myofascial trigger points may be in the right side of the neck. Likewise, a woman giving a history of low back pain after extensive labor and delivery may have strained a muscle or a number of muscles in the pelvic area or low back along the spine. Bilateral lower extremity pain in a vegan may be due to vitamin B12 deficiency.

Also, a detailed analysis needs to be carried out to assess all the types of treatments and care that have been used up to the point of present history taking. This is done to avoid unnecessarily repeating therapy that has already been given.

Histories and examinations performed by other therapists are reviewed so that previously applied diagnoses will be known and previously applied therapies that failed will not be repeated.

Previously taken X-rays and their reports are reviewed in detail and correlated with the present history and physical findings to assess the presence of radiological abnormalities that must be considered in the treatment plan. In the majority of cases, review of the old X-rays reveals no new information.

Surgical report(s) from surgeries that relate to the current pain problem should be reviewed so that previous surgical procedures will not be repeated. Also, review of the surgical report(s) is correlated with the current clinical picture to decide whether the person showed an adequate positive response to the surgery.

Sometimes evaluation can be done by one specialist who has some expertise in all the above-mentioned areas.

Review of Systems

In this part of the history taking the therapist gathers information relating to function of body parts and systems aside from the one related to the immediate pain problem. This may relate to questioning about the heart, gastrointestinal system, urinary function, hormone-producing glands, eyes, ears, and other areas to assess for the presence of other medical conditions that may affect the pain problem and the treatment of all factors relating to it. For example, if a patient with a chest pain problem also has a pacemaker, the use of a transcutaneous electrical nerve stimulator may be contraindicated in the treatment program.

Physical Examination

Physical examinations and evaluations may be carried out by a number of specialists on the "team." A general medical examination is used to assess the presence of general medical problems such as uterine dysfunction (endometriosis, etc.) or estrogen deficiency, thyroid problems, sinus or urinary tract infections, and other areas that may cause a chronic pain problem.

An orthopedic surgical consultation is used to assess for back, neck, or joint problems that may need conservative orthopedic or orthopedic surgical care. This evaluation assesses for problematic disc disorders in the neck and low back that may need surgery to provide a satisfactory end result. However, with respect to the chronic pain treatment team, the orthopedic surgeon acts as a part of the "team." His services are only a part of the total rehabilitation effort toward recovery.

A consultation about nerve and spinal cord function may be necessary to assess the presence of neurological dysfunction problems such as multiple sclerosis, neuropathies (nerve damage), etc. A neurological surgeon (neurosurgeon) may be needed to assess and treat a nerve- and disc-related problem that may need surgical treatment.

When available, the services of a physiatrist (physical medicine and rehabilitation doctor) may be of value in the diagnosis and treatment of chronic muscular pain and weakness. These specialists, or similar type therapists, assess muscle dysfunction and overall need for physical rehabilitation and reconditioning. They can use dynamometer or metric strength testing to assess muscle weakness. They can also document problems of range of motion restriction.

When evidence for the presence of atrophy is sought in people with chronic pain, only a few people will show it because the atrophy of unused muscles occurs bilaterally.

The pressure threshold meter is a very simple device that can be used to determine the presence of abnormal muscle tenderness and to help locate some of the trigger points in muscles.

Muscle strength testing can be carried out using a very accurate and sophisticated Cybex or other such machine. This equipment can be used to very accurately assess weakness in an affected extremity, the neck, or the back. However, a simple, inexpensive, hand-held dynamometer may be sufficient for some of the less complex analyses. Endurance can also be assessed using a Cybex or similar system.

A combined comprehensive evaluation can be carried out by skilled physical and occupational therapists to establish range of motion, endurance, lifting capacities, and dysfunction in the use of the arms or legs.

Myofascial evaluation can be performed by any specialist trained in the technique.

Rheumatology evaluation is conducted to assess the presence of degenerative joint disease, osteoarthritis, rheumatoid arthritis, fibromyalgia, and other reasons for chronic joint pain problems.

Blood Testing

Blood counts are performed primarily to analyze for infections and anemia.

Arthritis blood testing is done to assess the presence of rheumatoid arthritis, gout, ankylosing spondylitis, lupus, and other inflammatory joint pain problems.

Potassium levels are analyzed as they relate to myofascial pain syndrome, as are calcium, ionized calcium, magnesium, thyroid, and estrogen levels. A panel of B-vitamin levels is recommended for all patients with myofascial pain syndrome.

Special Tests

Psychologic Testing

The true emotional impact of chronic pain has not been totally spelled out. Nonetheless, the emotional impact of chronic pain is great and needs to be assessed. This may range from simply assessing the emotional incapacity that the pain problem has brought all the way to assessing "sick" patterns of behavior and interpersonal relationships that have developed because of the pain problem. Possible secondary gain factors that are preventing the person from getting well also need be assessed. An example of secondary gain factors may include a person who is on social security disability income and who fears that his or her benefits will be cut off by getting well.

There are numerous tests available for the evaluation of people with chronic pain. All testing must be properly interpreted to arrive at valid conclusions about the data gathered from the tests.

The most accurate clinical evaluation of a person with chronic pain is usually accomplished by a competent clinical psychologist or counselor who is experienced in assessing and treating chronic pain people and who is knowledgeable in the use and interpretation of the various tests mentioned below.

The Minnesota Multiphasic Personality Inventory is a lengthy test and is one of many tests available to assess emotional problems. A certain amount of abnormality is routinely found when testing any person with a chronic illness and will revert back to normal when the illness is terminated. Its use in chronic pain patients is limited.

Stress testing is another tool for assessing adverse conditions related to chronic pain. This is carried out with a test such as the social readjustment rating scale by a clinical psychologist. The impact of the pain problem on lifestyle may be assessed with the sickness impact profile.

The Melzack–McGill Pain Questionnaire is a short, simple, and easy-to-take test that was developed specifically for chronic pain people. It measures both psychological and somatic components of chronic pain people. The Beck Depression Inventory is a short and easy way to assess for the presence of depression.

There are numerous other tests available, and the therapist administering them should explain the scope and purpose of the specific test being administered to the patient.

Other factors that must be analyzed by the behavioral or functional assessment part of the diagnostic team are

1. Coping skills: How well are you coping with your chronic pain problem?
2. Pacing skills: Are you pacing yourself in such a way as to not antagonize your pain problem?
3. Cognitive function: Are you in touch with where you are at and what you are allowing your pain problem to do to you?
4. Degree of anxiety
5. Presence and degree of depression
6. Evaluation of interaction with spouse
7. Evaluation of interaction with family

Nerve Testing

Electromyography and nerve conduction velocities are used to test for evidence of nerve injury or nerve degeneration. These tests have to be closely correlated with the findings of the physical examination.

Activity Assessment Testing

One's physical capacity for various activities can be estimated by trained personnel, especially occupational therapists. Physical muscle strength can be measured by a physical therapist using weights or using a sophisticated piece of machinery such as a Cybex.

Sleep Analysis

Analysis for sleep problems may run the gamut of things from informal questioning all the way to a formal sleep lab evaluation. It is important to learn how difficult it is for the person to fall asleep and stay asleep. It is important to learn how often he or she awakens during sleep and how restful sleep is at night.

Local Anesthetic Injections

Trigger point injections can be used to establish the presence of a trigger point or trigger points. This consists of breaking up a trigger point with a needle and injecting a small amount of procaine (Novocain®) into any of the myofascial trigger points that are suspected of being problematic.

A specific nerve that may be thought to be a producer of pain can be deadened temporarily to determine its role in the pain problem. Spinal segments, containing many nerves, can be temporarily deadened with local anesthetic solutions to determine the role of the spinal cord in the pain problem.

Routine X-rays

People often present to the pain management therapist having had numerous X-rays of the painful part, including routine X-rays, CAT scans, MRI scans, and myelograms. The repetitive X-raying of the painful part is generally nonproductive and frequently shows only normal degenerative changes which are compatible with the person's age. A recent exception to this statement should be related. A 52-year-old woman had two whiplash injuries (1967 and 1973). By 1985 routine lateral neck X-rays showed a 2-mm slippage of C3 on C4. By 1995 this had sipped forward 5 mm and the patient complained of electric shocking sensations at times when she bent her neck forward.

Myelograms

A myelogram is an X-ray test in which special dye is injected into the spinal fluid to highlight the spinal cord and nerves. It is generally performed when looking for ruptured or degenerated discs or spinal cord tumors. It is also used to assess posttraumatic spinal cord damage, along with other worthy diagnostic procedures. However, be aware that myelograms are sometimes performed with questionable indications and have been noted by Hitselberger (1967) to have as high as a 20% incidence of false-positive results (something that appears to be there but really is not). This means that there may be the appearance of a huge defect (abnormality) in the test (dye column) that may be normal for that person. Unfortunately, these false-positive findings can result in unnecessary surgery, which may further antagonize the chronic pain problem.

Computerized Axial Tomography Scans

In this test the patient is passed through a circular opening and into an x-ray field that takes very sophisticated X-rays of the affected body part in a circular pattern. These X-rays are rearranged for viewing by a specialized computer and can give detailed analysis of body parts. This gives good images of the discs, spinal cord, and nerves. It also gives good images of many other vital body parts such as the brain, liver, kidney, etc. Sometimes the CAT scan is done after myelogram dye has been injected into the spine.

Magnetic Resonance Imaging

This test is accomplished with the person lying in a narrow tunnel. This is, in essence, an imaging process that is carried out with a powerful magnetic field instead of X-rays. The images obtained are rearranged for viewing with the aid of a very sophisticated computer. It can produce very accurate pictures of the spine, nerves, spinal cord, brain, and other vital body tissues.

Combination Tests

Sometimes a person's clinical condition is so difficult to diagnose that a number of the tests need to be combined. In that case a myelogram and MRI, a myelogram and CAT scan, or all three might be used as the clinician attempts to clarify the diagnosis.

Consultation with Other Pain Team Members

Usually one competent specialist in chronic pain problems can diagnose a pain problem, but the burden of diagnosing all the components of a pain problem and its related dysfunction is sometimes more than one therapist can handle. Therefore, a doctor, dentist, chiropractor, etc. may call upon the services of other specialists to further clarify the total picture. If the pain problem is being evaluated in an inpatient hospital-based program, there is usually a team of specialists that will be evaluating the total clinical picture.

Vocational Evaluation

This may be done when the person with chronic pain is getting ready to return to active employment. A great deal of this material is covered in Chapter 20 on job retraining. Once ready to return to active employment, the person will either return to his or her usual work or, if the former job is too demanding, may require a detailed evaluation to assess for which other types of less demanding work he or she is best suited. These evaluations are handled either by a special state agency or by a private vocational rehabilitation counselor designated by the employer. These agencies work in close conjunction with the professional who is treating the pain problem.

FORMULATING A WORKING DIAGNOSIS

After the evaluating processes are completed, the treating therapist or pain treatment team must formulate a working diagnosis. That means that a diagnosis or diagnoses must be made as to the person's condition(s) in order to determine what therapies will be utilized in the treatment of that (those) condition(s). The working diagnosis is the one that will dictate the direction that the treatment program will first take. Later on, other conditions that were of lesser impact when the evaluation was first made can be treated.

TREATMENT

Introduction: Complex Answers for Complex Problems

Chronic pain is usually a complex problem, with many areas to be considered in the treatment program. Therefore, the answers are complex. Treatment of persons with chronic pain is usually multifaceted and involves treating persons with physical, chemical, biochemical, emotional, and occasionally surgical therapies. These therapies may be used at the same time or in a sequential fashion to obtain a desired goal or end result. It is important to help the well-motivated chronic pain person keep going and maintain an improved quality of life. In addition to the use of numerous routine therapies, the benefit of strong pain-relieving opioids (narcotics) may be needed.

Getting Well is the Person's Responsibility

Each person is responsible for his or her own healing, for getting well. To accomplish this the pain person calls on therapists (M.D., D.D.S., Ph.D., MFCC) to supply treatments and to teach the steps to getting well and maintaining his or her health. Getting well is the responsibility of the person with chronic pain. In chronic pain treatment the therapist introduces the patient to the therapies to be considered, with an explanation of how they work, and the patient is responsible for using those therapies in getting well. This covers everything from instruction in home health care and diet to surgery. If surgery is decided upon as one of the therapies, the surgeon performs the necessary surgery, but the patient has responsibility for becoming as functional as he or she can after the surgery is performed. The chronic pain patient has a responsibility to give it his or her "all" and for as long as it takes. In the treatment of chronic pain, the patient has to shoulder the major part of the responsibility for his or her recovery. An individual must make up his or her mind to become an active participant in his or her overall recovery. The patient is the most important part of the treatment team. Since all this responsibility is the patient's, the patient must feel free to challenge the therapist(s) when he or she feels that something is not right in the treatment program. At the same time, the patient must also be ready to listen to the therapist he or she has chosen and follow his or her directives for helping to get well. The patient must ask questions and be ready to follow directions. He or she will have to monitor progress and accurately report progress and recovery to the treating therapist.

   The chronic pain patient must not expect a magic cure. It is likely that the pain will have ups and downs (see Figures 2.1 and 2.2 later in this chapter). Hopefully, the patient will learn to control the intensity, duration, and frequency of flare-ups.

Multifactoral

Multiple factors must be considered in the physical, emotional, and vocational rehabilitation of the person with chronic pain. Some of these factors include:

1. Pain severity
2. Severity of disability
3. Degree of muscle wasting and atrophy
4. Family dynamics
5. Degree of psychological preparedness (determines how aggressive the physical rehabilitation can be)
6. General health
7. Metabolic status
8. Level of stress
9. Motivation of the person
10. Motivation of the therapist(s)
11. Others

Multimodality

A "modality" is a method of therapy. Numerous therapies (modalities) may have to be used by the person with chronic pain to obtain the goals that are desired.

Modalities used by a physician may include:

1. X-rays
2. Medications
3. Biochemical therapy
4. Hormones
5. Correcting structural problems
6. Trigger point injections and nerve blocks
7. Hospitalization
8. Surgery
9. Others

Modalities used by the physical therapist may include:

1. Heat
2. Massage
3. Diathermy
4. Ultrasound
5. Exercise
6. Stretching
7. Back school program
8. Gravity traction
9. Transcutaneous electrical nerve stimulator
10. Joint mobilization
11. Others

Modalities used by a dentist may include:

1. Dental appliances
2. Stretch and spray
3. Trigger point injections
4. Electrical stimulation at trigger points
5. Correction of structural perpetuating factors
6. Correction of temporomandibular joint dysfunctions
7. Hard splint
8. Soft splint
9. Others

Modalities used by a psychologist or licensed marriage and family counselor may include:

1. Psychological and stress testing
2. Biofeedback
3. Cognitive therapy
4. Group therapy
5. Hypnosis
6. Others

Modalities used by a chiropractor may include:

1. Adjustments of the spine
2. Treatment of viscero-somatic reflexes
3. Myofascial therapy
4. Vitamin and mineral supplements
5. Normalization of leg length problems
6. Stabilization of the spine
7. Cranial or sutural manipulations
8. Others

Correction of structural problems includes:

1. Short leg
2. Short half-pelvis
3. Short upper extremity
4. Long second metatarsal (a bone in the arch of the foot)
5. Craniosacral complex
6. Cranial sutures
7. Craniomandibular complex

This is covered in Chapters 10 and Chapter 11.

Multispecialty

Either one specialist with broad knowledge from many areas of rehabilitation of the chronic pain person or a team of specialists with specialized knowledge in a number of pertinent areas of rehabilitation can be used. Usually, the overall rehabilitation of a chronic pain person cannot be accomplished by one therapist working alone. Some of the numerous modalities needed to accomplish the task are medical, dental, chiropractic, medicinal, biochemical, physical, emotional, and vocational therapies. This requires physical therapists, occupational therapists, vocational therapists, psychological therapy, family therapy, and numerous other interactive therapies and therapists. A physical therapist, chiropractor, physician, and psychologist or counselor may all need to work with the person over the same time frame. The physical therapist does mobilization, stretching, and progressive exercises; the physician does medication, biochemical, and hormonal work; the psychologist/counselor deals with the stress of chronic pain and abnormal family dynamics; the dentist deals with structural perpetuating factors in the head, neck, and mouth; and the chiropractor reestablishes spinal alignment and some of the joint dysfunctions.

Closely Supervised

In chronic pain treatment the patient needs one therapist to captain the "team" to facilitate and coordinate the care and management of his or her treatment. The "captain" is usually a physician, but in actuality any physician, dentist, psychologist/counselor, registered nurse, or chiropractor, with experience in proper management of chronic pain persons, can "captain" the rehabilitation team.

The person's progress needs to be closely supervised and adjustments in the application of therapy have to be made to fit the needs of the person as rehabilitation progresses. As healing progresses, dynamic changes in function, emotions, sleep, etc. occur steadily. More instruction is needed with each level of positive achievement as to how to progress to the next stage of recovery.

Structured

A definite program of adaptable structuring of all the therapies and goals indicated below is needed. The person with pain must be flexibly adapted to the structure of the program as progress is made.

Goal Orientation

The major goals of a structured pain rehabilitation program must emphasize:

1. Pain relief
2. Emotional restoration
3. Energy enhancement
4. Progression increments
5. Reassessment of progress
6. Return to work or productive activity

Pain Relief

Reassurance. One of the simplest techniques of promoting pain relief is education that informs the person of the nonmalignant nature of the pain process. Unfortunately, this technique may be relied upon too heavily by some therapists.

Personal education. This is carried out by having the pain patient become part of the treatment team.

Psychological therapy. Hypnosis, biofeedback, and stress reduction can all lower a certain amount of pain by encouraging relaxation and reduction of stress and tension.

Dental therapy. This includes the use of dental appliances, stretch and spray, trigger point injections, and other treatments.

Chiropractic. The chiropractor uses adjustments, spinal alignment, myofascial work, electrical therapy, and other forms of treatment.

Medications. One of the main medicinal approaches to pain relief is the use of anti-inflammatory and analgesic medication. Some muscle relaxers and tranquilizers will provide pain relief. This is further discussed in Chapter 21.

Vitamins and minerals. A number of people with chronic pain will obtain relief of pain symptoms and stress reduction by the use of oral and, in some cases, injectable B vitamins. This is covered in Chapter 10.

Injection therapy. Some of the numerous types of injections that can be used for pain relief include:

1. Trigger point injections
2. Epidural injections
3. Spinal blocks
4. Sympathetic blocks
5. Therapeutic injections (B vitamins, medications, etc.)
6. Injections of opioids

The injections mentioned above are further covered in Chapters 10, 11, and 29.

Surgery. In general, surgery is not advised in the treatment of chronic pain persons. However, there are a number of procedures that have merit if applied for the proper reasons and at the right time. These include:

1. Spinal cord stimulation (dorsal column stimulation)
2. Laminectomy and disc removal
3. Removal of lateral recess stenosis in the spine
4. Spinal fusion
5. Removal of endometriosis tissue
6. Deep brain stimulation
7. Others

Emotional Restoration

Getting well is a process and a challenge. Most people with chronic pain have seen a lot of therapists and run into many "blind alleys." This is frustrating. Also, once they find a therapeutic team to treat them, it may take months of great effort to recover.

Emphasis. The main emphasis is to decrease stress associated with chronic pain, restore proper family dynamics, direct people toward getting well, educate people about the nature of chronic pain, normalize sleep, give people hope, and let them see that there is a way out. In order to successfully create an ongoing process of physical healing, a positive mental attitude is necessary. With this attitude, one can develop the emotional stability and emotional tenacity required of a participant in a chronic pain rehabilitation program.

Behavioral adjustment techniques.   The emphasis here is on changing one's attitude about oneself and one's degree of disability, behavior modification, hypnosis, biofeedback, stress reduction, and medication management. More on these topics is covered in Chapters 15 to 17.

Prerequisites to obtaining emotional restoration (these also pertain to the physical part of the program) include:

1.   A decision to get well (move muscles; see Chapter 4)
2.   A decision to endure whatever it takes
3.   A decision to participate in the therapy program
4.   Goal setting. Without goals or reasons for getting well, the likelihood of achieving emotional healing and physical restoration is poor. Goals are reasons to get well. A person who does not have any goals will not get well. A goal can be as simple as calling an old friend on the phone or as complex as planning to climb a sizable mountain.

Patient education.   This is a constant, ongoing modality that should be used at every visit.

Cognitive therapy.   This is usually performed by a psychologist or a psychiatrist. This therapy deals with restructuring one's thinking processes about one's pain, suffering, and disability. The patient should be brought in touch with his or her pain so that he or she can learn how to turn attention away from it and onto more productive activities such as work and family. This is further explained in Chapter 15.

Behavior modification.   In reality, many chronic pain patients do not need their behavior modified; they need their pain modified. In many instances, once the pain is modified, the behavior is automatically modified back toward normal.

Small group therapy sessions may consist of up to ten people and spouses. This is good for support from and identity with other pain people. This needs to be at least partially structured (run by a therapist) to accomplish goals and for teaching purposes. A group that amounts to no more than a gripe session can be discouraging.

Family therapy.   All members of the person's family need to get involved in the treatment and support of the person. Antagonistic spouses can cause setbacks in progress and can act as a roadblock to healing.

Coping skills.   These are needed to help handle the pain, depression, grieving, stress, and physical disability associated with the chronic pain problem.

Pacing skills.   Learning how to pace oneself both at home and at work adds more to the overall recovery.

Relaxation training.   Some of the benefits of this therapy are help with sleep problems and lowering the effects of stress.

Guided imagery.   This modality helps divert attention away from the pain or helps the patient to imagine the pain is being relieved by what he or she imagines (e.g., dipping your hot back into a stream of cool water to douse the fire in your low back).

Hypnosis. One of the techniques that hypnosis offers is to help anesthetize one hand and then transfer the anesthesia from the numbed hand to a painful back. This can be used to aid onset of sleep. Another technique of hypnosis is regression analysis to decrease subconscious emotional blocks to becoming psychologically well.

Formal psychotherapy. This involves one-on-one therapy with a psychologist or psychiatrist to decrease depression or other psychological dysfunction due to the pain.

Medication management. The main medications that affect the psychological part of the pain problem are the antidepressants. Other medications of value are those that promote a better night's sleep. These are covered in Chapter 21.

Metabolic therapy. Metabolic therapy involves replacement of vitamins, minerals, hormones, and other essential chemicals that are insufficient or deficient to promote emotional enhancement and in some cases relief from depression.

Spiritual therapy. People of faith may look upon the painful ordeal that has come their way as being deserted by God or as a chance to gain new spiritual insights and growth with the Lord.

Energy Enhancement

Patient education. People who are taught where to properly put their recovery energies are more motivated and do not become exasperated by repeating therapies that do not "pan out."

Taking time to teach the patient with chronic pain valuable insights about the pain problem is the role for all the therapists on the pain treatment team. For example, when people get angry their pain problems flare up. Therefore, if patient and therapist work on controlling the patient's temper, the patient will have moved another increment toward recovery.

Metabolic therapy. Correction of vitamin, mineral, and hormone problems add to the energy and reserve of the person with chronic pain. This is partly covered in Chapter 10.

Goal-oriented therapy. Energy directed toward rewarding goals (work, home, hobbies, etc.) increases enthusiasm and recovery.

Injury prevention. Proper instruction (back school courses, instruction in proper use of the neck and arms, etc.) allows the person with chronic pain to prevent reinjury of the affected part.

Ergonomics. This involves study and correction of equipment design and placement in order to reduce operator fatigue and injury. If indicated, on-site review of the person's job should be done so that recommendations can be made for more efficient use of the arms, back, and legs to prevent fatigue or injury.

Biomechanics. This involves the application of mechanical laws and observations to living structures, specifically to the muscular system of the human body, to promote more efficient and effective use of the arms, legs, back, and torso.

Progressive mobilization. Tight muscles and joints cause excessive energy consumption when these structures are moved. Exercise that is too rapid or too vigorous can cause decreased energy, pain flare-ups, and discouragement. Slow, progressive mobilization gives freer movement and enhanced energy.

Treatment of physiological problems. This relates to treatment of abnormalities that occur in the person with chronic pain other than the pain problem itself. Some of these problems are allergies, sleep deficit, muscle weakness, emotional problems, hypoglycemia, premenstrual syndrome, decreased thyroid function, infections, and irritable bowel syndrome.

Progression Increments

The 5% rule. Each therapy that is attempted in the treatment of a moderate to severe pain problem has limits as to what it can contribute to the overall recovery of that person. Each modality of therapy, if it succeeds, may contribute as little as 5% to overall rehabilitation and healing. However, if there are enough 5% gains in the treatment program, the patient can end up with 50–100% overall improvement. Figure 2.1 illustrates the concept of progression increments and the theoretical improvement that can be realized when a number of modalities are sequentially applied to a person with a chronic pain problem.

The prerequisites to making progression increments are as follows:

1. A decision to get well (move muscles; see Chapter 4)
2. A decision to endure whatever it takes
3. A decision to participate in the therapy program
4. Goal setting
    a. Staying active
    b. Contributing to the financial support of the family
    c. Not letting the pain problem get out of control
    d. Becoming more physically active
    e. Less complaining about pain symptoms
    f. Others
5. A competent pain rehabilitation program

Progress: Two steps forward and one step back. In reality, progress in overall healing and restoration to normal function will look more like the graph in Figure 2.2. There will be good days and bad. The pace will seem like "two steps forward and one step back." The gains made will depend on the effectiveness of the therapy covered in the progression increments graph.

Reassessment of Progress

This is carried out every 6–12 weeks to assess the quality and quantity of recovery. Reassessment may be accomplished with testing which includes but is not limited solely to:

1. Sickness impact profile
2. The Melzack–McGill Pain Questionnaire
3. The Physiological Dysfunction Questionnaire
4. Review of the original review of systems to assess improvement of abnormalities
5. Any of the numerous tests of physical functioning recovery, including updating the abnormalities found on the original physical examination
6. Physical therapy and occupational therapy updating

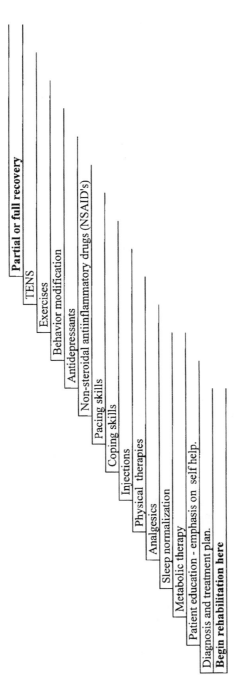

FIGURE 2.1 Progression increments: the 5% rule. "Begin rehabilitation here" denotes the "bottom of the barrel," the point at which many people in more severe pain begin their trek back to better health and better functioning. In actuality, the exact staging of the therapeutic steps is only approximate. Actual recovery with a specific therapy will vary from person to person and from therapist to therapist. Many additional therapies can be put into the slots indicated on the upward steps. Therapies must be tailored to meet each person's needs. Each therapy sets the stage for the next "step" up and adds to the overall rehabilitation of the person with pain.

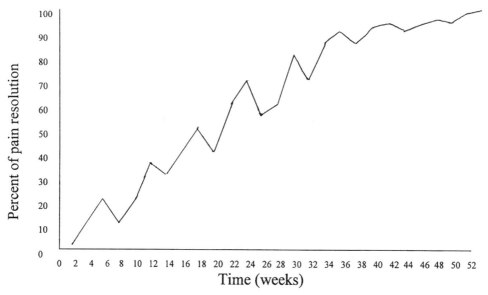

FIGURE 2.2   Progress of pain resolution: two steps forward and one step back. This graph represents the typical progression of recovery in a person with chronic pain. This is what occurs when proper therapy is administered. The progression is two steps forward and one step back, all the way to optimal recovery.

Vocational Rehabilitation

Progress is assessed by the vocational counselor and further goals are set to make further gains and progress.

Treatment Based on Principles

In some of the very complex cases there are no absolute principles of treatment. Therefore the patient's problem has to be broken down into treatable components. For example:

- If the patient has pain, use a pain-relieving medication.
- If the patient has decreased range of motion of a joint, use physical therapy, stretch and spray, Travell and Simons' myofascial trigger point injections, etc. to resolve the problem.
- If a vitamin-related neuropathy is present, treat it with vitamins orally or intramuscularly.
- If there is a sleep problem, use a method or medication to treat the problem. If a psychological problem is present, use psychotherapy. For an endocrine problem, use endocrine treatment.

THE FUNT ORTHOPEDIC SYSTEM: FUNT'S TRIAD

The Three Phases of Therapy

This system represents one of a number of approaches to incorporating all the materials in the first four parts of this chapter into a working model of dynamic application to the evaluation and treatment of people with chronic pain. The three phases as related by Dr. Funt (1991) are

1. Diagnostic phase
2. Treatment phase
3. Stabilization

Overview

The principles embodied here provide a brief overview, or condensation, of all the material that will be contained, in detail, in the sections to follow. It represents a condensed summary of what is involved in the diagnosis, treatment, and management of people with chronic pain. The three phases, diagnostic, treatment, and stabilization, overlap one another.

The very nature of chronic pain and related dysfunction, with its postural, functional, structural, psychologic, and metabolic components, makes it a very dynamic (ever-changing and moving) problem. Much of current therapy is based on conceptualizing a disease problem as static (unchanging). However, the Funt Orthopedic System (FOS) approaches dynamic diseases and disease processes with a sophisticated, dynamic, systematic, and sequential program that addresses all the nuances and frustrations of dealing with these complex and challenging patient problems. With the approach synthesized from the FOS, if the staging is followed and adhered to, the final goal is to produce pain-free relationships in the problematic body areas.

In the sections that follow the components of Funt's Triad will be broken down into finer detail and more precise steps.

There is a lot that goes on between all the phases listed below. For example, between the treatment and stabilization phases, a number of trigger point injections plus stretch and spray may be administered to improve the overall result for the right shoulder and arm or the low back pain problem.

Diagnostic Phase

The diagnostic phase is to gather information:

1. History (verbally)
    a. Prior or current history as it relates to the presenting pain problem
    b. Review of other systems of the body to assess for concurrent dysfunctions in other areas
2. Physical examination
3. Laboratory evaluation
4. Confirm the above signs and symptoms with diagnostic therapy
5. Evaluation for other contributory or perpetuating factors that are revealed by and during the diagnostic therapy

Part I: History

A person comes in and says, "Doctor M., this is what happened to me in December of 1978...I fell down. The next morning I woke up with pain in the right side of my face and pain radiating from my right shoulder to my right hand. After a while there was pain behind my right eye. Then I saw Dr. Y." The person tells Dr. M. what she experienced, and Dr. M. attempts to document the problem.

The person may tell Dr. M. that she had surgery 5 years ago for a jaw fracture, and the wires are still in place. On further questioning, the person may relate that she is seeing an ENT doctor for a sinus infection or a chronic inner ear infection. On review of other body systems, the person may relate that she has a malabsorption problem, a high-carbohydrate diet, or other metabolic messages that may spell poor nutrition.

All of the above historical data have a significance and interrrelate.

Part II: Physical Examination

On the physical examination, are the findings exactly where the person said they were? An attempt is also made to determine if there are physical findings in areas outside (away from) where the person said they were.

Consultation is also initiated with Dr. C., an independent medical consultant, who reports that additionally the person has an iron deficiency anemia.

During the course of the evaluation Dr. M. would want to take X-rays to document possible displacement of the condyle(s) of the fossa to rule out a dental perpetuating factor.

Other X-rays and/or laboratory testing is usually of value in evaluating the person with chronic pain.

Part III: Laboratory Evaluation

Laboratory evaluation (blood testing and urine analysis) is carried out according to the blood testing given in Chapter 10 and also in accord with the recommendations in Chapter 4 ("Perpetuating Factors") of Travell and Simons (1983).

Part IV: Confirm I and II with Diagnostic Therapy

Dr. M. begins diagnostic therapy by using noninvasive mechanical or physical therapy. This usually consists of a heel lift, a wrist splint, or the like. If the person plays tennis, and the shoulder–arm pain is a real problem, then a sling and rest for the right arm may be in order. Also, Dr. M. may want to suggest the person stay off of the tennis team. If the low back was a problem area, then a program that includes whirlpool treatments to the back might be considered.

Then, on a return visit, the person may say that since quitting the tennis team, the pain in the elbow has stopped. However, when Dr. M. examines the elbow, there is still problematic referral of pain from the elbow to the hand.

Or, the person may say, "As long as I have the lift in my shoe":

1.   My pain is better.
2.   My pain is unchanged.
3.   My pain is worse.

Up to this time Dr. M. has a hypothesis (working diagnosis) about what the diagnosis is. Once you institute diagnostic therapy and get positive (encouraging) responses you have an actual diagnosis.

During this phase Dr. M. may find out that the person's right shoulder and arm pain is responding well to the diagnostic therapy of using a sling and quitting the tennis team. However, once the therapy is stopped, the pain returns within half an hour. The facial pain may be responding well to the use of a dental appliance. However, half an hour after the splint is removed the facial pain comes back.

The next phase, the treatment phase, is not started unless the problems have been clearly documented.

Part V: Revealing Other Contributing Problems

Other contributory and/or perpetuating factors should be revealed as diagnostic therapy progresses. This usually relates to an unexpected or additional response to diagnostic therapy. For example, a heel lift applied to the right shoe, in the management of low back pain, may cause unexpected numbness in the anterior right thigh. The factors revealed may be mechanical (problems with a short arm or leg) or systemic. For example, after a problem becomes resistant to diagnostic therapy, it is discovered that the blood tests are still too low (less than optimal potassium level).

Also, the diagnostic phase may reveal problems that were minimal before or that the person did not realize before.

Treatment Phase

This phase is entered when Dr. M. wants to maintain the person's relief and progress for longer periods of time because the diagnosis has been confirmed by a positive response to the diagnostic therapy.

This phase may last 6–9 months. For example, it takes a person with a degenerative process in the temporomandibular joint a minimum of 6–9 months to heal with proper treatment. Another example is the person with chronic pain from myofascial pain syndrome. Treatment in the more severe cases may take up to a year or two, and even then the person may not be completely restored to normal function.

When the person gets comfortable in the treatment phase, then the stabilization work is considered.

Stabilization Phase

In this phase the treatment is converted to stabile corrections. For example, the shoe lift that was used to treat the low back pain problem is converted from a removable shoe insert to a permanent correction to the person's heel and sole of the right shoe.

Rapid Sequence: Diagnosis → Treatment → Stabilization

The following are examples of diagnosis, treatment, and stabilization that can occur rather rapidly:

1. A person gets a dental appliance for a headache pain problem. One week later the person is fine and does not have any more pain or headaches. The person returns in 3 weeks and is still doing fine. The person is seen 6 weeks later, and has not worn the appliance for 3 weeks and is still pain free. One dental appliance restored the dysfunctional headache problem.
2. An orthopedic dental (splint) appliance is made for a person with a clicking and painful temporomandibular joint problem and facial pain. Three months later the person wears it down to the point of being "tissue paper" thin. At that point the person throws the splint away and is doing fine. One doctor solved the whole problem with one type of treatment.

BIBLIOGRAPHY

Funt, L. (1991). Personal communication.

Pawlicki, R. (1980). Demographic and behavioral factors amongst female chronic pain patients from a rural Appalachian setting, paper presented at the Second Annual Meeting of the American Pain Society, New York, p. 14.

Sonkin, L. (1994). Myofascial pain due to metabolic disorders: diagnosis and treatment, in *Myofascial Pain and Fibromyalgia*, Rachlin, E. (Ed.), Mosby, St. Louis, pp. 45–60.

Travell, J.G. and Simons, D.G. (1983). *Myofascial Pain and Dysfunction: The Trigger Point Manual*, Williams and Wilkins, Baltimore, pp. 114–150.

3 Chronic Pain: What Is It?

Michael S. Margoles, M.D., Ph.D.

Those who wait for help; those who suffer in silence.

What you think your chronic pain problem is, is important.
What others think your pain problem is, is not important!

—The author (1995)

INTRODUCTION

When I talk about chronic pain, I am not talking about a headache that is relieved with two Bayer® aspirin. I am talking about a headache that will not respond to anything! That means a headache, backache, neck ache, or any ache that will not or has not positively and unquestionably responded to anything and anybody whose tried to do something for you or it.

Presently we have no model of chronic pain patients, or what they look and sound like, so that the public and professionals will know how to understand the problem and the patient. Progress toward understanding is being made in this area, but much confusion still remains.

In medicine we understand a lot about many diseases. Take, for example, rheumatoid arthritis. It deforms the people who have it. It is very easy to recognize. It is even painful. However, because we cannot yet "see" the "deformities" that chronic pain produces, it may be years before it is better understood.

So, what is the chronic pain patient to do in the meantime? The patient can take the material in this book to friends, family members, and medical professionals and try to educate them by getting them to read the chapters and sections that relate to his or her problem of pain and suffering. Education makes people wiser, and in some cases more compassionate. Go easy on those who are not interested in learning these important concepts.

Chronic pain is not just a pain in the back or neck. It is more than that. It is pain in the back plus disturbed sleep, depression, grieving, loss of job secondary to pain and disability, being humiliated and disgraced, accusations of faking, and more.

The usual model of recovery in these patients is not the usual 1 week or the 3- to 6-week recovery from acute sprains that is characteristic of the acute-type patient. The chronic type is a patient who is disabled from work after a mild to moderately severe injury. The recovery

1-57444-103-5/99/$0.00+$.50
© 1999 by CRC Press LLC

time can be 6–12 weeks or longer. Sometimes recovery requires 8–60 months. Some patients never recover and are left with residual pain and dysfunction that last for years! In some, the problem improves for 6–12 months and then gets slowly worse over the next 3–10 or more years.

It may start out with a severe diffuse low back pain problem, after a bending injury, and just remain with a residual of a low or midline mid-sacral pain in the years that follow the injury. These patients also recruit more areas of pain involvement as time goes on. With each new injury, more areas of pain involvement are added to the total picture. Their bodies do not resolve each flare-up completely, as do patients who heal according to the acute model.

More and more of the problems listed below are encountered as a pain problem becomes chronic and/or more complex.

COMPONENTS OF CHRONIC PAIN

Causes of Pain

Pain is an unpleasant sensation that occurs in varying degrees of severity and may be a consequence of a number of disease processes. By definition chronic pain is present for 6 months or more.

Pain may be due to:

- Injury: Accident, bowling, sprain/strain, falling
- Iatrogenic: This relates to scar tissue and other types of problems that are usually induced by various medical, dental, and chiropractic therapies
- Trauma: Hit with a bat, fall down stairs, automobile accident
- Infection: Acts as a perpetuating factor in myofascial pain syndrome
- Arthritis: Inflamed, swollen, and reddened joints
- Metabolic: Excess or deficiency of vitamins
- Tumor: When it expands internal organs or invades bones
- Psychologic: The agony of intense grieving can cause pain. Psychogenic is a much less common source of chronic pain than is commonly suspected. Unfortunately, a complex pain patient is brushed off as merely having a psychiatric problem as the cause of the pain.
- Structural problem: Short leg, short pelvis, abnormalities of feet, etc.
- Congenital: Dislocation of the hip

Descriptors for Pain

Some of the most commonly used descriptors for pain are

- Intensity of symptoms
  - Minimal: An annoyance, causes no handicap in the performance of activities of daily living (ADL) or job duties
  - Slight: Causes some handicap in the performance of ADL and duties that bring the pain on
  - Moderate: Causes marked handicap in the performance of ADL and duties that bring the pain on
  - Severe: Precludes the performance of ADL and/or job duties that bring the pain on

- Frequency of symptoms
  - Occasional: About 25% of the time
  - Intermittent: About 50% of the time
  - Frequent: About 75% of the time
  - Constant: 100% of the time
- Other modifiers
  - Intractable: Difficult to ease, remedy, or cure

Pain Assessment

Consider the statement "you can't measure chronic pain." It says there is no way to measure or assess chronic pain. However, you can assess and measure *the evidences of it.* The original statement can then be modified to say, *"You can't measure chronic pain, but you can assess and measure the evidences of it."* The statement can then be broken up into component parts and analyzed as follows:

You	(me, you, them, etc.)
can't	(are incapable of)
measure	(direct measurement or assessment)
pain	(the statement one makes about the discomfort of a hurt; it is a very subjective experience and may vary from person to person)
but	(however)
you	(me, you, them)
can	(are able to or capable of)
assess and measure	(being able to determine the quantity or amount and quality of)
the evidences of it.	

The obvious evidences of it are grimacing, decreased range of motion, tender myofascial taut bands, symptom-producing myofascial trigger points, local twitch responses, jump signs, discomfort during a properly executed physical examination, tolerance for sitting, sleep abnormalities, loss of employment, loss of enjoyment, decrease or absence of sexual function, and many others.

Models

"Bits and Pieces"

The following are a number of random statements about chronic pain from observations I have made over the past 21 years of pain management practice. Some are quotes from patients.

- Sometimes it is on the right. Sometimes it is on the left. Sometimes it is on both sides.
- Sometimes it's bad and sometimes it's good.
- The more you do, the more it hurts.
- As time goes on this gets worse.
- Most people with chronic pain look pretty good.
- Most women in chronic pain are compulsive about wearing makeup. Makes them look better than they really are.

- We look for expressions of pain in the face. It is usually not there in the chronic pain patient. It is generally more visible with acute pain, broken bone, acutely sprained back, etc.
- Chronic pain patients drop out of the social scene. Their absence is a message that they are hurting. They feel that the pain and suffering shown on their face is an embarrassment.
- Their sleep gets all messed up, and so does the patient. They are up numerous times each night, or just can't find a comfortable position to sleep in.
- It's embarrassing to say you have pain to another person who doesn't know what chronic pain is. And, all they can think of to say is "I'm sorry" or "My great aunt had pain once."
- "Good days and bad."
- Sometimes it's constant, day and night. This may go on for days, months, or years.
- Even those who love you stand by helpless, afraid, and embarrassed.
- Barbara D. said: "I'm just a pain away from feeling good."
- A disaster has occurred, and no one was prepared for it. Who ever heard of a pain preparedness list or pain insurance?
- It's hard to relate to others how grueling chronic pain goes on relentlessly day after day.
- How it shatters your dreams and hopes. How it takes over (or tries to take over) every fiber of your body.
- It's doubly hard, difficult, and embarrassing to attempt to relate your suffering to a medical professional who "turns his or her light out" (turns off his or her hearing ability and concern) after listening to you for 20 seconds or to one who has diagnosed you before you even open your mouth to explain.
- Those who have endured or experienced your pain problem with you may seem to understand you better than those who have not.

Emotions: They're Good for You, But...

We frequently hear that working out our frustrations and anger is good for the tension we have. Who knows, it may be good for pain symptoms, too.

There is a paradox in a chronic pain patient getting mad or angry. It may make the person feel better but may make him or her hurt worse because of the sudden tension that hits the muscles and nerves. This is not to say one should not get mad or angry; it is to say that a pain flare-up may result if one does.

Numerous emotions can trigger the pain centers of the brain and make the pain worse. These include intense:

- Hate
- Anger
- Anxiety
- Rage

Other emotions (situations) can make the pain feel better and more tolerable:

- Love
- Caring

- Distraction
- A diversion of your attention
- A good movie
- Talking to someone you like, love, or care about
- Forgetting about your needs and putting someone else's first

Centralist and Peripheralist

There are two basic but arbitrary divisions among therapists in the pain field: centralist and peripheralist. The centralist believes that all chronic pain is merely a memory in the brain's pain receptor area and that all the tissue injury responsible for the production of the original pain problem is gone by about 6–12 weeks after the injury has occurred. Some of the centralists tell their patients that their current perception of pain is nothing more than a "track" on the brain. In essence, they are telling the chronic pain patient that the whole problem is basically a reaction to the memory of pain. On the other hand, the pure peripheralist believes that all chronic pain is caused by damaged tissue that is chronically deranged, such as the effects of postoperative scarring that appears to be causing ongoing pain after an operation. Most pain management specialists can achieve a balanced thinking that incorporates material from both points of view. When a therapist is swayed too much in either direction, his or her thinking ultimately works to the disadvantage of the patient. This may cause problems in the delivery of medical care. The centralist, for example, will tend to avoid surgery at all costs, and the peripheralist may perform more than is needed. There are numerous other examples that can be cited. Ultimately, the decision to give (administer) adequate doses of pain-relieving medication and other care to a chronic pain patient will depend, to an extent, on whether a pain therapist physician is a centralist or peripheralist.

Chronic Pain: Who, What, When, Where, How

Chronic pain patients are walking about among us. They generally are not found to be in excruciating pain such as that which would be caused by a fracture of a bone. However, their pain can be that excruciating or more. These people are usually diligent workers and do well on a 30- to 40-hour workweek. They do not function well on workdays that are longer than 8 hours. They do rather poorly in overtime-type situations. Although there are millions of these people in the population of the United States today, it is very difficult to spot them in day-to-day situations. They generally become socially isolated and are not seen at social functions. Some of these patients, even though presenting to a physician while in their thirties or forties, may give a history of having pain, or growing pains, since the time of childhood. These patients are truly the silent sufferers in our society. Some women will date the onset of their illness to the birth of a child.

Patients with chronic pain are subject to being ostracized and rejected by the public. The most common present view of chronic pain is that it is a psychiatric problem or psychological illness. It then follows that the only type of therapy that will resolve this is behavior modification (psychotherapy). Chronic pain patients are viewed with skepticism by much of the medical and legal community and the public and are frequently treated as though they are hypochondriacs. The boss at work and the spouse are among the cadre of people who become suspicious that the patient has his or her pain complaints (problem) solely for purposes of secondary gain (to get something out of it such as getting out of doing work at home or on the job).

Some Methods of Coping

"Looking Good"

Coping is usually done to keep others from knowing that one is suffering or in pain. This can be done by:

1. Acting stoical
2. Using a "poker face"
3. Taking the attitude that "the show must go on"
4. Acting professional
5. "Wearing the mask"

Keep this in mind. When you use all these "tricks" to look okay, don't be surprised when friends and relatives find it hard to believe you are having pain problems with related physical dysfunction.

Mind Setting

Clayre R. offered the following insight: "If I let myself think I will always be this way, it upsets me, so I prefer to think there is a cure."

Comments

I've gone from enjoying life, to getting through each day.

—Maya A. (1993)

I often wonder if the people who allocate the money for research care about people in chronic pain. I feel that it isn't thought of as an urgent need, because we aren't dying or so they think. We *are* dying. It may be an inch a day, but we are dying and in the most painful, merciless way.

—Diane W. (1993)

My body has become a stranger to me.
What was my friend has become my enemy.
What was familiar is now foreign.
I cannot count on my body.
I cannot rely on my friend.
You've let me down.
You let me down daily.
You disappoint me! You make me angry!
You keep me from being myself.
Yet I am forced to dwell with you daily!
I must live with what I hate!
I war daily. My flesh and my will collide,
while I lay helplessly on the sidelines.

—Marilynn D. (8/13/95)

Sheri B. used the term "jerked around" when asked how Dr. Richard S. treated her at the Memorial Pain Clinic in the late seventies.

Norman G., in commenting on one of the "insurance company doctors" who had examined him, referred to that doctor as a "fiction writer" because of all the inaccuracies contained about him in that doctor's report.

Pain May Not Respond to Routine Therapy

Soft tissue pain problems may become a chronic resistant and progressive disease.

- Intensity of pain may progress as follows: minimal → slight → moderate → severe
- Frequency of pain may progress as follows: occasional → intermittent → frequent → constant

It may sound incredulous to say that some (a very few cases) nonmalignant, intractable, pain patients present with pain that is so severe that it is only moderately controllable with patient self-administration of Dilaudid® injection, Duragesic® patches, or a combination of the two. This has been found in 1–3% of my entire 4000-patient population. Obviously, there are others who respond to less powerful medications such as morphine, oxycodone, methadone, Levo-Dromoran®, Percodan®, Percocet®, Lorcet® 10, and others. About 9% of my patients have needed a schedule II medication to gain pain control and to regain adequate physical functioning.

Effects of Chronic Pain

Donna S. had the following to say about when severe pain strikes: "All I want to do sometimes is scream and yell."

Diane W. was having a psychological evaluation in January. The psychologist stated that she described her pain as not being entirely relieved by treatment (she had had two back surgeries, nerve blocks, and more, without any relief). The patient told the psychologist, "It's like having a terminal disease but you don't get to die." The psychologist concluded by saying, "She feels at this point the quality of her life is gone."

Ranjan P. (1989) had very severe facial, neck, and shoulder pain that has lasted for 10 years. She said the following about her pain: "Pain 'clings.' It feels like it enters my body and then it's like it's there to stay. It permeates me at the protoplasmic (a substance that constitutes the living matter of living cells and performs basic life functions) cellular level. It is completely unresponsive, totally resistant. Very resistant. Nothing can penetrate it. It is recalcitrant and unresponsive to anything I do. It is unresponsive to physical therapy, heat treatments, drugs, and more. It has a life of its own (it is like living and feeding off itself). It is almost like it lives apart from me. It is separate. It is the damnedest thing. It gets real bad around the time of my period, and that's when I lose it; I decompensate and regress when this pain comes on. That's when I get so desperate that I feel I've got to have a hysterectomy to solve the problem."

Pain Behavior

This refers to the body language (messages) that patients may display when they are hurting. The term may be a misnomer. It consists of grimacing and other facial expressions as the result of discomfort, twitching, limping, etc.

- It is less common in chronic pain.

- Some patients pride themselves on "looking good" and will not show they are in pain.
- The pain may cause groaning and abnormal walking patterns

Unfortunately, some physicians hold these actions against the patient. The patient may be labeled as being overly dramatic when showing "pain behavior," and the physician, nurse, etc. may interpret pain behavior as a form of faking to get attention.

Suffering

The Suffering Experience

Suffering is an emotional reaction to an unpleasant physical stimulus or event. Suffering is neither good nor bad. There is no right or wrong time to suffer.

Suffering is a reaction to the pain and is separate from the pain itself. It is an emotional attitude toward the pain. It can range from barely noticeable to very overt with moaning, intense guarding of the painful part or complaining loudly and bitterly about the pain problem and how it has devastated the person's life.

The problem of suffering may or may not have been initiated by the pain. It often becomes mixed together with the pain. The pain patient might say: "If only the doctors would get rid of the pain, then the other problems would go away. I didn't have any of these problems before." Individuals suffering from chronic pain must come to understand that the suffering is separate from the pain and that they must play a significantly larger role in the control and management of their suffering. This represents a much larger role than what is usually expected in the treatment of patients in the acute model. "Pain is inevitable; misery (suffering) is optional" (Paul F., 1990).

Suffering frequently accompanies pain. Suffering and pain are different. Pain is a physical sensation. Suffering is the anguish and emotional difficulties that accompany pain. Suffering can originate from a number of sources such as grieving over the loss of a job, upset about the loss of masculinity or femininity, and difficulty adjusting to the status of being in pain, disabled, and unemployable. Suffering is difficult to separate from the pain experience.

The following is a definition of suffering in chronic pain: To have sorrow, bitterness, remorse; external appearance that shows sorrow, pain, or discomfort; a facial expression of discomfort; a bodily attitude ("body language") of discomfort or being pained or in pain; to appear at a disadvantage.

Suffering may be judged as a sign of weakness, but this has not been borne out by appropriate medical studies.

Since an individual can control his or her feelings, emotions, and thinking processes, it is possible to modify the suffering response and some of the pain as well.

Pain and suffering are different. While a person may not be able to do something to reduce the pain every time it flares up, he or she can learn to decrease the suffering that frequently comes with it.

Mike M. (1996)

> Suffering — the longer it goes, the deeper it gets.

Kim S. (7/19/94)

Kim is a 41-year-old Caucasian female with burning sensory neuropathy (nerve damage) throughout all her limbs and all her torso. She also has subluxation of her eye lenses on both sides. She has college training in dietetics.

Until my pain problem became severe, life seemed good — I was working, getting together with friends, enjoying the outdoors, dating, and hoping someday to marry and have a family. Twelve years of chronic pain, beginning at age 29, completely changed life as I knew it, the impact reaching far beyond myself and physical suffering.

Because I hadn't yet learned how to minimize the pain, the first 3 years were the most difficult. The pain, overwhelmingly intense, consumed my every thought and all my energy. Necessary everyday activities, such as showering, dressing, or moving from one point to another, were extremely trying and in most cases worsened the pain. I wasn't able to focus or concentrate on anything but trying to reduce my pain. I struggled to maintain my usual lifestyle, but the pain was physically and mentally exhausting. As a result, my life gradually fell apart.

Unable to work, I began living with my parents. Ninety-nine percent of my life was spent in bed, living minute to minute in order to endure the pain. The only time I left home was for yet another doctor appointment, desperately hoping with each visit to find relief. However, the conclusion was always the same: there was nothing wrong with me, nothing more could be done, and no reason to follow up. The months turned into years, and I felt mentally tortured from constant pain, physically weak from prolonged bed rest, and depressed and despondent from repeated unsuccessful attempts to get help.

The above placed a heavy strain on all relationships, and eventually most were lost. I seemed to lose all sense of reality. All I knew or could relate to was pain. My most pleasant thought was dying. I couldn't stand to listen to anything or anyone, and could barely carry on a conversation. The little I had to say, no one wanted to hear. No one could understand how a perfectly healthy looking person could be in so much pain. The consensus was that the only thing wrong with me was my attitude, and I would feel better if I wanted to feel better; that I needed to see a psychiatrist because my depression was causing the pain. It wasn't long before I had no further contact with friends.

My family continued to provide support, but there were many bitter arguments and hard feelings. My parents spent a tremendous amount of time, money, and effort trying to help me either alleviate or ameliorate my pain. We have traveled long distances for doctor appointments, tried every treatment we could try on our own (to name a few, creams, full spectrum lights, herbal remedies, supplements of all kinds, yeast and allergy diets, mind/body exercises), purchased special soaps and detergents, sewn undergarments out of special material, moved to a new home, taken extraordinary measures to rid the house of anything that could cause health problems, spent time in a different environment (the Sierra Mountains) for which my father took off 3 months of work, and the list goes on and on. For the first 3 years it consumed my parents' lives, as well as my own, which in turn affected the lives of all the other family members. Arguments ensued from disrupted lives and everyone's tried patience. Though family relationships have never been quite the same, we are still a family.

I was 32 years old when we discovered that soft water provided significant relief from the pain. Since then I have tried to resume as normal a life as possible. The lengthy measures required to control the pain and the maximum level of comfort that could be achieved allowed me to complete 2 years of college work in 8 years. My life was spent at home with my parents or at school for a few hours a week when I felt well enough. Since graduating in May 1994, I have remained at home with my parents. On a good day, I accompany my parents to run an errand. On a bad day, I lie down most of the day. With my life situation, both then and now, I can't relate to other people my age, and therefore, I do not socialize with anyone outside my family. I attend family gatherings, but I spend most of the time daydreaming. I don't really belong anywhere or relate to anything or anyone. Making contacts and networking with people in my field of study is useless since any working future is at best unlikely. I have no future personal or working plans.

With time, the pain has become increasingly more difficult to control. I don't live, I exist. I am not afraid of dying, I'm afraid of living a tortured existence. I will NEVER again endure the pain and cruelty I experienced for the first 3 years. If the intensity of my pain reaches the level of the first 3 years, I will take my life.

Progression of the Pain

Some think that all chronic pain goes away over time. Chronic pain is defined as pain that lasts 6 months or more. If it has gone on that long, why think it will go away on its own in a longer period of time? I have seen it in patients for 10, 20, 30, 50 years and more. Mine has lasted 42 years and is now only about 80–90% resolved with 16 years of intense treatment.

Pain may become worse over time because of:

1.   Natural process (progress) of the disease itself
2.   Intense emotional stress
3.   Repeat traumas (injuries, assaults, accidents)
4.   Inappropriate physical activity (e.g., abuse of muscles)

Some Doctors Don't Understand Chronic Pain

Some doctors don't understand chronic pain, as manifested by some of the following statements or scenarios from patients:

- "Some spend as little as 5 minutes examining a patient with 10–20 years of pain."
- "It makes you wonder where this doctor got his pain training."
- "It's facing doctors who tell you that you have no basis for your pain complaints and they haven't even put their hands where it hurts."
- How can that doctor say that about me when that doctor 'never touched me!'"
- "Who is he? I'll bet he never felt my pain for a while. If he did, he'd change his mind."
- "If he could only feel my pain for 5 minutes, he would understand."
- "They can't feel what I am feeling."
- "He told me I'd have to live with it! What the hell does he think I'm doing now?"
- "They think I'm playing a game or something!"
- "Wow, those two are something else!"
- "The doctor said he had headaches too, and he couldn't understand why I had trouble coping with them."
- "The examination he put me through was pure torture, and then he had the nerve to tell me there was nothing wrong."
- "The doctor said the X-rays were negative and there couldn't be any cause for my pain."
- "I could touch my toes so he said there was nothing wrong with my back."
- "That doctor had an attitude!"
- "It's all in your head."
- Patient: "How long will it last?" Doctor: "I don't know."

- "Most doctors act like it's my fault they can't cure my pain".
- "I saw you walk in here yet you say you have to look at your foot when sitting or laying down in order for it to move…this doesn't make sense; you are too difficult to examine."
- "There is nothing more I can offer at this point. You can go back to work now."
- "Your life is slipping by. Don't you want to live it?"

Thomas B. (6/2/95)

Tom was a 37-year-old ex-police officer who was disabled in the line of duty in 1991. Pain occurred in the right chest and right side of back. Pain radiated to other side of the back and occasionally to the legs. He then became a commodities trader.

> 3/13/90 — Called to pick up a half-crazed, stoned on PCP, 275-pound man. During scuffle, suspect hallucinated, wanting to kill police officer, grabbing his holstered gun. They wrestled for gun when ambulance that was called pulled up behind, hitting Tom in the back of the right shoulder. Slammed against ambulance, never letting go of suspect. Never lost consciousness. Just felt sore all over, with pain in shoulder. Six or seven days later his right hand felt numb to fingers, turning blue and red; his whole right arm felt "dead." Went to orthopedist who took X-rays, treating with anti-inflammatory drugs. The anti-inflammatory medication irritated his gut. A week later hand became ice cold, became much worse. Saw neurologist, thoracic specialist. Doppler scan, EMG, all kinds of tests. His condition worsened. June 1991 first rib removed, right side to clear artery. Three days later, still in hospital, he threw up blood. He had bled for 2 days internally. Next day, thoracotomy done, lost three or four units of blood, replaced by his own that he had previously saved. Was in horrible shape with excruciating pain in right hand. Had 11 surgeries, including 5 laser surgeries, within 28 months. January 1992 diagnosed with reflex sympathetic dystrophy (causalgia) by Denver thoracic doctor. Two chest surgeries; sympathectomy performed — most of second rib was taken. Pleurectomy done, (neurolysis of TI nerve). He got feeling back in his fingers, then artery split. Had to have another surgery (concrete adhesions were found) — Dr. Soos. He moved to Arizona in January 1994 for weather — humidity and cold very bad for him. In Arizona a local medical doctor helped him out with Percocet® and MS Contin®. He went to trading commodities as a means of support. He still had severe pain in his right shoulder, chest and upper back. The pain limited his ability to function consistently in his commodities business, and in life in general. He had been in two to three behavior modification programs, stating "It was good while I was in the room."

William L. (8/96)

Saw several different HMO doctors. As we switched plans none did much at all (in their 5-minute "treatment"). I don't remember their names.

Maya A. (1996)

I can now do in one week what I used to do in one day!

Sally D. (4/1/96)

My pain is no longer confined to my knees, and the Alka Seltzer® with the Tylenol® #3 only make it barely tolerable. The other pain, especially in my left thumb, right elbow, neck, and back, seems to be worsening. I can no longer rely on crutches, a cane, or a walker during bouts of tendinitis because they aggravate some of the conditions. I do not know the answer, but more and more I see a time coming when I will not be able to tolerate the pain.

Separation

Severe pain is ultimate loneliness

—Rodenmayer (1967)

- Separation from God
- Feel punished
- Desire to get in the car and run away
- Leads to anxiety
- Separates you from what you want to do
- Loss of ability to work
- Loss of job
- Loss of credibility
- Loss of friends
- Loss of insurability for back and neck
- Loss of social life
- Loss of companionship
- Loss of sexual relationship
- Loss of hobbies and avocations

Giving a person a diagnosis of chronic pain, especially that of chronic low back pain, is like telling someone they have leprosy, only they don't know it until they go to look for a job or try to get health insurance. Either the person decides to separate himself or herself from others, or others decide to separate themselves from him or her.

Persons having back pain problems are routinely discriminated against. Most insurance companies will not issue insurance to cover a back or neck pain problem. Most employers will not hire individuals with a back pain problem. Individuals with back or neck injuries on the job are routinely discriminated against by their employers and frequently by the company that handles their worker's compensation insurance program. Such injured workers are frequently "swept under the carpet" and out of the way by independent medical examiners who make their living by providing this service to the insurance company. Over time these individuals learn to separate themselves from this system because the emotional abuse is too great and may cause extreme stress and distress.

Sometimes separation is only a feeling, but nonetheless it is there, whether artificial or real, and must be reckoned with. Separation may occur when a marriage is adversely affected by the pain problem of a spouse. More on this subject can be found in Chapter 30.

Elective separation. Some people may cause worsening of pain. In the long run, pain patients may want to avoid those (kinds of) people and their associated pain-provoking conflicts. It might spare them unnecessary physical and emotional pain.

Fear

- Unknowns
- Doctors and nurses

- Surgery
- More pain
- Pain won't go away
- Can't get enough medication to control the pain
- Fears, anxieties, apprehensions
- Fear of unknowns, being in the hands of strangers, at the mercy of insurance reps, loss of job, loss of family, loss of income, having to trust strange doctors and nurses

Marilynn D.

I don't use the energy to clean up (a mess I've made) for fear the energy won't be there when I need it (to do the next important task on my schedule).

Isolation

- Social
- Interpersonal relationships
- Feelings of loneliness
- A result of rejection

Some patients are an embarrassment to the medical community because (1) they do not fit standard diagnoses and (2) they do not get well with standard (usual and customary, conventional) therapy.

Patients with chronic pain may become inwardly directed and withdrawn. However, some will remain outwardly directed unless the pain becomes very severe.

Isolation is a major component of chronic pain and contains many levels. Isolation can be described on five levels (Ranjan P., 1989):

1. Social (from the human species): Avoidance of social situations such as parties, family gatherings, etc.
2. Interpersonal relationships (from friends, family, etc.)
3. External (from the outer surrounding world and environment)
4. Internal (from self): This is a significant and extremely provocative precipitant to the next stage of isolation; being and feeling isolated from oneself is a frightening entry into another realm of being
5. Absolute (from life): This is usually the stage when suicide is contemplated, when isolation from existence takes place

Marilynn S. is a hard-working mother of three children. She is a very spiritual and positive individual. Her faith in God has sustained her during the suffering from a merciless chronic pain problem. In the recent past, in addition to her severe bouts of pain and an uncooperative husband, she felt depressed and her memory began to malfunction. It was then that she almost lost her will to live.

The chronic pain problem leaves you feeling lonely, alone, rejected, and misunderstood, even by those who love you. Many chronic pain patients feel that they are a nuisance to others, which serves to precipitate isolation, hostility, etc. (Ranjan P., 1989).

Isolation is more often a feeling than a fact. The person with chronic pain is made to feel different from others. He or she is treated like an oddball, especially by well-intentioned professionals who frequently tell the person they do not know what the diagnosis is and/or he or she is going to have to learn to live with it. Once the individual finds out that there are millions of people who have similar problems, the feelings of isolation are put into a less dangerous and threatening category.

Richard S. (a 56-year-old man with severe pain following 20 surgeries) said: "Usually when the pain is so bad and you cannot get any medications, and the doctors refuse to give you any kind of relief, you get to feel like you're more of a burden to everyone around you. You feel more like a drain on society and others, and it would be better off for the doctors or family if you weren't here to hold them back. Then your pain would be over with." He also said: "Want to go off in a hole and pull it in on top of me.

Sally D. (4/1/96)

I have never really entertained thought-plans of suicide over this condition but once, here in my hometown, as I was driving on a country two-lane road I kept my foot on the gas pedal as I closed in on a railroad crossing where the signal was engaged. I finally stopped abruptly and watched how fast the train sped through. Another time, I had left my garage door closed after I had started my car and just sat there and sobbed. As I said before, I haven't really planned to take my life. I know I couldn't put the train's engineer through anything like that, and our garage does have some ventilation

I think these episodes were just pauses…A time to stop and say to myself how tired I was of this battle.

I am so tired of fighting the pain and even more tired of fighting the ignorance surrounding its management.

I love life. I love my life.

I need help.

Grieving and Anguish

Grieving and anguish are related to the losses mentioned under "Separation." Grief means deep mental anguish, as over a loss, such as loss of a job, limb, spouse, head of household status, companionship, and more. It implies sorrow, resentment over being harmed, deep hurt, and harm or hardship. An example would be how the patient feels after having been discredited or disgraced in a deposition or courtroom proceeding.

We usually think of grief as a limited process such as occurs when a spouse dies. In that instance it may last for up to 2 years. However, in chronic pain it may go on for years and years because the pain may go on for years and years.

A person has pain. Something is wrong. The person is grieving, but knows nothing about grief. This is somewhat like the loss of a loved one. What is the person feeling? Loss, loss and more loss — loss of a job, loss of consortium, loss of a marriage, loss of pride, loss of the ability to earn money and provide for oneself and one's family, loss of freedom of movement, loss of pain-free living, loss of self-esteem. The unfortunate thing about these multifaceted losses is that they may last for years.

Thoughts include: What am I feeling? Is this real or imagined? Am I just acting? Who can explain this to me? What do I feel? How can I explain it? How can I change the way I feel? I don't know. Something is wrong, but what is it?

Chronic pain patients have an ongoing grieving reaction composed of the following stages:

- Denial
- Depression
- Anger

- Searching
- Frustration
- Bargaining
- Acceptance

Steffeny T. (3/26/96)

Steffeny is a 40-year-old sales management executive for one of the large semiconductor companies. She had worked her way up the ranks and was netting $50,000 per year when she became disabled because of her chronic pain problem.

I left work on disability and they sent a rehab nurse to my house. She said I was on too many drugs, and narcotics were the worst thing for pain. The nurse said the narcotics were, in fact, creating the pain. I needed to go through detox.

I would have done anything for help. The pain pills did control the pain, but my pain and pain behaviors were getting bad. I did not know what else to do at the time. My personality seemed to be changing. Talking too much and trouble focusing on a subject. On the patches (Duragesic® patches) I do not have this problem.

In January of 1995 I decided this is not going to ever go away and I better make a life with it. I got out of bed, started working on my friendships with women. Have a few good friends and exercise every day. Soft aerobics to rock and roll. Yoga and meditation my way.

The university pain program took me off the meds, threw me in with people with eating disorders and street heroin addicts, forgot to tell me they understood I was there for pain and treated me like a crazy person who creates pain for attention. I went along with this. As soon as narcotics left my body my pain level jumped so high I was scared. I have been scared since. It seems to have progressed a great deal this year.

I gave the university pain program's way 100% for 5 months. After an 8-day run of a double head, eye, jaw, and neck ache that stayed an 8–10 pain level the whole run, I kept going in the garage with the door shut and starting the car. I then decided in October that even if narcotics were going to kill me, I would rather live with some pain-free time than live like this in any form. I am not really that depressed. I had never considered suicide in my life as an option. I started to experience sensations when in high pain, of actually losing my mind, my instincts, my faith. It is a hell inside, the hell of the pain.

I have lost my career, friends, money, self-esteem, and ability to study, read, use a computer, drive when I want, be reliable in dates, and make holiday dinners without problems. Making dinner every night is impossible. My sports (riding, skiing, jogging, tennis, softball, swimming) require warm water. All so far have had too much long-term pain to continue or try again. Not to mention I have lost my thirties, my looks, my figure. I can go

Recently my disability insurance decided I was not eligible for long-term benefits because it was in my mind and no objective findings that anything is wrong.

I have gained: time with my teenage daughter, strong interdependent marriage, less arrogance, more patience, a lot of humility, and more humanity.

I cannot even imagine being expected to handle this pain around the clock for the rest of my life. I am afraid about my future. I still seem to be losing things. My financial status is deteriorating and I will have three kids in college next year.

My major problems are pain and lack of sleep. They seem to go together or around each other. Can't sleep because of pain and insomnia, and when I don't sleep the pain is harder to handle and appears to be more severe. I also walk around very tired and spacey at times. I forget things I need to remember, like leaving keys in car, burners on, etc. I never did these things before. I also seem to forget what I am doing when tired.

I do not seem to be having any good days. I cannot remember the last day I finished saying, "Yes, I can do this." It has been since before Christmas.

I have so many symptoms besides pain, from itching to this mind-tormenting tingling that drives you crazy, and there is no way to handle it except stand in very hot water. But as soon as you turn off the water, it is back. It is worse than some of the pain.

I don't want to lose any more. This illness has taken so much away from me and my family. I am very willing to do my part to work on this and make it livable. I want not to feel like I live on a different planet than everyone else. I also am really tired of my mind and body never being in sync. Sometimes I am in a room full of people and I might as well be alone. I have gone from a life doer to an observer.

It may take as long as 2 years for many to get past the denial stage. Then the depression sets in, and suicidal ideation may become a problem. The depression is different from what occurs when a loved one dies in that it continues until the pain problem is resolved, and that may take a long time.

Pain Medication Issues

Whatever the cause of the chronic (intractable) pain, the patient may be depressed partly on the basis of not being able to obtain enough pain relief. In this respect, the use of opioids or opioid-containing analgesics may be viewed as an antidepressant for some chronic pain patients or for some components of a patient's pain.

Anger

The components of anger are

- Hurt
- Fear
- Frustration
- Disappointment

Georgianna S. (9/24/91)

Georgianna was a 63-year-old administrative aid who worked for her local government offices when her work accident occurred. One day she tripped while going down the office stairs, fell against a large file cabinet, and incurred pain in multiple areas of her body. She also experienced the onset of unremitting headaches, plus temporomandibular joint problems.

Yes, after 2 years of pain, I was angry. You should have recognized the outburst for that. You were right about the source of my anger. My subconscious had just been penetrated and assaulted by a statement against which I had built defenses for years. This stupid old Pollyanna had just been told, "There's nothing that can be done." And, unfortunately I chose your office to strike out in anger.

I agree I need counseling. My husband and I tried it together a few years ago. What problem does it solve if one of the parties to the problem wants a solution and the other refuses to admit there is a problem? One has to learn to accept or let go. The answer is one of decision, like one of my favorite poems: "God grant me serenity to accept the things that I cannot change, courage to change the things I can, and the wisdom to know the difference." I've always been the serene one who accepted everything life offered. When someone tries to control herself as I do, tries to help everyone else with their problems, keeps everything inside, and suddenly gets angry, speaks up, defends herself, then everyone is shocked. I'm suddenly the bad guy; I shouldn't behave like that. It is like the worm turning.

My other favorite poem is "Invictus." I quote the entire poem to myself, over and over in times of extreme stress, along with the Lord's Prayer. "Invictus" ends with my favorite words: "I am the master of my fate; I am the captain of my soul." My mother thinks this is sacrilegious, but I think God gives us the capacity to do things for ourselves. He gives us a brain to use as well as divine help, but He doesn't expect us to sit in a corner, doing nothing, and whining, "God help me." Nobody can help us if we do not strive to help ourselves.

Other Comments on Anger

The following comments are typical of how the chronic pain patient feels.

You do things; you break into a rage; you don't know why. You say, "This isn't me, but this is the way I feel." You become impatient. You're weary (and wary). You haven't rested well in months, and "The fools wonder why I'm all worked up!"

You're on edge and edgy. You become more vulnerable to criticism, especially from relatives who are close to you. You protect your painful part from being touched by others, even loved ones (this can be embarrassing).

A bra strap that has no mercy. Why doesn't somebody make one that doesn't hurt! You're compulsive about wearing a brassiere when out of the house. This compounds the agony. A belt puts too much pressure on your pain area, and slacks or shoes are too tight and constricting. An airplane seat feels like it was made for someone half your size. All these feelings contribute to the anger.

You begin to wish that many others had the same pain, for example, your doctor, your insurance company, or the insurance medical examiner they sent you to, so they might appreciate your agony. In fact, you have met others who have it and have read something that sounds like it in a magazine article. Then again, you may feel as though you are the only one who read the article.

Sensation Problems

This refers to abnormal sensations such as burning, prickling, tingling, pressure, tension, and tightness; jumping, jerking, and twitching of the muscles; and cramping in numerous areas. The person may experience sensations of tingling, burning, ants crawling on the skin, and other paresthesias.

Your leg feels "dead." Your hand is numb and you accidentally burn it on the stove but do not feel the burn. Your foot feels longer than usual. Your skin feels wet but is not. Your arm, leg, hand, torso, or abdomen feels swollen but is not. "Lightening" shoots down your back or extremities when you bend your neck or back. You swell in seemingly odd places.

- Paresthesias: Morbid or perverted sensation; an abnormal sensation, as burning, prickling, tingling, cramping, etc.
- Dysesthesias: Unpleasant abnormal sensation produced by normal stimuli. The straps or underwires of a brassiere can become very painful to muscles that have been injured in an accident.. Belts and tight clothes can cause pain.

- Routine activities can become more painful than expected.
- Unexplained sensations: Such expressions as "knifelike," "stabbing," "crushing," "burning," (less often, "freezing"), "a constricting band," "a storm," "a shock," "as if the flesh is being torn away," and "indescribable" are metaphoric attempts to describe a complex of totally unfamiliar sensory experiences" (Adams and Victor, 1981).

Dysfunction

Dysfunction is defined as altered or abnormal function, such as limping.

Emotional Dysfunction

Emotional impairment in chronic pain patients is manifested by:

- Decreased stress tolerance
- Presence of depression of mild to severe degree
- Various degrees of anger
- Showing "pain behavior"
- Impaired coping skills
- Impaired sleep
- Grieving reactions
- Suicidal ideation or the actual taking of one's life

Kathleen C., in her initial intake forms for our office, had this to say: "I have definitely thought sometimes that dying would be more comfortable than living with this pain — but I would never take my own life because it goes against my deeply held beliefs." Unfortunately some have already perished because they were given no hope or help.

More on these subjects can be found in Chapters 5, 15, and 16.

Cognitive Dysfunction

Cognitive refers to thinking, thought content, and the ability to use normal thinking processes. The more severe the pain, the more severe the impairment in thought and thought content may be. Coherent thinking usually calls for concentration. The distraction caused by pain that is severe and/or disabling provides enough distraction to compromise the employability of some individuals.

Physical Dysfunction

Examples include weakness of the hand or arm in upper extremity pain and weakness of the hip, knee, or ankle with lower extremity pain problems. Patients with low back and/or leg pain frequently state that their leg gives out, on the pain side, without warning. Many with low back pain state that they cannot walk on uneven ground. Low back pain sufferers experience sexual dysfunction because sexual activity aggravates their back pain.

When myofascial trigger points affect an extremity they often produce dysfunction in that extremity, such as weakness, giving way, or dropping things. A trigger point may cause loss of bowel control or may cause a knee to buckle unpredictably. Handwriting may change.

Chronic pain may also result in a change in a person's voice that reflects a strain caused by the pain. Tennis elbow, chronic tennis elbow, chronic bursitis, and chronic carpal tunnel syndrome adversely affect the function of the extremity.

Spatial Dysfunction

Spatial perception (where one is in time, place, and geographic location) is off and a person may bump into doorways or furniture or not be able to see in the dark or at dusk as well as he or she used to. The pain may feel as though it projects outside the leg or arm. A person's foot, hand, etc. may feel longer than usual.

A Theoretical Composite of the Various Terms Used Above

Sometimes people may choose to separate or isolate themselves from friends and family when back and leg pain flare up. They may go into a rage because of the inability of others to understand them and their situation. For example, you try to mow the lawn and your dysfunctional leg gives out. You fall to the grass on your pain side, causing an intense flare-up of your pain. Suffering is evident. Your pain flare-up makes you physically and emotionally dysfunctional. After you hit the ground, intense pain and paresthesias begin in your calf and heel. You realize your predicament and a strong sense of isolation hits you for 20–40 minutes. You grieve the loss of a normal life. You then grieve the separation and isolation. More and more of the above-indicated events are encountered as the pain problems become more chronic, more complex, and more severe.

Ignorance

Chronic pain patients are frequently confronted with ignorance that hurts.

"The Only Thing I Can't Do Is Bend Over"

Clayre R. is a very bright elementary school teacher. She is a very positive and upbeat person. Eight months ago she had a low back operation, and pain became progressively severe after her operation. Despite the severe pain, she continued to teach. Because of the severity of the pain, she used an electric cart to get to class and to move around within her classroom. She rode the cart from room to room and within the classroom. Because she used a cart to compensate for her severe postoperative low back pain, parents of her students and others assumed she was also hard of hearing and mentally retarded, both of which were untrue.

As Long as You Can Stand Up

As long as you can stand up, many people think there is nothing wrong with you, and if you can sit too, all the better! But if a person has to lie down wherever he or she goes, especially in the doctor's exam room, then the assumption is that he or she is either hurting or faking. Some professionals will not believe a person is in pain until they see a broken bone on an X-ray or blood oozing from a wound. Even then, some say, "You've got 6 weeks to hurt, and that's all!"

Penalized for Looking Good

One patient related this somewhat sad, but true, story. When she went to the emergency room in her nightgown and no makeup, complaining of pain, she could get a pain shot. When she appeared with the same complaint but was dressed and had makeup on, she was denied a pain shot.

A High Tolerance to Adversity

Some patients, through adverse situations such as physical abuse, have learned to have a high tolerance to adversity.

How to Reverse the Ignorance Problem

The following organizations have evolved since 1975 to resolve this problem:

- International Association for the Study of Pain
- American Academy of Pain Management
- American Academy of Pain Medicine
- American Pain Society
- Eastern Pain Society
- Midwestern Pain Society
- Western USA Pain Society
- The Arthritis Foundation
- National Chronic Pain Outreach Association
- Various fibromyalgia support groups
- American Chronic Pain Association

There are literally thousands of professionals and lay people who belong to these organizations, both nationally and internationally. It is apparent that these organizations are slowly reversing the ignorance problem. It is my impression that not many medical insurance companies are open to much of the knowledge that has been pouring out of these organizations for the last 20+ years.

Confusion

A person with back pain may be given numerous diagnoses, sometimes a different one from every therapist seen. This usually leads to confusion. Another variation of this occurs when a patient is given no diagnosis by the numerous consultants he or she sees.

There is also confusion about whether or not to operate, confusion about the presence of addiction and confusion about what medications can legally be given to someone with chronic pain.

In order for a therapist to diagnose chronic pain, he or she has to:

- Look
- Listen
- Touch

Look. The patient has to be studied, in detail, by the clinician. This takes time, if the patient has a grade 2–4 myofascial pain syndrome.

Listen. The therapist has to hear what the patient is saying. Too many times the therapist has decided beforehand what the patient's diagnosis is going to be and has difficulty hearing what the patient has to say that points to another diagnosis.

Touch. It is one thing to perform a "routine" physical examination on a person who complains of back pain. The touching, poking, and prodding can be rather limited in "routine" physical examinations. However, chronic pain patients require examinations that seek out specific tissues that may be causing or contributing to the pain. In patients with myofascial pain syndrome the examiner looks for specific muscles producing specific pain patterns. Frequently, the pain relating to myofascial pain syndrome can mimic the pain of numerous other conditions that cause the pain.

Recovery

Barbara D.: Thoughts on Getting Well

My first inkling that I might be improving came when I noticed that for brief periods (maybe only an hour) I felt better; not good, but better. When these tiny chinks in the armor of pain stretched into several days at a time, I became hopeful and felt, at last, that I was going to get better. However, the good days always ended, and the pain always returned. With that return came despair and intense depression. The hope of getting well was shattered over and over again. A psychiatrist who tried to help me with this told me that having good days meant just that. You had some good days. It didn't mean the pain was gone for good. I tried to make that work for me but I was not very successful. Gradually the pain seemed to be losing its grip on me, but I still went back and forth between good spells and bad spells, living on a roller coaster. I had a conversation with one of my doctors who said, "You're doing so well, you've come a long way." I replied, "Yes, but I still hurt." "But you've come so far." "I know, but I still hurt." I tried to explain to him that even though he might have various criteria by which to judge my progress, I only had one — pain — and *I still hurt.* I left his office giving mental assent to his claim that I was getting better, but I didn't *really believe* it in my heart. It is important to believe your doctor because when you doubt his judgment it is sabotage. I can't say enough about the importance of the doctor's positive encouragement. Sometimes it is all you have to hang onto. He says I'm getting better regardless of how I feel. These last few months, I noticed a gradual change in my attitude. A good bit of the time, I believe (emotionally) that I am better. When I have a bad spell I'll say to myself, "I'll feel better tomorrow," and I usually do. This is a big change for me. It comes after several months of experiencing some degree of stabilization in my body. I can begin to trust it again. I am beginning to feel able to plan my life again. I still experience physical and emotional setbacks, but they seem less terrifying and less severe. Chronic pain can never be fully understood by observation — only by experience.

Resolutions to Get Well

About 2 years before consulting me for a severe pain problem, Katrina F. had fallen down a flight of stairs. On one of her visits Katrina told me she was "sick and tired of being sick and tired." She had resolved to get back into the work force and had a job within 4 weeks of making that statement to me.

Pain Perception

The fact that a person feels pain results from impulses that come to the brain from sore, painful, or irritated nerves, skin, muscles, ligaments, joints, bones, and/or tendons.

Persons in acute pain may not have adapted to the pain and may not tolerate it well. They may show lots of "pain behavior" (grimacing, crying out with the pain, and feeling helpless). Some of this carries over to some chronic pain patients. Chronic pain patients, however, have had time to "learn" to adapt to and accept some or a great deal of their pain. The pain may become "familiar" and less threatening to them as time goes on. They frequently look "comfortable" despite the presence of ongoing pain that may be rather severe.

On the other hand, some chronic pain patients grew up having to "grin and bear it" or face the consequences. These children may have been abused or beaten by a relative. They grew up knowing that if they showed pain behavior after their abuse or beatings, they would be beaten harder or perhaps killed. They grew into adulthood showing little if any reaction to pain because of their childhood conditioning, as in the case of physical abuse.

Another patient, 49-year-old Sally G., looked comfortable despite the presence of significant pain. When I asked about her apparent indifference to pain, she said that she grew up in Seoul, Korea. As a child she had to be tough. There was lots of fighting between boys and girls when she was a child. She needed to be tough and show no evidence of pain. She had been an aggressive fighter.

Allodynia

One form of pain perception problem is allodynia, an unpleasant abnormal sensation produced by normal stimuli. For example, a woman has whiplash as the result of a car accident. Her neck, chest, and shoulders become painful and tender on both sides. When she puts on her brassiere, the pressure of the straps on her shoulders, the pressure of the side panels, or the pain caused by the underwire is so uncomfortable that she chooses not to wear the undergarment. Belts and other tight clothes might also become a problem.

Putting an average amount of pressure on the low back of some patients with low back pain may produce various degrees of pain and/or agony. Unknowing professionals may think this is a form of hysteria, but in fact it is allodynia, common in moderate to severe chronic back pain patients.

Myofascial pain syndrome patients frequently demonstrate this finding right at the trigger point or the reference zone (trigger point and reference zone are both defined in Chapter 10 and in the glossary). Patients with primary fibromyalgia syndrome (fibromyalgia, fibrositis) may demonstrate this finding at a tender point. Patients with neuropathic (damaged nerve) pain may have this finding when the skin about the affected area is stroked or palpated. There are numerous other medical conditions that will show similar abnormality.

Some Doctors Do Understand Chronic Pain

Some doctors do understand chronic pain, as manifested by some of the following statements from patients:

- "He believed me."
- "He believed what I said."
- "He listened to everything I said."
- "Someone who's been there."
- "He doesn't try to tell me how I'm feeling."
- "He cares enough about his patients to research any new developments they may have."
- "He doesn't believe in 5-minute patient examinations."
- "He didn't treat me like a dope addict looking for a legal 'fix'"
- "He understood what I was saying."
- "I was told, 'It's not in your head, this is a very real condition.'"
- "My psychologist said to me, 'I only treat patients with real pain.'"
- "He said, 'Your pain is severe.'"

- "I felt comfortable with him."
- "He knew what I was talking about."
- "He pulled out a book and showed me that my problems were in a medical textbook."
- "He told me I wasn't crazy."

Core Issues

Failure to adequately evaluate the patient is a very frequent problem. When the X-rays, magnetic resonance imaging, electromyography, and other tests are negative, there is sometimes a tendency to assume a psychological basis for the pain. The patient is put on an antidepressant and/or referred to a psychiatrist or psychologist.

A 5- or 10-minute examination of a chronic pain patient with intractable pain will never suffice. I have been saddened to see some doctors report findings to be normal when my examination of the same patient showed grossly abnormal findings. This relates to deep tendon reflex testing, pinprick sensation testing, and more. In general, I find that some doctors may not know how to interpret abnormal findings in the muscles, especially in patients with myofascial pain syndrome.

Even some of our sincere and most thorough physical examiners are frustrated by lack of findings that can link the patient's pain complaints with a physical abnormality. Perhaps we need a newer understanding or way to investigate or interpret some patients' pain complaints. This is needed in the area of soft tissue pain problems.

What is new in the area of soft tissue pain problem patient evaluations are the principles and practices embodied in the teachings and writings of Janet G. Travell and David G. Simons (Travell and Simons, 1983, 1992). These give us a whole new way to look at the largest organ system in the body, the muscles. Although complex, and difficult to learn, the wisdom of these two physicians provides an objective way of looking at muscles as a source of pain that can range anywhere from trivial to severe, incapacitating, and disabling.

BIBLIOGRAPHY

Barbara D. (1991). Personal communication.

Clayre R. (1989). Personal communication.

Margoles, M. (1983). Pain charts: spatial properties of pain, in *Pain Measurement and Assessment,* Melzack, R. (Ed.), Raven Press, New York, pp. 214–225.

Margoles, M. (1983). The stress neuromyelopathic pain syndrome, *The Journal of Neurological and Orthopaedic Surgery,* 4, 317–322.

Marie J. (1989). Personal communication.

Paul F. (1990). Personal communication.

Ranjan P. (1989). Personal communication.

Rodenmayer, R. (1967). *How Many Miles to Babylon?* Seabury Press, New York.

Travell, J.G. and Simons, D.G. (1983). *Myofascial Pain and Dysfunction: The Trigger Point Manual,* Williams and Wilkins, Baltimore, pp. 114–150.

Travell, J.G. and Simons, D.G. (1992). *Myofascial Pain and Dysfunction: The Trigger Point Manual,* Vol. 2, Williams and Wilkins, Baltimore, pp. 114–150.

4 Living with Chronic Pain

Richard Weiner, Ph.D.

INTRODUCTION

I have been in pain for over 24 years. I live pain every day. Pain is all I know.

I was in my early twenties when I had my first accident. I was a motorcycle policeman. It was hard work and low pay in those days. I was chasing a car and took a spill. I was laid up for a while and then I was able to get back to less demanding police work.

It was hard on my wife and kids, though, because I was laid up at home and not the nicest person. I was taking a lot of pain medication and it seems like I always had a headache.

The pain was getting worse, so I took an early partial disability and went to work for the state. In 1961 I was a passenger in a highway truck when we got hit by a tractor-trailer. My leg was torn off, and they had to put it back on.

It took a long time to get the right forms filled out for social security disability. There were times we did not have enough money to buy gas to go to the doctor.

I have seen several surgeons. They never seem to have enough time for my treatment. Their office is always filled up, without enough chairs to sit in, and I can not stand. Then they're never on time, and, well, I can't really complain because I do have my leg, but nothing they do for me really helps.

I have thought about killing myself so many times that the thought no longer scares me. To be rid of this pain would be worth it. I've already had six operations.

I can't sleep. I never find a position which doesn't hurt. The medicines don't even make all the pain disappear. It hurts to move, to stand up, and to brush my teeth. Everything hurts.

I've been in pain for 24 years. That's the life I have given my family. I either think about my pain or what life may have been."

—Mark (age 50)

The quotation above by Mark, one of my patients, illustrates just how terrible pain can be when it is chronic. It never seems to leave the person with a moment's peace. The pain affects the patient's ability to work and relate to other people. For many chronic pain patients the steady aches, burning, numbness, twisting, and stabbing sensations result in a severe loss of self-esteem, loss of interpersonal relationships, decline of family activities, curtailment of employment, and progressive loss of income.

CHRONIC PAIN DOES NOT DISCRIMINATE

Chronic pain is one of the great levelers. It cuts across race, religion, sex, and economic boundaries. As a case in point, Turk et al. described the treatment that Charles II, King of England, experienced:

> A pint of blood was extracted from his right arm, and a half-pint from his left shoulder. This was followed by an emetic, two physics and an enema comprised of 15 substances. Next his head was shaved and a blister raised. Following in rapid succession were more emetics, sneezing powder, bleeding and soothing potions, and plaster of pitch and pigeon dung was smeared on his feet. Potions containing ten different substances, chiefly herbs, as well as forty drops of extract of human skull, were swallowed. Finally, application of bezoar stones (gall stones from sheep and goats) was prescribed. Following the extensive treatment the King died!

HISTORICAL EARLY EXPLANATIONS FOR PAIN

Historians and anthropologists have found many records which prove that our earliest ancestors were afflicted by the ravages of chronic pain. Individuals in prescientific cultures felt less control over their environment and lives than we do today. Historically, men and women sought explanations and meanings for their problems in mystical, supernatural, or god-like concepts. The common frustration was a feeling of limited control or noncontrol over these events in their lives. Individuals who had chronic pain were thought of as bad, and their pain was viewed as a punishment. Pain was also attributed to evil spirits that invaded the body of an unworthy host. In different cultures various rituals were used to "exorcise" the evil spirits from the patient.

Early Egyptian Quest for Pain Relief

In 1983 Professor Turk and his colleagues, in a study about pain, wrote that the first recorded reference to remedies for pain was included in the Egyptian papyrus (1550 B.C.). In this document reference is made to the prescription of opium by the God Isis for Ra's headache. In the quest for the attenuation of suffering, Turk describes numerous and largely ineffective remedies for pain relief. These have included purging, puking, poisoning, puncturing, cutting, cupping, blistering, leeching, heating, freezing, sweating, and shocking.

Turk states that the physicians' pharmacopoeia included practically every known organic and inorganic substance. Patients have chewed, imbibed, supped, or suffered treatment with crocodile dung, teeth of swine, hooves of asses, spermatic fluid of frogs, eunuch fat, fly specks, lozenges of dried vipers, powder of precious stones, oils derived from ants, earthworms and spiders, feathers, hair, human perspiration, and moss scraped from the skull of a victim of a violent death.

CHRONIC PAIN MAY BECOME UNBEARABLE

There may be times in your life when the pain is almost unbearable. Pain that aches throughout your back, migraine headaches, or arthritis pains can keep you inactive. The fear of cancer pain and the anguish of phantom-limb stump pain from an amputation are daily realities for millions of people. Whether your pain problem was caused by an accident, injury, illness, operation, or unknown cause, one thing is for sure: if it has lasted 6 months or more, it is chronic and you may have difficulty coping with it from that time on.

Chronic Pain Is an Epidemic

Twenty million Americans have problems with migraine headache, six million Americans have back pain problems, and 800,000 have excruciating cancer pain.

Work injuries and motor vehicle accidents account for over 80% of the beginning nightmares for the chronic pain patient. Nonwork injuries and chronic illness make up the balance. Chronic pain has been linked to quicksand. It can become a vicious cycle, ruining the quality of life of the patient and his or her family.

Surgery May Not Be for Everyone

Two hundred thousand Americans (more than in any other country) will undergo back surgery each year. The success rate for back surgery is often like playing roulette. On a back not previously operated upon, the success rate for the first surgery is 33%. One-third of patients who have an initial back surgery will get better, one-third will have no change, and one-third will get worse. By the time the third back operation is performed in a given patient, the success rate is only 5%. Less than 30% of back surgery patients return to work. The financial loss associated with this type of chronic pain is well over a staggering $60 billion per year. The indirect costs in terms of lost work, time away from work, diminished output, devastated families, and ruined lives are untold.

Thelma (Age 56): Dashed Hopes

I was a guest at the club where I was injured. They were having a dance, and my husband and I love to dance. I had only two drinks the entire evening. We did a lot of dancing. After the party I was helping the people clean up when I fell down. I was in a lot of pain but I didn't think I was hurt. Actually, I was very embarrassed by the whole episode. At first the people at the club were very nice. They said that their insurance would pay for everything. It turned out that they had low coverage. They won't return my calls.

I have been to so many doctors that I don't know whether I'm coming or going. This disrupted everyone's life because my daughter had to drive me to all my appointments. I can only partially bend my leg and I walk with a limp. Cold weather drives me out of my mind with pain. About 2 weeks ago the doctor had to rebend my leg because it wasn't setting well. That was painful.

During the first month of my disability I couldn't do a thing. I was in the hospital part of the time. I couldn't sleep because I couldn't get comfortable. I had problems getting up to go to the bathroom and I had to use a bedpan. When the doctor took the cast off of my leg, the pain got intense.

I used to be so active, and now I can't. My husband and I have had no sex since my injury. I just can't bear the weight and pain. I have been horrible with my family. They bear the brunt of my temper. I can't clean. For example, I'm unable to kneel and scrub the floor.

I can't go ballroom dancing. I can't bowl. I just want to forget the whole injury. It's cost so much money, and the bills are overwhelming. I haven't worn a dress since the accident because I don't want anyone to see my scar.

My husband has been real supportive. He is concerned. I worry that he is doing too much for me because he has had a heart attack since my injury and is supposed to rest.

Changes in the weather make me worse. I can predict when it is going to rain now. The headaches start in my neck and go around my whole head. I get pain in my knees and the muscles get tight.

It's always hard to stand. I get a grating ache in my left thigh when I do. I won't swim due to the need to wear a bathing suit. My leg often feels like I have no support. It makes me feel so frustrated that I cry and cry. When will I get better? I feel like an old woman. I'm tired all the time. I smoke much more. It's been so hard to accept my pain. I want to get on with life. The kids are all gone and this is the time we planned to go out and enjoy life. I try to forget my disability and pain, but when I drop something and have to pick it up I hurt all over again.

The hardest loss is that I'm afraid to pick up my granddaughter now.

IS THE PAIN REAL? WHO DECIDES?

> Are you saying that the pain is in my head?
> I know that I hurt; this pain is real.

—Anonymous (but almost universal for all chronic pain patients)

Although chronic pain is an epidemic and a pervasive problem in society, it has only been within the last 20 years that we have really begun to scientifically study pain. Certainly we have always had treatments for patients who complained about pain, but for the most part complaints about pain were viewed as a side effect to some injury or illness. The medical scientific field has only recently begun to study and "see" pain as a problem in and of itself.

Until recently chronic pain has been considered a "nonissue" within our fragmented health care delivery system. Chronic pain has been considered a natural and unfortunate side effect which accompanied a primary illness (such as a heart attack or ruptured disc) or accident. It was the primary illness or injury that received the major emphasis in treatment of the patient.

There was also an accompanying assumption that if the effects of an injury did not show up on X-ray, electromyography, or other pertinent testing, then the patient was "faking it." Very few doctors ever questioned the state-of-the-art in our diagnostic ability to "measure pain."

CHRONIC PAIN: TWO CURRENT OPPOSING VIEWS

Among both health groups and the public, two opposing views currently exist regarding the understanding of chronic pain. These relate to what it is and how it got there.

The dominant (but changing) view is that chronic pain sufferers who continue to complain of pain 6 months after the onset are malingerers (fakers), social misfits, or (worse) frauds who are trying to "milk the system" for all they can get in the way of sympathy from the medical community and money from the insurance company.

A second and growing group see chronic pain sufferers as legitimate patients in need of appropriate medical treatment. This new perspective appears to be the motivating stimulus behind the emerging multidisciplinary pain therapy movement. It is the view of these therapists, researchers, and clinicians that the devastating impact of pain on the patient is unquestionable. Attention is being given to both new team approaches to treat pain, self-help, greater patient participation in pain control, and looking at policies and laws which serve as incentives or disincentives in the progressive recovery from chronic pain.

THE PRESENT VIEW OF PAIN IS NOT FREE OF BIAS

It is probable that one of the reasons why we have until recently failed to adequately study or understand the horrible impact and suffering experienced by many chronic pain patients has been the belief that science in general and medicine in particular was free of bias. With such a view, a doctor utilizes the best of his or her professional skills to diagnose a patient's condition. The fact that a diagnosis itself, such as syphilis, AIDS, or chronic pain syndrome, can carry a stigma has been little understood. In actuality, neither science nor medicine is void of bias, as can be seen in the following quotation by Illich (1976):

> Medicine is a moral enterprise and therefore inevitably gives content to good and evil. In every society, medicine, like law and religion, defines what is normal, proper, or desirable. Medicine has the authority to label one man's complaint as legitimate illness, to declare a second man sick though he himself does not complain, to refuse a third recognition of his pain, his disability, and even death. It is medicine which stamps some pain as "merely subjective," some impairment as malingering...morality is as implicit in sickness as it is in crime or sin.

VIEWS ON WHAT CAUSES PAIN

At any time our view of what causes pain, whether the pain is real, and how we will treat it depends on how we "see" the pain.

There are many reasons why pain may not be understood by doctors who do not work within a chronic pain-oriented practice or pain clinic setting. One reason is that the illness may not have progressed to the point where it will be discovered on a routine evaluation or standard diagnostic test. Another reason is that not all of the pain and related problems and symptoms will ever show up using our current technology. Because of these problems, science continually strives for better means of assessment.

A more fundamental reason why chronic pain is so often misunderstood and poorly treated relates to the need for a better definition of chronic pain.

The Current Definition of Chronic Pain

Chronic pain has only very recently been defined by medical practitioners as debilitating pain which has existed for at least 6 months. Due to its newness, this definition lacks richness and depth.

While acute pain is a warning signal that something is wrong, chronic pain needs further study to determine exactly what has gone wrong.

Drawbacks of Our Current Views

It is unfortunate that too frequently all pain is viewed as a problem that occurs because of tissue damage. The overemphasis of this type thinking, when trying to conceptualize the chronic pain patient, has led to misunderstandings about chronic pain and subsequent poor treatment of that group of patients. Chronic pain patients need a "whole person" approach to treatment of their problem, and an approach that attempts to treat only the tissue damage part of the problem denies chronic pain patients the totality of treatment that they really need.

A Better Definition of Chronic Pain

Chronic pain has multiple causes, each of which raises the stress dimension and impacts a patient's life. The components of pain are complex, requiring a comprehensive view and not concentrating on any single factor. The comprehensive model must consider the following areas:

1. Physical and organic
2. Emotional and psychological
3. The way a person perceives his or her pain and related disability
4. Environmental: Personal and domestic issues
5. The way a person reacts to his or her pain problem
6. Biochemical: Metabolic imbalances in the body that relate to the pain problem

Chronic pain is never static. It is not the same today as it was yesterday, even for the individual pain sufferer. It is neither black nor white. It is not an all or none phenomenon. It frequently occurs in a "nonanatomic" or "nonorganic" distribution. This means that it may not always fit into the anatomy that is considered for acute pain problems. However, the nonanatomic distribution of the pain and associated tenderness is one of the factors that may identify it as chronic pain. Chronic pain changes, and that is part of the basis for the model of chronic pain that follows.

A Model of Chronic Pain

Chronic pain is partially made up of a number of the following factors under each topic (all factors relating to chronic pain have not yet been discovered, and therefore this list remains incomplete at the present time). This listing is presented to demonstrate that there are factors relating to chronic pain that change with time and circumstances, and there are factors that do not change with time.

Physical factors (partial list)
- Disc disease
- Sciatica (pain down the leg)
- Headaches
- Facial pain
- Nerve disease
- Muscle irritation

Biochemical factors (partial list)
- Vitamin excess
- Vitamin insufficiency
- Mineral insufficiency

Location
- Frequently outside of common anatomical markers

Emotional factors (partial list)
- Irritable
- Depressed
- Sleep disturbance
- Loss of sex drive
- Weight change
- Financial problems
- Family problems

Time interval
- Pain and disability for 6 months or more

- Daily pain cycle changes in:
  - Intensity
  - Frequency
  - Duration
  - Location

All the above factors combine to spell out significant, commonly accepted components of the chronic pain problem. The following is a model of chronic disease which accompanies some of the more severe chronic pain problems.

Chronic pain is accompanied by stress and distress which lead to chronic disease. As defined by Hans Selye, distress always refers to an activity that is damaging. In 1936 Dr. Selye discovered the general adaption syndrome in which all stress producers, such as physical, chemical, and psychological damaging agents, will provoke a reproducible nonspecific body response. The body's defense system undergoes a three-level reaction in the general adaption syndrome:

1. Alarm stage: The body exhibits characteristic changes resulting from exposure to the stressor. The body's nonspecific reactions involve a three-phase response. First, the adrenal cortex (outer layer that produces hormones such as cortisone) becomes hyperactive and enlarges. Second, the thymus gland and lymphatic tissue shrink (these tissues relate to the body's immune system). Third, gastrointestinal ulcers appear.
2. Resistance stage: Body resistance will follow if continued exposure to the stressor (biochemical abnormalities, ruptured disc, depression, malocclusion, etc.) results in adaptation. The signs of the alarm stage will disappear and resistance will be maintained.
3. Exhaustion stage: Long-term exposure to the same stressor (such as chronic pain) to which the body had previously adapted will deplete the stores of adaptation energy. The signs of the alarm stage will reappear and may become irreversible, and if the individual or body fails to eliminate the causative factors, this may eventuate in extreme exhaustion, total emotional collapse, inability to function for even the smallest tasks, and overwhelming physical exhaustion.

Selye defined stress as a state within the body which produces observable symptoms, not just vague or general nervous tension. It was Selye's contention that each of us tends to respond to stress and distress with a particular set of signs. He believed that when these signs appear, it is nature's way of telling us to change our activity and find diversion. The following is a list of self-observable signs of stress:

1. General irritability, hyperexcitation, or depression
2. Pounding of the heart
3. Dryness of the throat or mouth
4. Impulsive behavior, emotional instability
5. The overpowering urge to cry or run and hide
6. Inability to concentrate
7. Feelings of unreality, weakness, or dizziness
8. Predilection to become fatigued
9. "Free-floating anxiety" (being afraid but not knowing exactly of what)
10. Emotional tension and alertness, feeling of being keyed up

11. Trembling, nervous tics
12. High-pitched nervous laughter
13. Tendency to be easily startled by small noises
14. Stuttering or other speech difficulties which are stress induced
15. Bruxism, clenching or grinding of the teeth
16. Insomnia
17. Hyperkinesia (increased tendency to move about without any reason)
18. Sweating
19. Frequent need to urinate
20. Diarrhea, indigestion, queasiness in the stomach, and sometimes even vomiting
21. Migraine headaches
22. Premenstrual tension or irregular menstrual cycles
23. Pain in the neck or low back due to muscle tension
24. Loss of or excess appetite
25. Increased smoking
26. Increased use of legally prescribed drugs
27. Increased alcohol or drug dependency
28. Nightmares
29. Neurotic behavior
30. Psychoses
31. Prone to accidents

The body reacts to any and all types of influences by entering into a state of stress. Whether distortions of biochemistry, psychology, or structural alterations exist, the three stages of symptoms are specific, as mentioned above. As these stress-related responses go beyond the physiological adaptive range of the body's ability to cope, a transition into distress occurs with clinical manifestations. Use of the above-mentioned models is important for devising a treatment plan that works.

The Nature of Suffering

The chronic pain patient might ask: "Must I really remain trapped by my pain, a victim of a never-ending nightmare? Does my future remain desolate, pitiful, and full of constant aches, burning, and numbness? Is there no way to relieve the steady twisting and stabbing sensations? And what of the toll that chronic pain has brought to my family?"

The answer is *no*! No, you don't have to surrender to the ravages of chronic pain. As bad as it may seem, you can learn to not only live with your pain, but through pain management skills can learn to reduce the toll of chronic pain.

The remaining chapters of this book will continue to draw upon the experience of therapists on the pain management team to help the chronic pain patient learn how to reduce the intensity, frequency, and duration of chronic pain and get back to the beauty of living a fuller life.

5 Chronic Pain Is a Family Problem

Michael S. Margoles, M.D., Ph.D.

INTRODUCTION

As far as health problems are concerned, you and your family have been very fortunate. The only problems you have had were never more than a day or two of stiffness in your back after doing too much housework, yard work, or playing too hard at tennis, baseball, or the like. Then, one day at work, you injure your back. After 1 month off work, bed rest, and physical therapy, you are no better. An magnetic resonance imaging study and myelogram are done and show that a lower lumbar disc is "out." Surgery is performed. The operation seems to work. However, when you return to work 6 weeks after your back surgery, the back pain, with associated leg pain and weakness, becomes unbearable. You have to stop working after only 3 days. A series of medications is used to try to get you going again. Corsets, physical therapy, traction, and even a transcutaneous electrical nerve stimulator unit are tried. Numerous blocks and spinal injections are given with only limited success. Before you know it, a year has slipped by.

Your insurance company begins to play games with you. They delay payment of your disability benefits on a fairly regular basis. This puts financial stress on you. Your creditors are demanding payments and harassing you and your wife. Unnecessary financial burdens fall on your spouse. They send you to consultants who make it look like you are playing games and faking it. All the above grates on your nerves. You become irritable. You are angry and depressed. You keep saying: "Why me? What did I do to deserve all this mess?" You lash out at your spouse and children. The situation at home gets tense and intense. Your social life begins to dwindle. Your friends and relatives grow weary of discussing your back pain problem over and over again. Your back pain problem interferes with your ability to sit for more than short periods of time. You can't even enjoy a movie without having to get up frequently. Your sexual relationship suffers because of the pain from the physical activity. The joy in your life seems to be fading. You experience some or all of the following feelings: hopelessness, helplessness, despair, bitterness, desperation, bewilderment, anger, resentment, hostility, or depression and many times abandonment, because the redundant complaints and medical activities involved in your illness are no longer getting sympathy.

Your pain symptoms are worsening. The pain medications are working less and less effectively. Your physician begins to bug you by telling you that you are taking too much pain medication. The doctor tells you that he does not know how long he can go on prescribing for you at your present rate of pain pill consumption.

You and your family have never been faced with a situation like this. Everybody in the family is trying to help you the best way they know how. They, too, are frustrated.

CHRONIC PAIN IS A FAMILY PROBLEM

Your chronic pain problem is a family problem. When you consider that you are part of a family unit, usually made up of you, your spouse, and one or more children, it stands to reason that what affects you affects them. Pause a moment and reflect on how your behavior, feelings, and emotions affect the other members of your family. Likewise, your pain problem has a similar impact.

When one member of the family is ill, it affects the whole family. Acute illnesses such as flu, broken bones, etc. impact the family for short periods of time. Everybody pitches in for a while in helping perform your usual duties, responsibilities, and chores. However, when you are chronically ill the burden of your usual responsibilities may be more than other family members can deal with. This puts a strain on the family unit. Family members tend to become less sympathetic to the continuing complaints, creating additional resentment and stress on the patient.

If you are the breadwinner, the impact may be great. If you are a young child, the impact may be small.

WHEN CHRONIC PAIN COMES TO DISRUPT THE FAMILY

When you go through an illness the whole family goes through it with you. Chronic pain is a problem that affects your whole family. If it occurs long enough, it becomes a "family disease," illness, etc.

At some point you may wonder how your pain problem has become a family disease. Your attitude and feelings about your pain problem affect other members of your family. A chronic pain problem can change your role in and contribution to the family.

You may find it hard to go out in public because of the pain and the energy that is expended trying to hide the pain. You know that people feel uncomfortable if they sense you are not feeling well. Your contact with the outside world may become, or has become, very limited and that may be very hard to deal with.

Before your back injury you may have been the main source of family income, transportation, and a major contributor to the family's emotional support system. As a result of your injury you may have become unemployed, irritable, and unable to provide your family the emotional support you used to freely give. Now you may spend a great deal of your time transporting yourself to doctors' offices and other related therapy appointments. These changes and others have a profound effect on you and your family.

RESPONSIBILITY

One can only realistically take "responsibility" for one's suffering, but *not* for one's pain (Patel, 1989). The majority of responsibility for dealing with your pain and suffering is yours. If it is my pain, then I can control my conception of my pain. No other family member can take that role for me.

If an activity or duty is within your capacity to perform, don't call on other family members to do it for you. While lifting heavy boxes may not be possible because you have a back or neck pain problem, that does not mean you cannot get up and get yourself a glass of water. Only when absolutely necessary should you call on a family member to help you with needs such as getting pain medications or massaging your painful areas. Instead of centering your thinking on the unfairness of the injury or illness, and what you cannot do, make an effort to persistently discover what you can do. A change in attitude, toward the positive, will go a long way toward the successful management of your pain and suffering. Reinforcement with inspirational tapes can be very helpful. Concentrate on turning your "lemons into lemonade."

Family members who do too much for you may be creating a dependence problem that may be harmful to the integrity of the family structure. They may be encouraging unhealthy attitudes that may interfere with your rehabilitation and recovery.

ISOLATION RESULTS FROM ATTITUDE AND BEHAVIOR PROBLEMS

Steps need to be taken to avoid the pain patient's tendency toward isolation. Family members who will love and care for you, despite your pain and suffering, are enhancing the integrity of the family structure. They are to encourage and strengthen you so that you can bear up to the rigors of your pain problem and your rehabilitation (recovery).

Their caring can take many forms, for example, avoiding unfounded suspicions, criticisms, and unnecessary arguments and quarreling about the pain and suffering problem. Encouragement to attend social functions is of value. At the same time, the rest of the family needs to be understanding when you say "enough!" Of equal importance is that the family be understanding when you have participated in social activities but can tolerate no more in a given week. They have to appreciated your limits.

Examine your household to see where opportunities exist. The family should encourage the patient to attend as many social functions as possible, but not become angry when the patient cannot go due to pain. Be patient here.

When mom is hurting a lot, dad needs to tend to the children. He also needs to teach them about what mom has, in language they can understand.

It is difficult for family members to feel that their concern and caring are enough. An act of caring, such as getting an important medication for a spouse, parent, or friend who is hurting, may be all that you can offer to the chronic pain patient. Your concern alone is usually very important in staving off some of the ravages of depression that so often accompanies chronic pain (Patel, 1989).

EFFECTS OF CHRONIC PAIN ON SEXUALITY

One of the major areas of impact of a chronic pain problem is in relationships. Pain impairs physical performance. It hurts to have sexual relations. During sexual activity, the patient is likely to forget and "let go," and possibly have to pay a price of a bad flare-up of the pain after the love making is over. There are many areas of sexuality that can be explored with a knowledgeable therapist.

Pain stifles the sex drive. It takes away the pleasure of orgasm. Chronic pain patients may have feelings of unworthiness and rejection (especially in women) when they cannot function adequately sexually. This is especially difficult if the spouse, lover, etc. is the blaming type.

The spouse, especially the husband of a female patient with a chronic pain problem, may fear causing unnecessary aggravation of an existing pain problem. This may inhibit the husband's potency. Loss of sex drive and interest in sexual activities may be partially remedied by alternatives such as fondling, intimacy, etc. This material will be dealt with more extensively in Chapter 17.

CHRONIC PAIN PATIENTS NEED TO BE ACCEPTED

Our present culture, with its emphasis on youth, beauty, muscle bulk, etc., treats chronic pain patients condescendingly. Sadly, medical professionals may also treat such patients as a bother when they cannot "cure" them (Patel, 1989). However, chronic pain need not get in the way of the important things in life.

The case of Maya A. points up some of this. Maya had been injured in an automobile accident in 1967. From that point on, things went downhill. Her back surgery in 1973 had not provided any significant gains. She finally had to give up her teaching position in Santa Monica and move back home to San Luis Obispo to live with her family in 1969. She was 27 years old at that time. She could have felt very embarrassed about the whole issue of moving back in with her folks. Her mom could have laid a real guilt trip on her. At one point the family physician suggested that the future was hopeless and that her mom put her in a nursing home. However, her mom had a different point of view which worked out to a wonderful advantage for Maya. Her mom told her that she wanted Maya to stay at home for the "pleasure of her company." Her mom did not care that Maya could not do the dishes; the pleasure of her daughter's company was good enough for mom. During the next 19 years that they lived together, with her father, Maya and her mom grew to have a beautiful and deeply caring relationship. A quality of interpersonal relationship developed that the two of them grew to really treasure. Disability brought growth and precious memories to the family.

The families of patients with chronic pain need to know that there is more hope than ever for the chronic pain patient and that keeping interpersonal relationships open and active will keep the chronic pain patient sharp and ready to get back into society and compete after recovery.

Keep in mind that the presence of a chronic pain patient in the household provides an opportunity to learn how to minister to and meet the needs of people who are suffering.

ATTITUDES AND ADAPTIVE FUNCTIONING

Your attitude and understanding about your pain go a long way toward understanding how to manage it. Chronic pain needs to be managed largely by the patient and occasionally by a team of pain experts.

While you may not be able to modify the physical aspects of your pain, you can frequently regulate your thinking and emotional response (attitude) toward the pain and thereby influence both your pain and suffering.

Understanding these points will help you to interpret and apply the materials in this chapter to your pain problem.

Types of Attitudes

Good attitudes
- Being self-sufficient
- Working
- Dressing your best

- Being optimistic
- Wearing makeup
- Group minded (think of the other person's needs)
- Independent
- Active
- Having friends
- Spending time with friends
- Self-reliant
- Taking walks
- Planning for the future
- Setting goals
- Exercising
- Taking responsibility

Bad attitudes
- Excess complaining
- Manipulation of others
- Secondary gain problems
- Not group minded
- "But knocking" (use "but" to devalue/negate progress)
- Moaning
- Pained sound to voice
- Inactive
- Dependent
- Withdrawing
- Irritable
- Negativism
- Pessimism
- Anger
- Despair
- Depression
- Crying

Bad Attitudes

As the pain and dysfunction of the chronic pain family member get worse, his or her usual attitudes and personality may change and be replaced by negativism, pessimism, anger, despair, and depression.

Attitude problems may be manifested by withdrawing, asking others for too much or too little help, irritability, doctor shopping, crying, moaning, unrealistic fears of becoming reinjured, avoiding responsibility, and overutilizing medication. Maladaptive (unhealthy) attitudes tend to promote being passive, being too dependent, depression, and feelings of loss of control.

You might argue and say: "I could change my attitude if only the doctors would take away my pain." However, they are not in control of your attitude; you are.

Good Attitudes

Adaptive (healthy) attitudes are manifested by being self-reliant, taking care of your own hygiene (bathing, brushing your teeth), taking walks, interacting with others in a positive fashion, planning for the future, setting goals, exercising, taking responsibilities, being tolerant of others, etc. Healthy attitudes encourage activity, independence, optimism, and a sense of self-control. Choosing the good attitudes is most beneficial to you and your family.

Patient Marie J. had this to say about her attitudes with respect to household duties:

> I had to give myself permission to not feel guilty about not having a clean house, having the laundry done, etc. I approached this subject with my husband and asked if we could have someone come in periodically and help clean the house. His reaction was a surprise to me. "We can handle it," he replied. And I responded, "No we can't. We have to accept that fact and get on with our lives." It was quite some time before I got help with the house, but after a few weeks, the whole family (Marie J., her husband, and five children) agreed it was worth it. I felt that my husband has always been a strong supporter of me and I feel he didn't want to admit that I might not get any better. I had accepted that fact, but he hadn't.

The best household environment is one in which responsibility for personal happiness is taken on by each person individually. This attitude is especially valuable in the home of a chronic pain patient. The reason for this is simply that good mental health will benefit all the people around you. Therefore, take time out for yourself, be kind to yourself, have friends for yourself, and spend time with your friends. Doing these little kindnesses for yourself will be uplifting and supportive of good attitudes.

A major problem that occurs with the development of chronic pain is a tendency toward attitude changes that are sometimes not adaptive. This includes irritability, depression, intolerance, anger, feelings of helplessness and hopelessness, despair, and remorse, to mention only a few. These problems tend to be less prominent with the milder degrees of chronic pain and more prominent in constant chronic pain that is severe and disabling.

Anxiety may be related to reliving the automobile accident that caused the onset of the pain problem.

Whining and audibly groaning only reinforce the message to yourself that you are in pain and you are suffering. You can benefit from making efforts to stop these audible reinforcers of your problem and plight. When patients who rely on this stop, they need a substitute outlet, which can be created in an adaptive way with psychotherapy (Patel, 1989). Personality regression may occur. This means that your manner of attitude and reaction to persons and events become that of persons younger and less tolerant of stress, distress, or situations that call for patience and waiting.

Improving Your Attitude (Is Your Responsibility)

Consider what Marie J. had to say about this:

> As my first year of treatment came to an end I was experiencing some backsliding at that time. I was very discouraged and so was my husband. The question I kept posing was, "What if I never get better than the way I am today?" I truly felt it was possible to still lead a happy life, by my choosing, even if I did not get any better than I was on that day. It simply meant restructuring my life and creating a "new normal life" for myself. Perhaps I would never be able to go backpacking, garden, play the piano, etc. ever again. Things that I considered part of my normal life were no longer possible, so it was time to create a new normal life.

Creating a "new normal life" is a useful concept and a potentially practical one for coping with chronic pain, but for some patients, this new way of living (via reconstructing new expectations and standards for oneself) may culminate in *resignatio*n to the pain, rather than *acceptanc*e of the pain. Acceptance is the prerequisite for creating a "new normal life," but resignation is defeating, futile, despairing, etc., all of which are precursors to suicidality (Patel, 1989).

PACING

Pacing is as important to you as it is to your family. There is nothing more frustrating to a person who once led a productive and fast-paced lifestyle than to be slowed down by a painful and disabling chronic pain problem. You have to restructure your lifestyle to accommodate your new, restricted, capabilities. Your family has to ease up by lowering the demands on you. Learning to "pace" yourself, according to the dictates and confines of your pain problem, can often produce a lifestyle that leaves you functional, productive, and still carrying on satisfactorily.

Marie J. had this to say:

> I am very selective about the things I do. I don't try to do it all. I've learned to pace myself and rest when I'm tired, and most important, I've learned how to say no when something is a little beyond my current capability. I do have a new normal life which allows me to do quite a few things I enjoy doing, but I need to follow the guidelines of my new normal lifestyle or I get into trouble.

DEPENDENCY

Before we embark upon the problems associated with too much dependency, I would like to address some of the problems with patients who are too *independent*. Some patients are so independent that they have trouble relying on anyone for:

1. Help
2. Medical advice
3. Direction

Dependency Problems

There are four types of dependency problems:

1. Excessive dependency on people
2. Excessive dependency on medications
3. Excessive dependency on the pain itself
4. Excessive dependency on yourself

Excessive Dependency on People

A certain amount of dependency on people and medications is normal and acceptable. However, when you use your pain problem to merely manipulate people into doing for you things you could do for yourself, your dependency on people is excessive. Consider the following case example.

Shortly after Jane married Dan, she suffered whiplash when hit from behind at a stoplight. It wasn't a problem at first. The pain migrated from her neck to her jaw, and then the excruciating headaches began. Eventually the pain medications stopped working. Dan did not seem to mind helping. Back and neck rubs appeared to relax Jane's neck, at least temporarily. Noises began to aggravate the pain. Any kind of noise aggravated the pain, so Dan hired a housekeeper to take care of the children and keep them quiet. Jane was thankful for the added help with the household chores because she felt dizzy when on her feet for any length of time. The weeks and months passed slowly. Jane became very frustrated by having to deal with the ongoing pain and suffering. Although she consulted many physicians, none could help relieve her pain. She became more and more irritable. Her anger spilled over to everyone around her. A sense of hopelessness began to grow within her. Despite that, Dan tried everything he could think of, but matters only got worse. Her attitude got progressively worse as the sense of hopelessness grew. The sense of hopelessness grew because she had relied on physicians to heal and change her and had not tried to determine what she could do for herself.

Excessive Dependency on Medications

When you use pills as a substitute for working through major psychological issues relating to your pain problem, you are depending on medications excessively. A certain amount of dependency on medications is okay, but be aware that abuse may occur. For example, suppose you and your physician agree that you may take up to six pain tablets per day in order to stay employed. If you do, that is following the directions. However, what if you cannot bear up to all the struggles of working and feel you have to take 10–12 pain pills to try to abolish all the discomfort of working? If you do this without permission from your physician, that is abuse of medication.

Excessive Dependency on the Pain Itself

Excessive dependency on the pain itself manifests itself as "being totally controlled by the pain (e.g., having conversations with people only when not in pain, revolving eating schedule around intensity of the pain, selecting clothes only according to level of pain, etc.) so that the pain is exclusively and dominantly relied upon to guide one's entire life. This, too, is a dependency (Patel, 1989). Some patients seem resigned to the role of a medical martyr. It is almost as though they enjoy their suffering more than they enjoy the thought of getting well.

Excessive Dependency on Yourself

While self-sufficiency is a necessary requirement to recover from a pain and dysfunction problem, too much stubbornness and self-reliance may cause you to "miss the boat" when it finally comes time to take you out of your misery. Attitudes of independence and submission are compatible.

PUTTING CHRONIC PAIN IN MEDICAL PERSPECTIVE

There are answers for the management of your chronic pain, but all the answers are not yet available. Your pain problem may only respond partially to current medical therapy. You can be assured that even though your chronic pain problem may not be curable, it is frequently manageable with competent help.

One patient offered the following:

I lived from one priesthood blessing to another, and little by little, over a long period of time, I did get better and am still working at getting even better. I have worked with a physical therapist to strengthen atrophied muscles. I went through orthodontia. I've used imaging a great deal to tolerate the pain. I started biofeedback, but didn't follow through because of money and scheduling problems. I still feel that biofeedback is a viable option. My husband and I went to a myotherapist and my husband now uses the myotherapy on me. I visit the chiropractor on a regular basis, which helps a great deal.

Marie J. said:

I remember the day I made the decision to get help from a pain management specialist. I was attempting to load the washing machine. I had to lay down on the garage floor several times and rest before I got the machine loaded. I knew I was in real trouble and needed help, so I made the call.

FAMILY MEMBERS AND FRIENDS

Family Members Can Help

An important role for loved ones is to offer support and encouragement. They may not understand exactly what the cause of your pain and suffering is, but they can encourage you to go through with the therapeutic program, especially when the going gets rough and discouraging.

Family members can help increase the good attitudes in two ways:

1. Realize that the chronic pain patient's attitudes (sense of well-being) may be adversely influenced by the pain and suffering.
2. Have compassion for the person with chronic pain.
   a. They have frequently been accused of having a purely psychological problem, with no real organic basis to their pain and suffering.
   b. They have been suspected by almost everyone of being able to work an 8- to 12-hour day if only they could get their act together, never giving them credit for already doing the best that they physically can during the 2–4 hours they can put in every day.
   c. They have been deprecated.
   d. They have been accused of faking.
   e. They have been denied disability benefits because the social security examiner did not have enough training to discern that they were really physically impaired.

When the person with the chronic pain problem is being indirect about the discomfort, for example by inferring that he or she needs a heating pad now, the person needs to be encouraged to be more direct with respect to expressing his or her needs and desires. Instead of a grunt or groan, encourage the person to say: "I need help" or "I would like a heating pad."

A chronic pain problem can strengthen a relationship and promote more togetherness and more sensitivity to the needs of each other. Remember that the caring goes both ways. A chronic pain sufferer *can* care about the needs of another person who is not in pain.

While open communication is important, too many negative attitudes and too much complaining about pain and suffering may be taxing to a spouse, family members, and others.

Suggestions for Handling Bad Attitudes

1. Do not recognize or give in to bad attitudes.
2. Question bad attitudes and be skeptical rather than unquestioningly believing them.
3. Give extra attention and interest to good attitudes.

Consequences of Bad Attitudes

If all you can do is moan about your pain problem, then you risk the loss of your friends. However, there are ways of communicating pain other than moaning, and for those patients who are overly independent, it is permissible to occasionally moan to close friends, thereby increasing vulnerability, self-disclosure, and intimacy (Patel, 1989).

The evolution of bad attitudes occurs gradually, over a long period of time. They occur subtly, in an almost unconscious fashion. It was not your intention to become a manipulator of those around you. There is no one worth blaming when this occurs. The main issue is that excessive attention, by you or your loved ones, promotes bad attitudes and is destructive to your overall rehabilitation.

The following is addressed to family members and friends of the patient. If you suspect that your spouse, loved one, or friend might be able to do the activity they request of you, say, "I feel that one of the best ways I can help you is to not do for you the things that you can obviously do for yourself." While such an explanation may evoke an angry response, the long-term effects may be beneficial to all family members.

At the same time attention is discontinued for bad attitudes, attention needs to be given to good attitudes. This area needs special mention because it is often overlooked. Any activities that show that the patient is moving his or her muscles in a positive direction (starting to provide for himself or herself) needs to be acknowledged with praise and excitement.

Your Pain Problem and the Family

Others in your family may believe that your pain experience is the cause of all the family's difficulties, but it is not that simple. Their beliefs and attitudes regarding your pain are usually part of the problem. Because of your pain, they may decide to worry or restrict their activity level. However, they need to realize that your pain is not a reason for them to stop living, nor do they need to use your predicament as a reason to stop growing. If they choose to do so, it could harm both you and them.

Marie J. stated:

> When the patient goes through all the ordeals of an illness, the whole family experiences it. It was very difficult for all of us. Financially, physically, emotionally, and spiritually. One son asked me if I would ever get well. I told him I did not know. He allowed that I had been sick for a very long time and he wanted me to get well so I could go on a school field trip with him.

Family Members and Friends May Do Harm by Encouraging Unhealthy Attitudes

These may include such varying attitudes as (Patel, 1989):

1. *Undermining* the reality of the pain
2. *Questioning* the existence of the pain
3. *Trivializing* the distress associated with the pain
4. Trying to *ignore* the pain
5. Constantly *tending to and inquiring* about the pain
6. *Psychologizing the pain* (i.e., attributing it to the nature of the patient, etc.)
7. *Accusing* the patient

THE SPOUSE AS AN AGGRAVATING FACTOR

Your spouse can act as a aggravating factor to your chronic pain problem. He or she can make your life a living hell. Some examples are as follows:

1. Physical abuse
   a. Beating
   b. Tripping
   c. Massage that is too hard and too insensitive
   d. Battering
   e. Driving a vehicle in a manner that is brutal to your pain problem
   f. Violence
2. Mental cruelty
   a. Deprecation
   b. Anguish
   c. Arguing
   d. Accusations of secondary gain
   e. Threats (of divorce, desertion)
   f. Antagonism
   g. Not helping when help is needed
   h. Threats of physical violence
   i. Jealousy
   j. Verbal abuse
   k. "Volatile" relationship
3. Sabotage
   a. Consorting with employer
   b. Consorting with other family members
   c. Consorting with friends
4. Manipulation
5. Sexual abuse

WHAT ABOUT THE CHILDREN?

Keep the communication open. Be open and tell them the truth. Get their support from the beginning.

Marie J. wrote:

> As my husband and I made the decision to see a physician pain management specialist, we had a family council with our five children, ages 15, 10, 9, 6, and 2, and explained that I was very sick and that the doctor was going to help me but that it would require considerable sacrifice and support from all members of the family. We asked if we could count on them for their help and support. They were all in agreement. That turned out to be the easy part. As the months passed and turned into years, I started to gain an understanding of what the sacrifice and support they rendered really meant. When the patient goes through all the ordeals of an illness, the whole family experiences it.

One patient with young children related the following as a method of coping with the needs of her children:

My youngest was 2 years old then and very busy. It was very difficult to keep her safe and cared for. There was no one to help, so I fashioned a long leash and attached it to her. I put diapers at the end of the couch and toys within her reach. I laid on the couch and raised her in this manner for the next year. When she would wander to the end of the tether, I would make a game out of dragging her back and we seemed to manage somehow (Marie J., 1989).

Today, Marie J. is an executive secretary. She works outside the home and cares for her family in a very active manner. It took 3 years of a very active program, involving specialists from many fields of medicine, dentistry, orthodontics, physical therapy, and chiropractic, and an aggressive myofascial program to bring her back to a very high level of independence and performance. No surgery was needed for her severe neck and back pain problem.

Children are naturally egocentric and tend to interpret others' (especially parents) behaviors and attitudes as reflections of themselves. A chronic pain patient may be quieter or more passive or withdrawn than usual. That individual's children may think that the parent is ignoring them because they have been bad, or they may think that the parent is punishing them or that mom or dad doesn't love them any more, It is important that patients reassure their children of their caring and love and patiently explain to them that they are acting different because they are in pain (Patel, 1989).

Use metaphors and/or drama to explain to your children what it means and how it feels to be in pain. For example, use the child's doll or toy soldier to demonstrate being hurt in a car accident or wounded, and use band-aids, red paint, etc. to illustrate the consequences of the accident. Then have the toy "come alive" by voicing its pain and feelings. Doing this will allow the child to better understand what the parent is going through (Patel, 1989).

When feeling neglected or deprived of adequate attention, children tend to "act out" their feelings by throwing temper tantrums, refusing to eat, demanding extravagant things, teasing other kids, and generally being difficult. This is the time when chronic pain patients may feel most stressed and frustrated and the time when children most need to be reassured and receive attention. In these instances children respond remarkably well to the parent's own self-disclosure about pain and kindness and attention (Patel, 1989).

WHAT ABOUT THE PARENTS?

Chronic pain patients who are also parents of young children or teenagers may feel guilty for not doing enough in attending enough to their children. They may blame themselves for being "bad parents" and hold themselves responsible for their children's failures or problems. At this stage some parents may not be able to tolerate such self-criticism and lash out in frustration at their children with verbal and physical abuse. After such an episode they may feel ashamed, repentant, and guilty. Other parents may delve deeper into their self-criticisms of their parenting and withdraw from their children. If any of these dynamics seem familiar to you, there are many options to pursue (Patel, 1989):

- Seek professional help.
- Call available hot lines in your community for referrals to appropriate measures.
- Try to talk to your children calmly, following the preceding guidelines, when *not* in severe pain (i.e., be sure to bring your pain level down using medications, physical therapy, etc. before communicating with your children). The rationale here is that when in marked pain, your frustration tolerance dips below normal and makes it more difficult to communicate and problem solve.

- Enlist the help of relatives and/or friends to take care of the children temporarily while you develop other more permanent resources.
- Hire live-in help or part-time help for child care or housework.
- Locate reading material on "parenting under stress" in your local library (Patel, 1989).

COMMUNICATION

Outside the Family

One patient decided to forsake her suffering to minister to others. In recent correspondence she stated:

> As I lay on the couch in incredible pain, day in and day out, I would call people who I knew were struggling with some aspect of their life, and I would listen and encourage them. I felt that I had been stripped of everything I used to function in life and that this was the only thing left that I could do that would have some positive effect. My voice never sounded sick, so no one ever knew that I was sick, and it allowed me to feel like there was still some purpose to my life (Marie J., 1989).

Within the Family

Marie J. stressed that communication within the family structure was crucial to her overall survival and recovery:

> Communication with each other was a key element in successfully handling mother being down all the time. I was very honest with everyone, including my five children, as to how I was feeling. They in turn felt comfortable in expressing their feelings, and together we could work out a solution to the problem.

GOAL SETTING IN PURSUIT OF CONTINUING LIFE AFTER PAIN SETS IN

Use goal setting as a means of planning a future and anticipating recovery of function if not recovery from physical suffering and pain.

Consider the case of Louise T. She is a 46-year-old woman who had been through 29 years of severe pain, 13 years flat on her back. She had been through one harrowing back surgery in 1975, and when that failed she was left with a husband who she eventually divorced because of his constant antagonism. She subsequently married a kind and considerate man who also had a chronic pain problem. In all their married years they had never had an "escape to paradise." I marveled at the way Jerre ministered to Louise. They both related well to each other. Despite her battle with pain, Louise always had a certain optimism about her that amazed me. She is a woman with a deep commitment to the Lord. Faith in God is a very big part of her day-to-day life. She recently had surgery on some residual bone spurs in her low back that were the cause of a great deal of her ongoing pain and disability. Before the surgery Louise made up her mind that she was going with Jerre to Florida to enjoy some fun things with him. Before the operation, she planned the whole trip, made the reservations, and bought the tickets. She still had quite a lot of pain after the surgery, but was determined to fly from California to Florida and enjoy some time with her husband. She was able to travel with the aid of some extra pain medication. She was even involved in two minor accidents on the trip, but remained steadfast in her pursuit of having a good time on her trip.

Goal setting is a very powerful and profound tool to cope with chronic pain. It is not a unitary construct or single action; rather, it is a multifaceted, complex, and layered set of means through which people gain more from pain and its miseries (Patel, 1989).

There are several types of goal setting, each one distinctly different and geared to serving people with varying needs:

- *Setting goals for life* (i.e., deriving meaning and purpose from one's experiences on earth as a part of the human species). Some people use religion and spirituality here in aiding them to make sense of something so unjust and chaotic as chronic pain.
- *Setting goals for career.* Some people may only become motivated at the prospect of financial reward, success, prestige, power, etc. From this they derive strength to continue battling their chronic pain.
- *Setting goals for society and/or others.* Altruism can be a very strong motivator for some people setting goals for self and family (Patel, 1989).

SEEKING COUNSELING AND GETTING HELP

Personal questioning regarding pain-related problems is difficult to deal with. You might be wondering: Do I inadvertently contribute to my suffering? Is there some subtle way in which I and my family benefit from my pain? Does my pain help my loved ones or me avoid some activity that I or they are uncomfortable with? Am I allowing myself to become more dependent because of my pain? How can I cope with this pain? Who would want to be near me like this? What is wrong with me for having this pain? I don't know what to do! These questions are not easy to answer because it is sometimes difficult to be objective.

If you think you need help, seek out a specialist. The specialist to look for is called a (1) marital therapist, (2) health psychologist, or (3) behavioral medicine specialist. It is best to find a specialist that combines all these therapies, but this is usually difficult to do.

The *marital therapist* can evaluate the complex interactions of your family and aid in understanding subtle changes influencing your family dynamics. Marital therapy is not only for families fearful of potential breakup. The marital therapist is also very appropriate for families undergoing continuous stress such as occurs with chronic pain problems.

The *health psychologist* or *behavioral medicine specialist* may have some differences between their fields of subspecialty, but there is enough overlap to use their titles interchangeably. When you look for one of these specialists, be sure to request one who specializes in chronic pain. Both of these fields combine health-related matters and psychology. Both of these specialists are primarily psychologists, and they understand how your pain influences your emotions and vice versa.

Where can these specialists be found? If you are fortunate enough to live in a city or town that has a multidisciplinary pain center, start there. You can also call your local hospital and/ or examine the yellow pages under the listings for counselors, psychologists, physicians, and other medically related listings. If this approach does not work, consult your local mental health center, and specifically request the specialists mentioned above. Do not accept specialists who merely emphasize medication usage or therapists unacquainted with chronic pain.

The emotional health of your family is as important as its physical health. Finding a good psychotherapist is not easy because there is no such thing as a "good" psychotherapist. What makes a psychotherapist good for you depends on whether or not you feel comfortable and understood by that therapist. The relationship between you and your therapist *is* the treatment in psychotherapy. If you have any doubts about the suitability of you therapist, discuss the issue with him or her. Feel free to shop around for another therapist. You would not dream of buying a car without looking at several and test driving each one. You realize there is enormous variability in price range, color, speed, size, durability, mileage, etc. Similarly, therapists come in many capabilities and need to be "test driven" before they are "bought" (Patel, 1989).

Ask yourself the following questions when looking for a psychotherapist:

- Does he or she really listen to what I have to say or have his or her own ideas about who I am?
- Is he or she patient in inquiring and eliciting information from me?
- Is he or she interested, attentive, and active in the session or distracted (i.e. phone calls, memory lapse, etc.)?
- Is he or she sensitive and compassionate to my situation and my pain?
- Does he or she make attempts to understand more about the nature, location, etiology (cause), prognosis, etc. of my pain?
- Does he or she try to explain my pain solely with psychologic jargon? If so, consider looking elsewhere.
- Does he or she subtly blame me for my pain?
- Does he or she try to dissuade me from my treatment plan by suggesting I reduce my medications,* quit medical supervision, etc.?
- Is he or she committed to helping me through my pain?
- Do I have feelings of warmth, caring, trust, genuineness, and honesty in the sessions? These are vital and necessary to the therapeutic relationship (Patel, 1989).

YOUR THERAPIST

Treating chronic pain patients is a very stressful job. Not many therapists have made the commitment to meet the needs of chronic pain patients as a full-time practice. Be supportive of your therapist. Be considerate and understanding. Give him or her "space" to make mistakes. In many areas of chronic pain therapy, the frontiers are still being pushed out. Be patient with your therapist. He or she needs extra time to listen to you and decide in what direction to take the program as you progress toward getting well. Give him or her as much support as you can. Send a thank-you card from time to time. As a chronic pain patient, you are a member of a team. The therapist is the captain, and you are one of the participants.

USING PAIN FOR OTHER GAIN

A special consideration is use of pain to avoid unwanted activities. For example, some individuals who are uncomfortable in social settings will find pain to be an acceptable excuse for staying home. Family members need to be especially alert to this situation. At these times the members of the support group (family, etc.) need to be firm in insisting upon your participation in the social event. They also need to be generous with their compliments when socializing occurs.

---

* Psychiatrists are licensed to dispense medications and alter medication treatment plans. Psychologists are not licensed to do so.

Secondary Gain

Secondary gain occurs when:

1. A patient exaggerates his or her pain complaints in order to get out of work duties or social activities.
2. Sometimes a wife or husband avoids sexual activity with his or her spouse by stating it will cause too much back pain.

No one intentionally wants loved ones to experience pain, but humans can sometimes unconsciously support a negative experience like pain because of the advantages that result. For instance, a husband who rarely displays affection (such as saying "I love you") now has a back or neck pain problem and is emotionally grateful for the assistance his wife gives him. This can be a very powerful force in his wife's unconscious support of his dependence on her. The wife, of course, would rather consciously not have her husband experience pain, but she simultaneously desires the affection and gratefulness that result from it.

Tertiary Gain

Tertiary gain occurs when:

1. An attorney advises a client against a certain treatment program, fearing that the patient will get well and ruin the attorney's chance for a good settlement amount.
2. A husband takes advantage of his wife's misfortune to improve the monetary gain from the injuries his wife received in an accident.

STOP BEATING A DEAD HORSE

Many chronic pain patients are self-sufficient persons who rarely let on about the presence of pain and/or dysfunction. Therefore, when a chronic pain problem strikes them down, they may have trouble getting relatives to acknowledge their disability. This can be detrimental to the patient's survival and rehabilitation.

Marie J. addressed this by saying:

> Even my own mother did not believe that I was really sick. I learned, along with my family, that few people understand what chronic pain patients and their families go through and they get tired of hearing that you don't feel very well yet. One friend never missed an opportunity to let me know that it was all in my head and that when I made up my mind to be well, I would be. I also experienced a significant weight gain during this time and had very unkind remarks made to me about being fat. One woman showed up on my doorstep and handed me a sack of clothes and said, "I just cleaned out my closet and I remember what it's like to be fat so I thought you could use these." She turned and walked away. I am still stunned. I donated the clothes to Goodwill. I wasn't that fat.

All of us seek to have friends and relatives who are compatible with us. When pain strikes, the field of possibles for this vital need may shrink dramatically. The pain problem can become an invisible barrier between you and those you want to include in your life. In your search to identify persons who will accept you, comfort you, and show you compassion, you may be "beating a dead horse."

There will be friends, family members, and professionals who do not believe you have a real pain problem. It really hurts when it's your spouse.

Joyce Landorf referred to these people (the "dead horses") as the "irregular people." These are persons, usually closely related (such as parents, aunts, uncles, brothers, sisters, etc.), who cannot give you the love, acceptance, and support you want and need.

These "other" people are emotionally handicapped. They never had it and they never will when it comes to lavishing emotions and understanding on you or anybody else. The truth is, they have no way to appreciate the pain and suffering you are enduring. This is true for three reasons:

1. They are emotionally handicapped. They lack the emotions that will allow them to relate to your problems.
2. The media have not presented an accurate picture of what chronic pain is.
3. Even if they do (did) have a pain problem, their emotional response, support system, etc. is different than yours. They are not you!

You have to pity the irregular people. Realize they are not on your side and never will be. Do yourself a favor and leave them alone. Think of them as an old junkyard dog. If you don't want to get mauled, leave them alone. The negative effects from provoking these persons too much can have a devastating effect on your emotional status.

Share your problems with those who understand and accept you, and leave the irregular people alone. Stay with the people who can give you positive input and caring and compassionate support. You may have to change friends, physicians, and jobs to get the mental peace and acceptance you desire.

CONCLUSION

Pain is more than a simple sensation of discomfort. Pain attitudes and suffering are determined by you and your family. What has happened to you and your family during the months and years of your pain problem? Have the changes in your life been constructive ? Have you become more dependent or less so?

With chronic pain, your goal is to *manage* your pain and suffering. Professionals you consult for help are there to steer you in the right direction. Proper control and management of your pain and disability are synonymous with being active and independent.

When you accept responsibility for handling your pain and suffering, you move away from unnecessary reliance on others, and this helps you take a more active position in deciding what can be done to improve your current situation. As a consequence, your thinking may become more hopeful and constructive.

BIBLIOGRAPHY

Baker B. (1987). Personal communication.

Margoles, M. (1983). The stress neuromyelopathic pain syndrome, *The Journal of Neurological and Orthopaedic Medicine and Surgery, 4*, 317–322.

Marie J. (1989). Personal communication.

Patel, R. (1989). Personal communication.

6 The Search for Help with a Chronic Pain Problem Can Be Frustrating

Sheri B.

One of the toughest parts of getting well, that I have faced, was getting a doctor to agree that I was sick!

In the beginning, about 8 years ago, the pain was mostly in my legs and hips, especially after strenuous exercise or stress. I would visit my family doctor, only to be told time after time that everything looked "normal."

The first clinic I tried was even more of a frustration. After waiting over an hour and filling out pages and pages of medical history, the doctor told me to "think warm" and try to keep positive thoughts in my mind. She did take some blood tests, but all of the results were "normal."

As the pain continued to get more intense and more frequent, I sought help from a specialist. Thinking arthritis might be the cause, I went for tests and X-rays. All the tests were "normal." The doctor suggested I consult a psychiatrist.

I was beginning to hate the word normal. It was obvious to me that what I was feeling could not possibly be normal or most of the population would be bedridden. Although I really did believe the pain was caused by something physical, I did have a lot of stress in my life and wondered if a psychiatrist could help. The result of the therapy sessions was significant progress in my personal problems, but absolutely no decrease in my pain. In fact, my therapist urged me to look for a neurologist.

I found not only the word neurologist intimidating, but also the expense. After already spending hundreds of dollars and many hours trying to identify the cause of my pain, and getting nowhere, it was difficult to commit to even more.

Instead of going to another doctor, I decided to try to improve my overall health by better diet and exercise. My hope was that a stronger body would surely not have so much pain. But no matter how gradually I increased my exercise or how many experts I consulted regarding correct form and scheduling, the pain would become overwhelming after only a few workouts.

Not only did exercise become impossible, so did many regular activities. Things like cleaning the bathtub, scrubbing the floors, any kind of shopping, or lifting would cause the pain to flair up within hours. It wasn't long before my work was severely affected.

A co-worker recommended a chiropractor. I had never been to one. Even though I did not feel very confident that this would help, I needed to do something right away. The doctor put me on a temporary disability leave from work and gave me adjustments three times a week. After about 3 weeks I was at least walking again and able to go back to work. But the pain was certainly not gone. My chiropractor continued to give me treatments for another month. When I insisted that the pain was not going away, he said he had done all he could and maybe I should lose 10 pounds to see if that might help. I was very sure my being 10 pounds overweight was not the cause of my pain and I never went back.

The following spring I developed allergies. While visiting a specialist for treatment, I described my pain problem. He recommended a neurologist and this time I went ahead and made an appointment.

Once again, there were many pages of medical history to be completed, followed by an extensive neurological examination. In the course of all of this, more symptoms developed.

I woke up one morning with very bad vertigo. It didn't matter if I was sitting, standing, or lying down — I was constantly dizzy. Even in my sleep. I actually dreamed of being dizzy. This was the most disabling symptom I had ever had because I could not hide it. Even walking across the room would result in bumping into furniture and walls.

After a 2-week leave from work and still no relief from the vertigo, I had to quit my job. In fact, I had to quit almost all activity. Even reading or walking caused the dizziness to increase and provoked nausea and headache.

It was as if my life had been jerked away from me. Of course, I was on the phone to the neurologist the first day. Unfortunately, he did not feel the urgency that I did. He saw me in his office within a few days and made an appointment for an EEG. It took almost 3 weeks to get this testing done and get the results. In the meantime, I had to just sit and wait. The results showed everything to be "normal."

There was that word again — "normal." Just what is normal, anyway? I decided it meant they were not looking in the right place because I was certain the way I felt was very abnormal!

I wasn't the only one frustrated by the constant dead ends. My husband, family, friends, and boss all tried to think of alternatives. Some, at times, surely believed it was "all in my head"; others never doubted the reality of a physical problem and dealt with their own feelings of helplessness.

It was then that I really learned the meaning of chronic illness. Most people are used to dealing with acute illness. In the case of flu, a broken bone, or infection, the doctor can usually diagnose the problem right away, prescribe medication to relieve most symptoms, plan a method of treatment, and give the patient an approximate time for recovery. That is acute illness. But in chronic illness, none of those things happen the way we are used to them happening. Instead, the patient may spend an endless amount of time and money just trying to get doctors to believe something is wrong. Then, a cure or estimated time of recovery is probably not forthcoming.

Chronic illness tries the patience and understanding of everyone, especially the person who is ill. It was very difficult to be a loving spouse, a fun-loving friend, or a responsible member of the family when I felt very sick and could not get any relief. Add to that the guilt and regret about what was happening to my life and my state of mind became more depressed by the day.

When my neurologist told me he wanted to do magnetic resonance imaging (MRI) to rule out a brain tumor or multiple sclerosis and that this would take several weeks to complete, I decided to see some other doctors in between the neurological tests to be sure I was covering all the possibilities.

I consulted an internist; ophthalmologist; a different neurologist; an ear, nose and throat specialist; a gynecologist; and a nutritionist. All but the last one found nothing abnormal.

The nutritionist took a lot of blood tests and pages of information and finally diagnosed several conditions. Most of them were complicated and difficult to understand. Some of them he said he would not explain until later, depending on how willing I was to use very unusual treatments. However, he assured me that he could help and proceeded to give me a very strict diet and many bottles of vitamins. As my husband and I drove away, we felt encouraged for the first time. At least someone was finally agreeing that something was wrong with me. It was a relief just to be believed.

The diet was very rigid. All foods except fish and some vegetables were forbidden. I also had to take 17–19 vitamin tablets six times per day. The doctor had been very specific about how I would feel and what effect the diet and vitamins should have on me. After 1 week none of the things he had described were happening. I was supposed to feel much worse while the toxins were being flushed from my body and be able to tolerate very high doses of vitamin C. None of this was happening.

When I called the doctor's office wanting to discuss my questions and reactions, he refused to talk to me unless I agreed to pay an $80 office charge for the phone conversation. He finally did get on the phone long enough to tell me to stay on everything and come into the office in a week. When I called back a few days later with further problems, the nurse could not find my file or remember who I was. She finally gave me some instructions that were the total opposite of what I had been told in the initial visit. At the end of 2 weeks, I did not feel any different and did not go back to that office.

This type of testing and experimenting went on for about 3 months while my neurologist completed the MRI, a sleep study, and a spinal tap. At the end of all of this I still had no answers.

Twice during that same 3-month period I was feeling so terrible that I went to the acute care center near home to see the doctor on call. My hope was that if someone could see me when the symptoms were at the worst, maybe something would show up that everyone else had missed. I was grasping at straws but all they told me was that I must have the flu. When I explained that it could not be the flu and what had been going on for the past few months, they accused me of being dishonest and lying to them.

At that time, the dizziness lessened enough that I could drive short distances and do simple activities. Although I had no idea why the symptoms were changing and could not predict when I would feel better or worse, I needed to get back to work, not only because depression and uselessness were driving me to the edge, but also because the expense of all the doctors and tests was very high.

I found a receptionist job and struggled through each day. Sometimes just sitting in the chair and answering the phone was too much for me. My co-workers were very understanding, but I knew it was difficult for them to have me feeling my way around the room and looking like I was about to collapse all the time. My self-confidence suffered too; I felt like such a burden to my husband, friends, and job.

Then I heard about a local orthodontist doing special work with pain patients. I called right away and got in the same day. The doctor explained his work with pain and temporomandibular joint problems. When he placed a tongue depressor between my teeth on one side, the dizziness decreased significantly. The technician made a plastic splint that fit over my bottom teeth. It repositioned my jaw to relieve the pressure.

The doctor did several tests on my muscles and was surprised at how much pain I had. The vertigo had became such a dominating symptom that I was not paying any attention to the increase in pain. By now, my whole upper body was extremely sensitive to any pressure. Headaches and neck pain were almost constant. Sleeping through a full night was impossible.

The doctor told me to wear the mouth splint for a couple of weeks and see what changes took place. It was difficult to get used to but well worth it. We had to try several different splints before finding the right size. With each change, my mouth would get very sore and I would have to learn to speak with the splint in place. As long as I could keep it in, the dizziness was virtually gone. The pain did not change very much. Although we all hoped we had finally found an answer, it became clear that we had only uncovered one piece of the puzzle.

To try to help relieve the pain, my orthodontist referred me to a physical therapist. With heat, ultrasound, and massage three times a week, some progress was made in my upper body. Unfortunately, the pain came back as soon as the treatments stopped.

The next step was another doctor specializing in pain therapy. Unlike my orthodontist, who could only treat my neck and head area, the new doctor would be able to treat my whole body.

Once again, I faced pages of medical history and information, an extensive and painful examination, many blood tests, and more expenses. I did feel much more confident this time than many of the previous exams. I was treated with respect and concern at all times. As with the orthodontist, this new doctor understood my need to find relief and get on with my life. Everything was done to make the initial exam as tolerable as possible, and as we proceeded, more pieces of my pain puzzle began to fall into place.

My treatment began with oral vitamins, vitamin injections, diet restrictions, and medication for pain and sleep. Also included was a stack of reading material to explain what was happening to me and what treatment was available. Finally, I began to feel like I was getting some control back of my own life.

A significant improvement was made almost immediately. The pain decreased and my energy increased. We had to stop the vitamin injections at one point to see how much of the progress was related to them and I sank back to a painful, tired condition. Once I resumed the injections my progress began again.

This meant it was time to learn to do my own injections. For a person who has never been able to watch a blood test being taken, this was a drastic step. I had to remind myself over and over how much better I would feel and how much I wanted my life back. I learned to give the injections.

I continued to feel better and was very encouraged. I found a more challenging and satisfying job and began to look forward to being well.

Then I got the flu. My husband was ill at the same time and it did seem to be a severe case. But mine settled in my arms, shoulders, and neck. The pain was so terrible that at times I could not even lift my arm to eat. After 4 weeks there was still very little change. Of all the pain I had had up to that point, this was the most frightening. How would I ever do anything if I could not use my arms?

The doctor was very supportive during all of this ordeal. He always had another alternative to relieve the pain and was understanding and encouraging when I felt like I couldn't fight it all any more.

I received intravenous colchicine injections and trigger point injections. The trigger points were very difficult and painful, but they gave almost instant relief. There was soreness for about 36 hours after these shots. That was a small price to pay for the end to any part of the pain.

My work schedule was more strenuous than usual at this time. I struggled to keep going even through the shots and the worst days. It was too much to ask of my body and I was losing ground again. Three months after being struck by the flu, the arm pain was back. This time I decided that rest was the only way to get back to a reasonable level of functioning. My body needed time to allow all the recovery to take place. It was very difficult to leave my job again, even temporarily. There was always a fear of letting go of too much and not being able to get it back. I wasn't ready to give up. This time was different, though, because I finally felt like the doctors were really on my side.

The first 3 weeks were slow and I worried that this would become my permanent situation. Then some changes started to take place. The pain was going away and my strength was increasing. After 6 weeks I was able to return to work.

Up to this time I had been giving myself vitamin injections every other day. The doctor decided to try once again to get me off the injections. This was great news to me since I was very sore and running out of places to give the shots. We decreased slowly until I was only taking one shot per week and then stopped completely. Within a few days the pain was beginning to increase again and my energy took a dive. The shots were still very necessary.

At the time of this writing, I still give myself vitamin injections and take some pain medication. I have hopes that one day I will be able to give that up. At least I am able to work a full schedule, have some kind of social life, and look forward to the future. The fear is always there of when the next setback might come. I try to enjoy the good days and remember on the bad days that I have come up from much worse. I think I'll be on the road to getting well for a long time, but now there are more days of health than days of hell. That's enough to keep me going.

Section II

Soft Tissue
Pain Problems

7 Soft Tissue Pain Problems: Introduction

Michael Margoles, M.D., Ph.D.

INTRODUCTION

The whole gamut of soft tissue pain problems, from simple back or neck (whiplash) strain/sprain to severe cases of fibrositis (fibromyalgia) or the complex and devastating problems of the severe myofascial pain syndromes, form a continuous pathway that may stop at any point of evolution or become more complex with the passage of time. Whereas numerous of these soft tissue pain problems are described in separate chapters of this book, be aware that a number of them can all occur in the same patient.

The following chapters will spell out what happens in numerous of these problematic clinical syndromes. The emphasis in this section is on the soft tissue pain problems mentioned above. These are problems that do not require surgery, but nonetheless may be mistaken for a surgical condition. Some of the highlights of diagnosis and management of these very common problems are discussed.

SOFT TISSUE PAIN PROBLEMS (STRAIN/SPRAIN)

Soft tissue refers to muscle, tendon, or ligament. Strains and sprains occur as a result of either overstretching or tearing a soft tissue structure such as a muscle, tendon, or ligament. They are mildly disabling and usually respond to simple therapies such as rest and/or mild medications.

Sprains and Strains (a "Pull") Are Very Common

A *strain* occurs when a muscle, ligament, or tendon is overworked or overstretched. It involves excessive effort or undue force. There may be localized pain and swelling in the area of the strain.

A *sprain* occurs when a muscle, ligament, or tendon is overworked and partially torn. There is usually localized pain and swelling at the area of the tear. It also refers to an injury to tissues about a joint in which some of the fibers of a supporting ligament (tissue that attaches bone to bone) are ruptured (torn away from the bone) but the continuity (integrity) of the ligament remains intact.

A common example of this is a "whiplash" injury, which may include either a strain or sprain or both.

Management

Strains and sprains are managed with simple measures. Analgesics are given for up to a few weeks to help control the pain. Anti-inflammatory medicines are used for up to a few weeks to decrease swelling and inflammation of tissues. Heat or ice plus massage and diathermy are used to soothe the injured tissues. A short period of resting the injured part is usually indicated, and this may involve the use of a splint, sling, cast, or bed rest for a week or two.

Prognosis

Most strains and sprains have a good prognosis and will resolve uneventfully in a maximum of 5–8 weeks.

What Next?

Myofascial Pain Syndrome

The following considerations are covered more thoroughly in subsequent chapters. A strain and/or sprain may result in a "force overload" to a muscle, or muscles, and create trigger points in that muscle(s). If a sufficient number of trigger points are activated, and there are perpetuating factors present, a myofascial pain syndrome can be generated.

Fibromyalgia

If the injury produces a diffuse aching and soreness throughout numerous body areas, fibromyalgia may have begun.

8   Jacki's Story

Jacki W.

Jacki is a 56-year-old lady and a very successful mother, real estate broker, and agent. One day, while on a tour of listed houses, she was involved in a severe automobile accident. She did not break any bones. However, the accident initiated a very bad pain problem. When seen at the lowest point in her struggle with pain and related matters, she wrote the following:

> My life since I was a passenger in an automobile accident 18 months ago has been a living nightmare for me and for my family. I will try to define it as best I can. There has never been one moment that I have been free of pain. My wonderful quality of life has been seized from me one ounce at a time until there is only a body trying to cope with being alive. I try so very hard to function with the smallest daily tasks. Before the accident, I was a "super mom" and a very busy professional lady in the whirlwind of everyday experiences. I was successful with my peers and had a very high esteem of my self-worth. I was very happy about life and all those around me.
>
> How I wish this vicious circle of pain and sleepless nights would end and I could become a whole and worthwhile person again! Sometimes I feel as though I'm walking into a beautiful meadow full of magnificent flowers and unbeknown to me the trail I am on is taking on a path of quicksand. The harder I try to get out to be among my beautiful flowers (life itself), the deeper I'm being pulled to the bottom of the barrel of quicksand!
>
> All my life I have been a survivor, having had cancer and won the battle against it. Somehow this one is so very different. I will continue to fight with all my being, to beat the wretched constraints that pain and weakness have thrust upon me.
>
> I have obtained help from my pain doctor and his lovely nurse. I now see hope and believe that there is a light at the end of the tunnel. I wish I had been referred to my pain doctor sooner after the accident, before my body had been weakened so much with this chronic pain. My pain doctor is my last hope after being treated or evaluated by close to 20 physicians, surgeons, and physical therapists.
>
> I have been caught up in the "bureaucratic web" of workman's compensation, which has been a living disaster. All I have ever wanted was to get well and to be able to get on with my life. I feel that in the 18 months since my injury, "they" (worker's compensation adjusters, attorneys, etc.) have broken my body and spirit.
>
> With the help of my husband and my pain doctor, my spirit is getting the strength I need to go on. There is a way out of the quicksand and I will be there to see all the beautiful flowers once more."

9 Fibromyalgia

Thomas J. Romano, M.D., Ph.D., FACP, FACR

"I hurt all over." "I'm tired all the time." "My bones ache." "I feel like I'm a hundred years old." All too frequently, these are the problems that are voiced by patients who come to their doctors in search of answers and some form of treatment that will ease their suffering. Often, reasons can be found for the patients' complaints. Fatigue might be caused by iron-deficiency anemia or an underactive thyroid gland (i.e., hypothyroidism), for example, and the problem can be dealt with to the mutual satisfaction of both patient and physician. However, for millions of Americans no easy or straightforward explanation can be found. Many such patients have been plagued by pain, fatigue, poor sleep, etc. and have seen doctor after doctor for many years in search of relief. They are not sure what is wrong with them and often begin to seriously doubt their sanity. Many have told me that they feel "like hypochondriacs," while others are convinced that they have contracted some rare, terrible disease that is escaping detection by even the most sophisticated tests. This is certainly understandable since the patients' symptoms are severe but routine physical examinations and laboratory testing fail to find objective evidence for the patients' subjective complaints. In all fairness to the doctors who encounter patients with such nebulous complaints, it is important to know that scores of diverse medical illnesses from cancer to heart disease can share the complaint of fatigue or lowered stamina. Thus the task of evaluating patients is a formidable one. However, this is little consolation to the patient whose symptoms have generated numerous doctor visits and myriad elaborate (and expensive) tests only to be told what he or she does *not* have. After being reassured that he or she is not dying of cancer or a failing heart or told that his or her blood profile is normal, it is only reasonable for the patient to ask, "Well, then, what *do* I have?" Sometimes, the response is a disquieting "I don't know," but more often the symptoms are explained by such phrases as "growing pains" if the patient is an adolescent or preteen, "your hormones are acting up" if the patient is a young adult, "you're getting on in years" if the patient is elderly, or "it's the change of life" if the patient is perimenopausal. Why these answers are given I don't know, but possibly it is because doctors feel they owe an explanation to their patients and this is the best they can come up with.

However, before dismissing the patients' complaints as being "functional," the doctor should consider the old adage "absence of proof is not proof of absence" and look further. The patient with pain, fatigue, and loss of motivation may be suffering from a chronic soft tissue rheumatism problem known as fibromyalgia syndrome (FS), formerly known as fibrositis. This is especially true if there are associated sleep problems, headaches, and feelings of numbness and tingling over the body. FS has been the subject of intense interest and much research in recent years, but a real breakthrough in understanding this interesting disorder came in the mid-1970s when Canadian researchers found that patients with FS had problems with deep sleep (i.e., stage four, non-REM, delta wave sleep) and had tender points at specific locations on their bodies (Smythe and Moldofsky, 1977; Moldofsky and Scarisbrick, 1976). These findings helped doctors to diagnose FS more accurately and helped to dispel the notion that FS was a condition of vague aches and pains. It was not until 1990, however, that the American College of Rheumatology (ACR) put its approval on criteria for the diagnosis and classification of FS (Wolfe et al., 1990). I was privileged to be a member of the committee that formulated the criteria (Table 9.1), which were intended to be both highly sensitive (88.4%) and highly specific (81.1%) as well as relatively easy to apply in an office setting. All that was necessary was for the doctor to obtain a history of widespread pain and then to carefully examine for tender points. If more than 11 of 18 tender points were found, then FS was diagnosed. However, knowing that a patient has FS does not automatically make the doctor aware of how it really feels to have FS. That is why patients with FS should join support groups to obtain the needed empathy and rapport that only fellow FS patients can provide. Moreover, obtaining literature written for patients and even by patients (Ediger, 1991) can provide insight into FS. A publication entitled *The Fibromyalgia Network* is a quarterly newsletter written and published by Kristin Thorson (7001 School House Lane,

TABLE 9.1 The American College of Rheumatology 1990 Criteria for the Classification of Fibromyalgia[a]

1. **History of widespread pain**

   Definition: Pain is considered widespread when all of the following are present: pain in the left side of the body, pain in the right side of the body, pain above the waist, and pain below the waist. In addition, axial skeletal pain (cervical spine or anterior chest or thoracic spine or low back) must be present. In this definition, shoulder and buttock pain is considered as pain for each involved side. "Low back" pain is considered lower segment pain.

2. **Pain in 11 of 18 tender sites on digital palpation**

   Definition: Pain, on digital palpation, must be present in at least 11 of the following 18 tender point sites:
   - *Occiput*: bilateral, at the suboccipital muscle insertions
   - *Low cervical*: bilateral, at the anterior aspects of the intertransverse spaces at C5–C7
   - *Trapezius*: bilateral, at the midpoint of the upper border
   - *Supraspinatus*: bilateral, at origins, above the scapula spine near the medial border
   - *Second rib*: bilateral, at the second costochondral junctions, just lateral to the junctions on upper surfaces
   - *Lateral epicondyle*: bilateral, 2 cm distal to the epicondyles
   - *Gluteal*: bilateral, in upper outer quadrants of buttocks in anterior fold of muscle
   - *Greater trochanter*: bilateral, posterior to the trochanteric prominence
   - *Knee*: bilateral, at the medial fat pad proximal to the joint line

Digital palpation should be performed with an approximate force of 4 kg. For a tender point to be considered "positive" the subject must state that the palpation was painful. "Tender" is not to be considered "painful."

[a] For classification purposes, patients will be said to have fibromyalgia if both criteria are satisfied. Widespread pain must have been present for at least 3 months. The presence of a second clinical disorder does not exclude the diagnosis of fibromyalgia.

Reprinted from Wolfe et al. (1990). *Arthritis and Rheumatism,* 33, 160–172. With permission.

Bakersfield, CA 93309, phone 805-833-8387). It offers information and encouragement for FS sufferers.

CAUSE

Primary or idiopathic FS (PFS) occurs in patients with no definable or demonstrable cause. These patients all seem to have a sleep disorder and many rheumatologists feel that it is a sleep problem that causes and/or perpetuates FS. FS is termed secondary or concomitant (SCFS) when it afflicts a patient who suffers from another illness such as arthritis, chronic heart disease, lung disease, or a hormone imbalance. It is thought that in the SCFS patient, the underlying illness sets the stage for the development of FS. The third type of FS, termed posttraumatic fibromyalgia syndrome (PTFS), occurs as the result of an accident, usually a fall or a motor vehicle accident. PTFS patients typically are healthy, productive individuals until their mishap, after which time they develop musculoskeletal pain, problems sleeping, headaches, etc. Leading rheumatologists have written about PTFS in textbooks (Smythe, 1989; Bennett, 1989). In fact, patients with "reactive fibromyalgia" (a term combining SCFS and PTFS) were shown to be more severely affected and more disabled than patients with PFS (Greenfield et al., 1992). Whatever the cause, FS can be an extremely painful debilitating disorder. Like arthritis sufferers, patients with FS can have either mild, moderate, or severe disease. Their symptoms can be modulated by the weather and there is no cure, although good treatment is available.

DIAGNOSIS

In the past, FS was diagnosed in many patients who had rheumatic pain but who did not fulfill criteria for such well-known diseases as rheumatoid arthritis or degenerative arthritis. It was a "wastebasket" term and a diagnosis of exclusion. This state of affairs was changed by the publication and application of the ACR criteria (Wolfe et al., 1990). FS can now be diagnosed reliably by a good history and physical examination. Regardless of the type of FS, patients who suffer with this disorder frequently have widespread pain that can change in intensity. Also, the patient may put more emphasis on a certain part of the body on one visit but another anatomic area on a subsequent visit. This can lead to confusion and misunderstanding. The pain of FS can be burning, gnawing, throbbing, tingling, aching, and/or smarting. It can be sporadic or constant. Flares of pain can be brought on by overexertion, weather changes, or stress. The pain can also be migratory and tends to be worse in areas of the body that are used the most. While pain is the prominent symptom in most FS patients, fatigue is the worst problem for some. Patients describe the fatigue as muscular exhaustion (like after strenuous exercise) or that the muscles refuse to work. An attempt to overcome the fatigue by sheer force of will (i.e., "mind over matter") often results in failure, frustration, and even guilt. Most FS patients are young women (female to male ratio is 10 to 1 nationwide) who "look healthy," and many have to overcome the temptation to perform despite the pain and fatigue (e.g., "no pain, no gain"). Difficulty in accepting the illness can lead to feelings of guilt, frustration, and anger. Some FS patients even suffer from a prolonged grieving reaction. Many FS patients have marital difficulties, especially if the spouse is unaware of the nature of the patient's condition.

Other problems frequently found in FS patients are headaches (in over 50%), irritable bowel syndrome, numbness and tingling of hands and feet, subjective feelings of swelling of hands and feet, and stiffness of the body's joints in the morning. This latter problem, often described as gelling in the tissues, can also be felt during the day when the body has been

TABLE 9.2 Conditions Often Occurring with Fibromyalgia

Some people with fibromyalgia may have *some* of these conditions, *some* of the time

Physical conditions

Allergies	Muscle spasms
Bruising	Nocturnal myoclonus
Clumsiness	Numbness and tingling
Dizziness	Photophobia
Dropping things	Premenstrual syndrome
Dry eyes and mouth	Sensitivity to environment
Feeling of swelling	Skin itch, mottling, rash
Hair loss	Sleep apnea
High or low temperature	Sore throat
Irritable bladder	Stiffness
Irritable bowel	Swollen glands
Lack of endurance	Tender lymph nodes
Migraine headaches	Tension headaches
Mouth sores	Vision changes and eye pain

Mental and emotional problems

Anxiety	Mood swings
Confusion	Panic attacks
Irritability	Trouble concentrating
Memory blanks	Word mix-ups

Adapted from Ediger, B. (1991). *Coping with Fibromyalgia (Fibrositis),* Fibromyalgia Association Texas, Inc., Dallas. With permission.

in one position for some time (e.g., sitting at a desk at work or sitting in a movie theater or concert hall). If a FS patient has such "gelling," it may be difficult for him or her to work, especially at a sedentary job. Other problems (Table 9.2) can also occur in FS patients, although not every FS patient has every problem listed.

It is imperative that the doctor do a "point count" on any patient suspected of having FS and that the examiner press with a force of approximately 4 kg. A dolorimeter (Figure 9.1) is an instrument for measuring the precise amount of pressure applied over an anatomic site. It can be used to quantitate sensitivity of tender points. This device is not needed to make the diagnosis of FS but is used to increase the level of objectivity of the examination.

DIFFERENTIAL DIAGNOSIS

FS needs to be clearly differentiated from psychogenic rheumatism and malingering, although malingering is only rarely encountered. In such cases, patients may report tenderness over almost every area palpated or pressed on by the examiner or may exhibit one pattern of tenderness on the first examination and a far different one on subsequent examinations. In contrast, patients with FS have tenderness over specific anatomic sites, and results of examination always tend to be similar. In fact, many patients with the syndrome help the physician by locating the exact area of musculoskeletal tenderness. Pressure over control points such as fingers, metatarsals, or forearm does not cause pain in the patients with FS but may elicit complaints of discomfort or cause withdrawal in the malingerer or patients with psychogenic rheumatism.

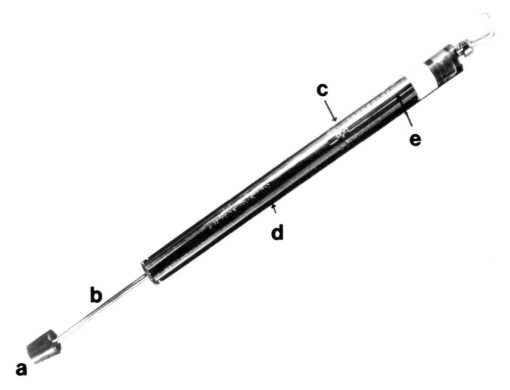

FIGURE 9.1   Hand-held dolorimeter. (a) Rubber stopper 1.54 cm^2, (b) metal rod, (c) scale in kilograms and pounds, (d) metal shaft, and (e) spring attached to rod.

Because the symptoms of primary FS are similar to those of other maladies, a careful search for other causes (Table 9.3) is needed in all cases. When warranted by additional history and physical findings in patients who complain of diffuse aching and stiffness, the following studies should be done: erythrocyte sedimentation rate (Westergren), rheumatoid factor with titer, antinuclear antibody, and complete blood count. Patients who complain of numbness, tingling, and burning need neurological evaluation; electromyography (classic needle EMG and/or surface EMG) and nerve conduction studies are done when indicated.

Additional laboratory procedures such as urinalysis, serum liver and muscle enzyme determinations, hormone studies, radiography, and nuclear medicine scanning should be performed if other signs and symptoms point to a disorder in a particular anatomic area or organ system. If the rheumatoid factor is of high titer and the patient has symmetric small-joint polyarticular arthritis, FS is considered secondary to rheumatoid arthritis. However, if results of all the standard laboratory tests are negative, as is often the case, then, and only then, can a diagnosis of primary FS be made.

The symptoms of malaise, fatigue, myalgia, and arthralgia accompany many connective tissue diseases. Patients with early rheumatoid arthritis may have a positive test for rheumatoid factor despite evanescent physical findings of synovitis or other evidence of articular inflammation. The response of the patient with rheumatoid arthritis to large doses of salicylates is greater than that of the patient with FS, although the latter may obtain some relief.

Patients with FS often complain of muscle achiness, and the diagnosis of polymyositis or dermatomyositis may be considered. However, these entities can be excluded if muscle enzyme levels and needle electromyograms are normal and objective evidence of proximal

TABLE 9.3   Conditions Other Than Fibromyalgia Syndrome to Be Considered in Differential Diagnosis of Patients with Chronic Aches and Pains

Metabolic problems	Bone disease (e.g., osteomalacia)
	Hypothyroidism
Inflammatory conditions	Early rheumatoid arthritis
	Polymyalgia rheumatica
	Systemic lupus erythematosus
	Polyarteritis nodosa
	Seronegative spondyloarthropathies
Infections	Viral prodromes
	Subacute bacterial endocarditis
	Sequelae of viral infections or vaccinations
	Brucellosis and other unusual infections
	Acute leukemias
Anatomic problems	Hypermobility syndromes
	Idiopathic edema
	Muscle overuse syndrome
	Paget's disease
Neurologic conditions	Early multiple sclerosis
	Early Parkinson's disease
Soft tissue problems	Myofascial pain syndromes
	Chronic myofascial pain syndrome
	Posttraumatic hyperirritability syndrome

Adapted from Romano (1988) and Travell and Simons (1983, 1992).

muscle weakness is lacking. Polymyalgia rheumatica is characterized by shoulder and pelvic girdle achiness and must be considered in elderly patients with these complaints. The erythrocyte sedimentation rate is elevated with polymyalgia rheumatica but normal in elderly patients with primary FS. Patients with polymyalgia rheumatica respond dramatically to relatively low doses of corticosteroid, while patients with FS do not improve.

Other entities, such as hypothyroidism, multiple sclerosis, and early Parkinson's disease, can be confused with FS, but these and other similar problems are accompanied by findings on physical examination or laboratory analysis that point to their existence.

At present, interest is intense in developing an objective test that is both sensitive and specific for FS. Although promising reports on objectively measurable abnormalities in FS patients have been presented at medical meetings and seminars (Fricton and Awad, 1990), no one test has been shown to reliably help diagnose FS in a given patient.

TREATMENT

The clinician who is aware of how FS presents can often make the diagnosis or suspect it at the patient's initial office visit. Workup can then be done promptly and a treatment plan initiated relatively quickly. Not only does this save the patient needless worry and expense, but it also renews the patient's faith in traditional medical approaches. If treatment is to be effective, this faith is essential, as is rapport between the patient and physician.

First and foremost, these patients need reassurance that their pain is real and that their problem is a cause for concern but not for alarm or worry. I tell my patients that FS does not kill or cripple but can cause pain that will be intense at times. They are advised that good treatment strategies are available. I stress that patients themselves can participate in their care. This is crucial because the patient must be an active partner in treatment and not merely a passive recipient of medical care. Support from family members, especially a spouse if the patient is married, is essential. If the spouse is carefully educated about the ailment and its treatment, he or she can often be included in the therapeutic effort.

No single "miracle drug" cures FS, and the approach to treatment varies from patient to patient. One must remember that FS is not a form of arthritis, although patients with arthritis may also have FS. Consequently, the rationale behind the use of nonsteroidal anti-inflammatory drugs (NSAIDs) for FS is different than that for arthritis. In FS, the NSAIDs are used for their analgesic rather than their anti-inflammatory properties because, as noted before, true inflammation is not present. Because many FS patients also have irritable bowel syndrome or other gastrointestinal disorders, I prefer to prescribe low doses (400–600 mg) of ibuprofen (Motrin, Rufen) orally three times a day with meals or 500–750 mg of a nonacetylated salicylate (Trilisate, Disalcid) orally three or four times a day.

In addition, the use of tricyclic antidepressants at bedtime helps prevent early morning awakening, partially inhibits REM sleep (thus allowing a deeper sleep), and has an indirect muscle relaxant effect. Most commonly used are amitriptyline (Amitril, Elavil, Endep) and nortriptyline (Aventyl, Pamelor), the active metabolite of amitriptyline. Both are effective, but I start with amitriptyline because it is less expensive in my area.

Amitriptyline is given at bedtime in an initial dose of 10–50 mg. If tachycardia (increased heart rate), visual blurring, or other anticholinergic side effects become a problem, I switch to 10–25 mg of nortriptyline, which has been reported to have a better side effect profile. The doses may be increased slowly as needed and as tolerated to a total maximum bedtime dose of 150–200 mg of amitriptyline nightly. Blood levels of these medications are monitored to avoid toxicity.

Other medications for bedtime use include doxepin (Adapin, Sinequan), trazodone (Desyrel), and imipramine (Janimine, SK-Pramine, Tofranil). I recommend starting at very low doses and making increments cautiously. Recent studies (Bennett et al., 1988) have advocated the use of cyclobenzaprine (Flexeril), a muscle relaxant that is structurally related to tricyclic medication, especially amitriptyline. Recommended doses are 10–20 mg as a one-time dose after supper or at bedtime. In addition to its sleep-promoting action, cyclobenzaprine also modulates efferent activity to muscle spindles, thus reducing muscle tension in a direct way.

Many patients who take these drugs have morning grogginess and sluggishness. I reassure them that these annoying but harmless side effects generally pass in less than a week. It is important that patients be told that although these medications are commonly used for depression, they are being prescribed for FS and not for depression. Patients with significant depression need to be referred for psychiatric help.

Muscle relaxants, such as 100 mg of orphenadrine citrate (Neocyten, Norflex) twice a day or 500 mg of chlorzoxazone (Paraflex, Parafon Forte) three or four times a day, may help selected patients.

Many patients with FS find it "hard to relax" and describe themselves as "worriers." They may be under stress either at work or at home and often push themselves to finish tasks even when they are in pain. These patient need to change their lifestyle and set aside time for relaxation and recreation. They must see to it that they "wind down" for an hour before bedtime.

If patients with FS cannot learn to relax on their own, psychological consultation may be necessary. I stress to patients that I am not sending them to see a psychologist because they are mentally unstable, but rather because I think that the psychologist is best suited to help with stress management and teach them relaxation techniques such as biofeedback.

Physical therapy modalities such as massage, acupressure, ultrasound, hot packs, and spray-and-stretch treatment are useful for some patients with FS but should be combined with pharmacotherapy for best results with few exceptions. Systemic corticosteroids and narcotics are to be avoided; they do not work, and the risk of undesirable side effects or dependence is too great.

Despite treatment, many patients continue to have active FS with tenderness of specific muscles or muscle insertions and muscle tautness and stiffness. These patients are good candidates for injection of a local anesthetic, with or without a glucocorticoid (i.e., "cortisone") preparation, into these areas. I usually inject the affected areas with 2 ml of 1% lidocaine (Xylocaine) or 1% procaine (Novocain), with or without 2–5 mg triamcinolone hexacetonide (Aristospan). This usually gives prompt, albeit temporary, relief and should be followed by local application of heat and avoidance of such aggravating factors as overuse of muscles and insufficient sleep. In some patients, the beneficial effects of these injections last for weeks or months, which far exceeds the half-life of the injected medications. Interruption of a pain–spasm–pain cycle is thought to be a mechanism of action of these injections.

SUMMARY AND CONCLUSION

FS is a common cause of musculoskeletal pain affecting young women most commonly. It is a physical problem that can affect many bodily systems including the muscles and the nervous system. The diagnosis of FS can reliably be made with the application of generally accepted criteria, and conservative outpatient treatment is frequently helpful, although not curative. Time must be taken to perform a directed physical examination; "laying on of hands" is essential for an accurate determination of the "tender point" count for an accurate assessment of the patient. More research needs to be done to determine not only the cause of FS but to develop better treatment. Since FS causes much pain and disability, it is imperative that more information about this common problem be forthcoming.

BIBLIOGRAPHY

Bennett, R. (1989). Fibrositis, in *Textbook of Rheumatology,* 3rd ed., Kelley, W.N., Harris, E.D., Ruddy, S., and Sledge, C.B. (Eds.), W.B. Saunders, Philadelphia.

Bennett, R.M. et al. (1988). A comparison of cyclobenzaprine and placebo in the management of fibrositis, *Arthritis and Rheumatism,* 31, 1535–1542.

Ediger, B. (1991). *Coping with Fibromyalgia (Fibrositis),* Fibromyalgia Association Texas, Dallas.

Fricton, J.R. and Awad, E.A. (Eds.) (1990). in *Advances in Pain Research and Therapy,* Fricton, J.R. and Awad, E.A. (Eds.), Raven Press, New York.

Greenfield, S., Fitzcharles, M., and Esdaile, J.M. (1992). Reactive fibromyalgia syndrome, *Arthritis and Rheumatism,* 35, 678–681.

Moldofsky, H. and Scarisbrick, P. (1976). Induction of neurasthenic musculoskeletal pain syndrome by selective sleep deprivation, *Psychosomatic Medicine,* 38, 35–44.

Romano, T.J. (1988). The fibromyalgia syndrome. It's the real thing, *Postgraduate Medicine,* 83, 231–243.

Smythe, H.A. (1989). Nonarticular rheumatism and psychogenic musculoskeletal, in *Arthritis and Allied Conditions,* 11th ed., McCarty, D.J. (Ed.), Lea and Febiger, Philadelphia.

Smythe, H.A. and Moldofsky, H. (1977). Two contributions to understanding of the "fibrositis syndrome," *Bulletin on the Rheumatic Diseases,* 28, 928–931.

Travell, J.G. and Simons, D.G. (1983). *Myofascial Pain and Dysfunction: The Trigger Point Manual,* Vol. 1, Williams and Wilkins, Baltimore.

Travell, J.G. and Simons, D.G. (1992). *Myofascial Pain and Dysfunction: The Trigger Point Manual,* Vol. 2, Williams and Wilkins, Baltimore.

Wolfe, F. et al. (1990). The American College of Rheumatology 1990 Criteria for the Classification of Fibromyalgia, Report of the Multicenter Criteria Committee, *Arthritis and Rheumatism,* 33, 160–172.

10 Myofascial Pain Syndrome: Clinical Evaluation and Management of Patients*

Michael S. Margoles, M.D., Ph.D.

INTRODUCTION

Myofascial pain syndrome (MPS) is a frequent basis of acute and chronic pain in any muscle location of the body. Awareness of its existence is growing. Specifics of clinical diagnosis are well defined and have been published in texts and magazines. Proper evaluation of the patient with MPS requires (1) a thorough history, emphasizing detailed analysis of the mechanism of injury; (2) physical examination employing analytic techniques that are specific for MPS; and (3) search for perpetuating factors. Perpetuating factors are mechanical, physiological, psychological, biochemical, metabolic, hormonal, and infectious elements that, if abnormal, promote chronicity in MPS and cause it to become resistant to many types of therapy. Management is a complex procedure that must be properly sequenced to ensure success in the recovery of the MPS patient. Clarification of International ICD-9-CM coding is presented. Grading of MPS severity is discussed to enhance professional communication and promote better understanding of MPS. Staging of therapy is broken into nine stages to simplify management sequencing.

The work that follows is intended to complement the seminal works of Travell and Simons (1983, in press). The reader is referred to their texts for more comprehensive reading about MPS (ICD-9-CM = 729.1).

A great deal of the most common, persistent, and disabling pains are of musculoskeletal origin (Fields, 1987). MPS is pain and/or altered sensation (tingling, numbness, burning, gooseflesh, swelling, tightness, tension, and other paresthesias) referred from active myofascial trigger points and may occur in the immediate area about a trigger point or as referred pain 1–3 feet away from the source. The pain of MPS can vary from mild to severe and incapacitating. MPS occurs most commonly in single muscles. However, it can spread to involve

---

* Adapted from *Pain Management: A Practical Guide for Clinicians,* 5th edition, Volume 1, CRC Press, Boca Raton, Florida, 1998, chapter 17.

many other adjacent and distant muscles. Myofascial trigger points may occur in any of the 500 muscles in the body.

Historically, MPS has been intermingled with numerous other terms used to describe soft tissue pain problems, such as fibrositis, fibromyalgia, fibromyositis, nonarticular rheumatism, paucy–articular rheumatism, psychogenic rheumatism, psychogenic pain, myogelosis, lumbago, and other clinical pain syndromes characterized by terms such as functional overlay, symptom magnification, etc. The result of all this varied terminology has been confusion.

Although MPS is common, and not too difficult to diagnose, many therapists are unaware of its existence (Fields, 1987). Some claim that there is a paucity of "objective signs." They say nothing of significance can be detected on X-ray, computed tomography (CT), and magnetic resonance imaging (MRI) scans and that diagnostic laboratory testing is lacking. This has the appearance of adding more confusion to confusion.

MPS is diagnosed by clinical assessment and augmented by appropriate laboratory testing. The criteria for diagnosing MPS have been published by Travell and Simons (1983).

In an era where "high tech" is "in," proper evaluation and management of MPS require astute comprehensive skills in clinical evaluation. The "hands-on" approach to MPS patients is still the only way that a proper diagnosis can presently be made. It is critical to determining the extent and complexity of MPS in order to decide what management approaches will be necessary to manage the patient.

Lack of an adequate physical examination, geared specifically to evaluation for MPS, is probably the most common reason that physicians fail to make the diagnosis. Diagnostic evaluation for MPS must be performed by clinicians with proper skills and training. The evaluations are arduous, technical, and time consuming.

While evaluating a patient with a soft tissue pain problem, keep the following formula in mind:

Myofascial trigger points + Taut bands + Perpetuating factors = Myofascial pain syndrome

CLINICAL POINTS OF IMPORTANCE

Clinical Examination

Adequate physical examination of the grade 2, 3, and 4 (see Appendix 3 at the end of this chapter for grading of severity and definitions) patients may require up to 1–2 hours. This is in addition to the history taking. With each increased grade of severity, the amount of time to complete an adequate history and physical examination (consisting of routine and myofascial elements) increases.

Preeminent Themes in the History

1. Mechanism of onset may be injury, trauma, strain, sprain, or spontaneous onset. The patient may be vague about the exact date of onset (Fields, 1987).
2. Etiology:
   a. Muscle overload (the muscle is usually strained in a shortened position) (Baker, 1986) may be one of a number of the important components here.
   b. Excessive or repeat traumas.
   c. Sleep disorder.
   d. Unknown.
3. Complaints of pain in a distribution that is regional and does not follow spinal segmental or single peripheral nerve distribution.

    a. Myofascial pain occurs in classic trigger point reference zones (Travell and Simons, 1983, in press).

    b. The referred pain of myofascial origin is frequently confused with radicular pain of spinal disc origin.

    c. The pain of MPS is deep and/or aching in quality and can be felt in joints, muscles, or any place in the body.

    d. Trigger points can generate paresthesias, autonomic symptoms (burning and gooseflesh), proprioceptive dysfunction, and weakness.

    e. The distribution of pain and/or altered sensations is usually not coextensive with the trigger points producing it.

    f. Symptoms from MPS may begin at the time of injury or may occur minutes, hours, days, weeks, or months after an initiating incident.

    g. Once initiated, an MPS can become progressively worse over a period or days, weeks, months, or years.

4. Complaints of dysfunction:

    a. Weakness of the affected limb.

       1. Unexpected giving way of the leg.

       2. Dropping things with the hand on the pain side.

5. The severity of symptoms from myofascial trigger points ranges from painless restriction of motion due to latent trigger points so common in the aged to agonizing incapacitating pain caused by very active trigger points (Travell and Simons, 1983).

6. Pain may be aggravated by:

    a. Changes in weather.

    b. Emotional stress.

    c. Physical stress.

    d. Premenstrual syndrome.

7. Difficulty finding a comfortable sleeping position is common in the more severe cases.

8. Dizziness may occur in cases where there is involvement of the head and neck.

9. Absence of other diseases to account for the symptoms.

10. Study of pain charts (also called symptom charts — the pain chart is an important diagnostic tool that helps determine the extent of the MPS and its severity), preferably filled out by the patient at each visit, provides clues to the location of trigger points causing the specific pain patterns (Margoles, 1983).

11. Pain may switch sides:

    a. Generally over a period of months.

    b. Occasionally within a few weeks.

    c. Rarely on a daily or every other day cycle.

12. Pain from one trigger point may mask that from another.

Physical Examination — Trigger Points

All patients with persistent pain or aching should be examined for myofascial trigger points and MPS (Fields, 1987). It must be emphasized that the evaluation of patients with MPS is not a casual endeavor. The clinician attempting to diagnose the more complex cases must be specifically trained in the evaluation techniques of MPS (Travell and Simons, 1983, in press) and/or should be supervised by a therapist expert in the proper techniques of evaluation and management. A "shot in the dark" approach is no substitute for training, skill, and acumen.

The essential aspects of the examination for myofascial trigger points consist of the following major and minor criteria which have been adapted from Simons (personal communication). To make the diagnosis, the findings should include five major criteria and at least one of the three minor criteria.

Major Criteria

1. Regional pain complaint.
2. Pain complaint or altered sensation in the expected distribution of referred pain from a myofascial trigger point.
3. Taut band palpable in muscles that are accessible. The accessibility to palpation of a taut band in a muscle is variable, depending on the thickness of adipose tissue, turgor and tension of the subcutaneous tissue, thickness and tension of overlying muscles, and tension on the muscle fibers being examined.
4. Exquisite spot tenderness at one point along the length of the taut band, in the muscle belly. This is usually the location of the trigger point.
5. Some degree of restricted stretch range of motion, when measurable, for the primary function of that muscle. For example, a trigger point in the levator scapulae muscle will cause decreased lateral rotation of the neck.

Minor Criteria

1. Reproduction of clinical pain complaint, or altered sensation, by pressure on the tender spot. The tender spot must cause referral of pain (or change in sensation) at a distance of at least 2 cm beyond the spot of local tenderness. Pain referral or altered sensation is elicited in response to pressure applied to the tender spot for 10 seconds before considered negative. "Altered sensation" may be described by the patient as a tingling, numbness, or "unusual feeling."
2. Elicitation of a local twitch response by transverse snapping palpation at the tender spot in the taut band.
3. Pain alleviated by elongating (stretching) the muscle or by injecting the tender spot (trigger point).
4. Restricted range of motion of the body part or joint affected by the myofascial trigger points bearing on it. Restricted range of motion of a joint gives clues to the location of trigger points. For example, decreased active abduction of the shoulder may be due to an infraspinatus trigger point or any of the five other muscles that can cause a similar problem about the shoulder.
5. Patients frequently give a startled response (jump sign) when sufficient pressure is applied to the trigger point (Travell and Simons, 1983) (see definition of a jump sign at the end of the chapter).
6. The trigger point occurs at a classic location (see Appendix 7).

Physical Examination — Other Myofascial

I routinely examine other body areas, unrelated to the patient's presenting problem(s), as part of my usual evaluation of MPS patients. I do this to determine the extent of the myofascial problem. I want to know if the patient has a simple (a single-muscle MPS) or complex (multiple-muscle MPS) problem. A quick and easy way to do this is to palpate an area that is easily accessible in all patients, whether thick or thin. The paraspinal muscles in the back, extending from the base of the occiput to the end of the sacrum, are ideal for this purpose.

To accomplish this:

1. The patient is prone on the exam table.
2. The neck is positioned in flexion by having the patient's neck and chin hang over a pillow at one end of the exam table.
3. The patient's arms dangle over the sides of the exam table to move the scapulae away from the paraspinal muscles.
4. All the paraspinal muscles from the base of the skull to the fifth sacral segment are palpated along both sides of the spine. Beginning 2–3 inches away from the midline, flat palpation (Travell and Simons, 1983) is used to check for taut bands, local twitch responses, trigger points, jump signs, and unusual tenderness.
5. In the more severe cases, I encounter an increased frequency of abnormal findings. Prognostically, this means slower response to appropriate management and a longer amount of time to recover.
6. Even if the back is the main area of involvement, it is rare that the entire back from C1 to S5 is involved. Therefore, the uninvolved areas can be examined to determine if overall involvement is greater than the presenting problem.
7. Results of this testing can be accurately logged onto the sheet marked "paraspinal muscle assessment."

Physical Examination — Problems Caused by Myofascial

Trigger points can cause dysfunction and other problems in the muscles they inhabit. This may manifest as weakness. The patient may have an abnormal JAMAR grip strength test. There may be decreased strength on manual muscle testing (MMT) in one or a number of muscles affected by any myofascial trigger points anywhere in the body.

Some muscles will demonstrate breakaway weakness (BAW) (Baker, 1986) when MMT is carried out. This occurs as the muscle is being resisted through its normal range of motion. About halfway through the muscle arc of motion, there is a sudden "breakaway." The muscle quickly loses strength, and the patient may experience pain in the muscle being tested. The suddenness of the breaking away addresses the presence of a trigger point. On the other hand, if the muscle being tested is diffusely tender and painful, the MMT procedure will show a generalized weakness throughout its entire range of motion. Functionally, the BAW can cause problems like dropping silverware, pots, dishes, and other potentially dangerous objects. It can cause the hip, leg, or knee to give way without warning.

Another manifestation of dysfunction related to trigger points is decreased range of motion of a limb or joint or the neck or back. At times, involvement of the shoulder(s) can be so severe as to cause a "frozen shoulder" that clinically looks identical to a bony fusion. The pain may be agonizing, especially when the patient attempts to move the shoulder.

Other dysfunction(s) may present as tendonitis and bursitis. The affected tendon, bursae, or joint may even appear slightly swollen.

Trigger points that are active cause pain and pain patterns that are frequently confused with arthritis. Careful study of the pain chart, physical examination, and X-rays usually reveals the myofascial nature of the problem. Even though the X-rays may show some degenerative changes, MPS may still be the cause of the pain and not the joint changes. One of my patients had fairly advanced rheumatoid arthritis of her hands. She did secretarial work. Typing activities caused pain in her hands. With proper myofascial management, her myofascial hand pain was resolved. Her hands became painless, but the rheumatoid deformities remained. Everyone who has a limp does not have arthritis of the hip or leg. A frequent cause of limping is trigger points in the gluteus minimus, medius, or maximus muscles. Limping can be caused by a trigger point in almost any muscle of the leg.

Paresthesias associated with active trigger points can be very distressing. At times, the numbness produced in the fingers and fingertips may cause the patient to get burned because of impaired perception to heat in the affected hand(s).

Proprioceptive dysfunctions are annoying. Trigger points in muscles cause faulty spatial orientation messages to be sent to the brain. Because balance is adversely affected, distances are misjudged. This is commonly manifested by bumping into furniture or doorways. In some of the worst cases, patients have reported walking into walls.

The net result of the dysfunctions caused by myofascial trigger points or MPS may be overall decreased physical functioning for activities of daily living such as job duties, bathing, hygiene, sleeping, sexual activity, etc. The greater the number of trigger points that scatter throughout the body, the more sizable the degree of physical impairment.

Physical Examination — Pressure Threshold Meter Test

As part of my routine examination of the grade 2, 3, and 4 patients, I perform a pressure threshold meter test (available from Pain Diagnostics and Thermography, Inc., 233 East Shore Road, Suite 108, Great Neck, NY 11023, phone 516-829-9469). This hand-held, pressure-sensitive gauge can be used quickly and easily. Testing is carried out in all or some of the muscles on the graph in Appendix 9. The meter can be used for three purposes:

1. To assess the presence of generalized tenderness in a patient who presents with what appears to be a localized problem.
2. To pick up trigger points in the classic MPS locations.
3. To document that the trigger point has been eradicated after being treated. After the trigger point is adequately treated, the abnormal tenderness changes back to normal.

Normative data are not available for all the muscles on the graph.

Perpetuating Factors and Laboratory Evaluation

This is a vital part of the evaluation and management of patients with MPS, yet many clinicians pay little or no attention to it. Perpetuating factors are a number of essential elements of MPS that prolong the pain and dysfunction. They make MPS resistant to "usual and customary" methods of management (Margoles, 1983, 1987, in press; Rask, 1980; Simons, personal communication; Travell and Simons, 1983; Travell, 1976, personal communication). They impede the patient's progress of recovery and confound the patient and the therapist.

If only short-term or incomplete relief is obtained after the application of an appropriate physical modality (trigger point injection, stretch and spray, Lewitt stretch, etc.), the patient has to be reevaluated for perpetuating factor problems.

In the more complex cases (grade 3 or 4), this must be done routinely as part of the initial comprehensive evaluation and management (see Figure 10.1).

The well-known perpetuating factors include:

    I.   Mechanical problems:
        A. Repeated injuries or accidents
        B. Structural problems (Travell and Simons, 1983)
           1. Short leg

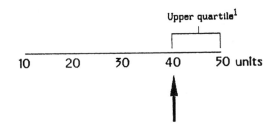

FIGURE 10.1 Blood testing for biochemical, metabolic, and hormonal perpetuating factors. If the patient's blood tests below the arrow pointing to the 40 units, he or she has a less than optimal blood level of that perpetuating factor. [1]This represents the optimal part of the normal range.

    2. Short hemi-pelvis
    3. Long second metatarsal(s) and short first metatarsal(s)
    4. Short upper extremity(s)
  C. Ruptured cervical or lumbar disc (Margoles, 1987)
  D. Brassiere straps that are too tight and/or support heavy breasts
  E. Persistent muscular overexertion (abuse of muscles)
  F. Abnormalities of dental structures including teeth, bones, joints, and/or muscles (Mackley, in press)
II. Physiological problems:
  A. The stress of a surgical procedure
  B. Chronic fatigue
  C. Lack of restorative and/or restful sleep
  D. Malabsorption syndrome
III. Psychological problems:
  A. Too much nervous tension and emotional stress
  B. Drug overdoses
  C. Chronic anxiety and/or worrying
  D. The MPS, with its associated pain and dysfunction, is a source of stress, anxiety, and depression
  E. Behaviors that promote abuse of muscles

Laboratory Assessments for Perpetuating Factors

Utilization of specific laboratory testing (Travell and Simons, 1983) and appropriate interpretation of results are some of the most important means of detecting perpetuating factors. Currently, many clinicians are skeptical about the role of correcting the metabolic abnormalities cited in Chapter 4 of Travell and Simons (1983). Correct adjustment of the biochemical, metabolic, and hormonal perpetuating factors is crucial to a satisfactory outcome in the management of patients with MPS.

IV. Biochemical:
  A. Vitamin problems:
    1. Too little (insufficient, less than optimal, or deficient) serum levels of:
      • B1 (thiamin)
      • B2 (riboflavin)
      • B3 (niacin)
      • B5 (pantothenate)

- B6 (pyridoxine)
- Bc (folic acid)
- B12 (cobalamin)
- C (ascorbic acid)
- D (cholecalciferol)

Less than optimal is deemed as a blood test level below the upper 75% of the normal range. For example, a blood test for a perpetuating factor has a normal range of 10–50 units. If the range is broken up into quartiles, the plotting would look like Figure 10.1. If the patient's result is below 40, the blood test level is less than optimal. A practical example would relate to a tire on a car. If its air content gets down to less than 75% of usual, the car does not handle well and may even be dangerous to drive. The tire functions best at between 75 and 100% of the manufacturer's recommended inflation. The same holds true for adjusting the blood test results in the management of patients with MPS.

    2. Too much:
      a. Vitamin A
        • Vitamin A toxicity from intake of vitamin A supplements or excess carotene conversion in the body to vitamin A (Margoles, in press)
        • Eating foods too high is vitamin A or carotene
  B. Mineral problems:
    1. Too little (less than optimal serum levels of)
      • Potassium
      • Calcium
      • Magnesium
      • Iron and ferritin
V.   Metabolic:
  A. Relative or absolute hyperuricemia (Travell and Simons, 1983)
  B. Low-grade or frank anemia
VI. Hormonal (Barnes, 1976):
  A. Hypometabolism (low thyroid function) (Travell and Simons, 1983)
  B. Insufficient estrogen supply
VII. Infections:
  A. Acute and chronic viral, bacterial, and other organismic infections of the lungs, kidneys, bones, sinuses, teeth, and gums

LABORATORY TESTING

I routinely order the testing listed below on all MPS patients with suspected biochemical perpetuating factors. Patients with grade 2, 3, or 4 are routinely tested before the first visit. Some of the tests take 7–10 days to get results back. In the grade 1 cases, the patient is first seen and examined to determine whether the blood testing seems necessary as part of the evaluation.

"PANEL" test (or equivalent)	*Additional initial testing to order*
Includes:	Ferritin
Hematology	Magnesium

"PANEL" test (or equivalent)	Additional initial testing to order
CBC	Calcium, ionized
DIFF	Endocrinology
ESR	T4 by RIA
Chemistry	T3 by RIA
Bicarbonate	12-vitamin panel from
Calcium	Vitamin Diagnostics
Chloride	Vitamin B12
Creatinine	Folic acid
Glucose	Vitamin B6
Iron	Thiamin
Phosphorus	Niacin
Potassium	Biotin
Sodium	Riboflavin
Urea nitrogen	Pantothenic acid
Uric acid	Vitamin A
Liver function	Vitamin C
Protein, total	Vitamin E
Bilirubin, total	Beta-carotene
LDH	RBC magnesium level
Alk phosphatase	AM and PM serum cortisol
SGOT (AST)	
SGPT (ALT)	
GGTP	
Lipids	
Cholesterol	
Triglycerides	
Urinalysis	

The ionized calcium test measures the unbound calcium in the blood. It is not the same as the routine serum calcium test. Many labs get the two tests mixed up.

Note: Special arrangements have to be made to ship the blood for vitamin levels to Vitamin Diagnostics. If you are interested in the specialized vitamin tests, contact Susan Feingold at Vitamin Diagnostics (phone 1-732-583-7773).

SPECIAL STUDIES

X-ray, CT, MRI, etc.

At present, there are no predictable findings in X-ray, CT, MRI, bone scan, or EMG studies that consistently support the diagnosis of MPS. Instead, it is the absence of significant bony, disc, and nerve pathology that helps point the clinician in the direction of MPS as the cause of the patient's presenting complaints. On the other hand, a positive result in any of the above-mentioned tests does not rule out MPS.

Figures 10.2 through 10.6 give the eight crucial stages of therapy in the management of MPS, plus the optional stage 9 for advanced therapeutic management. They are a summary of the text that appears in the section about management of MPS patients.

STAGING OF MANAGEMENT

Foundational Stages

Stage 1
Correct all perpetuating factors

- Structural, including dental
- Mechanical
- Endocrine
- Biochemical
- Physiological
- Infection

May require 6–26 weeks to accomplish. Titrate levels up with repeat blood testing. Some grade 1 and 2 patients recover spontaneously with correction of perpetuating factors.

Stage 2
Normalize sleep

Behavioral techniques are used first. Next, antihistamines, tricyclic antidepressants (Elavil®, Sinequan®, etc.), or mild muscle relaxers are utilized to induce and maintain sleep. Brand-name products are preferred. Wear sweats to bed to combat cramping by keeping legs warm.

FIGURE 10.2

STAGING OF MANAGEMENT

Foundational Stages

Stage 3
Correct psychologic perpetuating factors

Reduce tension, stress, and anxiety. Correct behaviors that promote abuse of muscles. Correct dysfunctional thinking. Cognitive restructuring of perpetuating factors. May require a minimum of 3 months in severe cases.

Stage 4
Medications to facilitate pain symptom control
and physical recovery

Medications are used to combat muscle soreness as physical activity increases. Begin with nonsteroidal anti-inflammatory drugs (NSAIDs) and/or Tylenol®. Progress to Darvon® and finally to the opioid-containing or opioid analgesics. Dosing is time contingent. Aim for 30–50% pain relief or to the point that the medication "takes the edge off" the pain. Using the analgesic medication, the patient is encouraged to increase all activities of daily living. Increased activity may activate latent trigger points. The resulting pain may necessitate stretch and spray or myofascial trigger point injections.

FIGURE 10.3

STAGING OF MANAGEMENT

Intermediate Stages

Stage 5
Facilitate recovery

This is important for the grade 3 and 4 patients. An occupational therapist expedites the activities of daily living. The patient is given a disabled-person parking sticker to encourage return to normal activity levels.

Stage 6
*Mobilization**

- Begin formal P.T.
- Stretch and spray
- Trigger point injections
- Lewitt stretch
- Williams and McKinzie exercises
- Partial range-of-motion stretching
- Chiropractic
- Tube exercises
- Massage
- Myotherapy
- Low-resistance stretching
- Low-impact aerobics

Begin to get rid of barrier trigger points. Nerve blocks and epidural injections can be attempted at this stage. If there is no response after three attempts, defer these to stage 7 or 9.

* Note: patients may only be able to tolerate therapy twice per week.

FIGURE 10.4

STAGING OF MANAGEMENT

Final Stages

Stage 7
Improve flexibility, strength, and endurance

- Back school
- Work-hardening program
- Trigger point injections
- Aggressive P.T.
- Work out barrier trigger points
- Medium-load stretching against resistance
- Chiropractic
- Stretch and spray
- Lewitt stretch
- Swimming
- Jogging
- Full range-of-motion stretching

Stage 8
Vocational rehabilitation

Vocational testing and vocational rehabilitation. Slowly work the patient back into the job market. In addition, a comprehensive ergonomic analysis is carried out to ensure compatibility with the patient's new or old employment.

FIGURE 10.5

STAGING OF MANAGEMENT

Advanced Stages

Stage 9
Advanced physical therapy

Note: This stage of the program is only for those patients wishing to pursue a career or avocation that calls for maximum physical performance. All of the listed components can be utilized.

- More aggressive work-hardening program
- Aggressive aerobic workouts
- Progressive weight or resistance training
- Parallel bar workouts
- Proprioceptive "fine-tuning"
- Jogging and running
- Work out all remaining barrier trigger points

FIGURE 10.6

MANAGEMENT

Introduction

The management of MPS may be an endeavor that is complex and challenging for both the therapist and the patient. There may be frustration for both sides of the management team. Certain of the perpetuating factors take time to correct. For example, muscles that have been thrown out of balance, along the spine, neck, and other areas, need time to come back into balance once the proper lift is prescribed for the shoe on the short leg side. Less than optimal serum potassium levels require time, effort, and retesting of the blood levels until the serum potassium reaches the optimal part of the normal range. The multiplicity of factors involved is shown in Figures 10.2 and 10.3, stages 1 to 3.

The patient may have a number of etiologies for his or her pain complaints. For example, there may be pain radiating down the leg. There may be trigger points about the low back, hip, or buttock which when stimulated reproduce the leg pain. The patient may also have an absent Achilles reflex and an MRI scan positive for a herniated disc on that side. The MPS can mimic the disc rupture. Therefore, in the absence of an acute paralysis from the ruptured disc, it is important to treat the MPS first.

Rehabilitation of the MPS patient is a progressive endeavor. Starting the therapy program for a grade 2, 3, or 4 patient with stage 9 (see Figure 10.6) physical therapy will fail. Prescribing a nonsteroidal anti-inflammatory drug to a grade 3 or 4 patient and injecting a single trigger point followed by stretch and spray to the injected muscle may net very limited results. Recovery is a "stepwise" undertaking (see stages 1 to 9, Figures 10.2 to 10.6).

At times, an interdisciplinary team of pain management specialists is necessary to treat the recalcitrant cases. This team needs to be coordinated by a physician knowledgeable in MPS.

Timing and staging of therapeutic interventions are crucial to the patient's advancement toward recovery. This is shown in Figures 10.2 to 10.5. For example, taking a grade 3 MPS patient and starting the therapeutic program with an aggressive, sports-oriented, physical therapy program (stage 9) will net disaster and frustration. It is unrealistic to treat MPS patients as purely mechanical problems. It is sad to see MPS patients condemned as malingerers when they fail a purely mechanical physical therapy rehabilitation program. This situation prevails with therapists who do not understand the limits and restrictions that MPS imposes on the myofascial muscles. Given proper management and management staging, the MPS patient can be brought to the stage where he or she can begin to work out the kinks and stiffness (stage 6). However, if that same patient is taken through all the proper stages and staging of therapy listed below, and then put into the same advanced physical therapy program, the patient is more likely to succeed and become rehabilitated. Stretch and spray or trigger point injections, if poorly timed, may appear to backfire, resulting in frustrating pain flare-ups and disappointment. When they are properly sequenced in the management staging, the results can be impressive.

When setbacks occur, if the clinician can comprehend that more perpetuating factors need to be sought out and corrected before further physical therapies are attempted, the situation is salvageable.

Foundational Stages

Stage 1 (Figure 10.2): Correct All Perpetuating Factors (Travell and Simons, 1983)

A. This must be done, in most cases (some of the grade 1 and 2 patients and all of the grade 3 and 4 patients), before the physical therapies of stages 6, 7, 8, and 9 are attempted.

B. Special attention must be given to meticulously "cleaning up" all the perpetuating factors (Travell and Simons, 1983).

C. When all these are corrected, the MPS will either resolve spontaneously or will become more responsive to the next stages of management.

D. Special note about some of the biochemical problems:

1. An easy program of oral replacement therapy is given in Appendix 5. It can be implemented, without the use of recommended blood testing, in all of the grade 1 and some of the grade 2 patients. Patients can order the products from Bronson, or you can stock the products in your office. It can be used in the grade 3 and 4 patients, but I recommend that the complete panel of blood testing be ordered first, because once the patient is on oral B-complex vitamins for as little as 3 days, it distorts the blood test results. If you think you may need a panel of vitamin tests, to orient your management regimen, have the testing done before you begin to supplement whatever the patient is taking.

2. Taking vitamins by mouth does not guarantee an optimal blood level. There is no way to guess the vitamin nutriture from the clinical picture and complaints. Currently, the only accurate way to assess this is to get the 12-vitamin panel from Vitamin Diagnostics (see section on blood testing below). Vitamin Diagnostics also offers cellular vitamin assays. Consult Goodhart (1980) for listings of the symptoms of deficiency and inadequacy of the various vitamins.

3. Some patients need a course of high-potency (Margoles, 1989) B-complex injections. The composition of the injections is

   Syringe #1

Fortaplex or B-Plex 100	$^1\!/_2$ cc
Riboflavin, 50 mg/ml	$^1\!/_2$ cc
2% Xylocaine® (lidocaine) or Novocain® (procaine) w/o epi	$^1\!/_2$ cc

Syringe #2

DPAN (dexpanthenol, 250 mg/ml)	1 cc
Hydroxycobalamin, 1000 mg/ml	¼ cc
Folic acid, 5 or 10 mg/ml	¼ cc

Separate syringes are used because folic acid precipitates the B1 and B6 in the Fortaplex or B-Plex 100. Depending on the vitamin blood test results, patients are given the above injections once or twice per week. Patients with the lower blood test levels are given the injections twice per week. In the severely depleted patients, the contents of each syringe can be doubled during the second and following weeks, to increase the effectiveness of the B-complex injections. See Appendix 1 for suppliers of the recommended products.

4. Some of the low normal hemoglobin, hematocrit, red blood cell, and ferritin levels are resistant to many of the commonly available iron tablets. The therapist may have to resort to Feosol elixir and, if that fails, a short course of low-dose iron–dextran injections may be necessary to bring the hemoglobin, hematocrit, and red blood cell count up to a satisfactory part of the normal range.

5. Some patients are intolerant of the magnesium tablets that will be used to bring their serum magnesium levels into the optimum part of the normal range. In those cases, giving 3 mg of boron p.o. may help (Travell and Simons, 1983).

6. Some patients may require up to 60–100 meq of oral potassium per day. The need for potassium seems to vary directly with the severity of the disease. The low normal serum potassium levels are responsible for both the cramping and charley horses these patients complain of and much of the myofascial muscular irritability. A simple formula for oral replacement is found in Appendix 6.

Stage 2 (Figure 10.2): Normalize Sleep (Margoles, in press)

A. MPS patients need six to eight uninterrupted hours of restful and restorative sleep.
B. Therapy is initiated with behavioral techniques.
C. Medications are added as the need arises.
   1. Tailored to meet the needs of the patient.
   2. Tricyclic antidepressant, Benadryl®, muscle relaxer (Soma®, Ativan®, Klonopin®). Brand-name medications are preferred. Intermittent use is preferred. The more severe grades of MPS patients have a higher tolerance for these medications. I believe this is a reflection of their altered biochemistry and usually corrects as the patient progresses through all the stages of recovery (Margoles, 1989).

Stage 3 (Figure 10.3): Correct Psychological Perpetuating Factors

A. Reduce tension, stress, and anxiety.
B. Correct behaviors that promote abuse of muscles.
C. Correct dysfunctional thinking.
D. Cognitive restructuring.
E. Correction of "good sport syndrome" behavior (Travell and Simons, 1983).

Stage 4 (Figure 10.3): Medications to Facilitate Pain Symptom Control and Physical Recovery (Margoles, 1984, in press)

A. Tricyclic antidepressants, such as Elavil® (amitriptyline) and Norpramin® (desipramine), in grade 2, 3, and 4 patients may be of help in normalization of sleep abnormalities. This may produce as much as 20–30% pain relief.

B. The use of oral and injectable B-vitamin preparations decreases the irritability of the myofascial trigger points. With the use of the recommended vitamin program, most patients slowly develop a negative tolerance to narcotics, narcotic-containing analgesics, and other controlled substances as management progresses (Margoles, in press).

C. Grade 1 MPS patients need no medication for pain symptom control.

D. In grade 2 MPS patients, some of the pain and stiffness will benefit from the use of Tylenol®, nonsteroidal anti-inflammatory drugs* (NSAIDs), or the milder opioid-containing analgesics such as Darvocet-N® 100, Tylenol® or aspirin and codeine (30 mg), Ultram®, or Vicodin®.

  1. Use of NSAIDs for more than 6 weeks is not recommended. Long-term use of NSAIDs can be considered potentially dangerous to numerous vital organs of the body.

E. For grade 3 and 4 MPS patients, the goals of medication usage are to decrease pain symptoms, increase range of motion of the joints affected by the MPS, increase walking tolerance, increase up time, improve the quantity and quality of restful sleep, increase social activity level, and maintain or restart employment. In some of these patients, exercise and physical rehabilitation may have to be facilitated by blocking pain symptoms with appropriate analgesic medication.

  1. The NSAIDs as a whole may be of limited value in the management of this patient group. Too much reliance on the NSAIDs can produce gastric bleeding and other undesirable side effects. Switching from one of these weak analgesics to another, instead of using a true analgesic medication such as Vicodin®, Tylenol® and codeine, Percodan®, or morphine, can be a significant factor in delaying the patient's recovery.

  2. In some cases of NSAID intolerance, it is possible to use small doses of oral and intravenous colchicine (Margoles, 1988, in press; Rask, 1980, 1985). Intravenous colchicine can produce dramatic pain relief and improved physical function in some of the grade 2, 3, and 4 patients. It can be given intravenously once or twice per week for 3–6 weeks or more.**

  3. It is somewhat surprising to find that the opioids and opioid-containing analgesics in many grade 3 and 4 cases will control postexercise stiffness better than the NSAIDs.

  4. Analgesic medications are given on a time-contingent basis, by the clock and not according to the pain. Begin with the least potent analgesics (such as Tylenol®, NSAID, or Darvocet-N® 100) and then progress up to the stronger analgesics as the need arises (Vicodin®, Anexia 7.5, Vicodin ES®, Lorcet® 10, Percodan®, Demerol®,*** morphine, etc.) (Margoles, 1984; Meyers and Meyers, 1987; Tennent and Ulemen, 1983; Smith, 1981, 1989; Jaffe and Martin, 1985; Foley and Portenoy, 1986; Gilmann et al., 1980; Houde, 1974; Porter and Jick, 1980; Stimmel, 1985). Use of these medications is contingent upon the clinician's

---

  * These include, but are not limited to, Advil, ibuprophen, Anaprox, Ansaid, Butazoladin, Clinoril, Dolobid, Feldene, Indocin, Rufen, Meclomen, Medipren, Tylenol, acetaminophen, Motrin, Nalfon, Naprosyn, Orudis, Lodine, Tolectin, Toradol, Voltaren, Disalcid, Trilasate, and others.

 ** Available from College Pharmacy, 833 Tejon, Colorado Springs, CO, phone 800-888-9358. Order: colchicine 1 mg/2 cc, preservative free; 2-cc vials, RX#473290.

*** For reasons unknown to me, Demerol® tablets have not been very effective in this group of patients. Injectable Demerol® is not desirable for long-term administration because the buildup of normeperidine can worsen the pain.

"comfort level" in dealing with them and the patient's pain severity, cooperation, initiative, complexity, chronicity, tolerance, psychologic status, and motivation toward appropriate goals.

5. Doses of Percodan®, Percocet®, or oxycodone as high as 10–14 tablets per day are occasionally needed in grade 3 and 4 patients. Blood testing for clotting time and liver and kidney function is needed to properly follow up the patient at these doses of medication. Serum levels of narcotic may or may not correlate with the amount of relief or toxicity. Blood testing for the narcotic itself is usually unreliable as an indicator of expected clinical effectiveness.

Intermediate Stages

Stage 5 (Figure 10.4): Facilitate Recovery

A. Registered occupational therapist is called in
   1. Comes in to facilitate activities of daily living with respect to household work, work outside the home, driving automobile, etc.
   2. Facilitate hygiene:
      a. Bathing
      b. Showering
      c. Use of bathroom and toilet
      d. Other
   3. Makes recommendations for adaptive devices:
      a. Toilet
      b. Shower and bath
      c. Kitchen
      d. Gardening
      e. Automobile
      f. Dressing and undressing
      g. Other
B. Disability parking sticker:
   1. Helps with banking, shopping, getting to work, etc.
   2. If in doubt, the physician should give one to the patient to see if it encourages increased functioning
   3. Encourages the patient to get out and get back into society
   4. Effective in return to work
C. Correct abuse of muscles:
   1. Avoid excessive bending, lifting, and twisting
   2. Avoid lifting loads that are too heavy
   3. Avoid the "good sport syndrome" (Travell and Simons, 1983)
   4. Don't carry luggage or bags that are too heavy
   5. Avoid clothing that is too tight
   6. When traveling long distances, get up every 20–30 minutes to stretch and relieve tension on muscles

Stage 6 (Figure 10.4): Mobilize (Margoles, in press)

A. To improve range of motion
B. To decrease dysfunction
C. To improve pain by getting muscles back to normal resting length

D. This is accomplished by:
1. Stretch and spray (Travell and Simons, 1983)
2. Trigger point injection (Travell and Simons, 1983)
3. Begin to work on BARRIER trigger points (see Appendix 10)
4. Lewitt stretch
5. Chiropractic
6. Specific physical therapy:
a. Low-impact aerobics
b. "Tube" exercises (Margoles, in press)
c. Williams flexion exercises
d. McKinzie extension exercises
e. Low-load stretching (against resistance)
f. Partial range-of-motion stretching
g. Low-resistance stretching
7. Swimming
8. Nerve blocks, epidural injections, and sympathetic blocks can be attempted at this stage; if no positive results with two to three procedures, these can be attempted again at stage 7 or 9

Final Stages

Stage 7 (Figure 10.5): Improve Flexibility, Strength, and Endurance (Margoles, in press)

A. Back school program
B. Work hardening
C. Aggressive physical therapy
D. This is enhanced by:
1. Stretch and spray (Travell and Simons, 1983)
2. Trigger point injection (Travell and Simons, 1983)
3. Lewitt stretch
4. Chiropractic
E. Swimming
F. Jogging
G. Full range-of-motion stretching
H. Medium-load stretching (against resistance)
I. Get rid of more BARRIER trigger points (Appendix 10)
J. Manipulation under anesthesia

Stage 8 (Figure 10.5): Vocational Rehabilitation

A. Vocational testing
B. Ergonomic analysis
1. Relates to energy requirements to perform specified tasks
a. Example: measurement of the amount of energy and range of motion to perform a strenuous work task, which could then be compared to the patient's current work capacities
2. At present, this is not an exact science
C. Vocational counseling
D. Vocational training and rehabilitation
E. Vocational placement

Prognosis

A. Grade 1 and 2 MPS patients should be able to get back to either their usual work or modified usual work.
B. Grade 3 patients will have to be retrained to lighter work, and only if they can tolerate it.
    1. If the patient can be retrained, he or she should be phased back into active employment slowly. This is advised because of unavoidable muscle atrophy when off work for 8 weeks or more. An approximate return-to-work schedule would be 4 hours/day for 2–4 weeks, 6 hours/day for 2–4 weeks, 8 hours/day for 2–4 weeks; then the patient can begin to do overtime work.
    2. Patients who have been off work for a year or more would be the ones who need the 4-week intervals for shifting up to longer work hours.
C. There is no predictable recovery for grade 4 patients at the present time.

Advanced Stage

Stage 9 (Figure 10.6): Advanced Physical Therapy (Margoles, in press)

Note: This program is only for those MPS patients who have a professional career or avocation that calls for maximum performance. This relates to athletes, dancers, and the like. It may necessitate extra "fine-tuning" of all perpetuating factors that were picked up on in the initial and subsequent exams.

A. Work-hardening program
B. Aggressive aerobics
C. Progressive weight training
D. Parallel bars
E. Proprioceptive reeducation
F. Aggressive rehabilitation of neuromuscular timing and coordination
G. Fine-tuning of muscular coordination
H. Running
I. Improving cardiac endurance
J. Use of pressure threshold meter to measure progress and set further goals
K. Use of Cybex or similar to set aggressive goals to spur recovery
L. Work out all remaining BARRIER trigger points

Conclusion

The speed of recovery at each stage must be adjusted to the patient's fortitude in achieving each level of accomplishment.

Some patients will respond to the simplest of interventions, such as massage or gentle pressure applied on the trigger points. The more severely afflicted patients will require an extensive and complex therapy program that requires a number of years to accomplish substantial recovery. Some of the grade 3 and grade 4 patients will only obtain partial recovery with a year or more of therapy. Some of the more complex cases, such as grade 3, will not be able to make it past stage 6. Most of the grade 4 patients will not be able to make it past stage 5.

Many of the MPS patients will not tolerate physical therapy at three times per week. These patients will do better if the physical therapy is kept to twice per week.

As management progresses, the metabolic, biochemical, mineral, and hormonal perpetuating factors need to be rechecked at least every 6–12 weeks. This will ensure that the blood levels remain in the optimal part of the normal range. In most cases, the potassium needs to be rechecked every 10–14 days during the first 8–12 weeks of therapy. In many of the grade 3 and 4 patients, difficulty may be encountered in attempting to bring the serum potassium level to the optimal part of the normal range (Margoles, in press).

Some of the grade 1 patients will have to be on their vitamin and mineral supplements for the rest of their lives. All of the grade 2, 3, and 4 patients should be on permanent (ongoing) correction of all perpetuating factors for the rest of their lives.

The effectiveness of sleep normalization should be assessed every 2 weeks. Patients' needs for behavioral techniques and medications change frequently during the first 6 months of management in the grade 3 and 4 cases. As they improve, it takes less and less medication to effect an adequate sleep pattern. There is no one technique or medication that works for all MPS patients.

For most of the grade 4 cases, perpetuating factors that have yet to be discovered may help reclaim these most challenging cases.

At every stage of recovery, extensive teaching of patients must be carried out so they can learn self-management techniques. This will help them "stay out of trouble" in the future. They must be taught "early warning signs" to know when to return for help. Some of these include:

1. Return of pain
2. Disrupted sleep patterns
3. Can't find a comfortable sleeping position
4. Persistent aches
5. Unexplained weakness

PROGNOSIS

Once a myofascial, always a myofascial. Myofascial pain patients are not treated and cured, they are managed (Travell, personal communication). In some patients, after the initial incident in which the MPS became active, the tendency for recurrence of trigger-point-related problems remains for life. The second, third, and fourth episodes of MPS may occur in areas different from the original problem and differing from each other.

Many of my patients relate that a close relative, such as their mother, father, sibling, and in some cases their child or children, has problems that sound like MPS. To date, there has been no conclusive proof that the problem is genetically transmitted or that the tendency to generate an MPS predated any given accident. However, I believe the tendency to MPS is inherited. I also believe that some people are predisposed to it for an as yet unknown reason. Future studies (Texidor and Margoles, in press) will assess some of the genetic problems that are thought to be relevant to MPS.

Some patients will discontinue the treatment(s) used to correct their perpetuating factors. For most of the grade 1 and 2 patients, this may not have an adverse effect. However, this may be different for some of the grade 3 and 4 MPS patients. After a few months or years pass, they may trigger another flare-up of MPS pain and dysfunction that is worse than the original problem. With prompt treatment, these subsequent episodes can usually be managed quicker than the original problem.

Many of the grade 1 patients will respond to just the correction of the perpetuating factor problems. The higher the grade of severity (i.e., grade 3 or grade 4), the more complex and prolonged the management program becomes.

Overall prognosis for full recovery and return to normal lifestyle is as follows:

- **Grade 1**: Excellent — up to 100% of pre-MPS functioning
- **Grade 2**: Good — up to 75% recovery
- **Grade 3**: Fair — up to 50% recovery
- **Grade 4:** Poor — up to 25% recovery

The following are some relative timetables for response to appropriate therapy:

- **Grade 1**: Usually 2–4 weeks of treatment. One to four office visits.
- **Grade 2**: Up to 12 weeks of therapy. Visits are every 1–2 weeks.
- **Grade 3**: Six months to 3 years. Weekly visits for the first 6 weeks, every 2 weeks for the next 6 weeks, and every 2–4 weeks after that. Even after 3 years, patients may have to be seen every 1–6 months for an indefinite period of time.
- **Grade 4**: These patients will require all the therapy indicated for the grade 3 patient, and the management may need to go on indefinitely. After the first 6–12 weeks of therapy, patients need to be seen at 2-week to 3-month intervals. This group of patients is prone to mishaps, such as falling when a weak leg gives out. A minor auto accident can cause an acute flare-up that may last 6–12 weeks, requiring weekly or every other week visits for 6–12 weeks.

TREATMENT COSTS

The cost of management for grade 1 and 2 patients is usually no more than that incurred in the treatment of acute arthritis or an acute back or neck strain.

The cost of treating grade 3 patients is similar to that of treating an acute arthritis problem that goes on to chronicity. Medication costs would be less expensive for the MPS patient.

When grade 4 patients are analyzed for cost of therapy, two issues must be kept in mind:

1. This type of patient has historically been an MPS patient who was mistaken for a patient with a ruptured disc. At present, all costs associated with lumbar or cervical surgery run about $20,000. This cost is unfortunate. Had the patient been recognized as having a referred pain of an MPS instead of radicular pain of a ruptured disc, the savings are obvious. The surgery compounds the MPS problem by possibly adding scar tissue and other surgery-related problems.
2. The cost of chronic ongoing therapy in treated versus untreated patients:
    a. Without treatment, grade 3 and 4 patients may become increasingly disabled. The problem may remain static for years or until adequate therapy is instituted.
    b. The best hope for recovery and relief of disability is an active treatment program. In the long run, this is a less expensive way to treat grade 4 MPS patients.

CONCLUSION

MPS should be suspected in all cases of unexplained pain. It is relatively easy to diagnose once the clinician has proper training.

MPS is a complex problem, but it is a manageable condition. Proper procedures must be followed in the staging of therapy. In the treatment of MPS, resolution of the perpetuating factors is a critical step of prime importance to the rest of the recovery program.

MPS is broken up into gradations of severity in this chapter. The prognosis for complete recovery decreases as the grade of severity increases.

Suggestions are made for minor changes in the ICD-9-CM coding of MPS (Appendix 4) to enhance the overall ability to record and report MPS.

BARRIER trigger points are presented as one of the many unique features of MPS. The concept of BARRIER trigger points explains some of the more frustrating aspects of treating patients with MPS.

GLOSSARY OF TERMS

Dysfunction. Lack of proper function. Abnormal function. Weakness of a limb. Dropping things with the hand on the affected side. The leg gives out unpredictably on the affected side.

Jump sign. A general physical response to an unanticipatedly painful stimulus. Like a recoil, flinch, or startle. The patient may unexpectedly wince, cry out, withdraw, or "jump" in response to the painful stimulus. This is frequently a response that occurs to pressure applied to an active trigger point. It may also be noted when a taut band in a muscle is snapped either by pincer palpation or flat palpation (Travell and Simons, 1983). A general response that occurs so rapidly and spontaneously that the patient has no time to prepare for it.

Local twitch response. Transient contraction of the group of muscle fibers that contains a trigger point. The trigger point is usually in a taut band. Palpation must be specific. The muscle is palpated at right or oblique angles to the trigger point containing a taut band. The contraction of fibers is in response to stimulation (usually by snapping palpation or needling) of the same or sometimes of a nearby trigger point (Travell and Simons, 1983). The contraction may occur locally at the site of the trigger point, such as occurs in the infraspinatus muscle. It may occur up to 1 foot away from the trigger point, but within the fibers of the muscle, such as occurs when the iliocostalis thoracis is strummed by flat palpation at T9 and causes a "twitch" in the iliocostalis lumborum at L2, L3, L4, or L5.

Myofascial trigger point — active. A focus of hyperirritability in a muscle or its fascia that is symptomatic with respect to pain; it refers to a pattern of pain at rest and/or on motion specific for the muscle. An active trigger point is always tender, prevents full lengthening of the muscle, weakens the muscle, usually refers pain on direct compression, mediates a local twitch response of muscle fibers when adequately stimulated, and often produces specific referred autonomic phenomenon, generally in its pain reference zone. To be distinguished from a latent myofascial trigger point (Travell and Simons, 1983).

Myofascial trigger point — latent. A focus of hyperirritability in a muscle or its fascia that is clinically quiescent with respect to spontaneous pain; it is painful only when palpated. A latent trigger point may have all the other clinical characteristics of an active trigger point from which it is to be distinguished (Travell and Simons, 1983).

Paresthesias. Abnormal sensations in the affected area such as tingling, numbness, sense of ants crawling on or in the area of problem. Is broadly defined as an abnormal sensation, but will in the present context be restricted to mean an altered quality of sensation other than allodynia and dysesthesia. It is usually difficult to describe paresthetic sensations, because specific words are lacking, and the patient uses metaphorical expressions like "crawling," "running water," "tingling," "tightness," etc. or, simply stated, "different from normal" (Lindblom, 1985). Refers to crawling, burning, or "pins and needles" feelings that arise spontaneously (Dorland's, 1985).

Proprioception. Sense of position. Spatial orientation. Perception mediated by proprioceptors or proprioceptive tissues (Dorland's, 1985). Receiving stimuli within the tissues of the body, as within muscles and tendons (Dorland's, 1985). Sensory nerve terminals which give information concerning movements and positions of the body; they occur chiefly in the muscles, tendons, and the labyrinth (Dorland's, 1985).

Taut bands (palpable band or nodule). The group of taut muscle fibers that is associated with a myofascial trigger point and is identifiable by tactile examination of the muscle. Contraction of the fibers in this band produces the local twitch response (Travell and Simons). This is an objective finding. The patient has no control over the presence or absence of the taut band. These are present up to the point of onset of rigor mortis.

"Trick." Substituting or using unaffected muscles and/or joints for (instead of) movements rather than the ones that are painful or restricted by the presence of an active or latent trigger point.

APPENDIX 1: SUPPLIERS OF INJECTABLES

Suppliers of B-Complex Injection Products

Because of FDA intervention, products listed below are not always available from the listed distributor. You may have to contact a number of distributors listed in order to obtain the indicated product.

Product	Brand Name	Distributor
Riboflavin (B2)	Various @ 50 mg/ml	(4) (6)
Dexpanthenol (B5)	D-PAN 250 mg/ml	(1)
	Dexpanthenol	(2) (5)
Folate (Bc)	Folvite 5 mg/ml	(3)
Folic acid, 10 mg/ml		(1)
Hydroxycobalamin		(4) (6)
B-Complex Products		
B-Plex 100 (30 cc)		(1) (2) (5)
Thiamin (B1)	100 mg	
Riboflavin (B2)	2 mg	
Pyridoxine (B6)	2 mg	
Panthenol (B5)	2 mg	
Niacinamide (B3)	100 mg	
27-gauge 1- or 1½-inch needles		(5)
30-gauge 1- or ½-inch needles		(5)

(1) Merit Pharmaceuticals
      2611 San Fernando Road, Los Angeles, CA 90065
      Phone 213-227-4831

(2) Henry Schein, Inc.
      5 Harbor Park Drive, Port Washington, NY 11050
      Phone 800-772-4346

(3) Obtain through local drugstore

(4) Central Avenue Pharmacy
      133 Fifteenth Street, Pacific Grove, CA 93950
      Phone 800-501-9715

(5)   Family Pharmacy
       2053 Lincoln Ave., San Jose, CA 95125
       Phone 800-939-DRUG

(6)   Santa Clara Drug
       2453 Forest Ave., San Jose, CA 95128
       Phone 408-296-5015

APPENDIX 2: TERMINOLOGY/ABBREVIATIONS

Manual muscle testing (MMT):

1. Muscle testing that is done manually by the evaluating therapist
2. Does not refer to Cybex, etc. testing

Range of motion:

1. Can be done visually with an estimate
2. Can be done with a goniometer or flexometer
3. Can be done with electronic goniometer

Breakaway weakness (BAW) (Baker, 1986):

1. Refers to sudden giving way of the part being manually tested
   a. Usually points up the presence of a trigger point in the muscle being tested

APPENDIX 3: CLINICAL CLASSIFICATION OF SEVERITY

MPS includes persons in whom pain is soft tissue in nature. MPS refers specifically to trigger point problems relating to muscles, and not other types of soft tissues such as ligaments, tendons, and skin. The following is a classification of MPS based on (1) extent of geographic involvement, (2) severity of pain and altered sensation, (3) presence of perpetuating factors, and (4) extent of physical impairment.

Format followed for each grade of MPS:

1. Extent of or geographic involvement
2. Presence of perpetuating factors
3. Severity of pain and altered sensations

Pain severity is graded as follows:

P1:   Physical impairment: Minimal
         Intensity: Mild
         Patient appears uncomfortable: No
         Pain affects psyche: No
         Frequency of pain: Intermittent
         Patient is aware of pain during activity: No
         Pain is aggravated by activity: Minimal
         Need to change position for comfort: No
         Pain is present while resting: No

Pain interferes with sleep: No
Other: Pain is forgotten during activity

P2: Physical impairment: Minimal
Intensity: Mild
Patient appears uncomfortable: Occasionally
Pain affects psyche: Mild
Frequency of pain: Intermittent
Patient is aware of pain during activity: Mild
Pain is aggravated by activity: Occasionally
Need to change position for comfort: No
Pain is present while resting: None
Pain interferes with sleep: No
Other: Mild interference with activity

P3: Physical impairment: May prevent some activities
Intensity: Moderate
Patient appears uncomfortable: Occasionally
Pain affects psyche: Mild
Frequency of pain: Intermittent and frequent
Patient is aware of pain during activity: Yes
Pain is aggravated by activity: Yes
Need to change position for comfort: Yes, occasionally
Pain is present while resting: Mild
Pain interferes with sleep: No
Other:

P4: Physical impairment: Prevents patient from doing many activities
Intensity: Moderate to severe
Patient appears uncomfortable: Frequently
Pain affects psyche: Moderate
Frequency of pain: Constant and varies little with activity
Patient is aware of pain during activity: Yes
Pain is aggravated by activity: Yes
Need to change position for comfort: Frequently
Pain is present while resting: Bothersome
Pain interferes with sleep: Frequently; can find no comfortable sleeping position
Other: Marked handicap; pain may cause outcries

P5: Physical impairment: May prevent almost all activities
Intensity: Severe
Patient appears uncomfortable: Frequently to constantly
Pain affects psyche: Severe
Frequency of pain: Constant
Patient is aware of pain during activity: Yes
Pain is aggravated by activity: Constantly
Need to change position for comfort: Frequently
Pain is present while resting: Constantly

Pain interferes with sleep: Constantly
Other:

4. Degree of physical impairment. This consists of evaluation of physical functioning in the following categories:
    1. Routine job-related activities
    2. Work around the home
    3. Socialization activities
    4. Getting up or down out of a chair
    5. Sports activities
    6. Hobbies
    7. Sexual activity
    8. Sleep function
    9. Hygiene (shower, grooming, shampooing, toilet, etc.)
    10. Eating and feeding functions
    11. Chewing (food, etc.)
    12. Dressing and undressing
    13. Driving a vehicle
    14. Overall strength and endurance
5. Other pertinent comments

Figures 10.7 to 10.9 were derived from an analysis of my first 333 patients with these characteristic MPS findings. What is depicted is a composite of what I assembled in the stereotypical case of each type of patient, mild, moderate, and, severe. In contrast, Figure 10.10 is derived from an analysis of one patient who had all the findings that are characteristically seen at each grade of severity.

Grade 1: Mild (see Figure 10.7)

1. A single muscle (see Appendix 7 for trigger point locations). Unilateral.
2. None.
3. Frequently P1 and on occasion may go to P4.
4. General impairment is mild. May preclude heavy lifting.
5. Altered sensations are low intensity. Once treated, there is usually no recurrence of symptoms.

Example. A 32-year-old female patient presents with pain in the shoulder and arm. She is found to have an infraspinatus trigger point of the shoulder. It causes a slight decrease of range of motion with accompanying pain when she brushes her hair to a point past her ear on the ipsilateral side. The problem is easily relieved with a trigger point injection plus stretch and spray.

Grade 2: Moderate (see Figure 10.8)

1. Bilateral involvement of the same muscle (e.g., deltoid on both sides, gluteus maximus on both sides, etc.).
2. A few are active; for example, a short leg or arm, and a less than optimal serum potassium level.
3. Frequently P2 and on occasion may go to P4.

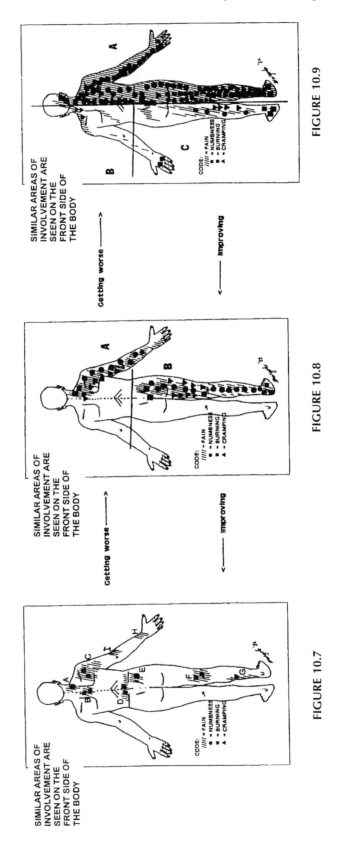

FIGURE 10.9

FIGURE 10.8

FIGURE 10.7

FIGURE 10.7 Grade 1 (mild) MPS. If seen on the rear surface of the body, it might be diagnosed as A = cervical strain or cervical arthritis; B = thoracic strain; C = shoulder strain, bursitis, or rotator cuff syndrome; D = lumbar strain/sprain, lumbar disc disease, lumbar facet syndrome, or arthritis of low back; E = low back pain or sacroilitis; F = pain in the back of the knee or arthritis of the knee; G = arthritis of the ankle, neuritis or neuropathy, or Achilles tendinitis; H = arthritis of the wrist, carpal tunnel syndrome; Dequervain's disease of the wrist, or strain/sprain of the wrist; I = lateral epicondylitis. If seen on the front surface of the body, it might be diagnosed as B = costochondritis; C = shoulder strain, bursitis, or rotator cuff syndrome; D = pelvic pain of unknown origin; E = groin pain, hernia pain, or interstitial cystitis; F = arthritis of the knee, chondromalacia of the patella, or internal derangement of the knee; G = shin splints; H = arthritis of the wrist, carpal tunnel syndrome; Dequervain's disease of the wrist, or strain/sprain of the wrist; I = tennis elbow.

FIGURE 10.8 Grade 2 (moderate) MPS. Nonanatomical recruitment (progression of pain areas occurs as the severity of the disease progresses. If seen on the read surface of the body, it might be diagnosed as A = cervical disc disease or a pinched nerve; B = lumbar disc disease, a pinched nerve, or sciatica. If seen on the front surface of the body, it might be diagnosed as A = cervical disc disease or a pinched nerve; B = lumbar disc disease, a pinched nerve, sciatica, or femoral neuropathy. Areas of symptoms may be present as A, B or A + B. Presentation may also occur with the A-type pattern, running down both arms and neither leg, or the B-type pattern, running down both legs and neither arm. An isolated A or B symptom pattern is most likely to be confused with a ruptured cervical, lumbar, or cervical and lumbar disc. In an occasional case there is an A-type pattern in the upper extremity on one side and a B-type pattern in the lower extremity on the contralateral side.

FIGURE 10.9 Grade 3 and 4 (severe and severe + complex) MPS. With further progression there is a spread of the symptoms in the upper and lower parts of the body, as seen here between the shoulder and buttock on the right side. There may be the appearance of a "spillover" of the pain, paresthesias, and dysesthesias (altered sensations) onto the side opposite the original pain problem, as seen in the left shoulder and left leg. Areas of involvement may be present as A, A + B, A + C, or A + B + C. There may be an A-type pattern on both sides, and this will also involve the anterior aspects of all four limbs, including the anterior shoulders and hips and usually sparing the abdomen. In general, physicians caring for such patients generally do not know what to make of all the broad areas of symptomatology. Therefore, one area, such as the back or neck, with its accompanying pain referred down the arm or leg, is focused on to the exclusion of the other areas of involvement. In these latter instances the referred pain of MPS is mistaken for radicular pain of a ruptured cervical or lumbar disc.

4. As much as 50% for physical work. Precludes heavy lifting, repeated bending, and stooping. Occasional absence from work (1–2 days of missed work per 6-week period).
5. One of the trigger points usually produces more of the total symptom picture than the mirror image partner. Both must be treated to obtain a successful outcome. A moderate amount of problems with altered sensations.

Example. A 27-year-old male patient presents with dizziness and headache after a rear-end automobile accident. He has a "whiplash" injury of the neck. The headaches and dizziness occasionally prevent him from driving to work. Examination reveals symptom-producing trigger points in the sternocleidomastoid muscles on both sides. He has a short hemipelvis on the left. The problem is corrected with a 1-cm butt lift under the left buttock and trigger point injections to both of his sternocleidomastoid muscles, followed by stretch and spray. There is no recurrence of symptoms.

Grade 3: Severe (see Figure 10.9)

1. Multiple-muscle MPS in numerous areas of the body. Some are active unilaterally, and some are active bilaterally (see Appendix 7).
2. Many perpetuating factors are detectable, both from the physical examination and comprehensive blood testing.
3. Severity may vary with different regions of the body. Some may be P1, some P2, some P3, and some P4. P3 and P4 are most frequent.
4. Impairment of activities of daily living is severe, resulting in limited employment (either unemployment because of the pain problem or limited to very light type of work) and hardship. Depending on the overall clinical picture, some of these patients will be limited to light work, whereas others may only be able to do sedentary work.
5. In the instances of bilateral activation of trigger points, one of the pair usually produces more of the total symptom picture than the mirror-image partner. Both must be treated to obtain a successful outcome. There is a moderate amount of altered sensation and dysfunction related to the trigger points. The numerous perpetuating factors complicate the recovery.

A grade 3 patient may present with a moderate to severe, intermittent, myofascial low back pain. It may appear that only one muscle, such as the longissimus thoracis or one of the glutei is responsible for the problem. However, in reality, in grade 3 patients, any of a number of the following muscles may be contributing to the problem (the contribution of symptoms usually comes from paired muscles, such as right and left longissimus thoracis, right and left iliocostalis lumborum, and right and left quadratus lumborum, to mention only a few):

Coccygeus
Gluteus maximus
Gluteus medius
Gluteus minimus
Iliocostalis lumborum
Iliocostalis thoracis
Iliopsoas
Levator ani

Longissimus thoracis
Lower latissimus dorsi
Multifidus
Obturator internus
Piriformis
Quadratus lumborum
Rectus adominis
Rotatores brevis
Rotatores longus
Serratus post. inferior
Soleus
Sphincter ani
Vastus lateralis

The grade 3 complex may produce a significant physically disabling clinical picture. Mild to moderate reflex sympathetic dystrophy may occur in any of the painful extremities. Intense referred extremity pain may be mistaken for the radicular pain of a ruptured disc.

Example. A 45-year-old woman is struck on the driver side of her car while going through an intersection. Impact is greatest at the driver's door. The door is caved in, breaking her left pelvis. Her seat belt is torn away, and she is thrown about in the front of the car. She sustains muscle trigger points in the right trapezius, sternocleidomastoid muscle, scalenus anterior muscle, muscles acting upon the jaw, both infraspinatus, both quadratus lumborum, right gluteus medius, right pyriformis, and right gluteus minimus muscles. She has constant headaches on the right and radicular pain down the right arm and leg. She has not been able to work for 2 months since the injury. She also has postconcussion syndrome and posttraumatic stress disorder. She spends 6 weeks in a pelvic sling in the hospital to heal the pelvic fracture, which also disrupted her pubic symphysis. Once ambulatory, all the above pains are still problematic. Examination reveals 1 inch of shortening of the left leg. This is corrected with a shoe lift of 1 inch. Her pelvis is now short on the left side, and this is corrected with a butt lift. Blood testing reveals less than optimal levels of serum blood count, potassium, ionized calcium, iron, magnesium, thiamin, pyridoxine, pantothenate, folic acid, and cobalamin. The biochemical problems are corrected with oral supplements and a few weeks of twice weekly balanced B-complex injections. She is put through a program of stretch and spray, trigger point injections, Lewitt stretch, and limbering and strengthening exercises. By 6 months postinjury, she has 50% recovery of physical function and 50% relief of pain. At that point, she can return to her routine secretarial work, but finds that she cannot work any overtime and misses up to 2 days of work per week because of pain and fatigue problems. She is able to do only 50% of her usual housework.

Grade 4: Severe and Complex

All of grades 1 to 3 are seen in this group. Restricted range of motion of a joint gives clues to the location of trigger points. For example, decreased active abduction of the shoulder may be due to an infraspinatus trigger point or any of the five other muscles that can cause a similar problem about the shoulder. However, because the referred pain of MPS has been mistaken for radicular pain of a ruptured disc or a surgically treatable mechanical back problem, these patients will have had one or more surgical attempts to remedy the problem. In my practice, I have seen such patients who have had as many as 20 surgical attempts to remedy the pain and dysfunction. One patient had five cervical disc removals and fusions, five lumbar disc removals and fusions, and five surgeries on each of his shoulders to attempt to remedy his myofascial pain and dysfunction problems.

1. Same as for grade 3.
2. Numerous and extensive.
3. Moderate to severe in most areas. Constant in most areas. Varies between P4 and P5.
4. Totally disabled for all work.
5. The multiple surgeries add another dimension to the overall problem — sizable amounts of scar tissue. This often makes it impossible to obtain meaningful remedies to the problem. Moderate to severe reflex sympathetic dystrophy may occur

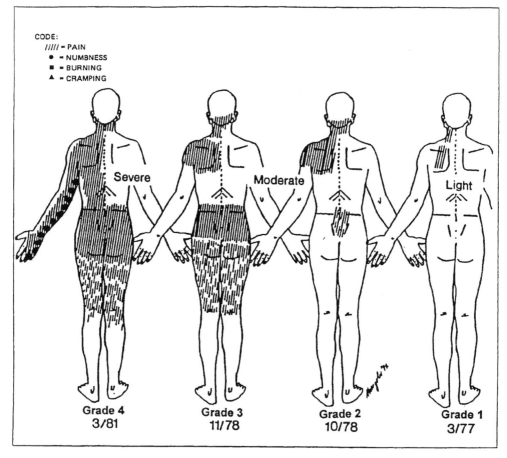

FIGURE 10.10   MPS grades 1 to 3. This is a 23-year-old woman who had cumulative trauma to her left shoulder in March 1977. Her pain progressed following reinjury (an automobile accident in August 1978). Her symptoms progressively worsened. Following a myelogram in March 1980, an L4–5 disc was removed laterally. Three months postoperatively all the patient's pain returned and became progressively more severe, involving additional body areas. Although the patient is different, the spread of pain and resistance to surgical intervention are similar between the two cases.

in any of the painful extremities and may significantly compound the problem of management. These patients are totally disabled.

Example. For our example here, we pick up on the 45-year-old woman from the example given in the section on grade 3. Twelve months posttrauma, becoming weary of the unrelenting pain radiating down her right leg, she searches out a reputable neurosurgeon for a second opinion. A CT and a myelogram show a "bulging disc" at L4–5 and L5–S1. She is desperate and pleads with the surgeon, "Do something — the pain is driving me crazy!" Surgery is performed. Pain is significantly relieved for 3 months. Then the pain returns "with a vengeance." She asks for further surgical options, and a fusion is performed. This time there is no relief of the pain at all. She is left an invalid who cannot work at any gainful employment.

APPENDIX 4: ICD-9-CM CODING OF MPS

I propose that the following be adopted for coding MPS:

Under 729.1 "Myalgia and myositis, unspecified"
    729.10 = is specific for MPS

The following fifth-digit subclassification is used to designate site of involvement:

0 = Head and neck
1 = Shoulder region
2 = Upper arm
    a. Elbow to humerus
3 = Forearm
    a. Radius to the wrist
4 = Hand including fingers
5 = Pelvic region and thigh
    a. Low back, buttock, hip, femur
6 = Lower leg
    a. Knee joint to just above the ankle
7 = Ankle and foot
    a. From the ankle to the toes
8 = Other specified site
    a. Ribs, trunk, vertebral column, upper back, mid-back
9 = Multiple sites

The following sixth-digit subclassification is used to designate grade of severity:

1 = Mild
2 = Moderate
3 = Severe
4 = Severe and complex

The following seventh-digit subclassification is used to designate whether the MPS is occurring on only one side or both (MPS that is bilateral represents a more complicated and difficult to treat condition):

1 = Unilateral
2 = Bilateral

Therefore, if a patient is coded as 729.1532, it means that the patient has a severe bilateral MPS of the low back.

APPENDIX 5: ORAL REPLACEMENT PROGRAM

It must be kept in mind that the use of vitamin and mineral therapy acts as a complement to a well-planned management program.

The management suggestions made here are based upon answers obtained in a study within my practice (Margoles, in press), clinical experience with 1500 patients, and recent medical literature on the subject (Jeppsson and Gimmon, 1983; Margoles, 1983, in press; Travell and Simons, 1983; Travell, 1976; Farmer, 1985).

Individual variability may exist from patient to patient with respect to absorption of orally administered vitamins and minerals.

The body does not recognize any differences among vitamins that are "organic," "natural," or "synthetic" in origin. They all work equally well.

The various vitamins and minerals are all interdependent. To attack the deficiencies and insufficiencies one by one, in a consecutive series of time frames, would be impractical, expensive, and time consuming.

A trial of vitamin and mineral supplements is initiated for 6–12 weeks. It usually takes that long to decide whether the therapy will have a positive effect on the patient's MPS.

I recommend vitamins and minerals from Bronson Pharmaceuticals for oral use because the products are

1. Pharmaceutical grade
2. Hypoallergenic
3. Well formulated by recognized authorities and biochemists
4. No unusual ingredients used
5. Inexpensive
6. Available throughout the world by mail or telephone order from the following location: Bronson, 1945 Craig Road, P.O. 46903, St. Louis, MO 63146-6903. If ordering from countries outside the United States, put "Attention Ellen" on your correspondence. The toll-free telephone number is 1-800-235-3200. When answered, place your order. Specify your name, address, and country. You will be given additional instructions by the person at Bronson.

Product Recommendations (Bronson)

The oral vitamin products recommended below are a basic program that replenishes most of the vitamin problems encountered in this patient population. Vitamin A is left out because it can provoke pain in those who run a high normal to high blood level of this vitamin. If blood testing shows the vitamin A level is low or low normal, it can be added as part of the supplement program. The program below is for starting and maintenance of vitamin replenishment.

The following must be kept in mind. If a patient is started on this program and has a good clinical response (less MPS pain, better energy, less irritability of the myofascial trigger points, to mention only a few), this program and others (replacement of potassium, thyroid, etc.) should be adhered to for life.

ORAL VITAMIN DIRECTIONS SHEET

Name _____

Date _____

Bronson product	#[b]	Number items to take per day[a]				
		Week 1	Week 2	Week 3	Week 4	Thereafter
B complex with C and E	4	1	2	3	4	4
Mineral insurance formula	12	1	2	3	3	3
Folic acid, 800-μg tablets	97	1	1	2	2	2
Vitamin C, time release, 1000 mg	78	1	2	2	2	2

[a] When more than one per day is indicated, it is best to split the dose and take one dose in the morning and one dose at night. If three are indicated, take them with breakfast, lunch, and dinner, If four or more are indicated, break up the dosing any way you like.

[b] This is the unique number assigned to each Bronson product. For instance, #4 is assigned to nontime-release B complex with C and E. If you call Bronson and say you want 250 bottles of product #4, they know it is a nontime-release B complex with C and E.

B Complex with C and E (Nontime Release)

Note: Nerve regeneration may occur with the recommended dosing of the B-complex vitamins.

If you do not want to work with the Bronson product, obtain a B complex with C, but without zinc or iron, that has the following formulation or close to it:

Per tablet:

B1 (thiamin mononitrate)	15 mg
B2 (riboflavin)	10 mg
B6 (pyridoxine hydrochloride)	10 mg
B12 (cobalamin concentrate)	5 mg

Niacin amide	100 mg
D-Calcium pantothenate	20 mg
Folic acid	0.4 mg (400 mg)
Biotin	200 mg
C (ascorbic acid)	500 mg
E (alpha-tocopherol)	30 IU

Mineral Insurance Formula

Per three tablets:

Calcium	250 mg
Phosphorus	250 mg
Magnesium	200 mg
Iron	15 mg
Zinc	15 mg
Copper	2 mg
Iodine	150 mg
Manganese	5 mg
Molybdenum	100 mg
Chromium	200 mg
Selenium	20 mg

Although it is generally recommended to take vitamins with meals or food, some people can take them on an empty stomach without problems.

APPENDIX 6: MANAGEMENT OF POTASSIUM PROBLEMS

Potassium is replenished based on the serum potassium level. This is demonstrated in Figure 11.11.

Potassium is replaced at a dosing of 10 meq for each quartile away from the optimal part of the range. Therefore, if the patient has a blood test level of 3.8, 30 meq of potassium is the initial dose, given in divided dosing throughout the day. When the serum potassium is repeated 7–10 days later, the same formula is used to bring the blood test level to the optimal part of the normal range. If the patient retests at 4.5 meq/liter, 10 more meq of potassium is given per day, for a total of 40 meq of supplemental potassium per day. Time-release products are preferred, but KCL-Elixir or K-Lyte type products do equally well. Some of the more complex cases may eventually need as much as 50–100 meq/day.

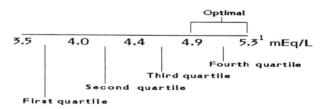

FIGURE 10.11   Blood testing for serum potassium level. [1]Values for serum potassium may vary from lab to lab.

APPENDIX 7: CLASSIC TRIGGER POINT LOCATIONS (SIMONS, 1984)

Figures 10.12 to 10.18 are from Basmajian, J.V. and Kirby, L. (1984). *Medical Rehabilitation,* Williams and Wilkins Company, Baltimore. Reproduced with permission.

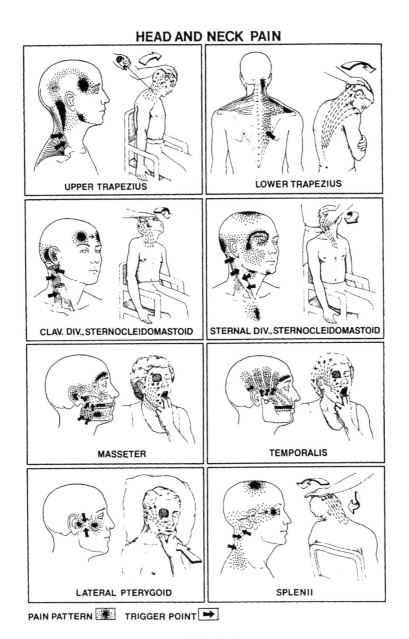

HEAD AND NECK PAIN

UPPER TRAPEZIUS

LOWER TRAPEZIUS

CLAV. DIV., STERNOCLEIDOMASTOID

STERNAL DIV., STERNOCLEIDOMASTOID

MASSETER

TEMPORALIS

LATERAL PTERYGOID

SPLENII

PAIN PATTERN   TRIGGER POINT

FIGURE 10.12

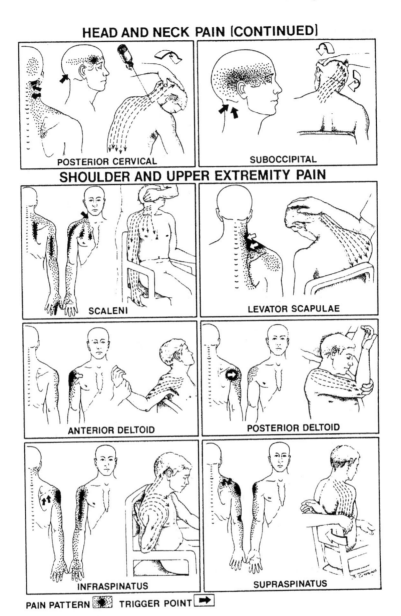

HEAD AND NECK PAIN (CONTINUED)

POSTERIOR CERVICAL

SUBOCCIPITAL

SHOULDER AND UPPER EXTREMITY PAIN

SCALENI

LEVATOR SCAPULAE

ANTERIOR DELTOID

POSTERIOR DELTOID

INFRASPINATUS

SUPRASPINATUS

PAIN PATTERN ▓ TRIGGER POINT ➡

FIGURE 10.13

SHOULDER AND UPPER EXTREMITY PAIN (CONTINUED)

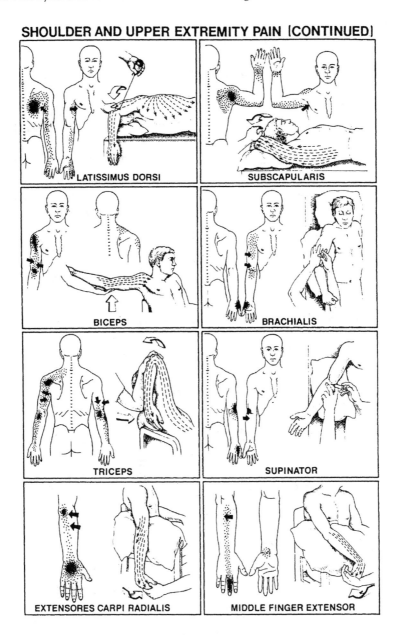

FIGURE 10.14

SHOULDER AND UPPER EXTREMITY PAIN [CONT.]

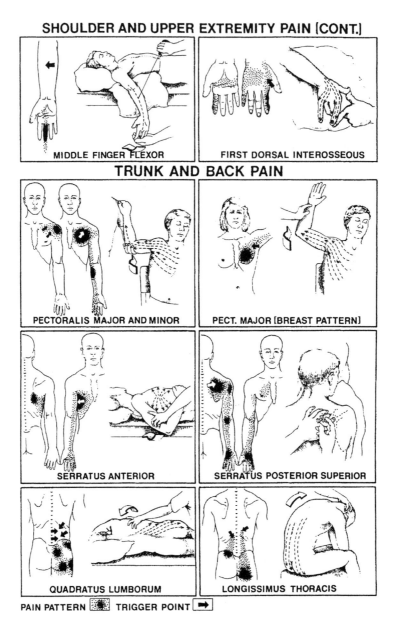

MIDDLE FINGER FLEXOR

FIRST DORSAL INTEROSSEOUS

TRUNK AND BACK PAIN

PECTORALIS MAJOR AND MINOR

PECT. MAJOR [BREAST PATTERN]

SERRATUS ANTERIOR

SERRATUS POSTERIOR SUPERIOR

QUADRATUS LUMBORUM

LONGISSIMUS THORACIS

PAIN PATTERN   TRIGGER POINT

FIGURE 10.15

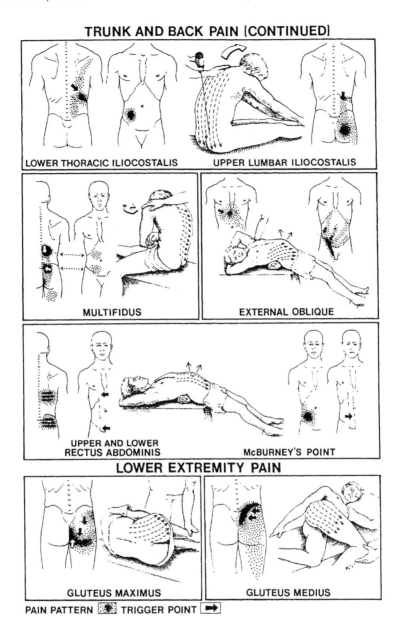

FIGURE 10.16

LOWER EXTREMITY PAIN (CONTINUED)

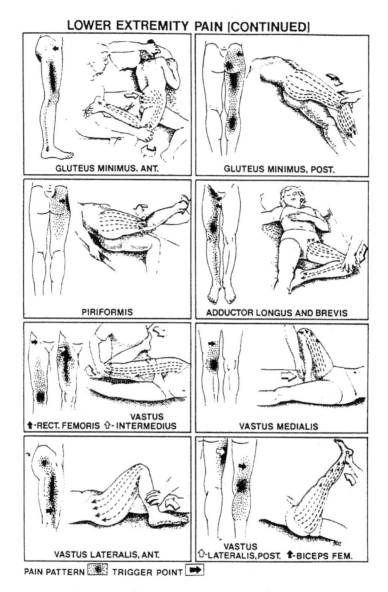

FIGURE 10.17

APPENDIX 8: MUSCLES THAT MAY BE AFFECTED BY TRIGGER POINTS

Abdominis obliqui
Abdominis transversus
Adductor pollicis
Anconeus
Biceps brachii
Brachialis
Coracobrachialis
Deltoid
Digastric, posterior
Extensor carpi radialis

Extensor carpi ulnaris
Extensor digitorum
Extensor indicts
Flexor carpi ulnaris
Flexor digitorum
Flexor policis longus
Frontalis
Gastrocnemeus
Gluteus maximus

Gluteus medius
Gluteus minimus
Hamstring
Iliacus
Iliocostalis lumborum
Iliocostalis thoracis
Iliopsoas
Infraspinatus
Interosseus of the hand

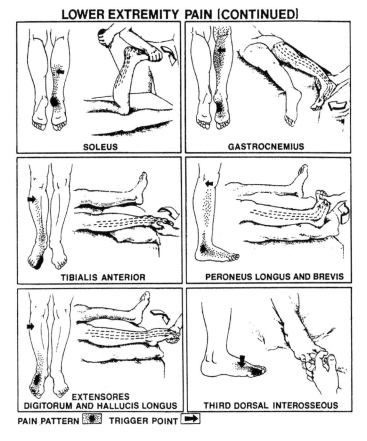

FIGURE 10.18

Lateral pterygoid	Piriformis	Sphincter ani
Levator ani	Platysma	Splenius capitus
Levator scapulae	Pronator teres	Splenius cervicis
Longissimus thoracis	Psoas	Sternalis
Lower latissimus dorsi	Pyramidalis	Sternocleidomastoid
Masseter	Quadratus lumborum	Subclavius
Medial pterygoid	Rectus abdominis	Subscapularis
Multifidus	Rectus capitus post maj.	Supinator
Obliqi inferior	Rectus capitus post min.	Supraspinatus
Obliqi superior	Rotatores longus	Temporalis
Obterator internus	Scalenus anterior	Teres major
Occipitalis	Scalenus medius	Teres minor
Omohyoid	Scalenus minimus	Tibialis anterior
Opponens pollicis	Scalenus posterior	Trapezius
Orbicularis oculi	Semispinalis capitis	Triceps brachii
Palmaris longis	Semispinalis cervicis	Upper latissimus dorsi
Paraspinal muscles	Serratus posterior inferior	Vastus lateralis
Pectoralis major	Serratus posterior superior	Vastus medialis
Pectoralis minor	Soleus	Zygomaticus major
Peroneus longus		

APPENDIX 9: PRESSURE THRESHOLD METER LOG SHEET

PRESSURE THRESHOLD TESTING

x = average
y = minimum

m = male
f = female

R = right
L = left

Kilograms/cm^2

Sternocleido. R L

Scaleneus Ant. R L

Biceps R L

Triceps R L

Deltoid R L

Upper trap. R L

Levator scapu. R L

Supraspinat. R L

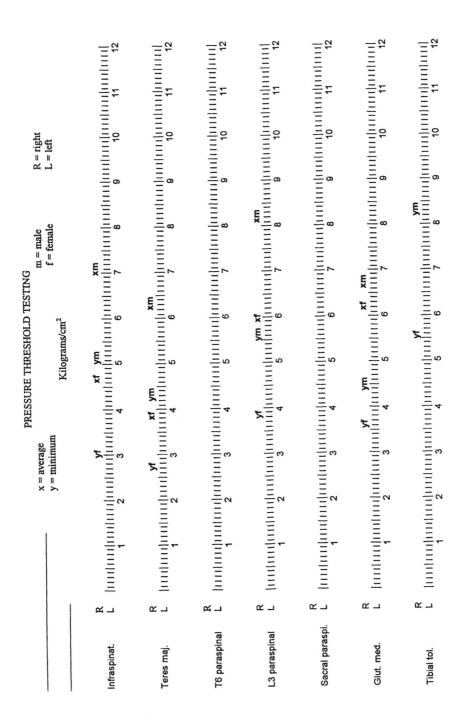

APPENDIX 10: BARRIER TRIGGER POINTS

To highlight one of many problems that are unique to MPS, I have employed the term BARRIER trigger point. BARRIER trigger points produce trigger point barriers. A BARRIER trigger point is any trigger point, active or latent, that prevents an MPS patient from obtaining desired physical activity goals. They appear as a silent encumbrance. They are perceived by the patient as a wall, snag, or impasse. It is a message that the patient gets in the back of his or her mind — if a patient pushes his or her physical activity level too far, he or she may suffer and pay dearly, possibly for a long time. At times, BARRIER trigger points have the appearance of a boundary that must not be crossed. It is part of the stress and frustration that exasperate many MPS patients.

Along the way from step to step and stage to stage of recovery, BARRIER trigger points may be encountered. As soon as one myofascial trigger point is gotten rid of, it paves the way for more action, motion, and activity. However, other trigger points may be activated as the MPS patient tries out his or her new freedom.

When asked how they are doing, established patients will frequently say they are doing fine. New patients, when asked if their pain problem is getting better, worse, or staying the same, may say that the pain problem is presently unchanged. What they are frequently saying is that as long as they do not try to traverse their BARRIER trigger points, they have no problems.

Patients give the appearance of being back to "business as usual." However, if you ask a few more questions, often you will find out that they are holding back for fear of bringing on an attack of pain and disability by triggering a BARRIER trigger point.

For example, before the onset of her MPS, one woman who likes to bowl could bowl five games before getting tired or feeling a bit achy Now she says that if she bowls more than one game, she will experience a pain flare-up for 3 weeks. That is something she cannot risk because of her job and family responsibilities. This woman may have a problem with trigger point BARRIERS. One company executive no longer flies in a plane for more than an hour because of the fear of triggering a disabling low back pain problem.

Not all BARRIER trigger points will become painful when activated. Some may only appear to the patient as mild stiffness or a short-lived ache as the patient steps up his or her activity level and breaks through a barrier.

A case example will be used to illustrate the concept of BARRIER trigger points. The case assumes that all perpetuating factors have been brought under control in order to keep the focus on the BARRIER problem.

Case Example

Before management, 32-year-old Mary Smith had a painful and totally frozen right shoulder for 6 months because of subscapularis trigger points. This problem resulted from a fall at work. It represented the first, or major, BARRIER to her recovery from MPS. She also had pain in the right side of her neck and interscapular area from T3 to T7. She was graded at a 3.

Pain prohibited her from work, housework, bowling, and skiing. Management resolved the problem. She was then left with an atrophied right shoulder. In reality, however, many muscles throughout the body had atrophied because of her overall inactivity.

A combination of trigger point injections, stretch and spray, and physical therapy got her on her way. At that time, she could actively abduct the shoulder to 135 degrees and the neck problem was clearing.

One day, she reached up to the third shelf of her cupboard (150 of forward flexion and 160 of abduction) to pick up a 5-pound bag of flour. Over the next 3 days, progressive and severe pain began to radiate down her right arm. This activated the second BARRIER.

Evaluation revealed that she had activated a latent trigger point in the infraspinatus muscle. This trigger point and the others that will be mentioned were all generated by her accident. The infraspinatus trigger point was relieved with appropriate therapy, and she was able to do her housework.

Feeling encouraged, she booked a night of bowing with some of her friends. By the time she finished her second game, she noticed a pulling sensation in her posterior right flank and some mild discomfort just above the waistline on the right side. The bowling, a routine activity for her, had activated the third BARRIER to her recovery. Upon retiring that evening, she took two aspirins and applied moist heat. At 5:00 the next morning, she was awakened by sharp pains and muscle spasms in the same area. She had difficulty walking because of the pain. She saw her myofascial therapist, who diagnosed trigger points in the right quadratus lumborum. This was quickly remedied by trigger point injections, followed by stretch and spray to the affected muscle.

She was then feeling fine. She could do all of her activities of daily living and was getting along fine.

Then the ski season came around. She booked a weekend with a few friends. She was an intermediate skier, but stuck to the beginner runs the first day. After doing a number of easy runs, with a lot of right turns, she noticed the onset of cramping in the lateral right hip and radiation of pain down the outside of her right leg from the hip to the ankle. She began to limp and needed to rest often. The pain and cramping were distressing and discouraging. The skiing, a routine activity for her, had activated the fourth BARRIER to her total recovery. Her friends took her to the nearest town, where they found a physician familiar with MPS. He diagnosed a gluteus minimus trigger point. He used trigger point injections, stretch and spray, moist heat for 10 minutes, and sent her on her way.

Since that last BARRIER was removed, her recovery has been complete. She has returned to a fully active lifestyle without any residual pain or restrictions.

REFERENCES

Baker, B. (1986). The muscle trigger: evidence of overload injury, *Journal of Neurological and Orthopedic Medicine and Surgery,* 7, 31–43.

Barnes, B. (1976). *Hypothyroidism: The Unsuspected Illness,* Thomas Crowell Company, New York.

Dorland's Illustrated Medical Dictionary (1985). 26th ed., W.B. Saunders, Philadelphia.

Farmer, T. (1985). Neurological complications of vitamin and mineral disorders, in *Clinical Neurology,* Vol. 4, Baker, A. and Joynt, R. (Eds.), Harper and Row, Philadelphia, pp. 1–8.

Fields, H. (1987). *Pain,* McGraw-Hill, New York, pp. 209–229.

Foley, K. and Portenoy, R. (1986). Chronic use of opioid analgesics in non-malignant pain: report of 38 cases, *Pain,* 25, 171–186.

Gilman, A., Goodman, L., and Gilman, A. (Eds.) (1980). *Goodman and Gilman's the Pharmacological Basis of Therapeutics,* 6th ed., Macmillan, New York, pp. 494–583.

Houde, R. (1974). The use and misuse of narcotics in the treatment of chronic pain, in *Advances in Neurology: An International Symposium on Pain,* Bonica, J. (Ed.), Raven Press, New York, pp. 527–538.

Jaffe, J. and Martin, W. (1985). in *Goodman and Gilman's the Pharmacological Basis of Therapeutics,* Goodman, L. and Gilman, A., (Eds.), 7th ed., Macmillan, New York, p. 516.

Jeppsson, B. and Gimmon, Z. (1983). Vitamins, in *Surgical Nutrition,* Fischer, J. (Ed.), Little, Brown, Boston, pp. 241–282.

Lindblom, U. (1985). Assessment of abnormal evoked pain in neurological pain patients and its relation to spontaneous pain: a descriptive and conceptual model with some analytical results, in *Advances in Pain Research and Therapy*, Fields, H., Dubner, R., and Cervero, F. (Eds.), Raven Press, New York, p. 412.

Mackley, R. (in press). The role of trigger points and myofascial pain syndrome in the management of head, neck, and face pain, in *Conquering Chronic Pain*, Margoles, M. (Ed.).

Margoles, M. (1983). The stress neuromyelopathic pain syndrome, *Journal of Neurological and Orthopedic Medicine and Surgery*, 4, 317–322.

Margoles, M. (1983). Pain charts: spatial properties of pain, in *Pain Measurement and Assessment*, Melzack, R. (Ed.), Raven Press, New York, pp. 214–225.

Margoles, M. (1984). Opioid usage survey of the members of the American Pain Society, unpublished data.

Margoles, M. (1987). Cervical discs as perpetuating factors in chronic moderate to severe myofascial pain syndrome and SNPS, *American Back Society Newsletter*, 2, 3–4.

Margoles, M. (1988). Colchicine usage in the treatment of patients with pain, *Journal of Neurological and Orthopedic Medicine and Surgery*, 10, 913–918.

Margoles, M. (1988). Breaking colchicine tablets to make them more palatable, *Journal of Neurological and Orthopedic Medicine and Surgery*, 9, 95.

Margoles, M. (1989). Vitamins by mouth and by injection in the treatment of patients with chronic pain, *Journal of Neurological and Orthopedic Medicine and Surgery*, 10, 341–343.

Margoles, M. (1989). Comprehensive evaluation and treatment of the patient with myofascial pain syndrome, *Journal of Neurological and Orthopedic Medicine and Surgery*, 10, 344–346.

Margoles, M. (in press). The stress neuromyeloencephalopathic pain syndrome (SNPS), in *Conquering Chronic Pain*, Margoles, M. (Ed.).

Margoles, M. (in press). The stress neuromyeloencephalopathic pain syndrome (SNPS): update, *Journal of Neurological and Orthopedic Medicine and Surgery*.

Margoles, M. (in press). Vitamin A toxicity in chronic pain patients, in *Conquering Chronic Pain*, Margoles, M. (Ed.).

Margoles, M. (in press). Vitamin and mineral problems in patients with chronic pain, in *Conquering Chronic Pain*, Margoles, M. (Ed.).

Margoles, M. (in press). Medication management in patients with chronic pain, in *Conquering Chronic Pain*, Margoles, M. (Ed.).

Margoles, M. (in press). Sleep problems in patients with chronic pain, in *Conquering Chronic Pain*, Margoles, M. (Ed.).

Margoles, M. (Ed.) (in press). *Conquering Chronic Pain*.

Margoles, M. (in press). Some important aspects of clinical and laboratory evaluation and treatment of patients with myofascial pain syndrome.

Margoles, M. (in press). Advanced physical therapy techniques in the rehabilitation of patients with chronic pain, in *Conquering Chronic Pain*, Margoles, M. (Ed.).

Margoles, M. and Margoles, M. (1984). The use of narcotic analgesics in the treatment of chronic orthopedic pain patients (COPP) — an informal and retrospective study of 95 patients, *Pain*, Suppl. 2, S31.

Meyers, F. and Meyers, F. (1987). Management of chronic pain, *American Family Physician*, 35, 139–146.

Porter, J. and Jick, H. (1980). Addiction rare in patients treated with narcotics, *New England Journal of Medicine*, 302, 123.

Rask, M. (1980). Colchicine use in 500 patients with disk disease, *Journal of Neurological and Orthopaedic Surgery*, 1, 351–369.

Rask, M. (1985). Colchicine use in 3,000 patients with diskal (and other) spinal disorders, *Journal of Neurological and Orthopedic Medicine and Surgery*, 6, 295–302.

Simons, D. Personal communication.

Simons, D. (1984). Myofascial pain syndromes and their treatment, in *Medical Rehabilitation*, Basmajian, J. and Kirby, R.L. (Eds.), Williams and Wilkins, Baltimore, pp. 312–320.

Smith, D. (1981, 1989). Personal communication.

Stimmel, B. (1985). Pain analgesia and addiction: an approach to the pharmacologic management of pain, *The Clinical Journal of Pain,* 1, 14–22.

Tennent, F. and Ulemen, G. (1983). Narcotic maintenance for chronic pain, medical and legal guidelines, *Postgraduate Medicine,* 73, 81–94.

Texidor, M. and Margoles, M. (in press). The evaluation of vitamin/electrolyte for the management of chronic low back pain of myofascial origin.

Travell, J. Personal communication.

Travell, J. (1976). Myofascial trigger points: clinical view, in *Advances in Pain Research and Therapy,* Vol. 1, Bonica, J. and Albe-Fessard, D. (Eds.), Raven Press, New York, p. 921.

Travell, J. and Simons, D. (1983). *Myofascial Pain and Dysfunction: The Trigger Point Manual,* Williams and Wilkins, Baltimore.

Travell, J. and Simons, D. (in press). *Myofascial Pain and Dysfunction: The Trigger Point Manual,* Vol. 2, Williams and Wilkins, Baltimore.

11 The Role of Trigger Points in the Management of Head, Neck, and Face Pain*

Ronald J. Mackley, D.D.S., M.S.

In order to treat something, we must first learn to recognize it.

—Sir William Osler

HEAD, NECK AND FACE PAIN — YOU MAY NOT HAVE TO LIVE WITH IT!

Pain is a common experience for everyone. While everyone suffers pain at one time or another, it is important to understand that normal, healthy muscle tissue does not hurt. Ninety percent of the pain experienced in a lifetime is muscle pain.[2] None of this pain should be considered "normal" or "untreatable". With the understanding of what causes muscle pain, solutions and treatment become evident, resulting in control of most muscle related pain experiences.

PAIN AND ITS ORIGIN

There are two types of pain: acute and chronic. Acute pain is informative to the body. It signals important health problems: a toothache, an earache, appendicitis, a broken bone, a burn, a sprained ankle, etc. This type of pain indicates that we have a problem which needs attention. Usually, determining the source of the problem is relatively simple. The treatment needed is well known and accepted. You know what you have, and that there is a predictable end to it.

Chronic pain is likewise connected to disease. It is often caused by a condition in the muscles. Most chronic pain has a definable cause. To say that a pain caused by such actions

---

* Chapter reprinted from Mackley, Ronald J., The role of trigger points in the management of head, neck, and face pain, *Functional Orthodontist,* September/October 1990. With permission. Pain referral patterns reprinted by permission of Janet A. Travell, M.D., David G. Simons, M.D., and Williams and Wilkins from *Myofascial Pain and Dysfunction, The Trigger Point Manual.*

as turning to lift a book or bending over to pick up a baby ignores the true source of the discomfort. The act is merely a triggering mechanism for the underlying problem, **MYOFASCIAL TRIGGER POINTS**.[3]

MYOFASCIAL PAIN (PAIN FROM MYOFASCIAL TRIGGER POINTS)

MYO means muscle: FASCIA (pronounced fasha) is the connective tissue that holds us together. Therefore, myofascial pain is pain that comes from the muscle or the fascia covering the muscle. Pain can also come from the skin, ligaments, tendons, and tissue covering the bones.

Muscle comprises the largest tissue mass in the body. Myofascial pain is a very common problem. It has been estimated that twenty percent of the population experiences myofascial pain problems, and ten percent are restricted in normal physical activity because of muscle pain.[4] Myofascial pain comes from hypersensitive areas in the muscles called trigger points or trigger areas. These trigger points hurt when pressure is applied to them, or when the muscle is overused or abused.

A trigger point may cause restriction of movement and weakness of the affected muscle or body part (arm, leg, jaw, etc.). It may also "refer" pain to other areas of the body, producing symptoms that are often misdiagnosed, such as bursitis, ruptured vertebral discs, and earache.[5]

THE REFERRAL OF PAIN

Dr. Janet Travell, a pioneer in myofascial pain treatment, was President John F. Kennedy's personal physician. She relieved his back problems, and made it possible for him to perform his day to day duties. She has noted that it is not uncommon for pain to be referred a distance away from the muscle that caused the pain. Dr. Travell explains that the referred pain comes from a small zone of hypersensitivity known as a trigger area or trigger point which is located within the affected muscle. She has demonstrated that **EACH SKELETAL MUSCLE HAS A SPECIFIC PATTERN OF REFERRED PAIN**. That is, a trigger area in a muscle will produce pain in another part of the body when this trigger area is activated. When activating stress is applied to this area, through pressure or active use of the muscle, the pain travels by the same pathway between the trigger area and the distant site where the pain is experienced.[5]

SPECIFIC MUSCLES PRODUCING REFERRED PAIN

To illustrate some of the pain referral patterns of the head, neck, and face areas, the following muscles have been included.

The **trapezius** is probably the muscle most often beset with myofascial trigger points. It comprises most of the shoulder muscles (Figure 11.1).

The **sternocleidomastoid** responds clinically like two separate muscles, each having its own characteristic referred pain pattern (Figure 11.2). It is involved in rotating the head to the side, and maintaining the head in an upright position when we are sitting or standing.

The **masseter** is one of the primary muscles that closes the jaw. It can be felt by placing your finger on the angle of your lower jaw, and by clenching your teeth (Figure 11.3).

The **temporalis** muscle is a broad, fan-shaped muscle that fits on the side of the head in the "temple" (Figure 11.4). It is important for chewing your food, and can be a frequent source of headaches.

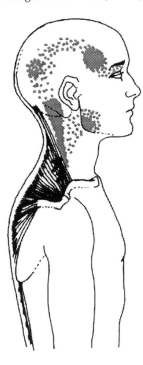

FIGURE 11.1   Referred pain pattern and location (X) of trigger point 1 in the upper trapezius muscle. Solid area shows the essential referred pain zone; stippling shows the spillover zone.

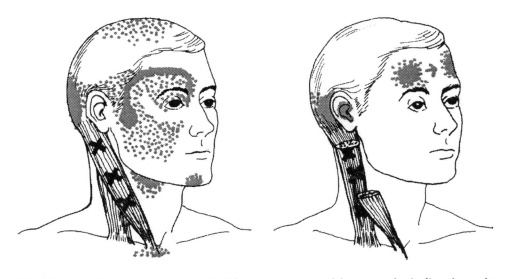

FIGURE 11.2   Referred pain patterns (*solid area* shows essential zones and *stippling* shows the spillover area) with location of corresponding trigger points (Xs) in the right sternocleidomastoid muscle. (Left) The sternal (superficial) division. (Right) The clavicular (deep) division.

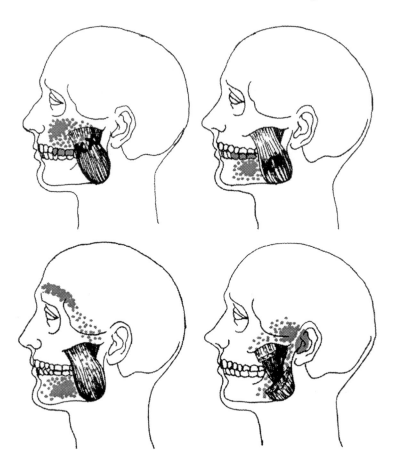

FIGURE 11.3   The (Xs) locate trigger points in various parts of the masseter muscle. *Solid area* shows essential referred pain zones, and the *stippled areas* are spillover pain zones.

The **scalene** muscles are found on the side of the neck. They serve as prime movers for side bending of the head. Their trigger points can refer pain all the way down the arm into the hand (Figure 11.5).

The pain referral patterns illustrated all originate in muscles of the jaw and neck. These muscles represent only a limited number of the muscles in this area. Muscles in other parts of the body can refer pain into the shoulders, arms, hands, chest, low back, and legs.

PERPETUATING FACTORS

Perpetuating factors are what keep the pain problems going. It is essential to successful myofascial pain management to identify what they are and to eliminate them, if possible. Perpetuating factors make the muscles more susceptible to myofascial pain and irritability.

That it is important to correct perpetuating factors is illustrated by the apocryphal story of the man who stepped in a hole in the sidewalk and broke his leg. He was treated and the bones of his leg healed, but two months later he stepped in the same hole and again broke the leg. *No one had patched the hole.* If we treat myofascial pain syndromes without "patching the holes," that is, by not correcting the multiple

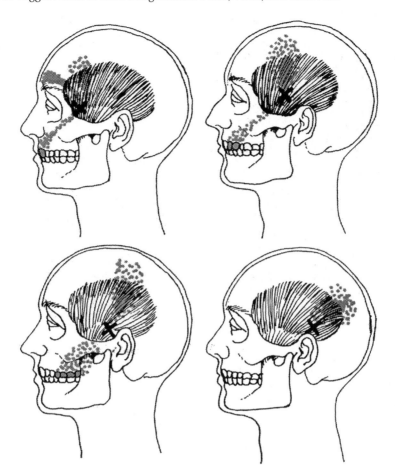

FIGURE 11.4   Referred pain patterns from trigger points (Xs) in the left temporalis muscle (essential zone, solid area; spillover zone, stippled). A, anterior "spokes" of pain arising from the anterior fibers (trigger point one region) B and C, middle "spokes" (trigger point two and trigger point three regions). D, posterior supraauricular "spoke" (trigger point four region).

perpetuating factors, the patient is doomed to endless cycles of treatment and relapse. For patients who have suffered myofascial pain for many months or years, we find it necessary to spend most of our time patching holes.[5]

The answer to the question, "How long will the beneficial results of specific myofascial therapy last?", depends largely on what perpetuating factors remain unresolved. In the absence of such factors, the muscle with fully inactivated trigger points (TPs) should be no more susceptible to TP activation than the normal muscle was originally.[5]

In some patients, these perpetuating factors are so important that their elimination results in complete relief of the pain without any further treatment of the muscles.[5]

There are four general types of perpetuating factors:[5]

A. Mechanical Stress

These may come from:

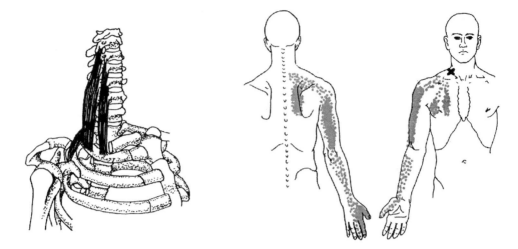

FIGURE 11.5 Composite pain pattern (solid areas are the essential, and stippled areas are the spillover pain reference zones) with location of trigger points (Xs) in the right scalene muscles. Scalenus; anterior, medius and posterior. Some trigger points may have only one essential reference zone.

1. Body structure inadequacies, i.e., one leg shorter than the other, a long second toe (which affects the way one walks), or short upper arms;
2. Postural stress, i.e., misfitting furniture, poor posture when standing or sitting, abuse of muscles through too many repetitions of the same action (hobbies and/or occupation);
3. Dental malocclusion (teeth that don't meet properly) and;
4. Constriction of muscles by such things as bra straps, heavy purses, tight shirt collar or necktie, tight belt or garter straps.

B. Nutritional Inadequacies and Excesses

Nutrients of special concern in patients with myofascial pain syndromes include Vitamin B1, B6, B12, Folic acid, and Vitamin C. Many patients with chronic myofascial pain require resolution of vitamin inadequacies for lasting relief. Several minerals, especially calcium, potassium, iron, and magnesium, are essential for individual muscle fibers to contract normally.[5] Too much Vitamin A in the diet can irritate muscles.[9]

C. Hormone Inadequacies and Diet

There are three or four times as many women who report myofascial pain problems as there are men. There appears to be a least three significant reasons for this:

1. Women's hormone balance is constantly changing. Dr. Larry Funt has observed that "at least 15–18 percent of female patients with myofascial pain visiting my office during a month will develop premenstrual headaches even after their chronic headaches are under control. The headache usually will start three days before the patient's period, and may or may not be relieved temporarily by aspirin. Yet, in a day and a half, many of the old symptoms of the chronic headache reappear and aspirin has no effect at all."

2. "Food plays an important role in the onset of headaches. Women are more affected by this factor than men since they are more frequently on diets that do not afford proper nutrition."[8]
3. Inadequate levels of thyroid hormone can completely frustrate attempts to eliminate myofascial pain. Hypoglycemia is a perpetuating factor related to impaired energy metabolism. Allergies can be another perpetuating factor, as can diets with too much refined sugar.

D. Acute or Chronic Infection

It is commonly known that pain and aching can accompany viral illness, such as "Flu". The activity of myofascial trigger points tends to increase during any systemic viral illness, or other active infections.

IT IS ESSENTIAL TO THE SUCCESSFUL MANAGEMENT OF MYOFASCIAL PAIN PROBLEMS THAT THE PERPETUATING FACTORS BE IDENTIFIED AND CORRECTED. OTHERWISE, THE "PATIENT IS DOOMED TO ENDLESS CYCLES OF TREATMENT AND RELAPSE."[5]

TMJ DYSFUNCTION SYNDROME

TMJ stands for temporo-mandibular joint, the jaw joint. It is located just in front of the ears. The lower jaw (mandible) fits into a socket in the temporal bone, the bone where the ear is attached.

TMJ dysfunction may typically make itself felt in various areas of the head, and can be involved with the following: recurrent headaches, migraine-like pain on one or both sides of the head or face, earaches, dizziness, ringing in the ears, toothache, difficulty in swallowing, and neck spasms. TMJ sufferers frequently hear a clicking or popping sound when they open or close their mouth. Symptoms often increase when chewing. The muscle close to the ear may be tender, and jaw movements are frequently limited and/or irregular. Stiff neck and limited ability to bend the neck are frequently associated with TMJ dysfunction.

A MULTIDISCIPLINARY APPROACH IS NEEDED TO MOST EFFECTIVELY RESOLVE MYOFASCIAL PAIN

Health professionals of all disciplines have received excellent training in their particular area of expertise. It is not possible for one person to be an expert of internal medicine, ear-nose-throat, neurology, orthopedics, neurosurgery, chiropractic, osteopathies, dentistry, and physical therapy. Yet, it may require the expertise of several of these disciplines to adequately manage chronic pain

It is important to keep in mind that 90 percent of all headaches are muscle contraction headaches, 8 percent are vascular (migraine-type), 2 percent is from other causes. Muscle pain is very resistant to relief from medication alone (muscle relaxants, "pain killers," tranquilizers). However, it responds quickly to treatment that allows these affected muscles to relax, and return to their normal resting lengths.

Frequently, the most effective method of relieving head, neck, and face pain is to start treatment with an orthopedic mouth splint that is worn on the lower teeth to reposture the lower jaw. Unless the jaw is balanced properly, allowing the head, neck, and shoulder muscles to return to their appropriate resting position, pain will tend to reoccur. Dental malocclusion can be a potent perpetuating factor of head, neck, and face pain.

Chronic myofascial pain can usually be relieved and effectively managed. It is not uncommon to hear statements such as one offered recently by a long suffering patient who exclaimed, "This is the first time in 42 years that I have not had a headache."

CASE HISTORIES

The following case histories have been included to illustrate the variation of myofascial pain problems.

Case History 1

13-year-old girl. She has complained about throat, neck and head pain for about a month. At first we thought it was the flu. Then she started coming home from school with headaches and neck pain. She does have reading glasses, but doesn't wear them enough. The pain goes away with aspirin, but it comes back off and on. Finally, she realized the soreness was in her lower jaw, and below her ears on both sides. I felt maybe there was some infection in her back teeth, so l took her to my dentist. He referred to the phrase TMJ and recommended having something done for it.

An orthopedic mouth splint was constructed. Within a week of wearing it, the jaw pain was gone. It returned when she left the splint out, and chewed bubble gum. Consistent wear of the splint, spray and stretch treatment with Fluori-methane, and exercises to increase the range of motion of the neck, jaw, and shoulder muscles provided her with relief of her pain.

Case History 2

26-year-old receptionist. 16 years — I fell from my bicycle onto the pavement and struck my chin against the curb. I saw my family physician who cleaned and dressed my scrapes. My chin and jaw were very sore and stiff so she recommended that I see my dentist to rule out any damage to my jaw.

17 years — I began experiencing a locking sensation and a tired feeling in my jaw, also a "popping" or shifting. I saw my regular dentist and he took x-rays. He said that he didn't see any breaks or cracks in my jaw, but that all four of my wisdom teeth were impacted. I had all four teeth removed at the same time by an oral surgeon. I had an adverse reaction to the surgery and was out of school for over a week. I was badly swollen and bruised to the point that my sister didn't recognize me. This went away after about two weeks. The sutures were removed the third week and I had great difficulty opening my mouth beyond an inch. Soon after my teeth were removed I began to have frequent indigestion and headaches. I was the editor of my high school yearbook along with carrying a full load of classes, so much of it was attributed to over-exertion on my part. I did see my family physician for my indigestion, and she ran several tests including an upper G.I. series. I was diagnosed as having a hiatal hernia and told to take antacids and try bland foods. I noticed at this time that seemingly "bland" foods such as bread and macaroni made my indigestion worse.

21 years — I don't recall anything in particular between the ages 17 to 20. The summer that I turned 21 I came down with what I thought was the flu. I had extremely bad headaches and my neck was stiff to the point I could not rotate it more than an inch or two in either direction. I saw a doctor towards the end of the illness (which kept me home from work for seven days) and he felt that I might have spinal meningitis. He stated that if I was not better in a few days that he would like to admit me to a hospital to run some tests, including a spinal tap. Luckily, my headaches decreased, although I did not regain full mobility of my neck muscles. I did not enter the hospital.

22–26 years — My headaches began increasing, both in frequency and severity. By the time I was 24 I was having at least one severe headache per month. These would coincide with my monthly cycle, starting 3–4 days prior to the onset of menstruation and lasting 2–3 days. They would be accompanied by an upset stomach, although I never vomited. By the time I was 26, I was having headaches at least twice per week. If I would catch the headaches before they became too bad I could control the pain by using Alka-Seltzer Plus. Regular aspirin or Tylenol would not affect them.

Also, at this time, I noticed that when I would tilt my head back to look up it would cause a great deal of pain. If I kept it back for a prolonged period of time, such as watching a movie or fireworks, I would develop a very bad headache.

In February of my 26th year, I began work in an orthodontic office as a receptionist. By now my headaches were constant and accompanied by severe neck, shoulder and back pain. My orthodontist gave me a thorough head and neck pain examination, then took an impression and fit me with a diagnostic splint. A week later my headaches were virtually non-existent, although I still had a great deal of pain in my neck, shoulders and back. My orthodontist then began to use a stretching technique accompanied by a Fluori-methane spray to relax my muscles. This, in conjunction with the splint, helped my muscles to relax and eased some of the tension from them. I still could not attain a full range of motion and tilting my head back was still quite painful. At this time, he recommended that I see an allergist and a physical therapist.

I saw the allergist first and some of his findings truly surprised me. While I am allergic to many environmental items, it was the food items that caused my greatest distress. Trying to remove such basic items as wheat and milk from my diet was difficult, but once accomplished, the change in my facial appearance was dramatic. My eyes have always been red streaked and irritated, which I've attributed to wearing hard contact lens. Within one week of eliminating these foods from my diet, my eyes cleared considerably, my nasal passages cleared and the dark circles under my eyes lightened.

27 years — I began seeing the physical therapist twice the first week, then reducing the treatments to once a week for six weeks. At each session my muscles were first heated and relaxed with moist heat, then an ultrasound unit was used to heat the deeper muscles that the moist heat could not reach. The therapist then manipulated my muscles with light massage. Afterwards, I was instructed on proper posture and given stretching exercises to do at home.

By the end of the six weeks I was virtually pain free. I must continue my stretching exercises at home and I have joined a gym to help strengthen and tone my muscles. I also continue to wear my splint at night to avoid clenching and grinding my teeth. I must watch my diet continually and read labels to avoid hidden additives.

On the whole, I feel 100% better. I have more energy, more flexibility, and I am a happier person, less cranky and more fun to be with. I do not feel I'll ever be "cured" but I have the pain under control rather than letting the pain control me.

Case History 3

51-year-old male dentist.   2 years — I broke my leg near the hip joint. I was in a cast from under my arms, and down both legs. Only my toes were not covered. There was a board between my legs to keep my legs apart. I had "charley horses" in my leg muscles for several years after when I did anything that was very active.

11 years — I had a pain in my lower back that would switch from the right leg to the left leg. It finally settled in my right leg. When I would go up stairs, I would need to put my hand under my right thigh muscles and lift to make it up the next step. A chiropractor adjusted my back, and the pain went away.

15 years — I was playing tackle football in a P.E. class. I was tackled after catching a pass and I landed on my back. I couldn't straighten up because of the pain between my shoulder blades. This was relieved with a chiropractic adjustment. That same fall, my mother took me to an optometrist to get my eyes checked. I was taking aspirin every afternoon as soon as I got home from high school, because I had a headache in both temples. The glasses helped, but I still have a headache in the temples in the afternoon.

16 years — I ran the 440 yard dash for the high school track team. The spikes on the shoes would make the arches of my feet hurt so bad I could hardly walk.

17 years — In the middle of the basketball season, I pulled a hamstring muscle in my left leg while playing on the high school varsity basketball team. I lost my starting position and had to sit on the bench while my replacement was very instrumental in our team winning the state basketball championship.

18 years — After graduating from high school, I played in a church basketball league once a week. I would be so stiff and sore a couple of days after that I could hardly walk. I would get better just in time to play the next game.

23 years — I developed a click in my left jaw. To open my mouth all the way, I would need to shift my lower jaw to the right to get it to pop. Then I could shift back to the left, and open the rest of the way.

25 years — I went deer hunting with my father-in-law. I shot a small deer. We decided to put a pole between its legs and carry it out. My right shoulder had a deep, dull, constant ache for the next year.

30 years — I developed pain in my left TMJ that became severe when I chewed anything hard. I quit eating meat and french bread. I couldn't chew them. I went to a dentist who determined I had a tooth that was out of position, so my other teeth couldn't fit together properly without shifting my jaw to miss that tooth. The dentist reshaped the chewing surfaces of my teeth so all the back teeth came together at the same time. The pain in the joint went away.

33 years — The spinous process on my first thoracic vertebrae was fractured. I wore a neck brace for six weeks. Without being able to bend my neck, I had to bend my back a lot to continue working. This caused severe low back pain. A physical therapist was able to keep me going.

45 years — There was an almost constant burning sensation between my shoulder blades. Sometimes, the pain in this area would become so severe that I would lie down on the floor to relieve the pain. It wasn't unusual to awaken in the morning with a stiff neck. When I had a severe stiff neck, muscle relaxants didn't help much. It would get better in a few days.

47 years — My right elbow had bothered me for several years after being in a bowling league. One time I reached for a carton of milk that was on the table. I couldn't lift it, because of the pain in my elbow. The elbow developed an almost constant ache. I had it injected with cortisone twice. It didn't help.

48 years — I was attending a three day seminar. I sat on the front row the first day. On the second day I sat in the same seat. After an hour, the back of my neck was hurting enough that I went to the back of the room and stood up so I wouldn't need to lift my head to look at the lecturer. Standing caused my lower back to ache.

49 years — My neck was really stiff one morning. It kept getting worse as the day progressed. I went to a chiropractor. I couldn't raise my right arm up onto the table. He tried to adjust my neck, but he wasn't able to. It was too painful. He gave me a soft neck brace to wear. It got better in a few days. The back of my neck would really hurt when I drove a car any distance, so I kept the neck brace in the car. Whenever I drove I would put it on.

During a twelve month period, I was treated by an osteopath, two chiropractors, and a homeopathic physician. None of them provided me with any lasting relief of my problems.

In addition, I took some muscle relaxants. They didn't help. The relief I obtained as a teenager from chiropractors was really dramatic. Now they don't help very much.

We went to Europe for four weeks that summer. I carried a camera case that contained two cameras and several lenses wherever we went. My shoulder and back would really ache. When we returned home, my neck and upper back were very uncomfortable. In November, I attended a seminar on myofascial pain and trigger points. Since that time, I have been getting progressively better, because the problem has always been in the muscles. The therapy I have had since that time has been directed at the muscle pain problems. Two years later, I am significantly improved. I still have to be careful, but I am no longer in almost constant pain.

These case histories have been included to illustrate the fact that **MYOFASCIAL PAIN PROBLEMS ARE CUMULATIVE AND PROGRESSIVE.** Unless the trigger points are relieved, the problems tend to become more complex and more difficult to treat as additional muscles are involved in the muscular adjustments that must occur when a muscle remains in a state of irritation. These problems will not just go away by ignoring them. There is much that can be done to relieve the discomfort. The earlier the symptoms are treated, the easier it is to get lasting relief.

MYOFASCIAL PAIN IS CUMULATIVE AND PROGRESSIVE

Myofascial pain comes and goes, but with each recurrence it tends to become more severe, limits muscular function more, and become more painful. Dr. Larry Funt and Dr. Bruce Kinnie, both of whom are orthodontists, have developed a chart illustrating the progression of pain and disability from age 4 years to 70 years[1] (Chart 11.1).

THE GOOD SPORT SYNDROME

One of the unfortunate things about myofascial pain problems is the general lack of understanding regarding what it is, how it begins, and how to get rid of it. There is a common statement that is made, "I've tried everything, and nothing helps. I have concluded that I will just have to live with it." Another common feeling is that if the pain is ignored, it will go away. This leads to what is referred to as the "Good Sport Syndrome."

The "good sport" is the opposite of being a hypochondriac. Hypochondriacs tend to complain about every little ache and pain, and worry that it may be something serious. "Good sports" are determined to ignore pain, and charge ahead in whatever activity they are engaged in with total disregard to the pain they are experiencing. They seem to believe that giving in to their pain would be a sign of "weakness". There are some problems with this type of reasoning:

1. The activities they are engaged in may be an important perpetuating factor to their particular problem,
2. Abuse of muscles irritates trigger points,
3. Myofascial pain is cumulative and progressive (refer to chart). If new ways of doing things are learned that will safely allow them to perform the activities that are important to them, their lives will be more comfortable. It may be necessary, for a period of time, to discontinue that particular activity.

SELF EVALUATION

The Kinnie–Funt (K-F) Chief Complaint Visual Index for Head, Neck, and Facial Pain and TMJ Dysfunction form has been included to assist you in identifying problems that may be troubling you. All of these symptoms can be myofascial in origin (Chart 11.2).

The Funt Symptom (F-S) Index *

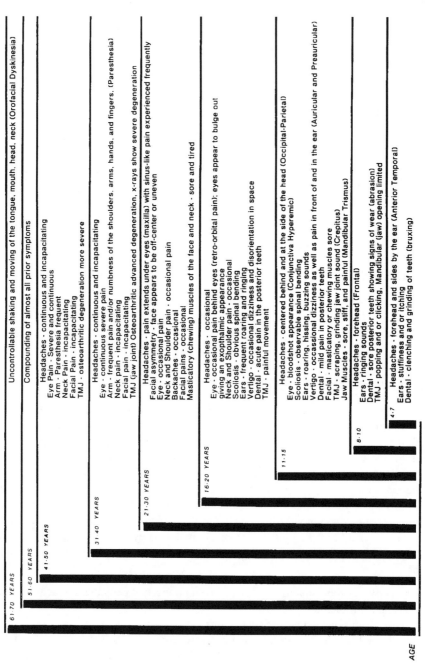

AGE	

61-70 YEARS — Uncontrollable shaking and moving of the tongue, mouth, head, neck (Orofacial Dyskinesia)

51-60 YEARS — Compounding of almost all prior symptoms

41-50 YEARS
Headaches - continuous and incapacitating
Eye Pain - Severe and continuous
Arm - Paresthesia frequent
Neck Pain - incapacitating
Facial Pain - incapacitating
TMJ - osteoarthritic degeneration more severe

31-40 YEARS
Headaches - continuous and incapacitating
Eye - continuous severe pain
Arm - frequent pain and/or numbness of the shoulders, arms, hands, and fingers. (Paresthesia)
Neck pain - incapacitating
Facial pain - incapacitating
TMJ (jaw joint) Osteoarthritic advanced degeneration, x-rays show severe degeneration

21-30 YEARS
Headaches - pain extends under eyes (maxilla) with sinus-like pain experienced frequently
Facial asymmetry - face appears to be off-center or uneven
Eye - occasional pain
Neck and Shoulder pain - occasional pain
Backaches - occasional
Facial pains - occasional
Masticatory (chewing) muscles of the face and neck - sore and tired

16-20 YEARS
Headaches - occasional
Eye - occasional pain behind eyes (retro-orbital pain); eyes appear to bulge out giving an exophthalmic appearance
Neck and Shoulder pain - occasional
Scoliosis - obvious spinal bending
Ears - frequent roaring and ringing
Vertigo - occasional dizziness and disorientation in space
Dental - acute pain in the posterior teeth
TMJ - painful movement

11-15 YEARS
Headaches - centered behind and at the side of the head (Occipital-Parietal)
Eye - bloodshot appearance (Conjunctiva Hyperemic)
Scoliosis - observable spinal bending
Ears - roaring, hissing, buzzing sounds
Vertigo - occassional dizziness as well as pain in front of and in the ear (Auricular and Preauricular)
Dental - mild pain in posterior teeth
Facial - masticatory or chewing muscles sore
TMJ - scraping, grinding jaw joint sound (Crepitus)
Jaw Muscles - sore, stiff, and painful (Mandibular Trismus)

8-10
Headaches - forehead (Frontal)
Ears - ringing sounds
Dental - sore posterior teeth showing signs of wear (abrasion)
TMJ - popping and or clicking, Mandibular (jaw) opening limited

4-7
Headaches - forehead and sides by the ear (Anterior Temporal)
Ears - stuffiness and or itching
Dental - clenching and grinding of teeth (bruxing)

*An evolutionary, progressive and cumulative clinical index patterned from symptoms documented in craniomandibular pain patients by Lawrence A. Funt (Bethesda, Maryland) and Dr. Bruce Kinnie (Columbia, South Carolina).

©1984, The Kinnie-Funt (K-F) System of Referred Pain of the Head, Neck, Face and Temporomandibular Joint, Page 40.

CHART 11.1

The Kinnie-Funt (K-F) Chief Complaint Visual Index for Head, Neck, and Facial Pain and TMJ Dysfunction

Name: _____

Age: _____

Date: _____

1. Please circle the number in front of the symptoms you regularly or occasionally have.

2. Indicate your main or chief complaints in order of their current importance.

(A). _____

(B). _____

(C). _____

3. Please draw areas of pain or distress on the picture below.

A. Eye Pain and Eye Orbital Problems:
1. Eye (orbital) pain: above, below, behind.
2. Bloodshot eyes (hyperemia)
3. Blurring of vision
4. Bulging appearance (exophthalmia)
5. Pressure behind the eyes (retro-orbital pressure)
6. Light sensitivity (photo-phobia)
7. Watering of the eyes (lacrimation)
8. Drooping of the eye lid (ptosis)

B. Head Pain, Headache Problems, Facial Pain:
1. Forehead (frontal)
2. Temples (temporal)
3. "Migraine" type headache
4. "Cluster" headache
5. Maxillary sinus headache (under the eyes)
6. Posterior back of head headaches with or without shooting pains (occipital headache)
7. Hair and or scalp painful to touch (parietal headache)

C. Mouth, Face, Cheek, and Chin Problems:
1. Discomfort
2. Limited opening
3. Inability to open smoothly, evenly
4. Jaw deviates to one side when opening
5. Inability to "find bite"

D. Teeth and Gum Problems:
1. Clenching, grinding at night   (bruxism)
2. Looseness and or soreness of back teeth
3. Tooth pain (toothache)

E. Jaw and Jaw Joint (TMJ) Problems:
1. Clicking, popping jaw joints
2. Grating sounds (crepitus)
3. Jaw locking opened or closed
4. Pain in cheek muscles
5. Uncontrollable jaw, tongue movements

F. Pain, Ear Problems, and Postural Imbalances:
1. Hissing, buzzing, ringing, or roaring sounds (tinitus)
2. Diminished hearing (subjective hearing loss)
3. Ear pain without infection (otalgia)
4. Clogged, stuffy, "itchy" ears, feeling of fullness
5. Balance problems: "vertigo" (disequilibrium)

G. Throat Problems:
1. Swallowing difficulties
2. Tightness of throat
3. Sore throat without infection (coryza)
4. Voice fluctuations
5. Laryngitis
6. Frequent coughing or constant clearing of throat
7. Feeling of foreign object in throat
8. Tongue pain (glossalgia)
9. Salivation (intense)
10. Pain in the hard palate (posterior areas)

H. Neck and Shoulder Problems:
1. Lack of mobility-reduced range of movement
2. Stiffness
3. Neck pain
4. Tired, sore, neck muscles
5. Shoulder aches
6. Back pain upper and lower
7. Arm and finger tingling, numbness and or pain

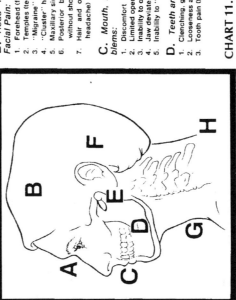

CHART 11.2

A visual clinical index correlated from the most frequently seen symptoms documented in head, neck and facial pain patients by Dr. Bruce H. Kinnie (Columbia, South Carolina) and Dr. Lawrence A. Funt (Bethesda, Maryland)

© 1984. The Kinnie-Funt (K-F) System of Referred Pain of the Head, Neck, Face and Temporomandibular Joint. Page 38

Reprinted by permission of Lawrence A. Funt, D.D.S.

POSTSCRIPT

People need to know that someone knows they are hurting — that it is not terminal, that it is not in their head, and that they are not making it up or faking it.

BIBLIOGRAPHY

1. Kinnie, B.H., and Funt, L.A.: *Anatomy of a Headache,* published by European Orthodontic Products, Inc., 1984
2. Gelb, H., and Siegel, P.M.: *Killing Pain Without Prescription,* Harper and Row, 1980
3. Prudden, B.: *Pain Erasure, The Bonnie Prudden Way,* M. Evans & Co., 1980
4. Funt, L.A.: Personal communication
5. Travell, J.G., Simons, D.G.: *Myofascial Pain and Dysfunction, The Trigger Point Manual,* Williams and Wilkins, 1983
6. Kinnie, B.H., Funt, L.A.: Patterns of Pain Referred by Muscles of the Head, Neck, and Face, unpublished
7. Gelb, H.: *Clinical Management of Head, Neck and TMJ Pain and Dysfunction, A Multidisciplinary Approach to Diagnosis and Treatment,* W.B. Saunders Company, 1977
8. Funt, L.: A New Approach to Chronic Headache, *The Female Patient,* Vol. 5, May 1980
9. Margoles, M.S.: Vitamin A Toxicity Symptoms, *J.A.M.A.,* 1984.

12 A Patient's Guide to Trigger Points

Jay Bayer D.O.

The following information is presented as general information on trigger points (TrPs) and to provide some understanding of a commonly overlooked diagnosis. It is beyond the scope of this chapter to present all aspects and details of the diagnosis and treatment of trigger points.

TRIGGER POINTS

I refer to them as tissue "hot spots." They are usually found in muscle but also tendons (attach muscle to bone), ligaments (attach bone to bone), fascia (cover or envelope muscles), some joint surfaces, periosteum (lining on bone), enthesopathies (the transitional area where ligaments attach to bone and becomes inflamed), and skin or scar tissue. For facilitation, I will use muscle in the discussion, but the above-mentioned structures may be substituted.

CAUSE

Muscle may sustain damage from direct injury, falls, fractures or sprained joints, excessive or unusual exercise, or wrenching movements, as well as general overuse such as doing chores or activities to which you are not conditioned or accustomed. Other mechanical factors include repetitive overuse, muscle overwork and fatigue, and vocational stresses of poor work habits while standing or sitting with slouched posture (chair too high or too low, back not supported) for extended time spans (i.e., shoulder or arm elevation, head forward position [computer work], repetitive or sustained grasp, working assembly line, etc.). They may also appear after certain viral illnesses and posttraumatic or postsurgical scarring.

TYPES

There are active TrPs which are of recent origin and cause pain. Latent TrPs are active TrPs on semi-retirement. They may remain silent but reactivate with muscle stain. Usually producing stiffness and restricted motion, they are less irritable than active TrPs, but maintain the same symptoms. Secondary, associated, or satellite TrPs may appear. This is true in adjacent muscle groups where more workload is placed on them due to the major TrP. These groups may present with "protective spasms."

ONSET

Sudden onset is usually associated with a well-remembered muscular strain or injury. Gradual onset is not as easy to pinpoint. It results from repeated physical stress or overuse. TrPs can be found in all ages. Active ones are more common in athletes and younger persons. Latent ones are more common in older persons, especially more sedentary middle-age persons.

TRP MAIN CHARACTERISTICS

1. It is a localized, focused area of pain within a tight muscle band. Patients may refer to this area as "ropey," "knots or knotted," "spastic area," etc.
2. They are activated by direct pressure or compressive forces, misuse, or strain on the muscle. This reaction may cause a noticeable twitch (perceived as a spasm) and travels to another part of the body, called a reference zone, which is specific for the involved muscle. It not only refers pain, but tenderness. Note that instead of pain, altered or distorted sensation such as numbness or anesthesia may occur. Commonly described sensations are deep achey, dull (constant or variable intensity), shooting, stabbing or jabbing pain; numbness; sometimes burning; etc. Bizarre things like local sweating, paleness, and gooseflesh may accompany the reaction. When a gun trigger is pulled, the bullet hits a distant target. When a painful point is compressed, it triggers a response to a referred area.

   It is this very characteristic of TrPs that is so confusing to physicians of any specialty unfamiliar with chronic pain. Because TrPs do not follow specific anatomical patterns (i.e., like the sciatic nerve), the response may be labeled as an "abnormal or exaggerated pain response" or nonorganic. This type of misinterpretation produces a furthering pattern of confusion to insurers and attorneys and ultimately contributes to frustration of the patient.
3. Weakness and restricted motion in the involved muscle. When maximum effort (of contraction) is attempted, there is less than normal strength. Muscle strength is unreliable due to the guarding action of the TrP. The person may drop things, like when trying to put a carton of milk away. Another example is encountered when working in the yard. There is a sudden low back pain, bringing the person to the ground. They cannot get up due to the pain. The ambulance whisks them away to the emergency room, where X-rays and such are negative. They are sent home with a pain medicine and muscle relaxant and told they will be better in a few days. Low back strain is the common diagnosis, and unsatisfactory treatment results ensue.
4. The event of the original injury may be long gone, even faded into memory, but the TrP activity may be present for months, years, or decades. When traumatized, muscles "guard" the injured area while healing for about 6 weeks. (Note: Initially pain is a message with the purpose of healing. The guard may remain with no biological reason to continue the pain. The muscle obeys by limiting its use with resultant weakness, limited motion, and chronic stiffness. Further loss of power due to reduced ability to use the muscle is added with time.)

5. An active TrP can vary symptoms in the same day or day to day. The threshold of pain is not constant. It may vary from a minor discomfort to a major impairment. A latent TrP can be activated at any time.
6. Special note: TrPs may be related to underlying problems such as a herniated disc, neurologic illness, gall stones, internal organ disease, etc.

Due to the nature of muscles, emotional or nervous tension may activate a TrP. Muscles react by tightening up. In psychiatry, anxiety is noted to be manifested in neck and upper shoulder "tightness," while depression is more characteristic in the low back. Stress prepares you for "fight to flight" even when that is not possible.

After reading the above, it is no wonder why conventional medicine is confused by this.

GENERAL COMMENTS

1. During examination, when the TrP is felt and compressed, this may cause a "jump response." Patients often try to pull away or cry out ("ouch" is common).
2. TrPs, for legal reasons, are objective findings with specific characteristics.
3. TrPs are soft tissue diagnoses, based on a good interview (history) and a hands-on examination. They cannot be found on X-rays, MRIs, CTs, blood tests, or nerve studies.
4. Following the natural course of healing, this type of chronic pain serves no useful function to the body. Every patient experiences a physical and emotional response to pain disorders, or any illness for that matter. Left undiagnosed, misunderstood, and inappropriately treated, there is no mystery to the confusion, frustration, and suffering a chronic pain patient endures.

TRPS ARE MYOTONIC NOT PSYCHOGENIC

Patients who have suffered for months or years with a chronic undiagnosed pain develop psychological pain coping behavior. They experience secondary depression and sleep disturbances (lying on a TrP while asleep will activate it). They are anxious, frustrated, and exhibit a sense of hopelessness. It affects their work, home, and social life, restricting pastime activities and exercise. At some point, they may lose control of their life to the point that the pain controls them.

In my review of such cases, commonly the patient has undergone multiple specialty examinations and numerous tests with the result that "no organic cause for the pain can be found." It all means that a soft tissue diagnosis was overlooked. Insurers, employers, and sometimes the patient question the patient's state of mind (psychogenic — "It's all in your head"). Insurers also press examining doctors to comment on symptom magnification, which if not understood and answered with qualification can ruin a patient's life. It also indicates the insurer believes the patient's pain is psychogenic. In realty, this type of patient does have pain which creates psychological concern. The latter can add to the pain state. Patients with psychogenic or psychiatric pain states feel intimidated by improvement. They will either want assurance they will be pain free or exhibit all types of mannerisms to avoid getting better. TrP patients want restored function. They accept the fact that they may never be restored to a 100% pain-free state, but that they can restore control of their lives.

The good news is that (1) TrPs are eliminated when treated appropriately and (2) the pain medicine field understands the chronic pain patient, which provides a therapeutic foundation upon which the chronic pain patient can rebuild his or her life.

CONCLUSION

We are still learning about pain. The above is merely one piece of the great jigsaw puzzle. Unless the health care worker has experience and training in this field, the diagnosis will be overlooked. It requires no fancy tests, just the basic skills of medicine. This type of chronic pain has taken its toll on patients' lives and cost to the health care system.

13 In Defense of a Trigger Point Patient: Trigger Points Are Myogenic, Not Psychogenic*

Jay D. Bayer, D.O.

The following pointers and suggestions, based on the author's experience, may provide insight to any practitioner in the pain management field who is asked to give a deposition, perform an insurance medical examination (IME), write a narrative report, or champion the validity concerning a patient suffering with chronic pain.

It is amazing if not amusing that insurers and their attorneys cannot believe that a patient who has suffered an injury can continue to experience symptoms of pain months or years after the injury.

The insurance industry has convinced this author that it chooses an ignorant and unenlightened approach (by choice) concerning chronic pain patients and trigger points (TrPs). Rather than relying on rational diagnoses, the insurance industry instead chooses to blame the patient's aberrant psyche. This blame is unfounded by wisdom to understand that chronic pain patients do not knowingly or willfully choose this lifestyle of suffering. Rather, the system has failed — even victimized — the chronic pain patient. Instead of fixing the problem, energy and funds appear focused on placing blame.

Contrary to the insurance industry's unethical position, this chapter will provide several medical/legal points for the reader's consideration.

The first part of any practitioner's job is to consider the total patient. Physicians of pain medicine may often be the last professional to evaluate the patient. Here is a person who has been examined by countless health professionals, undergone extensive and expensive testing, participated in all kinds of therapy programs from biofeedback to physical therapy, and taken a polypharmacy of medication, yet continues to have pain. At this level, patients feel no one believes them and they may even question their own sanity! Wouldn't you be frustrated, anxious, apprehensive, depressed, and even feel a sense of hopelessness? And now they are

---

* While the chapter focuses on trigger points alone, applicable myofascial pain terminology may be substituted for trigger point.

1-57444-103-5/99/$0.00+$.50

in the hands of another health professional who probably is unknown to them, and unless rapport is established, the patient will undergo the examination with an apprehensive, discouraged, or even angry demeanor. The insurers and attorneys read reports that contain such statements as (1) no organic cause for the pain can be found, (2) the subjective complaints of the patient are not substantiated by objective findings (implying a functional, not organic, cause), (3) tissue healing would have been completed in at least X weeks or months including failure to respond to standard medical treatment, or (4) Waddell's or psychosocial signs indicate the patient is overreacting to the amount of pain stated. Their conclusion, based on the above, is that this patient's pain must be psychogenic. They turn to physicians for IMEs, with questions like "symptom magnification," a little gem which insurers and attorneys must insert. It is perhaps a key "magic word" to which too much emphasis in decision making is given.

POINT #1A

Avoid inappropriate or misapplication of terms that are subject to observer bias. The layman's understanding is rarely on the same level as the physician's, and misapplication may devastate a patient's case or life.

The two terms that can cause the most damage to an honest patient when misapplied are *symptom magnification* and *malingering* (see, for example, *Udvasi v. W.C.A.B.,* 667 A.2d 433 [Pa. Cmwlth. 1995]). The latter term should be avoided in a medical report as it is a legal term, not a medical one, and implies intent to fraud. If used, the physician must assume the burden of proof. Malingerers are rare, but when you do suspect one, convey the information in your records (i.e., "Mr. E. exhibits nonphysiologic pain), but avoid the term malingering; that is for the legal system to establish. When questioned about whether Mr. E. exhibited signs of malingering, an appropriate answer is that you (the examiner) do not determine malingering, as it is a legal not a medical term. Explain the meaning of certain patient responses (see below), when necessary.

Symptom Magnification

Remember the clinical state of the patient. Know your skills. Chronic pain patients are apprehensive and may exhibit pain avoidance based on past examinations on or about TrPs or other soft tissue areas. Pain coping behavior is a product of chronic pain syndromes. The skilled, knowledgeable clinician avoids the implications of symptom magnification by describing its clinical significance specific to the patient being examined. After the laying on of too many hands, pain anticipation and avoidance behavior can be expected. Without interpretation, lay people (insurers, lawyers, hearing officers, judges) may reach suspicious, unfounded conclusions, only because the medical system has failed to provide accurate information.

When reporting nonorganic or psychosocial signs, explain the significance or purpose of the sign, how you performed the examination technique, and if the results translate into meaningful clinical significance for that specific patient. That is, the examiner's skill to render a chronic myofascial pain patient's response to nonorganic signs as valid is a requisite.

The following has been done: Consider a person with no low back or leg problems or past history of injury. An MRI is performed, reporting a herniated nucleus palposis at L5 S1. Isn't it curious that no clinical signs either in the history or physical can be found? In this situation, the translation is that of an objective finding on CAT scan with no clinical objective findings. Do we treat the test or the patient?

Clinical Wisdom

Medicine's foundation is the physician's clinical examination (history and physical) and supersedes tests which are meant to serve and support.

All tests, clinical or laboratory, are subject to yielding false positives or false negatives. Psychosocial or nonorganic signs, such as Waddell's, can be influenced by many variables, which, in turn, reduce the sensitivity, leading to over- or misinterpretation by the examiner and inaccurate conclusions by the inquisitors.

POINT #1B

Many of us are familiar with Waddell's signs for nonorganic pain. If a patient has three of the five signs, it is suggestive that the pain is not organic; however, further investigation is warranted. My experience has been that many patients' reactions are *misinterpreted* by examiners unfamiliar with chronic pain patients and TrPs. A simple example of a commonly encountered misinterpretation is the "jump response." Patient verbalization and physical withdrawal from palpitation of a TrP are a response well known and documented in the pain literature.

An unknowing, biased, or untrained physician may report:

1. An overreaction (one of the five Waddell signs).
2. The patient's pain response diverges from accepted neuroanatomy.
3. The pain described by the patient does not follow the normal nerve or dematome patterns. Exactly! A characteristic of TrPs. They follow a reference zone unique to the involved muscle or tissue.
4. Patient exhibited "exaggerated pain behavior."
5. Bizarre pain response of functional pain reactions.
6. Exhibits signs of nonorganic pain or Waddell's signs are positive.

Hopefully, the above comments will cause the reader to focus more clearly when asked, "Does the patient exhibit signs of symptom magnification? The answer should not be a misunderstood label but descriptive of your unbiased findings. Insurers and attorneys have difficulty in determining the difference between a chronic pain patient with psychological pain coping behavior, one with pain of psychiatric origin, or those seeking secondary gains. It is our job to provide clinical facts, not terms or labels, to explain, without bias, the rationale of the patient's reactions.

An Issue on Clarification

Increasing numbers of cases and reports are applying and misinterpreting Waddell's and other nonorganic signs as being diagnostic of psychogenic pain or malingering, with devastating consequence to chronic pain patients. These signs are clinical tools and are diagnostic of nothing. They aid in understanding the patient. A clinician must determine: "Why is the patient reacting like this?" "What is he or she trying to tell me?" "What does it really mean?" Isn't it curious how truth dies so easily yet a lie lives forever? Because of the confusion associated with their usage, a quick review is in order.

The most familiar grouping of nonorganic or psychosocial signs is Waddell's, which consists of five types of physical signs. The article was published in *Spine* magazine in 1980, entitled "Non-Organic Physical Signs in Low Back Pain."

If three or more of the five signs are reported, it helps separate the physical from the nonorganic and clarify assessment of physical pathology. The paper suggested that these nonorganic signs could be used as a clinical screen for patients requiring further psychological testing. The paper emphasized that these signs are only one part of an assessment and should not be overinterpreted or substitute for a complete clinical examination or psychological profile.

In summary, if the patient has three or more of the five signs, it is suggestive that the pain is not organic; however, further investigation is warranted.

It has been this author's experience that many patients' reactions are misinterpreted by examiners unfamiliar with chronic pain patients and/or that they were untrained or unfamiliar with the examination technique of Waddell's signs (clinical validity). A simple example of a commonly encountered misinterpretation is the "jump response." The patient's verbalizations and physical withdrawal from palpation of the TrP are a response well known and documented in the pain literature.

POINT #2

Failure to discover an organic cause of pain when the past medical workups are noncontributory may be due to:

1. Overlooked tissue diagnosis (greatest probability).
2. The medical profession has not yet discovered the knowledge to understand this patient's cause of pain.
3. No health professional encountered had performed an adequate, in-depth history or examined the soft tissue.
4. An adversarial relationship existed.
5. Observer bias. Failure of the examiner to maintain neutrality.

In this author's exposure, some if not many IMEs fail to provide specific clinical details upon which a *working* diagnosis is based. Unless performed by a physician familiar with, experienced in, and trained in pain medicine and chronic myofascial pain syndromes, the diagnoses are vague and records review frequently exposes observer bias and misconceptions concerning the patient. The actual clinical condition of the patient can rarely be appreciated from medical records alone.

Numerous encounters with other specialties involved in pain cases reveals that some disciplines refuse to take soft tissue pain and diagnoses (notably TrPs with their nonanatomical reference zones and fibromyalgia) seriously or acknowledge their existence. Unawareness or lack of training is excusable but easily corrected with current pain medicine knowledge.

Grave concerns arise when physicians who examine, report, or testify regarding pain patients manifest their dogmatism, close-mindedness, or special interest by arriving at incorrect conclusions. Labeling or diagnosing a chronic pain patient as psychogenic, unsubstantiated by overwhelming evidence, will bring disaster, devastation, and potential irreversible damage to a patient's life and family. "If you can do no good, do no harm."

POINT #3

Reviewing Past Records: Some Clinical Hints

From experience, if I read all the patient's records, test results, and/or discuss the case to any extent with others, including the insurer, prior to my examination, it was difficult not to rely on previous findings or focus my attention in that direction during my evaluation and report writing, with a neutral approach (IMEs, legal referral, or first encounters with private patients).

My suggestions:

1. Avoid reading records or discussing the patient until after the initial examination is complete. Make your own diagnoses based on your examination findings and judgment. Do not allow prejudice to alter your neutrality and introduce observer bias.
2. Approach the patient as one who has chronic pain, not the patient's legal issues. It is the patient who has pain, not the pain that has the patient.
3. Practice the art of medicine. Hold the patient's hand if you have to. Establish rapport. If legal/insurance issues are involved, assure the patient that you are seeking answers that may have been overlooked. Your purpose is not to be adversarial, but to believe the patient.
4. Legal/insurance examinations. Since many chronic pain patients have been "through the system," their presentation may be one of suspicion, hostility, or frustration. Explain that some confusing issues exist and your intent is to conduct an examination, in a neutral manner, to determine the patient's present clinical condition. Make the patient part of the exam by petitioning him or her to provide details in his or her medical interview. Concerning the physical, ask the patient to indicate any specific areas or movements that are particularly painful or sensitive. (Representative of a prime example is the patient with reflex sympathetic dystrophy.) Reassurance that you will examine gently and be considerate of the patient's problematic areas while conducting the examination is a beneficial clinical tool to reduce "examination apprehension." Finally, tell the patient that the information derived from the examination will be presented to the interested parties to provide better understanding of the case.

In depositions, creating this habit provides credibility when your report or testimony conflicts with that of a colleague.

POINT #4

TrPs are objective, reproducible findings. Watch an attorney's facial expression when you deliver a "yes" to "Were there objective findings?"

The TrPs are:

1. Focally tender.
2. Palpable taut band of muscle.
3. Compression of the TrP by palpation:
   a. Reproduces patient's pain.
   b. Produces local twitch response.
   c. Produces referred pain or sensory zone specific to the involved muscle or soft tissue structures.
4. Pain of the TrPs is highly variable from day to day, week to week, etc. TrPs may be active, latent, secondary, etc. There can be single muscle myofascial pain, a chronic myofascial pain syndrome, or chronic enigmatic pain.
5. TrPs resolve when treated.

6. "Soft" objective or secondary findings are found, such as decreased range of motion, muscle weakness, decreased muscle tone, altered sensory responses, etc.

7. Emphasize that TrPs do not follow neuroanatomical pathways. They have their own zones or reference regions and their "mapping" is documented. This unique characteristic of TrPs is objective in itself. The above is well supported in the pain literature.

POINT #5

Pain Behavior

The opposing attorney will point out that you are not a psychiatrist. But, armed with Point #4, you can state with a "relative degree of medical certainty" that this patient does have *pain*.

1. Yes, the patient may exhibit overreaction or bizarre pain behavior that could be a sign of nonorganic or functional pain. Prior to your examination, due to an overlooked diagnosis, it seemed that the objective findings did not support the subjective complaints. It can be reemphasized that TrPs do not follow standard nerve, sensory, or anatomy pathways. They have their own unique reference zone, as mentioned above.

2. Some patients will present with dramatic pain behavior (i.e., nearly falling upon rising, swaying from one piece of office furniture to another, or "walking funny" [author prefers this over antalgic gait]). Why? After a long, devastating, undiagnosed pain state, these patients are subconsciously (sometimes) reaching out in desperation trying to prove that they do suffer pain. With previous workups being negative, they themselves question their mental state. They do experience an emotional reaction with pain coping behavior that in turn fuels the pain. Add that any patient in this situation experiences a physical and emotional component. One goes hand in hand with the other. Their pain state creates a reaching out with these "hands" seeking help, someone who will believe them.

3. Emphasize the therapeutic relationship derived from establishing physician/patient rapport. For the reasons above, the experiences the chronic pain patient has endured have left him or her a victim. The patient has lost control of his or her life. A physician need not be a psychiatrist to practice humanitarianism, understanding, and kindness, to recognize true suffering in a patient with pain — "the art of medicine."

4. Explain the validity of the chronic pain patient's response to nonorganic signs or overreaction to examination techniques. Their pain coping behavior is a known adaptive process, increasing and changing with time. With some variables, it is predictable. Perhaps as pain knowledge increases, clarifying this adaptive process could become an objective finding in the clinical history. Remember, this type of pain has no useful biological function to the body.

5. Finally, review the patient's work attitude and reaction to the possibility that function may be restored. These patients do want to get better and to return to a productive lifestyle and improve their quality of life. Those with psychiatric pain, seeking secondary gain, "malingerers," etc. are intimidated by the thought of restored functions. They may only agree to further treatment if they can be guaranteed to be "pain free."

Stress that the true chronic pain patient will display hope, and exhibit a positive attitude, based on your findings. When asked, "What do you wish to achieve from this relationship (doctor/patient)?" the responses of such patients may include that they want to return to some type of work, normal daily living, recreational activities, etc.

Key Point

Chronic pain patients will not open up and share their thoughts and concerns unless the examiner believes them. Belief is the foundation for restoring their lives; it is therapeutic. Belief sows the seeds of faith in themselves and trust in the examiner. Trust provides the hope of improvement. Hope breeds the willingness and encouragement to do whatever possible to find a new career and participate in their care. Finally, hope, faith, and trust restore the patient to the first step in regaining control of his or her life.

Such patients readily accept the probability that they may not be totally pain free, but exhibit hope of some restored function. When the first response is that they need someone to fill out an insurance form, well...

POINT #6

Focus on your findings and being unbiased, rather than a specific diagnosis. Questions that contain key "magic words" are often posed by insurers and attorneys, and the practitioner may be trapped into an answer. Qualify your response based on the findings of your medical interview, physical exam, and any records reviewed. If your conclusion is rendered hastily or not based on sound judgment and medical wisdom, you will be doing the patient a disastrous injustice. When a lawyer asks you, "Dr., is it possible?" keep in mind that anything is possible but it has to occur at least 51% of the time to be probable. A good answer would be, "Yes, it's possible, but not probable in this case."

Your description of the TrP, the characteristics found by palpation, coordinated with a history of the pain's onset, restricted motion, muscle-specific weakness, and pain distributions are the objective findings important to the case. The diagnosis should not be a misunderstood label, but descriptive of your findings. Diagnosis codes are limited in the pain field and require updating. Remember that the average lay person may be familiar with such terms as chronic fatigue syndrome and fibromyalgia, but will lack understanding. Remember, words are the tools of a lawyer.

Note: Fibromyalgia does have two objective findings:

1. Reproducible multiple tender points (literature states at least 11 of 18). They are sometimes erroneously referred to as TrPs but do not meet the clinical criteria. Patients with fibromyalgia can have TrPs, in addition to the tender points.
2. Stage IV disrupted sleep established by a sleep history and/or sleep study.

POINT #7

When asked if you disagree with other experts who have also examined the patient, use diplomacy. Rather than disagree with a colleague's findings, note that:

1. Medicine is an art, not a science. There is much to discover about pain, but like artists, we each have different approaches and techniques, different experiences and training.

2. Other medical experts conducted their examinations according to their training and expertise, as you did. Your reported opinion is based on the clinical data documented in your records, on which you based your conclusions.

3. Clinical medicine is a jigsaw puzzle, chronic pain is a multifaceted problem, and your conclusions just added one more piece. The previous examinations and reports, although negative, did provide you with information about organic diseases or pathophysiologic mechanisms that were not the cause of the patient's pain. Because their expertise and specialty excluded more serious problems, you were able to provide new conclusions using the tools of your training and experience, adding to the global evaluation of this patient.

Pain is a message, and you are the interpreter.

Be aware that throughout history experts have been wrong.
Those with open minds learn from nonexperts as well as their own experience.

Who the H__ wants to hear an actor talk?
—Harry M. Warner
Warner Brothers Studios, 1927
(an expert in motion pictures)

Knowledge is a Principle thing
but with all thy knowledge get thee understanding.

—Proverbs

The mere knowledge of a fact is pale;
but when you come to realize your fact
it takes on color. It is all the difference between
hearing of a man being stabbed to the heart
and seeing it done

—Mark Twain

You get a little too much costumery out of your statements.
Always dress a fact in tights, never an ulster (long loose heavy coat)
—Life on the Mississippi

On Specialists:
Given one well trained physician of the highest type
He will do better work for a thousand people than ten specialists.
—William J. Mayo

14 Reflex Sympathetic Dystrophy

Michael S. Margoles, M.D., Ph.D.
Sylvia H.

Reflex sympathetic dystrophy syndrome (RSDS) is a multisymptom, multisystem syndrome that affects one or more extremities, but may affect any part of the body. RSDS is a disabling disease with simultaneous involvement of nerve, skin, muscle, blood vessels, and bones. The sympathetic nervous system affects all tissue levels — skin, subcutaneous, fascia, muscle, synovium, and bone. The only common denominator in all reflex sympathetic dystrophy (RSD) patients is pain. All other symptoms or changes may or may not occur.

> RSD is an all inclusive term applied to a great variety of seemingly unrelated disorders. A clear concept of this disorder has been frustrated by the myriad of terms applied to the syndrome, lack of clear diagnostic criteria, the absence of proven therapeutic modalities and our poor understanding of its physiology.
>
> —G. Forde, M.D. (10/20/95)

Recently, the name of this syndrome has be changed to complex regional pain syndrome (CRPS).

In the past, numerous names have been used to describe the all-inclusive term RSDS (CRPS). These include minor causalgia, posttraumatic pain syndrome, posttraumatic spreading neuralgia, posttraumatic spreading arthrosis, Sudek's atrophy, shoulder–hand syndrome, sympathalgia, chronic traumatic edema, posttraumatic dystrophy, reflex neurovascular dystrophy, reflex dystrophy, and others.

What follows is a condensation of the literature on RSDS. However this "syndrome" is not as clear-cut as one might believe, based on the material presented. There are few absolute criteria for RSDS, and many of the findings to be discussed can be found in other clinical syndromes, such as fibromyalgia, myofascial pain syndrome, some of the arthritis conditions, and other medical disorders.

DIAGNOSIS

Some of the abnormalities that are seen in patients with RSDS are sensory abnormalities, abnormal blood flow, abnormal sweating, and weakness. It may manifest days, hours, or weeks after an injury. Pain is present in 90% of patients. Manifestations include increased hair growth, abnormal nail growth, and associated spasm of muscle or dystonia. Pitting or nonpitting edema is usually present and localized to the painful and tender region. It usually occurs in one or more extremities. The patient may demonstrate tremor and difficulty initiating movement. Vasomotor instability may be manifested by Raynaud's phenomenon, cool–pallid appearance, mottled discoloration, vasoconstriction, warmth, erythematous appearance, vasodilatation, or increased sweating.

Some patients experience periods of remission and exacerbation. Periods of remission may last for weeks, months, or years. A small percentage of patients have developed generalized RSD affecting the entire body. Minor injuries, such as a sprain or a fall, are frequent causes of RSDS. It can start immediately after the injury or up to 10 days later. One characteristic of RSDS is that the pain is more severe than expected for the type of injury that occurred. RSDS may subside for years and then recur with a new injury. The recurrence should be treated immediately.

Sympathetically maintained pain (SMP, the type found in cases of RSDS and some of the more severe cases of myofascial pain syndrome) is different from ordinary pain and should be suspected when the following occur (RSDS/SMP):

- It usually does not respond to conventional narcotic analgesics.
- Patient is in more pain than can be explained by physical abnormalities.
- The pain lasts longer than the expected healing time.
- These patients will frequently use characteristic words to describe their pain. The most commonly used are burning, hot, stabbing, and shooting. Others will describe feelings of aching, tightness, numbness, and tingling sensations.
- The pain is usually nondermatomal, except in cases of causalgia, where the pain follows the course of the injured nerve.

A number of precipitating factors have been associated with RSDS, including:

- Developed after visceral disease
- Developed after central nervous system lesion
- Trauma (often minor) ranks as the leading provocative event
- Ischemic heart disease and myocardial infarction
- Cervical spine or spinal cord disorders
- Cerebral lesions
- Infections
- Surgery
- Repetitive motion disorder or cumulative trauma, causing conditions such as carpal tunnel
- In many of the patients a definite precipitating event cannot be identified

Pain symptoms include:

- Severe
- Constant
- Burning
- Lancinating
- Frequently begins distally

- Follows neither a dermatomal nor plexus distribution
- Occurs in one or more extremities
- Pain is the most troubling feature of this illness (for most patients)
- Bilateral in 18–50% of cases
- Spreads in 70% of cases

Other symptoms include:

- Abnormalities in the motor system (weakness)
- Trophic changes in the superficial tissues (skin)
- Trophic changes in the deep tissues (muscle and/or bone)

The full-blown syndrome, which is easy to recognize, consists of:

- Distal extremity pain
- Diffuse swelling
- Smooth shiny skin with abnormal color
- Allodynia
- Joint pain and tenderness
- Juxta-articular osteoporosis
- Pitting or nonpitting edema is usually present and localized to the painful and tender region
- Decreased range of motion of the affected part; eventual development of dystrophy (hair loss, increased nail growth) and/or atrophy, tremor, difficulty initiating movement, focal dystonia (abnormal tissue or muscle tone), or skin changes:
  - Skin atrophy
  - Deep tissue atrophy
  - Dryness
  - Increased hair growth in involved area
  - Increased hair loss
  - Abnormal nail growth
  - Changes in skin temperature
  - Vasomotor instability
  - Raynaud's phenomenon
  - Cool–pallid
  - Mottled
  - Vasoconstriction
  - Warm
  - Erythematous
  - Vasodilatation
  - Increased sweating

When the hand is affected, there also appears to be a significant incidence of palmar fasciitis. There are numerous diffuse areas of abnormal tenderness. A small percentage of patients have developed generalized RSD affecting the entire body, manifested by abnormal blood flow, trophic changes in the bone, and increased uptake on radionuclide bone scan. Some patients with mechanical allodynia suffer slow temporal summation of burning pain when given mechanical stimuli at three strokes per second.

Specimens of synovial tissue are histologically abnormal. Varying degrees of synovial edema, proliferation of the capillaries, fibrosis of the subsynovium, and slight perivascular infiltration with chronic inflammatory cells (chiefly lymphocytes) are noted.

TREATMENT

RSD can be an extremely difficult and frustrating syndrome to treat. Avoiding immobilization after injury or surgery will clearly reduce the incidence of RSD. Other treatments that may be of value include:

1. Drug therapy
   - Local or systemic corticosteroids
   - Muscle relaxants
   - Alpha-adrenergic blockers
   - Beta blockers
   - Analgesics (weak or strong)
   - Nonsteroidal anti-inflammatory drugs
   - Tricyclics and related compounds
   - Tranquilizers
   - Calcium channel blockers
2. Blocks
   - Nerve blocks
   - Sympathetic blockade
   - Intravenous regional blocks
3. Physical therapy
4. Transcutaneous electrical nerve stimulation
5. Sympathectomy
   - Surgical
   - Cervical
   - Radiofrequency
6. Implantable devices
   - Dorsal column stimulator
   - Infusion pump
   - Peripheral nerve stimulator

COURSE OF THE DISEASE

Duration of RSDS varies. In some cases, the pain continues for at least 2 years and in some cases indefinitely. RSD spreads in 70% of patients. The usual pattern of spread is up the same extremity and then it may continue to spread on the same side of the body or to the opposite extremity. In stage 3 RSD, some patients may have RSDS spread throughout the whole body. The etiology and the underlying pathophysiology of RSDS are poorly understood. Both central and peripheral processes contribute to the clinical manifestations of RSD.

SYLVIA H.

Sylvia H. had many classic RSDS clinical findings, and the diagnosis had been established through examination by many clinicians over the years. When first seen, Sylvia was a 39-

year-old mother of two teenage daughters and a housewife. She had burning and pain that involved most of her body. She was quite helpless, because of her disease, and was very frustrated. The fingers of her left hand were rigidly flexed into the palm of her left hand. The fingers of her right hand were deformed and pointed in numerous directions. They had a bluish discoloration to them. They were useless. Her fingernails were uncut and looked like claws. The muscles of her forearms were extremely atrophied, but the muscles of her left forearm and upper arm were less so. One of her daughters accompanied her to help her with all activities she needed to do with her hands. She had classic finding of stage 3 RSD (see chart at the end of this chapter). She appeared very stressed, older than her stated age, and was downcast.

This is what Sylvia wrote about her disease and its course:

> I am a 40-year-old white female from Colorado Springs, Colorado, who sought last and final hope of medical attention with Dr. Michael of San Jose, California, for the first time in July of 1996.
>
> Oh my…where do I begin to describe what Dr. Michael's treatment has done for me?…
>
> As I referred to in my opening sentence, Dr. Michael was my final hope for any kind of medical treatment, as I had been informed by countless physicians here in Colorado that
>
> - I'm a hopeless case with zero hope.
> - Learn to accept and deal with what I have with the outlook only to worsen with more and more pain, fibrosis, atrophy and deteriorating with each passing day and then die.
> - However, even given all that, I would still live to be a ripe old age…
>
> For me this was not a viable option. I was already 95% bedridden with inhuman pain to the point of insanity; had to be fed, bathed, dressed, groomed; ostomy needs tended to; deteriorating/wasting nerves, tissue, muscles, and bones with atrophy and fibrosis; barely walking, sitting, or standing; in no way, shape, or form able to be a "wife," "mother," or "housewife." I couldn't/can't hold a job, was unable to do any kind of hobbies (which also were a source of income for this household) such as sewing, pottery, ceramics, woodwork, metalwork, macramé, meticulous beading, animal training (for obedience, police work, show/confirmation, etc.), horseback riding, skiing, swimming, gymnastics, buying/selling/trading art, etc. I became literally 100% dependent on family and friends for my every need, which damn near cost me my marriage and relationship with my teen children, as well as losing countless friends as they speculated that this disorder was/is contagious.
>
> Here I was now, 34/35 years of age, couldn't comprehend *what* was happening to me. The "pain" and migraine headaches were so intense, whereby it hurt to blink my eyes, cry, breathe, move, and so much as even to be touched. The fresh breeze from an open window whisking across me put me into hell. Just simple thought processes were an effort. Laying completely still was my only option to maintain an even insane pain level of a screaming 9.5 level (10 being the worst). Through not moving around, being active, or being a productive human being, because of all the pain, the tissues, muscles, and bones have literally deteriorated, rotted, and wasted, become fibrotic and atrophied…to the point where I became a breathing carcass. It was only a matter of time before I would become nonexistent.
>
> In 1991 I sought medical attention for the massive pain and the various deformities, tremors, spasms, etc. Little did I realize that my nightmare from hell would begin

when I was diagnosed with the letters R-S-D (reflex sympathetic dystrophy), and I was utterly *clueless* to what that was!!

Reflex sympathetic dystrophy gives physicians and the medical community the right to "humor" you with sugar tabs, ridicule you, refuse you as a patient, and/or kick you to the curb and bail out by simply stating, "This patient is above and beyond my capabilities and there is no known medical treatment existing for this disorder."

Reflex sympathetic dystrophy gives physicians and the medical community the right to "label" your medical records with "This patient is crazy, mentally ill, unbalanced, disturbed, a serious psychiatric case — recommend long-term extensive lockup psychiatric inpatient care; patient needs serious structured programs; consequences for her attitude and/or behavior"; etc. "The patient is making herself sick, making her body deformed, spasm etc.; it's childhood trauma, etc." It's unbelievable what I've been put through with physicians in Colorado. The icing on the cake came earlier this year at a university hospital, when after an extensive review of records and physical exams that were done by reflex sympathetic dystrophy "specialist" clinics/doctors, a "research" center...proclaimed that there was "nothing" they could do or have to offer; pain meds was not the answer, yet they didn't have any other answers, suggestions, options, etc. other than live with it, deal with it, come to terms with it, and get on with your life...This is the way you are. It's a sad case; the entire disorder will progressively take over *but* I should live to a ripe old age...

My thoughts were, I had no more thoughts. I was completely outraged with myself for not succeeding in snuffing myself off this planet; when the pain was sporadically severe for days or weeks or months at a time; when the movement, range of motion, and dexterity wasn't there sporadically for days, weeks, and months; when migraines were endless and the tremors and spasms were beating me up. All in the mid to late '80s, when I was completely bedridden. When the episodes passed, I would be fine once again for several days or weeks. Sore, but fine until the next time.

Upon the diagnosis of this reflex sympathetic dystrophy in '91 and everything that was attempted failed...I was determined to snuff myself off the face of this planet, as I was *not* going to go through life like this, as I wouldn't put my own dogs, horses, bird, cat, or fish through it. However I failed at that too because of the lack of movement, energy, dexterity, etc. and I was being supervised too closely.

After the medical community bailed out right and left, I proceeded to consult a Dr. Kevorkian, as I now needed assistance in what I needed to do. However, family kept intervening with the telephone number and address, as well as this doctor was in high demand and very hard to get ahold of.

Family and friends kept pleading with me to keep looking for a resolution. A friend told me of a show being aired on TV and encouraged me to watch it. That was in '94; Dr. Harvey Rose had addressed some real breakthroughs in pain management, but he wasn't from Colorado, he was in northern California; Nonetheless, I contacted the TV station to obtain Dr. Rose's telephone number and address.

I contacted Dr. Rose, explained my situation, etc. However, because of the airing of the show featuring the doctor, he had been inundated with telephone calls and was not accepting any more patients, but he did have the name and telephone number of a lady in Denver, Colorado, who was in a similar situation and was coming to California for medical treatment and was putting something together to try to change Colorado physicians' attitudes and Colorado laws about pain management.

I contacted this lady and we spoke for several hours about each other's situation. Two hours into our conversation, she told me of a Dr. Michael and what he's done for her and gave me his telephone number.

I contacted Dr. Michael, explained my dilemma, and was scheduled with an evaluation appointment. One thing led to another and Colorado doctors committed themselves with promises, treatments, etc. Thus I scrapped the appointment with Dr. Michael. All the promises of treatment, etc. by Colorado doctors were nothing more than false hopes and empty promises.

Desperate people do desperate things. I was informed of great hope down in Mexico for very inexpensive rates; very innovative, latest and greatest medical technology without the process of the FDA that the United States has. So off to Mexico we went. It's unbelievable the number of Americans down in Mexico in the same crisis that I was. Incredibly, to make a very long story short, Mexico is not the place to go. The name of the game down there is the American greenback. Needless to say, those trips ceased within 6 months.

By the end of the first quarter of 1996, almost 6 years into the diagnosis of this reflex sympathetic dystrophy, 15/16 years since the first symptoms and onset of "pain"...medical treatment that stretched from standard conventional to nonconventional to Chi Gong to T'ai Chi to that TV pain button to herbs to homeopathic meds to teas to therapy (occupational and physical), I was finished, beaten to the ground like a wild severely injured animal. I turned to my husband, pleading for him to assist me in ending my life. Let me go where there is no more pain and suffering, where there's light (as I've remained in dark to very dim rooms), where there's life and noise, etc. He found my request unfair, selfish, a cop-out, and cited our wedding vows — "in sickness and in health, for better or worst, rich or poor." Because of "love," he didn't want to let me go...Needless to say, we seriously butted heads, as I strongly feel that as an intelligent, bright, thinking, rational, thinking human being you have the right to a "quality" life. When that's gone, you should have the right to terminate yourself.

Although I saw absolutely no more hope and everything was all too late to turn around, family and friends encouraged me to call and set an appointment with Dr. Michael. Give him a chance, see what he has to say, offer, diagnose, etc.

Reluctantly, I did set an appointment with Dr. Michael with the attitude, "Yeah, right! There we go again. Yet another doctor who will bail out and say, 'Gee, I'm so sorry. It's above and beyond my capabilities. There's no treatment. I have nothing to further offer you.'" Yes, I had a negative attitude that wouldn't quit, but I did go and attempted to have an open mind; humor my family and friends by going. I had long since given up any kind of hope, treatment, improvement, etc. I was being punished by fate and was destined to die a very horrible way fully knowledgeable, as this reflex sympathetic dystrophy doesn't affect the mind. The only reason you're "touched" is because of the pain, and nobody but nobody sees it or hears it.

Anyway, I did fly to San Jose, California, with a great deal of assistance from my oldest daughter, and I went to see Dr. Michael.

On the very first two back-to-back visits, Dr. Michael had fully reviewed my medical records. I had filled out a very extensive questionnaire for the doctor. We spoke in great detail and did a full exam from head to toe. Truly, it was the exam from hell, and all I kept wishing for is that Dr. Michael would put me out of my endless misery. Which he did upon the completion of all his exams, but not in the way I had hoped for. He discovered that I had severe pain. After the examination, Dr. Michael injected a heavy-duty dose of narcotics (4 mg of Dilaudid®, a very powerful pain-relieving medication) into my hip. As God is my witness, within 8–10 minutes, for the first time in *years* I was virtually almost totally "pain" free. I never imagined in all my wildest of dreams (and I've had many) that this was ever possible.

Between July '96 and August '96, I went back out to California for another 2-day back-to-back appointment with Dr. Michael and a telephone conference in between the two trips; various adjustments were made with meds, further researching, goal setting, and so forth.

Upon the second trip and appointment, Dr. Michael performed another very extensive physical exam, making measurements and so forth. Further adjustments were made with meds, vitamins, occupational and physical therapy, etc.

In summary, from July 1996 (the first trip and set of appointments with Dr. Michael, arriving with an 8.9–9.5+ "pain" level) through mid-November 1996 (4 months), Dr. Michael's treatment, concept, and approach have done more for me than any doctor's previous attempts. Before, I was only getting worse with each passing day because of the narrow attitudes of those attempting to treat me.

In just 4 months, Dr. Michael has begun to give me my life back and has added "quality" and "meaning" back into life.

You know, you don't know what you got until it's gone and just how much we take for granted and simply demand and expect.

It has been all uphill; by no means am I saying it's been overnight...With the treatment from Dr. Michael, the following leaps and bounds have taken place since July '96:

- I have more endurance and energy. I am up at about 7:30 a.m. and out of bed by 10:00 a.m. Resting mid-afternoon and back up by 4:00 p.m.; slowing down by 8:00 p.m.
- Sleeping by 1:00 a.m. Before seeing Dr. Michael, I was 95%+ bedridden in a dark/dim bedroom with little to zero noise, in constant agony, tears rolling uncontrollably because of the pain. Not sleeping, unless it was out of pure exhaustion and crashing, etc.

Before I continue, my "pain" on a scale of 1 to 10

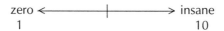

Before, it was a *constant* 8.5–10+. After seeing Dr. Michael, it's down to 0.5–1.5 with the meds, which has produced the following effects:

- The tremors, spasms, etc. are down to a minimum. Before, they were beating the crap out of me, causing the pain to go to 10+.
- I am able to do light housework such as dusting, sweeping, mopping, vacuuming, laundry, microwave cooking, grilling, cooking (when it's all prepped and set up), wiping down the bathroom and home, watering the garden and yard, rounding up trash throughout the home and relining all the trash cans with plastic liners, pressing and ironing clothes and towels (and sheets with assistance); feeding the dogs, cats, bird and wildlife; walking the dogs and horse; *drive*; take care of errands; light shopping. Before it was *zero.*
- As for personal things for myself, I am feeding myself food and liquid with utensils, pedestal mugs, and glasses and am able to serve myself. With some assistance I bathe, shave, do my hair, dry myself, tend to my ostomy needs, get dressed, and put on makeup. I am able to sit, stand, lay down, walk, and go up and down stairs without assistance 85% of the time. I am doing simple sewing and crafts; learning the computer; playing with the dogs, bird, and horse; ride the horse once or twice per week in the round pen on an easy walk; am able to sit, stand, walk, and lay for 1½ to 2 hours at a time; and

can make love once every 7–10 days or so. Before: *zero*. (Editors' note: Because of her hand deformities, Sylvia had to obtain special voice-sensitive equipment for her computer.)

I now have a reason and a purpose to live...there's some form of "quality" to my life. I'm not this angry, bitter, enraged, snappy, demanding, hostile little bitch anymore. I have regained patience, reasoning, endurance, self-esteem, self-worth, etc. I can now be touched, hugged, and cuddled without going to hell and beyond. I can feel attractive again, as I can polish and groom up with nice outfits, makeup, *and* my fingernails can be cut (without anesthesia), filed, and polished! I don't feel ashamed, embarrassed, humiliated, and like a burden so much anymore, as I don't have to be tended to for my every need, whim, wish, and desire. I can now do for myself again! And it's great! *No one* can even begin to imagine unless they've been where I was at just a tad over 4 months ago.

All this doesn't come without tremendous effort, cost, meds, and opioids. Dilaudid-HP® (1 cc) plus lidocaine 2% with 2 cc injected every 3 hours along with a Duragesic® patches (100–150 µg/hour every 3 days) and oral and injectable vitamins are some of the major ingredients that have been very influential in turning my severe pain problem around. These all combine to bring my "pain" down to damn near nothing, enabling me to do therapy, water therapy, occupational/physical therapy throughout the day, sleep/rest, and progress back into life whereby I do for myself, tend to my personal needs, and do for others. It's great to be able to clean again, garden, and interact with people, animals and life again — be a part of life again. What a feeling!

Without Dr. Michael, I wouldn't be where I'm at today. For that matter, I don't believe I'd be alive right now, that I could have guaranteed you. Truly, the dreams that I'd had were believed to be impossible. It was all too far gone. Never in a million years did I dream that anything was ever possible for me again — *only* to be shot down and stomped on. It only goes to show that dreams and hopes are never not obtainable. It takes a lot of determination *and* most of all the right physician who is innovative, open-minded, and not afraid to take all higher education, research, and knowledge and follow through on his/her "oaths" to heal the sick and make them well again, to relieve pain and suffering, etc. Between state and federal laws and health insurance companies, today's physicians aren't allowed to be doctors anymore. They're practicing "legal peer group" medicine and the hell with the patient. Let's just leave it at that and not get me started. The past is best left in the past. As I firmly believe had I been treated properly and the "pain" more aggressively addressed, this reflex sympathetic dystrophy would never have progressed the way it did. On the road of a destructive, deforming, agonizing path. However, I would have lived to be a ripe old age. Oh goodie!

Anyway, my goals and plans are to continue to make the trips to San Jose, California, to see Dr. Michael to continue with the program. I look forward to becoming more and more independent and regaining movement and dexterity to as close to 100% as possible. Through usage, I hope that the muscle atrophy and joint deformities go away. If not, I'll have the hands reconstructed so they'll work and be attractive again and it is hoped that someday no meds will be needed to function and that the body can stay out of pain on it's own.

ASSESSMENT CRITERIA

If you think you have or your client/patient has RSDS, use the criteria below to assess the stage of involvement.

Code: check mark = present or done, blank = absent, ? = probably present, X = intermittent.

Stage 1 (acute stage)
___ Onset of constant severe burning pain closely limited to the site of injury
___ Hyperesthesia
___ Localized edema
___ Muscle spasm
___ Stiffness and limited mobility
___ Vasospasms: at onset, skin usually warm, red, and dry and then changes to cyanotic, cold, and sweaty
___ Average duration of stage 1 is 3 months; in mild cases, this stage lasts a few weeks and then subsides spontaneously or responds rapidly to treatment
___ Hyperhydrosis
___ Allodynia (pain is produced by stimuli that do not normally induce pain, such as touch, pressure, and warmth)
___ Hyperpathia
___ Hyperalgesia
___ X-rays reveal no bony changes
___ Bone scan with ^{99}Tc shows uptake by the small joints
___ Can last 6 weeks to 6 months

Stage 2 (dystrophic state)
___ Pain becomes even more severe and more diffuse
___ Edema spreads and changes from soft to a brawny type
___ Hair becomes scant; nails become brittle, cracked, and heavily grooved
___ Spotty osteoporosis occurs early but may become severe and diffuse
___ Increased thickness of joint
___ Muscle wasting
___ Stage 2 may last 3–6 months
___ Marked allodynia
___ Marked hyperalgesia (increased sensitivity and lowered threshold to painful stimuli (such as occurs in a superficial burn of the skin)
___ Diffuse osteoporosis or periarticular demineralization may be visible on X-ray
___ Bone scan shows increased uptake

Stage 3 (atrophic stage)
___ Marked trophic changes become irreversible
___ For many patients, the pain becomes intractable and may involve the entire limb
___ Atrophy of the muscles, in particular the interossei of the hand or foot, is marked
___ Interphalangeal and other joints of the foot or hand have become extremely weak; have limited motion and may finally become ankylosed
___ Contraction of flexor tendons occurs and occasionally subluxations are produced
___ Bone deossification has now become marked and diffuse
___ Burning pain and allodynia may become less severe
___ The skin becomes smooth, glossy, drawn, and pale or cyanotic and the skin temperature is decreased
___ The nails become increasingly brittle and ridged, with lateral arching
___ Subcutaneous tissue is very atrophic, with marked decrease in the fat pads, and the digits thin and pointed
___ The interphalangeal and other joints of the foot or hand are extremely weak, having limited motion and finally become ankylosed

GLOSSARY OF MEDICAL TERMS

Allodynia. Pain is produced by stimuli that do not normally induce pain (such as touch, pressure, and warmth).

Ankylosis. Stiffening or fixation of a joint.

Atrophy. A wasting of a normal developed organ or tissue due to degeneration of cells. This may be due to disease, aging, or undernutrition.

Autonomic nervous system. The part of the nervous system responsible for the control of bodily functions that are not consciously directed, including heartbeat, intestinal movements, sweating, etc.

Bone deossification. Demineralization of bone.

Brawny edema. Thickening and dusky discoloration of edematous tissue.

Causalgia. Severe burning-type pain following injury to a nerve.

Cyanotic. Blue color due to decreased oxygen in blood or decreased blood flow.

Dystonia. A state of abnormal tissue or muscle tone.

Dystrophy. Progressive changes that may result from defective nutrition of tissue.

Edema. Excessive accumulation of fluid in body tissue.

Etiology. Cause of a specific disorder.

Fascia. Connective tissue forming membranous layers of variable thickness in all regions of the body.

Fibrosis. Thickening and scarring of connective tissue.

Flexor tendons. Tendons that bend.

Hyperalgesia. Increased sensitivity and lowered threshold to painful stimuli (such as occurs in a superficial burn of the skin).

Hyperesthesia. Oversensitivity to touch and light pressure.

Hyperhydrosis. Excessive sweating.

Hyperpathia. Excessive reaction to painful stimuli. The pain increases too rapidly and lasts longer than usual.

Interphalangeal. Pertaining to the joints of the fingers.

Intractable. Resistant to treatment.

Ischemia. Pertaining to an inadequate blood supply.

Neurovascular. Relating to the nerves of the walls of blood vessels.

Osteoclastic. Breaking down bone tissue.

Osteoporosis. Thinning of the bone.

Palmar fasciitis. Thickening of the tissue in the palm of the hand.

Pathogenesis. The mode of origin of any disease.

Pathophysiology. Derangement of function seen in disease.

Periphery. The part of the body away from the center.

Perivascular infiltration. The abnormal entry of a substance around blood vessels.

Raynaud's phenomenon. Spasm of the arteries of the toes or fingers with paleness and numbness of the fingers.

Reflex. A reaction, an involuntary movement or response to a stimulus applied to the periphery and transmitted to the nerve centers in the brain or spinal cord.

Stimulus. Anything that arouses action in the muscles, nerves, or other excitable tissue.

Subcutaneous. Beneath the skin.

Subluxation. An incomplete dislocation.

Sympathetic nervous system. One of two divisions of the autonomic nervous system (the other is the parasympathetic) having fibers leaving the central nervous system via a chain of ganglia close to the spinal cord.

Syndrome. A combination of signs and/or symptoms that form a distinct clinical picture indicative of a particular disorder.

Synovium. Lining of a joint that produces lubricating fluid.

Thermography. A study to measure heat produced by different parts of the body.

Trophic. Resulting from interruption of nerve supply.

Vascularity. Relating to blood vessels.

Vasoconstriction. Narrowing of blood vessels.

Vasodilatation. Widening of blood vessels.

Vasomotor. Causing widening or narrowing of blood vessels, denoting the nerves which have this action.

Vasosapasm. Contraction of the muscle coats of blood vessels.

BIBLIOGRAPHY

Forde, G. (1995). RSD lecture to the Pain Interest Group, University of California San Francisco Medical Center.

Reflex Sympathetic Dystrophy Association pamphlet, pp. 1–15.

RECOMMENDED REFERENCES AND READING

Barolat, G., Schwartzman, R., and Woo, R. (1987). Epidural spinal cord stimulation in the management of reflex sympathetic dystrophy, *Applied Neurophysiology,* 50, 442–443.

Bonica, J.J. (1990). Causalgia and other reflex sympathetic dystrophies, *Postgraduate Medicine Journal,* 6, 53–145.

Bonica, J.J. et al. (1990). Causalgia and other reflex sympathetic dystrophies, in *Management of Pain,* 2nd ed., Lea & Febiger, Philadelphia, pp. 234–235.

Cronin, K.D. and Kirsner, R.L.G. (1982). Diagnosis of reflex sympathetic dysfunction. Use of the skin potential response, *Anaesthesiology,* 37, 848–852.

Database RSDSA.

Ficat, P. and Hungerford, D. (1977). Reflex sympathetic dystrophy disorders of patello femoral joint, in *Reflex Sympathetic Dystrophy,* Williams & Wilkins, Baltimore, chap. 9.

Hannington-Kiff (1992). Reflex Sympathetic Dystrophy Is Triggered by Failure of Natural Opioid Modulation in the Regional Sympathetic Ganglia, P.S.N.S., a publication on Pain and the Sympathetic Nervous System, Winter 1992.

Hendier, N., Uematsu, S., and Long, D. (1982). Thermographic validation of physical complaints in "psychogenic pain" patients, *Journal of the Academy of Psychosomatic Medicine,* 23(3).

Hunter, Schneider, Mackin, and Callahan (1983). Reflex sympathetic dystrophy. Rehabilitation of the hand, in *Reflex Sympathetic Dystrophy,* 2nd ed., Lankford, L. (Ed.), C.V. Mosby, St. Louis, chap. 47.

Kajander, K.C. (1990). Dynorphin increases in the dorsal spinal cord with a painful peripheral neuropathy, *Peptides,* 2, 719–728.

Knobler, R.L. (1992). The Pathogenesis of RSD: Immune and Viral Mechanisms, lecture presented at Thomas Jefferson University Medical College, April 10–11.

Kozin, F. (1979). Painful shoulder and the reflex sympathetic dystrophy syndrome, in *Arthritis & Allied Conditions,* 9th ed., Lea & Febiger, Philadelphia, pp. 1091–1120.

Kozin, F., McCarty, D.J., Sims, J., and Gonant, H. (1976). The reflex sympathetic dystrophy syndrome. 1. Clinical & histologic studies: evidence for bilaterality, response to corticosteroids and articular involvement. *AWMad,* 60, 321–331.

Malament, L.B. and Glick, J.B. (1983). Sudeck's atrophy, the clinical syndrome, *Journal of the American Pod. Association,* 73(7), 362–368.

Mays, K. et al. (1981). Stellate ganglion blocks with morphine in sympathetic type pain, *Journal of Neurology, Neurosurgery, and Psychiatry,* 44, 189–190.

Poplawski, Z.J., Wiley, A.M., and Murray, J.F. (1983). Post-traumatic dystrophy of the extremities, *Journal of Bone and Joint Surgery,* pp. 642–655.

Price, R.W. et al. (1975). Latent infection of the peripheral ANS with herpes simplex virus, *Nature,* 257, 686–688.

Raja, S. and Hendier, N. (1990). in *Sympathetically Maintained Pain, Current Practice in Anesthesiology,* 2nd ed., Rogers, M. and Decker, B.C. (Eds.), Mosby Year Book, St. Louis, pp. 421–425.

Raja, S.N. et al. (1991). Systemic alpha-adrenergic blockade with phentolamine: a diagnostic test for sympathetically maintained pain, *Anesthesiology,* 74, 691–698.

Roberts, W.J. (1986). A hypothesis on the physiological basis for causalgia and related pains, *Pain,* 24, 297–311.

Schwartzman, R.J. Submitted to the *Handbook of Clinical Neurology.*

Schwartzman, R. and McLellan, T. (1987). Reflex sympathetic dystrophy, a review, *Archives of Neurology,* 44, 555–561.

Schwartzman, R.J. et al. (1990). The movement disorder of reflex sympathetic dystrophy, *Neurology,* 40, 57–61.

Spebar, M.J., Rosenthal, D., Collins, G.J., Jarstfor, B.S., and Walters, M.J. (1981). Changing trends in causalgia, *American Journal of Surgery,* 142, 744–746.

Teeple, E. and Ghia, J.N. (1983). Considerations in the treatment of causalgia, *Anes,* 58, 294.

Uematsu, S., Hendler, N., Hungerford, D., Long, D., and Ono, N. (1981). Thermography and electromyography in the differential diagnosis of chronic pain syndromes and reflex sympathetic dystrophy, *Electromyography in Clinical Neurophysiology,* 21, 165–182.

Waiz, M.A. et al. (1974). Latent ganglionic infection with herpes simplex virus type 1 and 2: viral reactivation in vivo after neurectomy, *Science,* 184, 1185–1187.

Section III

Psychology

15 Psychological and Behavioral Management Approaches to Chronic Pain

David A. Devine, Ph.D.

The fact that psychological approaches could have an impact on chronic pain relates to the reality that what we do, think, and feel has an effect on our experience of chronic pain. For instance, we know that when we tense up our muscles to pain, we intensify our pain experience. This occurs for several reasons. For one thing, tensing cuts off the blood supply and flow of nutrients to an area in which they are much needed in order to heal. This is called dysponesis or "faulty bracing." We also know that when you think negative thoughts regarding your pain experience and other life experiences, your perceived pain will increase. Lastly, when you feel anxious or depressed, you are much more likely to perceive painful stimuli.

In describing the theories and techniques which I feel are useful in conquering chronic pain, I think it is important to place the comments in context. In my practice as a fee-for-service outpatient psychological health service provider, patients are referred primarily by other health service providers (i.e. physicians, dentists, nurses, chiropractors, and psychotherapists). If the patient comes in without a treating physician, I insist that he or she establish a relationship with one and obtain a complete medical examination. The next step in my office is obtaining a complete evaluation of the patient's pain situation. This includes, but is not limited to, a review of medical and psychosocial history and records, a description of any physical and/or psychological traumas, medications taken, surgeries, brief life history, and current psychosocial status. Psychological aspects of the problem may be evaluated additionally by paper-and-pencil questionnaires and tests.

The next step usually involves the application of biofeedback and relaxation-based therapies to counteract the effects of dysponesis (faulty bracing) and autonomic overarousal. As noted above, dysponesis involves abnormal tensing up or bracing the muscles in response to external or internal stimuli. The effect of releasing dysponesis can be to decrease pain. The most direct approach to decreasing faulty bracing is through the use of electromyography biofeedback. This biofeedback modality involves the placement of electrodes directly over the affected level of tension in the muscle. With proper training, the patient is able to learn how to consciously let go of muscle tension. With conscientious practice both at home and in the office, this process soon becomes automatic.

1-57444-103-5/99/$0.00+$.50
© 1999 by CRC Press LLC

Autonomic overarousal refers to the overactivation of that part of the nervous system which controls respiration, heart rate, constriction of the blood vessels, and other body regulatory responses. An example of this process would be the way adrenalin is released into the body when a threat is perceived. A charge of energy known as the "fight or flight" response is immediately felt throughout the body. This primitive response causes the heart rate to accelerate, the sweat response to increase, and the pupils to dilate. These responses increase a person's chance for survival in a life or death situation by preparing him or her to combat an enemy or run away. However, in modern times, the threat is usually something that the autonomic response won't help us deal with (e.g., a critical boss, rush hour traffic, or perhaps pain). Biofeedback approaches teach the self-regulation of overarousal usually using either temperature training and/or GSR training. By learning to increase the amount of peripheral circulation through hand-warming or to decrease the amount of sweat response, autonomic balance is achieved. This learning process is enhanced by the patient completing about 20–30 minutes of home stress management exercises on a daily basis.

As the patient begins to acquire the skills of self-regulation, the next level of skill to develop is that of cognitive restructuring. This refers to helping the individual shift or change his or her ways of thinking away from those thoughts which promote pain perception. Examples of pain-promoting thoughts would be: "I can't be happy as long as I experience pain." "I'll never get better." "What did I do to deserve this pain?" "I can't stand it!" These negative thoughts can be controlled by identifying them and then making an effort to change them. Sometimes these thoughts are readily apparent in the person's thinking and conversation. At other times they exist as part of the individual's unconscious messages and must be identified through interaction with a skilled psychotherapist. A process of inquiry on the part of the patient and the psychotherapist is often helpful in identifying where in the patient's history he or she first came to believe the negative and pain-promoting statements. Once this has been done and worked with, it becomes possible to let go of these entrenched and harmful ideas.

People often pick up painful pain scripts in childhood as a result of experience with pain personally or with a family member. For example, a patient may have been sick as a child from either trauma or disease. In coping with sickness, the parents may have been oversolicitous. Because of this, the child may have started to use pain or disability for attention. This type of situation is most likely to develop in a family where one or both of the parents have problems with personal inadequacy and guilt. In such a situation, parents may try to make up for their inadequacy or guilt by doing too much for the child and making him or her too dependent. Gradually the child learns that he or she can get his or her needs met not by functioning in a normal assertive active way, but by functioning in an abnormal passive and dependent way. Such learning may also take place vicariously when a parent is chronically ill. In such a situation, where the parent may tend to be overconcerned about his or her own health status or where the parent is operating at a regressed dependent level, this serves as a model for the child, which is learned and quickly internalized. Of course, adults can also learn maladaptive behavior from chronic illness and their treatment by those around them. As Pawlicki so vividly points out in his chapter on pain and the family, sometimes family members reinforce maladaptive pain behavior on the part of their members. Usually this is done with the best of intentions.

Psychotherapy can be particularly helpful in assisting the individual to work through the grief and feelings of loss generated by chronic pain. Chronic pain usually involves the loss of some physical and/or psychological ability. The reaction one has to this loss is similar to the loss of a loved one. Just as we invest emotional energy in loved ones, we also invest psychic energy in our physical body and psychological self-image. When either or both of these are damaged or diminished, we experience loss if the loss is ongoing and a chronic grief process may ensue.

In the case of acute pain, which by definition is limited in duration (technically less than 6 months), one does not undergo this grief process because the loss is not perceived as permanent. An individual therefore may be anxious when in acute pain and fearful, but not depressed or grief stricken.

In the case of chronic pain as in the loss of a loved one, the first task of working through the loss is accepting the reality of the loss (Worden, 1982). This process may be blocked, however, by denial. Denial is believing there is a magical cure for the pain problem, when in reality there is none. The patient enacts this denial by going from doctor to doctor attempting to find an external and complete cure for the problem. Psychologists refer to this psychological attitude as one of external locus of control. This means believing that one's behavior and destiny are controlled by forces outside one's control. One of the major tasks for the psychotherapist in attempting to help chronic pain patients is to help them change their locus of control from external to internal. This involves the confrontation that they are going to have to take primary responsibility for dealing with effects of the pain. It is at the point at which the patient becomes an active participant in the healing process that a shift in behaviors and attitudes takes place. The patient no longer is searching from doctor to doctor in hope of a magical and total cure. He or she may consult a variety of health care specialists, but with a different attitude than before. This new attitude may be demonstrated by the question, "How can we work together to improve my situation?" rather than demanding "Fix me" or "This is all your fault."

If the patient does not face his or her situation and deal with his or her loss, he or she is very likely to become depressed. Depression is a clinical condition which is manifested by the following: depressed mood, markedly diminished interest in almost all activities, significant weight loss or weight gain, insomnia or sleeping too much, agitation or slowing down, feelings of worthlessness, diminished ability to think or concentrate, indecisiveness, and recurrent thoughts of death. Most chronic pain patients go through a period when they are depressed. This could be mistaken by an unsympathetic observer as some process or "disease" which resides inherently in the patient. Quite the contrary however. We must understand that depression is the result of a complex interaction of biological, behavioral, cognitive, and emotional factors. In order to deal with it, interventions can take place in any of these domains. From the biological level, antidepressant medications may be prescribed. From the behavioral level, exercise and other physical activities may be recommended. For the emotional and cognitive components, cognitive restructuring and psychotherapy may be necessary.

EMOTIONS AND PAIN

Depression is usually associated with the emotion of sadness encountered in the chronic pain patient. Two other basic human emotions are also usually present at some point in the chronic pain experience: fear and anger. Let's look at each.

Fear is often more predominant and obvious in the acute pain situation. Immediately after the shock of injury has subsided, the individual may be fearful of death or further injury. This fear produces the autonomic arousal of the fight or flight response. Prehistorically, and in life or death situations such as an accident or battlefield situation, fear would be an adaptive emotion because it would motivate the individual to do something to remove himself or herself from the situation and give him or her the wherewithal to do so. However, if the fear continues over a period of time (e.g., months), it can change into what is commonly known as anxiety. Anxiety is a state of chronic fear. It can take the cognitive form of worry about the future in terms of health, finances, relationships, family, or any number of other concerns. Patients may begin to fear that they will never get well, that their spouses will leave them, that they will lose many if not all the material assets that they have acquired, and social rejection will occur (i.e., the fear that others will condemn them for being lazy or faking). Of course, some of the physical components of anxiety are those of tight bracing muscles, shallow breathing, and cardiovascular changes noted earlier.

Anger is often the least obvious emotion present in the chronic pain situation. This is because it is often camouflaged by resentment and as such seems to smolder rather than to be actively exhibited. The resentment is basically chronic anger that has become more passive and latent rather than active and overt. It may manifest as resentment against an employer, a family member, or some other external entity. It may also appear as anger toward one's body or a body part. Anger is a very powerful emotion and in an acute situation may adaptively mobilize the individual toward action, as does fear. However, in the chronic form of resentment, it leads to the long-term stress-producing reactions of fight or flight in much the same manner as fear.

As noted above, cognitive therapy, psychotherapy, and biofeedback-based relaxation therapy are effective techniques for changing these emotions. They address the cognitive, physical, and behavioral components of these problematic emotions. Another way to deal with negative emotions is to increase one's "happiness response." There are a number of ways to bring this about, but one of the simplest and most straightforward ways is to increase one's "serum fun level." Dr. Richard Kroenings created the concept of serum fun level as a logical extension of conventional medical measurements like serum cholesterol levels — an important indicator of well-being. Dr. David Bresler (1979) followed up on this idea by prescribing to his patients that they complete a number of fun activities each week. Often these activities are ones which patients used to do but no longer engage in as a result of being stuck in a chronic pain situation.

SEX AND CHRONIC PAIN

It has been estimated that "over half of the patients with chronic pain will have a deterioration in the frequency and quality of sexual activity — a percentage equal to the highest rate of sexual problems seen in any group of nonpsychiatric patients" (Maruta, 1982). This problem has often been overlooked by health providers, and many times patients are reluctant to discuss it as well. Specifically, the pain patient is less likely than the spouse to identify sexual dysfunction in the marriage as a problem. This may be due to the difficulty in acknowledging a problem which may have a psychological component. If the problem is not acknowledged and dealt with, however, it may lead to further resentment on the part of the spouse. In a circular fashion, the buildup of resentment leads to further sexual dysfunction.

The onset of a chronic pain problem changes the relationship of the marital pair. In doing so, the couple is called upon to use communication skills to cope with the change. If communication skills are underdeveloped, coping may suffer, hence diminishing the sexual relationship. The place to start in dealing with the problem is assessing each spouse's needs and desires for sexuality. Then feelings about these needs should be explored in a constructive nonblaming atmosphere. Ways can then be developed to meet the needs for sex and intimacy while preserving self-esteem in each partner.

It should be noted that prescription drug use and dependency are major causes of sexual problems in chronic pain patients. The use of sedatives and analgesics may negatively affect sexual functioning. Once an individual has withdrawn from sedatives, narcotics, and tranquilizers, there may result an increase in sexual functioning.

HYPNOSIS AND IMAGERY

Hypnosis and imagery are extremely useful procedures in healing and pain control. Individuals with hypnotic talent are able to develop numbness in parts of the body through self and hetero suggestion. One such procedure is called glove analgesia. After induction of a hypnotic state, the patient is asked to imagine a bucket full of a powerful transparent anesthesia being placed in front of him or her. The patient is then asked to dip his or her hand in the bucket slowly, absorbing as much of the anesthesia as possible. This results in a numb, woodenlike sensation. Next the patient is asked to place his or her hand on the painful area and allow the sensations of numbness to flow into the area and allow the painful sensations to flow into the hand. Subsequently, the hand is dipped as many times as necessary to obtain maximum relief.

Hypnosis may be used for other effects as well. It may be used to expand the sense of the passage of time so that the patient may experience an increased period of pain relief, or it may be used to decrease the subjective sense of how long a pain episode has lasted. Hypnosis combined with imagery may be used to uncover any psychological needs or issues which may be inhibiting pain relief. These may be such issues as resentment, grieving, perfectionism, or others. The process may be further expanded to include hypnotic regression to abolish repressed anger and pathologic, self-degrading messages. Any roadblocks to cooperating with the therapeutic team may also be removed.

Also, hypnosis may be used for imaginal rehearsal to increase desired behavior. For instance, a patient who is trying to change a behavior is much more likely to succeed if he or she can produce it in the imagination first. Hypnosis and imagery have a direct effect on the healing systems of the body and may be used to imagine the painful area getting better. This technique has been used successfully with both benign and malignant pain (Simonton et al., 1978).

GROUP TREATMENT FOR CHRONIC PAIN

During the past few years, group treatment for chronic pain has become an increasingly accepted modality. When chronic pain patients are treated in a group, many advantages accrue. As a group, they face common problems such as addiction to pain-killing drugs and recurrent depression. They also face similar social problems such as overdependency on family members, hassles with insurance companies and employers, and learning to live and cope with disability.

One of the most pervasive negative psychological states among these patients is the sense of being alone. The sense that "no one understands me" and "others can't possibly know what I'm going through" adds to whatever depression and feeling of loss of control already exists. By being together with others who face similar types of problems and issues, a context is provided to deal with them from a position of support and empowerment rather than isolation and helplessness.

From a therapeutic point of view, patients are often able to absorb new ways of looking at old problems if they receive credible feedback from peers. The same message may be accepted if heard from someone else who has a similar chronic pain problem, which would otherwise be rejected if heard from someone who was perceived as "well." Furthermore, the effect of hearing the message from more than one person is usually more powerful. The issue of dependency on the part of the patient is also more effectively dealt with in a group context where there is not so much psychological pressure to rely on one person (the doctor) for having all the answers or performing a miracle cure. As patients rely more and more on each other and less and less on the group therapist, a sense of group cohesion and social support builds up. As it does, members of the group are better able to assimilate confrontation of "pain games."

Pain games are maladaptive coping strategies which take place in an interpersonal context. They are set up on the part of the patient to achieve certain payoffs from the external social environment. Usually they rest on a psychological assumption that denies the existence of chronic pain. Where there is a denial of chronic pain there are great "efforts on the part of patients (both cognitively and behaviorally) to avoid partially or totally the harsh unwelcome reality of chronic endless pain" (Gentry and Owens, 1986). As Gentry recently argued, "denial–is the primary motivating factor behind 'pain games,' for example, doctor-shopping, addiction, excessive disability, litigation, focusing on the past in day-to-day communications, and externalization of one's pain experience (referring to pain as 'it,' something outside the otherwise healthy self)."

INTEGRATIVE MODEL OF PSYCHOLOGICAL PAIN MANAGEMENT

Pain patients often find themselves caught in a medical–legal system which attempts to separate mind and body phenomena. In this system the location of the cause of the pain is assumed to be either in the mind *or* the body. This dualistic approach has been labeled by some as the traditional "medical model." When this approach is taken, evaluators attempt to establish how much if any of the problem is physical and how much is mental. This approach may leave the patient in a problematic position. The patient may find that doctors' and insurance company reports are conveying the impression that the pain problem is mostly if not completely "in the patient's head." This is because today the discrimination of psychophysiological disorders (illnesses where abnormal psychological processes play a major role) from physically based disorders is accomplished almost entirely by the exclusion of physical explanations of the patient's body complaints. "This procedure unrealistically assumes that physical and psychological processes that result in somatic (physical) symptoms must be mutually exclusive. That is, if a physical process is found that explains the symptoms, then psychological factors must not be involved. If a physical process is not found, then psychological factors must be involved, even if no specific psychopathological process that can independently account for the symptoms is identified and to which therapy can be directed" (Wickramasekera, 1988). The medical model approach may lead to traumatic experiences for chronic pain patients. They may feel accused of making their complaints or faking pain.

A more useful and empowering approach to evaluation and treatment could be called the "integrative model." This model seeks to integrate mind and body dynamics into a unified whole. Chronic pain is not seen as a mutually exclusive mind/body problem. It is not even seen as summational, that is, so much body component and so much mental component equals the whole of the problem. Mind and body dynamics are seen as an interactive dynamic whole which cannot be broken down into quantifiable parts. The integrative model acknowledges that both mind and body are important parts of the problem and must be treated within the context of one another. More specifically, one could readily see that chronic physical pain causes real psychological depression and that psychological depression (psychic pain) can cause real physical pain. Therefore, in order to successfully treat the chronic pain patient, health service providers must address both the mental and physical aspects of illness, for either alone will lead to ineffective treatment at best and iatrogenic (doctor-induced) illness at worst.

ASSESSMENT OF CHRONIC PAIN WITH PSYCHOLOGICAL TESTS

Chronic pain patients are sometimes puzzled when they are asked to complete psychological questionnaires, inventories, and tests. They may be concerned that these tests will be used to determine if the pain is "real" or "just in their head." It is true sometimes that these tests are used in the context of the medical model and legal settings to make such determinations. However, in the context of the integrative model, they are properly used to assess the psychological component of the problem in a nonjudgmental way. This is important for several reasons. These assessment devices enable the psychologist to key into specific areas which need work, thus saving time and increasing clinical accuracy. Second, they can provide benchmarks for improvement when readministered at a later date. Third, they can validate for the patient the actual extent of his or her suffering on an objective basis, which can provide a measure of relief in and of itself.

The question which arises is how one knows how the test results will be used. The answer hinges on the context in which they are administered. If they are administered in a treatment context which ascribes to the integrative model, then they will most likely be used in that way. If they are used in a medical model setting or a forensic setting, then they will most likely be used accordingly.

CHOOSING A PAIN PSYCHOTHERAPIST

Choosing a psychotherapist is a very personal decision. The therapeutic relationship is an intimate one in which the patient should feel comfortable. Also, the therapist should be licensed to practice psychotherapy by the state. Currently in California, the following professionals are specifically licensed to practice psychotherapy independently: doctoral-level psychologists, medical doctors, medical doctors with a specialty in psychiatry, clinical social workers, and marriage, family, and child counselors. The latter two groups usually hold master's degrees in their fields. Lastly, the psychotherapist should have specialized knowledge, training, and experience in the chronic pain area. The extent of expertise is difficult to ascertain in this relatively young but growing specialty area. Perhaps the most direct method would be to discuss with the provider his or her treatment model (medical, integrative, etc.) and to ask about memberships in relevant professional organizations. Such organizations may include local and national pain societies, biofeedback societies, hypnosis societies, behavioral medicine societies, etc. Also ask which specific therapeutic modalities are used in treating chronic pain and the extent of training and experience using each. Although there are no specialty boards certifying individual practitioners, such boards are now being organized and should be operational within the next several years.

From the foregoing discussion it is clear that chronic pain is a multidimensional, complex problem. No one person or professional specialty has all the answers. Also, the patient's search for the answers is just as important as the professional's. It is imperative that all of us, professional specialists and patients, pool our resources to advance our understanding and treatment of the challenging problem of chronic pain.

BIBLIOGRAPHY

Bresler, D. and Turbo, R. (1979). *Free Yourself from Pain,* Simon and Schuster, New York.

Gentry, W.D. and Owens, D. (1986). Pain groups, in *Pain Management,* Holzman, A. and Turk, D. (Eds.), Pergamon Press, New York, 1986.

Maruta, T. (1982). Chronic pain patients: expect marital and sexual disruption, *Sexual Medicine Today,* pp. 20–23.

Simonton, O.C., Mathews-Simonton, S., and Creighton, J. (1978). *Getting Well Again,* Bantam Books, New York.

Wickramasekera, I. (1988). *Clinical Behavioral Medicine,* Plenum Press, New York.

Worden, J.W. (1982). *Grief Counseling and Grief Therapy,* Springer, New York.

16 Chronic Pain and Stress

Richard Weiner, Ph.D.

INTRODUCTION

It is now widely believed that stress plays a major role in the onset of illness, although the process is not fully understood. Stress produces an imbalance that requires a changing chemical and emotional response.

Both lay public and health care providers acknowledge that our lives are stressful. We should take measures to reduce the negative impact of stress on our health.

Many investigators are perplexed by the lack of an accepted definition of stress. As a result, they have been handicapped in the development of reliable assessment instruments and, to a lesser extent, in devising effective treatment programs.

There is a growing interest in holistic and organizational approaches to health problems. The treatment for chronic pain and its related stress requires a multidisciplinary team approach as is currently embodied in the chronic pain clinic treatment of chronic pain.

This chapter explains the models of cognitive learning principles and discusses environmental, behavioral, and physiological roles in stress management. A combination of social forces is occurring that will both escalate research efforts in and serve as an important catalyst for stress management treatment centers. As public policy decision makers embrace cost containment reimbursement methods, health care providers are forced to pay more attention to preventive medicine.

This chapter covers the following points:

1. Introduces a definition of stress
2. Describes stress triggers
3. Outlines some of the current assessment techniques
4. Introduces the emerging role of molecular biology for state-of-the-art research
5. Highlights stress reduction techniques that each individual can use to help himself or herself

THE DEFINITION OF STRESS

Change causes stress. The change can be positive, such as a job promotion, or negative, such as chronic pain. The process that occurs during change requires the individual to adapt to new

1-57444-103-5/99/$0.00+$.50
© 1999 by CRC Press LLC

demands and new roles. When the degree of change is intense, and this is frequently the case, or it may be of long duration, stress may be damaging to the individual's health.

Hans Selye (1974) defined adaptation to stress as follows:

> ...the specific response of the body to any demand made upon it....All agents to which we are exposed produce a non-specific increase in the need to perform adaptive functions and thereby reestablish normalcy....It is immaterial whether the agent or situation we face is pleasant or unpleasant; all that counts is the intensity of the demand for readjustment or adaptation.

Utilizing the method of case review, Professor Meyer, at Johns Hopkins University, demonstrated that illness became a problem when clusters of major change events occurred for a patient in a short time span. In later research in 1968, Wolff demonstrated that rapid and escalating societal stress contributes to a high incidence of psychosomatic disease.

In spite of the many outstanding achievements of modern medical science, it is now clear for the first time that the major cause of death and disease is due to stress-related disorders.

SOCIAL VERSUS INDIVIDUAL STRESS

Stress is a cumulative by-product of rapid social change and individual life circumstances. Examples of social stress may be triggered by economic instability, such as occurs when a pain patient has to quit gainful employment due to pain and related disability. Another stress comes in the economic area when a patient who has a back or neck pain problem finds that it is no longer easy to find a job now that the stigma of having a chronic neck or back pain problem has been tacked onto his or her work record and/or job interview forms. Major social changes occur with patients in chronic pain. They find that they no longer have empathetic friends left to talk to, and they generally withdraw from most social activities and confrontations. The effects of change in the work environment have been written up by Weiner and Hendricks (1985).

Individual responses to these stressors may include one of the following:

- Chronic pain
- Sleep disorder
- Migraine
- Peptic ulcer
- Heart attack
- Impotence
- Weight change
- Nausea
- Vomiting
- Diarrhea

ASSESSMENT TECHNIQUES

Self-Awareness

Assessing stress can start with self-awareness by an individual. He or she may be having marriage difficulties or interpersonal problems at work or in other relationships.

An evaluation to determine a type A personality assessment should be considered when the pressure of work deadlines begins to take a toll on the individual and relaxation is difficult to achieve (Price, 1982).

Holmes–Rahe Evaluation

Stress Test Comments

In 1977, Thomas Holmes and Richard Rahe, professors at the School of Psychiatry at the University of Washington School of Medicine, developed a brief screening device titled the Schedule of Recent Events. In this study investigating the relationship among social readjustment, stress, and susceptibility to illness, they noted a correlation between intensity of life change and onset of severe illness. From their retrospective study they assigned a numerical value to events, such as divorce, marriage, death in the family, job change, pregnancy, large mortgage, etc. Although some of these might be considered happy events, according to Hans Selye's theory of the nonspecific response, they all are capable of evoking a neurophysiological and biochemical reaction. This is exactly what Holmes and Rahe found to be true. Several additional studies by Rahe (1973) and Holmes and Masuda (1973) have used this simple assessment instrument with a high degree of success in predicting illness.

Stress Testing

Social Readjustment Rating Scale

Event	Value
Death of spouse	100
Divorce	73
Marital separation	65
Jail term	63
Death of close family member	63
Personal injury or illness	53
Marriage	50
Fired from work	47
Marital reconciliation	45
Retirement.	45
Change in family member's health	44
Pregnancy	40
Sex difficulties	39
Addition to family	39
Business readjustment	39
Change in financial status	38
Death of a close friend	37
Change to different line of work	36
Change in number of marital arguments	35
Mortgage loan over $10,000	31
Foreclosure of mortgage or loan	30
Change in work responsibilities	29
Son or daughter leaving home	29
Trouble with in-laws	29
Outstanding personal achievement	28
Spouse begins or stops work	26

Event	Value
Starting or finishing school	26
Change in living conditions	25
Revision of personal habits	24
Trouble with boss	23
Change in work hours, conditions	20
Change in residence	20
Change in school	20
Change in recreational habits	19
Change in church activities	19
Change in social activities	18
Mortgage or loan under $10,000	17
Change in sleeping habits	16
Change in number of family gatherings	15
Change in eating habits	15
Vacation	13
Christmas season	12
Minor violation of the law	11

Scoring

Select all of the above events that relate to you and that have occurred in the last 18 months. Then total them up.

    300+ points   = High risk
    200–299 points = Medium risk
    150–199   = Low risk

Studies have shown that there is a direct correlation between the magnitude of the life change score and the onset of illness. The higher the score, the greater the probability of the onset of illness. Likewise, the higher the score, the greater the need for the institution of preventive and holistic measures to counteract the effects of stress. Holmes and Masuda (1973) postulated that these life events enhance the probability of disease by lowering bodily resistance.

Epilogue on the Holmes–Rahe Test

These simple assessment instruments could and should encourage preventive measures. A counseling intake interview, social factors, and physiological factors need to be considered in conjunction with these test results.

As health care dollars become scarce and there is a shift to a holistic health model, these tools (i.e., the Holmes–Rahe test) will become as fundamental to diagnostics in the stressed chronic pain patient as the stethoscope is to the modern practice of medicine.

PALLIATIVE MANAGEMENT

Palliative management (the treating of symptoms) is more widespread today than preventative medicine. It is possible to assess the diagnosis and treatment of a stress disorder at many stages. For example, many physicians recognize and treat hypertension. They accomplish this by utilizing standard examination techniques and ordering routine laboratory tests. If this confirms their diagnosis, they often place the patient on medication. The attendant physician may even advise the patient that he or she should adapt to life's stress triggers by stating, "I will place you on medication for stress. However, it would be better if you changed your lifestyle and learn how to cope with your problems."

THE PHYSIOLOGY AND BIOCHEMISTRY OF STRESS

Most physicians recognize that there is a mind–body interaction by an individual and his or her environment, even though the exact process is little understood. Stress disorders develop over time and occur only after repeated exposures to stressful situations. Each stressful situation adds to the last in a cumulative fashion. Other environmental and metabolic factors may play a role in stress-related disorders. For example, a migraine headache may be initiated by a dietary imbalance, psychological stress, various other factors, or an interaction among all of them. Which of the related factors came first becomes an academic argument since the interaction among all the related factors takes a mild headache and escalates it up to the severity of a "migraine."

Perhaps the most promising area presently under investigation involves research into the biochemistry of health. In 1973 scientists discovered the endorphin. Endorphin is a naturally occurring narcotic within the brain that not only shields the body from pain, but is thought to influence emotion and mood. It is part of the "fight or flight" response to stress. Some researchers claim that endorphin and other such chemicals may actually be the molecular basis of emotion. It is believed that peptides such as endorphin relay messages between the hormone system and the brain and are called "neuropeptides." Little is known about which emotional mood neuropeptides foster. Although endorphins have only recently been discovered, efforts to map their location in the brain will help determine how they impact clinical symptoms. They are tentatively offered as one mechanism to explain the relation of stress to disease. In the future, an endorphin count may be used to determine a person's tolerance to pain and may play a role in the diagnosis and treatment of any stress disorder an individual may have.

NEW DIAGNOSTICS

Magnetic resonance imaging, in addition to positron emission transaxial tomography, computerized axial tomography, and computer-enhanced electroencephalography, is providing new information about the structure and metabolism of the brain.

TREATMENT

Awareness of the problem is the first step in treating any illness. Stress reduction education will become a high priority when we learn more about mind–body interactions.

Holistic approaches will allow the patient and the clinician to become partners in the prevention and treatment of stress disorders. Using this approach, the individual must assume greater personal responsibility for his or her health care. This requires emphasizing changes in lifestyle and will necessitate both patient and physician education.

Time has to be taken by the physician to talk with the patient about an illness episode to evaluate his or her diet, amount of sleep, exercise, and other important relevant factors.

Intervention requires coordinating palliative modalities and preventive strategies. Medication and surgical techniques need to be supplemented with biofeedback training, autogenic positive imagery, and relaxation techniques.

A multidisciplinary clinic can be a valuable resource in this effort.

PRESENT NEEDS

We need to create an approach to health care that includes a health hazard appraisal that estimates future risks along with the patient's physical examination. This kind of appraisal needs to be routine with the modern clinician.

CONCLUSION

Stress plays a major role in chronic pain problems. A response to stress triggers that are intense and prolonged can throw the body off balance. As the body attempts to adapt to the load of a stressful situation or series of events, it may pass the point of being able to adapt, and further illness may be added to a chronic disability.

Treatment needs to emphasize early recognition rather than waiting for the disease process to worsen and become more debilitating. Treatment requires a blend of both traditional medicine and holistic behavioral modalities.

17 Touching and Being Touched

David D. Robinson, Ph.D.

Of all the primary emotions, sex is the most difficult one to talk about. It may cause more people more sadness, embarrassment, and ill feeling than almost any other facet of life. To many, it is a source of satisfaction, contentment, and connectedness, however.

It is so difficult to talk about because it is so personal and because the cultural values of the majority of Americans are so strongly influenced by New England puritanism and Victorian values. The basic difference between the Puritans and the Victorians is that Puritans considered almost any kind of pleasure as inherently sinful. Victorians acknowledged sexual need in some men, but not in respectable women. Actually, respectable men were not supposed to have sexual need either. A prayer found among the effects of a Victorian gentleman asked the Lord for help in subduing his "impurity." To both Puritans and Victorians, sex had one function: procreation. The Puritans believed that we are conceived in sin, we live in sin, and we die in sin. The New England Puritans were not the only puritans. The Jansenists were French Catholic heretics who taught that sex is sinful. The Jansenists influenced the Irish, and Irish priests have strongly influenced American Catholics. Thus puritan traditions have influenced many Americans.

Major changes in American values came in the 1920s after an unimaginably horrible war in which our society and also many European societies were said to have lost their innocence. President Woodrow Wilson urged American participation in a "war to end all wars." The grim realities and the aftermath of World War I proved Wilson's idealism naive. The result of our loss of innocence was erosion of traditional values. In the 1920s some women began wearing revealing bathing suits, smoking cigarettes, driving cars, and "going with men." Yet, most Americans retained conservative views of what behavior was permissible between the sexes.

As late as the 1930s there were strange prohibitions on touching. For example, child care books advised not to pick up, touch, or feed babies when they cried because it would spoil them. Popular literature of the 1930s and early 1940s, except that of Henry Miller (*Tropic of Cancer* and *Tropic of Capricorn*) and D.H. Lawrence (*Lady Chatterley's Lover*), contained nothing sexually explicit (which contemporary readers would have considered obscene) and little profanity. Miller's works were banned in the United States. In the movies, kisses were brief and married couples were never shown in the same bed. Movie dialogue contained no profanity until a dramatic scene in *Gone with the Wind* in which Clark Gable told Vivien Leigh, "Frankly, Scarlet, I don't give a damn."

World War II took men away, and women gravitated into virtually every job that men had been doing. The war years were a very sad and lonesome time for many people. Sexual behavior that occurred under the stresses of war probably would not have occurred in more stable times. Brief encounters took place. Strangers married or otherwise slept with strangers. Under the stress of loneliness, relationships broke up, and servicemen got "Dear John" letters. With the further breakdown of traditional patterns caused by World War II and mass migrations away from hometowns and families, many felt free to experiment sexually and otherwise.

The war brought a tremendous spurt of energy and productivity, more technologic innovations, and a strong sense of progress to American life. In the postwar years, scientific and technical advances continued at a fast pace, and America welcomed these changes. The future held incredible promise. During this period, in 1948, Alfred Kinsey, an Indiana University professor of invertebrate biology, conducted a survey of male sexual behavior and published his famous *Kinsey Report* (Kinsey et al., 1948). It was the first scientific study of what men actually do sexually — or say they do — and it was a best seller. A few years later, Kinsey published a second book reporting sexual behavior in women, and it flopped (Kinsey et al., 1953). People in the 1950s still were not ready to hear or believe that women have sexual feelings and needs. It was one of the last signs of widespread sexual restraint in American culture.

In the 1960s William Masters, a middle-aged gynecologist, and Virginia Johnson, a social worker who was about his age, began to conduct scientific studies of the anatomy and physiology of both male and female sexual response and of sexual dysfunction in couples. Masters, and possibly Johnson, waited until they were middle aged to begin their research in order to avoid probable accusations of impropriety. Presumably, sexual urges of middle-aged men and women were mellow enough that raging youthful hormones would not contaminate their research. They kept completely quiet about it until they were ready to publish. They wrote *Human Sexual Response* (Masters and Johnson, 1966) in the driest, most technical way they could, in order to avoid provoking criticism and charges of sensationalism. Based upon their scientific understanding of what they had been seeing, they developed behavioral techniques for alleviating, and in many cases curing, sexual dysfunctions that had resisted conventional medical or psychiatric treatment. They understood sexual functioning well enough to relieve pain on intercourse or lack of orgasm in women and premature ejaculation and erectile failure (impotence) in men. They were the first to do so.

One of the most important findings of Masters and Johnson is that men and women receive different messages about sex from our culture. Men tend to encourage each other to express their sexuality. In our culture, except in fairly recent years, women have not tended to expect or encourage other women to feel or need sexual pleasure. The basic cultural message that most women have tended to receive is, "Nice girls don't do 'it' or talk about 'it' or express any curiosity about 'it' or satisfaction with 'it.'" Among respectable women, it was as if there were a conspiracy of silence about sex. Women talk about sex among themselves much less freely than men do — at least traditionally they have, but the times they are a changin' — at least for a while they changed. In the 1970s, because of the pill, the Vietnam war, Masters and Johnson's work, and a number of other influences, many women recognized their sexual needs and changed their behavior. Some of these changes have been far from beneficial, as we can see by the current epidemic of sexually transmitted diseases, especially AIDS. In the late 1990s we have seen a return to traditional values that many men and women never left. Regardless of value changes or not, it is hard for a great many people to talk about sex. Aside from tradition, one of the reasons for difficulty in talking about sex is that we are not taught the names of body parts and what they do. The reason is simple. Our parents were as ignorant about these topics as we are.

Why is sex all that important in the first place? It might help to put it into human perspective by considering its three legitimate functions. The first is procreation, which everybody knows already. The second is recreation, which we recognize leads to so much difficulty in the way that some people lead their lives. The third function of sex is what Masters and Johnson called "pair bonding," and its discovery was somewhat of a surprise to them. They found that when couples who had otherwise strong relationships resolved sexual dysfunction, their relationships became immensely stronger. When both members of couples experienced the complete, normal sexual response cycle from beginning to end, they bonded even more strongly. Some animal species mate for life: Canada geese and wolves, to name two. Humans who pair bond are more likely to stay together than if they do not bond. In other words, pair bonding strengthens families. Stronger, closer families enhance individual survival and improve society.

You may notice that I said "legitimate" functions of sex, because there are people who misuse their sexuality by behaving in sexual ways that another person finds obnoxious. "Obnoxious" is a relative term, and the way I am using it, it ranges from rape or child abuse to a married couple in which one party absolutely insists that the only way he or she can possibly be fulfilled is for the partner to do something that results in his or her humiliation, degradation, physical discomfort, anxiety, etc. In many stable relationships, one partner finally gives in to the other partner's pleading, promises, threats, etc., because it is easier to give in than to experience the pressure. I am calling that kind of sex illegitimate, in order to focus on the extremely important and legitimate functions of procreation, recreation, and pair bonding.

Masters and Johnson's findings are consistent with the well-regarded research of Harry Harlow and his associates at the University of Wisconsin and that of other primate researchers. For example, Harlow and Zimmerman (1958) found that touch and being touched are absolutely necessary for normal development in monkeys. Harlow raised infant monkeys in individual cages under one of two conditions. In one, they were able to cuddle with a soft, mother-sized terry-cloth object. In the other, they lacked the terry-cloth "mother" and had only a mother-sized wire frame on which they crouched with miserable expressions on their faces. Monkeys who were able to cuddle the terry-cloth object were able to socialize with other monkeys when they got the chance, but those who were stuck with the wire frame were socially unresponsive. Eventually, Harlow and his associates were able to rehabilitate some of these monkeys, but they were socially retarded. Other studies of primates (Simonds, 1974) seem to reveal a four-channel system of social communication: two channels are audio-visual and two are tactile. They use one audio-visual channel in routine communication when all is well. They use the other audio-visual channel to warn intruders against encroachment on personal territory or other circumstances that threaten to break the peace. The animals chatter excitedly and assume specific postures and facial expressions. The inefficient aspect of audio-visual communication is inaccuracy. The target of the communication may not receive it, or a party to whom the communication is not directed may receive it *as if* it were directed that way. One channel of tactile communication is clawing, biting, hitting, etc. that takes place when a warning is not heeded. They use the other channel of tactile communication to demonstrate care and positive feelings. The efficiency of tactile communication is its directness and accuracy. It is difficult to mistake the meaning of tactile communication if it is delivered directly. Tactile messages can be inefficient because it is hard to deliver a tactile message to more than one receiver at a time, but tactile messages are harder to misinterpret than messages expressed in audio-visual channels.

In other words, touch is probably the most important way to send critically important messages to people about whom we care and to receive their replies. Touch can convey reassurance, kindness, and warmth — as well as sexuality. In recent years, the catholic mass has included expression of a sign of peace to others nearby, and this is usually a handshake. Not all Catholics like this, though. Some express discomfort at being expected to touch strangers.

Couples who are strong and healthy can exchange messages of affection and love in traditional sexual ways, although they might define sex strictly as intercourse. When pain interferes with sexual performance and enjoyment, many people stop having sexual relations — including touching — and this is a big mistake. In order to keep important "I care" or "I am cared about" messages flowing, it is necessary to keep (or resume) touching. Even though you may like to have intercourse according to your usual pattern, pain may keep you from enjoying it. Whatever your strength and endurance and/or range of motion, it is important not to give up on touching, even though intercourse in your usual manner may be painful. You may find that some other positions for intercourse, with or without pillows, bolsters, or other supports, may work out fairly well. If pain interferes with intercourse to such an extent as to seriously diminish the pleasure, alternatives still exist. Any form of touching that both parties enjoy is permissible, and mutual interest and acceptance are the sole criteria of what's okay.

An alternative to intercourse is giving or getting a massage with warm oil or talcum powder. It is good to do this on a big towel, in order to avoid getting oil on bedclothes or carpeting. Another alternative is washing your partner's feet. That's right, *feet*. Put a basin of warm water on the floor in front of the chair your partner is sitting in; you can sit on the floor. Put your partner's feet on a towel. Pick up one foot and hold it over the basin, and dribble warm water over it. Set it down, and work up a lather of soap on your hands. Wash your partner's foot and spend time on each toe. Rinse the foot, and wrap it up in a towel. Do the other foot. Unwrap the first foot and wet it down again. Rub some 20 Mule Team Borax on the tough skin on the ball of the foot and on the heel in order to rub off some old used skin. Avoid rubbing Borax on the arch. Rinse off the Borax, and rub a little salt on the places where you rubbed the Borax. The salt gets into the tiny abrasions caused by the Borax and creates a pleasant tingling sensation. After the first foot has been Boraxed, rinsed, salted, rinsed, dried, and wrapped in a towel, it's time to rub oil (baby oil or perhaps scented oil) into each foot. This foot-washing process should take a long time and gives plenty of opportunity to give or receive touch, depending upon whether you are the washer or the washee. It can be done in the most comfortable position a person with chronic pain is able to assume. The important thing is to give and get tender, caring touch, and the only way to find out if these alternatives are satisfying is to try them.

About half the battle of getting and giving satisfying touch is in setting the climate for it. Often, communication failure or accumulation of emotional garbage keeps loved ones at an uncomfortable distance. Conflict between intimates is inevitable, and it is necessary to establish a workable means to resolve it. Many people do not resolve conflict; they ignore it and hope it will go away. Sometimes it will go away, but too often, it just smolders. Avoiding or ignoring conflict may seem like a good thing to do, but bad feelings accumulate, and then finally, they all pour out in a rush. When this happens, it may cause a destructive fight in which people say hurtful things to one another. One of the most useful books for helping people to understand and avoid the many pitfalls of poor conflict resolution is by George Bach and Peter Wyden (1981): *The Intimate Enemy: How to Fight Fair in Love & Marriage*.

If you are feeling the agony of alienation from your partner because chronic pain has caused you to avoid touching, it is important to try to express what you need and want and to do some constructive problem solving. When people have chronic pain, innovation is extremely important. It may take considerable time, patience, and experimentation to work out a mutually satisfying pattern of touching and getting the touching you need, but it is certainly worth trying.

BIBLIOGRAPHY

Bach, G.R. and Wyden, P. (1981). *The Intimate Enemy: How to Fight Fair in Love & Marriage,* Avon, New York.

Harlow, H.F. and Zimmerman, R.F. (1958). The development of affectional responses in infant monkeys, *Proceedings of the American Philosophical Society,* 102(5), 501–505.

Kinsey, A.C. et al. (1948). *Sexual Behavior in the Human Male,* W.B. Saunders, Philadelphia.

Kinsey, A.C. et al. (1953). *Sexual Behavior in the Human Female,* W.B. Saunders, Philadelphia.

Masters, W.H. and Johnson, V.E. (1966). *Human Sexual Response,* Little, Brown, Boston.

Simonds, P.D. (1974). *The Social Primates,* Harper & Row, New York.

Section IV

Physical Therapies and Rehabilitation

18 Massage Therapy in the Treatment of Chronic Pain

Beverly Breakey, R.N., C.M.T.

The healing power of touch is probably the oldest treatment method known to mankind. Even so, it is often overlooked in chronic pain management due largely to our Western medical model, where compassionate human touch has been displaced by technology.

Some argue that massage therapy, or bodywork as it is often called, has no medical value, but merely "feels good." Others realize this very quality plays a vital role in rehabilitating the person who must learn to live with pain. Going to bed in pain only to arise in pain weakens the spirit of even the most hearty. Massage therapy can help to restore body awareness and at the same time promote healing through both physical and psychological change.

WHAT IS MASSAGE THERAPY?

When we hear the term "massage therapy," it conjures up a milieu of images, often including one of a hefty Swedish female pounding on a partially shrouded body, draped helplessly over a narrow table. This of course relates to Swedish massage, developed in the early 1700s by Peter Heinrick Ling. Swedish massage in its traditional form is much too vigorous for the chronic pain patient, but its basic concept has given rise to other techniques which are very beneficial.

Massage therapy, or bodywork, refers to hands-on methods which facilitate change within the muscles and fascia that surround them. It does not include the manipulation of joints as performed by doctors of osteopathy or chiropractic. It does include rocking or supported movements of the head or limbs and applications of heat or cold in the form of hot packs, ice, or a rapidly evaporating spray.

Having one's muscles worked is similar to any other type of physical workout. When done by a therapist, however, the specific problem areas are first identified, then coaxed into releasing their excess tension. The strokes must be appropriate for the shape of the muscle, its location, its type of tension, its composition, and response factors of the tissues and the patient as a whole person.

1-57444-103-5/99/$0.00+$.50
© 1999 by CRC Press LLC

Exercises are introduced at a point in time when the muscles have regained sufficient elasticity to benefit from strengthening or stretching. However, improved health of the muscles and fascia comes from a combination of whole person therapy, including not only bodywork and exercise but also good nutrition, medication management, and behavioral adjustment. The latter three elements are discussed elsewhere in this volume.

PROBLEMS AND SOLUTIONS

Pain

Pain is the number one complaint of the chronic pain patient. Since muscles are not equipped with an early warning sensory system, tension and irritation may accumulate before pain is perceived.

The first session of bodywork may be quite uncomfortable as the therapist probes and manipulates muscles, sourcing out problem areas. After several sessions, tension-related pain begins to diminish. Before this, however, sleep improves, as does one's sense of well-being.

Along with improved sleep comes increased energy. This is confusing when pain persists. Psychotherapy can be very helpful at this stage. The patient must develop methods of keeping pain in perspective while living a life that involves compromise and adjustment. A realistic goal is managing the pain, not eradicating it.

Muscle Spasms

When the chronic pain patient complains of pain, frequently its origin is spasoming or intense contracting of a muscle or groups of muscles. This may occur randomly, often unprovoked. A person may be sitting watching television or waiting for a traffic light to change when suddenly gripped by a cramp-like pain. This tendency for the muscles to contract without warning not only is physically disabling but creates a conditioned edginess in the person's behavior.

Massage therapy reduces muscle spasms, helping the tissues to relearn their resting length or intended pattern. This is accomplished by a variety of muscle manipulations called "strokes." An oil or lotion is used on the therapist's hands to prevent irritation to the patient's skin. The quality of the painful tissue is first assessed. It may be ropey (fibers stretched lengthwise), knotted (small lumps), grainy (as if containing sand), or armored (thick and unyielding). Once this is determined, appropriate strokes are used to soften and lengthen the fibers, thereby helping restore them to a smooth and elastic state.

Trigger Points

Pain within the muscles is also related to "trigger points." They are so called because they trigger a chain reaction in the muscles which results in contractions, spasms, and pain referred to other areas. A person is not consciously aware of these sensitive points but will complain of an achiness or heaviness in a nearby area. Direct pressure on one elicits severe pain that may cause a person to jump or feel nauseated. Working with them requires special techniques and a competent therapist.

The "spray and stretch" technique is effective in desensitizing active triggers. After a rope-like band of muscle fibers has been identified, it is slowly and gently stretched by the therapist. At the same time, a rapid coolant spray is applied to the area in a prescribed pattern. The coolant shocks the muscle into remaining in the stretched position. It is then thoroughly warmed using a moist hot pack. If the tissue is sufficiently healthy, it will retain its resting length. If not, the procedure is repeated. This technique is described *Myofascial Pain and Dysfunction, The Trigger Point Manual* (Travell and Simons, 1983)

Both latent (soreness on direct pressure) and active triggers (highly sensitive upon pressure) may by reduced by creating hyperemia or increased blood flow in the tissues. There are three basic ways to do this.

The first is to press deeply into the point of pain, causing an ischemia, or absence of blood. The patient is asked to breathe slowly and deeply as the pressure is applied and then quickly released. This method is described by Bonny Pruden (1980) in *Myotherapy*. It is also part of an oriental method called Shiatsu" (Namikoshi 1981). Even though this procedure is painful, the patient will often say it is a "good hurt," as the focus of the problem is addressed. Once the pressure is released, blood rushes into the area, bringing with it a supply of oxygen and nutrients.

The second technique is called "cross-fiber friction," which is a modification of Swedish massage stroke "petrissage." Ropey bands of muscle are worked across their fibers, where they change texture and attach to bones or other muscles. The goal of this technique is to send a message along the muscle fibers to "let go."

Muscles have a built-in defense mechanism of contracting to protect or bring stability to an area. Sometimes this stability is necessary, as in conditions of deteriorating bones and cartilage. When this is not the case, muscles can be reeducated to lengthen or relax. In their normal state they have a maximum capacity to expand and contract. During this process of relearning, trigger points become less active and gradually disappear.

The third method is an Esalen Swedish massage technique called "small circles." The thumb or fingers slowly inscribe small circular movements first in one direction, then the other, in and around the trigger point. Pressure is gradually increased until the area becomes reddened with increased circulation.

Manual work by itself will not reduce the irritation of trigger points. A person's general health and nutrition also play an important role. These other treatment aspects are discussed elsewhere in this volume.

Poor Circulation

There are various physiological effects of slow, deep muscle manipulation, one of them being improved cardiovascular circulation. The tiniest blood vessels, called capillaries, dilate through mechanical action which in turn stimulates a dilatation of the slightly larger blood vessels. This improves blood flow, bringing nutrients to the tissues and removing waste products of metabolism. It also increases warmth to the skin and an improvement in its condition. Any sign of progress helps to restore the chronic pain patient's faith in the body as a system that can heal.

Another benefit is the reduction of swelling or painful inflammation. As the muscles are worked, uric acid and other by-products of normal muscle activity are moved into the surrounding tissue fluid. This is picked up by the lymph system, carried to the general circulation, and then eliminated from the body. It is important to drink plenty of water following a session of massage therapy in order to facilitate this process. Active movement and good fluid intake are two general health habits of critical importance to the chronic pain patient, as the muscles and thicker layers of connective tissue that enclose them may remain in a state of inflammation for long periods of time.

Applications of heat such as hot tubs, saunas or heating pads warm and weaken the muscles, helping them to relax. As they soften, they also expand. Too much heat, however, will aggravate already swollen tissues.

Applications of cold such as ice packs or a coolant spray will reduce swelling but at the same time irritate trigger points. Alternating heat and cold stimulates the circulation and is the best procedure for muscles that have both swelling and trigger points.

Different Strokes for Different Folks

This old adage is an especially important factor in massage therapy for the chronic pain patient. There are three basic body compositions relative to muscle development: soft muscles, which are found in bodies that have a rounded shape with round bones; long high-tension muscle fibers, found in tall bodies with long bones; and the dense muscle type, which belongs to a more rectangular body shape.

Chronic pain patients rarely are in the denser, more well-developed muscle type. These thick muscle fibers absorb shock better than the others and are less likely to become injured or unhealthy.

In the soft muscled body, shock is largely absorbed by the joints. Muscles tend to be rather loose in texture and contain more fat in their natural state. People with these bodies generally do not like to exercise, and because of this their muscles are more prone to irritation and slow healing.

High-tension muscle is also a prime target for chronic irritation. Already taut, as in a sensitive stringed musical instrument, jarring or poor nutrition sets up a response of contraction that is difficult to unwind.

A competent and experienced therapist will know how to both assess body types and choose appropriate combinations of bodywork for them. Early diagnosis and treatment is important to interrupt inappropriate patterns of contraction and thereby prevent scarring and adhesions. Bundles of muscle fibers can actually lose their elastic plastic quality. When this happens they become tough and fibrous, remaining tender and forever lost to the body's system of free movement and strength.

Postural Compensation

Anyone who experiences continued pain develops postural compensations or patterns of guarding affected areas. This is an unconscious activity performed over months or years in an attempt to get away from pain. There are two methods of learning that involve hands-on work and movement which benefit the chronic pain patient: Feldenkrais and Trager®. They are best introduced following a series of massage therapy where muscle tone has improved and some degree of joint mobility has been restored.

Moshe Feldenkrais, an Israeli physicist who dedicated his life to the study of human development, realized that once we begin to stand and walk we develop inappropriate patterns of movement. His method focuses on relearning movement through gentle, painless bodywork and exercises. This is of special benefit to the patient with chronic pain because repetitive movements that contradict the body's natural posture can cause irritation of the muscles, which in turn causes pain. These inappropriate patterns, however, become so familiar that the body feels they are correct. Before they can be changed, the natural movement must be programmed back into the system through a reeducation process.

For example, a person can work at a desk that is too high and set up an unnatural sequence of muscle movements involving the hands, wrists, arms, shoulders, neck, and head. The first pain warning may be a headache. What will the person do? Treat the headache, of course. The situation may continue for months or years, creating more and more inappropriate stretching or contracting of various muscles, until the body forgets what is natural and what is not.

In his book *Awareness for Movement,* Dr. Feldenkrais (1972) discusses his theory and gives examples of helpful exercises to unlearn such patterns. This is accomplished by repeatedly experiencing appropriate movement. The work begins on the floor, where one literally learns to turn, crawl, stand, and walk all over again. A Feldenkrais practitioner acts as teacher, bodyworker, and coach throughout this process.

Trager® is another method that uses gentle, painless body movement and exercises suited to the physical problems of the chronic pain patient. Developed by Milton Trager, M.D., the teaching involves a system of gentle rocking motions that elicit positive feelings of light, effortless mobility (Trager, 1987). These feeling responses enter the central nervous system and begin to trigger changes by means of the many sensory–motor feedback loops between the mind and muscles.

The Trager® practitioner does not change the condition of the tissue through mechanical action but rather uses the work to communicate a quality of feeling to the nervous system. The message the body receives is, "Oh yes, I can move freely, easily and painlessly." This is an important message for the person who has chronic pain and has been hearing quite another voice: "Contract, be on guard. Pain can strike at any time." This work is especially suited to people who have poorly developed or soft muscles since it sets in motion the entire system, bringing a sensation of aliveness to the body and mind. The chronically contracted or high-tension muscle system also benefits from these gentle rocking patterns of movement which are difficult to consciously resist.

WORKING WITH OTHER DISCIPLINES

At one time or another, most health professionals encounter patients with chronic pain. The complexity of what has come to be known as myofascial pain syndrome is always difficult to treat. The massage therapist adds a dimension to the multidisciplinary team that serves several roles.

Medical Practice

For the typical medical physician whose schedule allots 15 minutes per patient, the massage therapist can be of invaluable support for observation and assessment. Massage therapy sessions last 1–2 hours. During that time a therapeutic alliance develops between patient and therapist that is based on trust arising from intense, focused work.

A skilled massage therapist can differentiate subtle changes in the quality of the skin, muscle, or connective tissue. This helps to measure progress or regression, health or ill health, and the massage therapist is often the first to see it.

Because massage therapists are trained to observe the person as a whole being, attention is paid to much more than the areas of complaint. Voice, gait, skin color, hair texture, mood, attitude, dietary habits, exercise routines, sleep patterns, work interest, recreational life, spiritual pursuits, creative expression, and relationships are either observed or discussed during the hours of work. Changes in these are as important to whole person healing as taut bands of muscle and trigger points. These data can be very helpful to the physician as he or she coordinates medication management and other treatment methods.

Progress is always slow when working with the chronic pain patient. Any slight improvement such as being able to tend the flower garden or sleeping through the night is celebrated as a major milestone and viewed as renewed hope. Someone on the team needs to spend time with the chronic pain patient to be the detailed observer and provide emotional support. Often the physician does not have that time, and the massage therapist can fill part of that need.

Physical Therapy

Physical therapists view massage therapy as an important aspect of their practice and often include massage therapists on their staff. Massage is a physical therapy, but it goes beyond the physical to the emotional and spiritual through its nurturing, relaxing effect.

Chronic pain patients often view the technological modalities of traditional physical therapy such as ultrasound, galvanic current, or traction as too impersonal. Physical therapists and their assistants are not trained in bodywork as is a massage therapist; therefore the two practices complement each other.

Chiropractic

Joint manipulation is the most significant aspect of traditional chiropractic treatment. Chiropractic doctors know that muscles move bone, and the reverse is seldom true. Schools of chiropractic differ in approach; some teach massage, and others do not.

Many chiropractors use brief massage, ultrasound, moist heat, or galvanic current before attempting to manipulate bony structures. When these methods are insufficient to induce adequate relaxation, massage therapy may be ordered. Massage therapists often work in the chiropractic office.

Psychotherapy

Massage therapy can support psychotherapy in most situations, especially if the patient has been deprived of touch. Dr. Ashley Montagu (1971) has written extensively on touching and the human condition. In his book *Touching,* he concludes that inadequate tactile experience results in an inability to relate to others. The chronic pain patient is often viewed as "needy" by family members and professionals. Massage therapy provides a positive tactile experience so that the patient can once more accept the body with its limitations rather than view it as a failure.

Dentistry

Myofascial dentistry and orthodontia are both relatively new fields of health care. In support of this work, massage therapy serves to release face, scalp, neck, and shoulder tension that contributes to malocclusion or improper alignment of the jaw.

Restoration of temporomandibular joint (TMJ) function can be aided by massage therapy when trigger points and muscle spasms are alleviated prior to the application of splints and appliances. Massage therapy is also very helpful to patients before surgery to the TMJ. It induces a deep relaxation response in the body which helps to dispel fears associated with anesthesia and surgery.

EDUCATION AND TRAINING OF MASSAGE THERAPISTS

Eleven states in the United States have licensure and standards of practice for massage therapists. Others have school curriculum standards, and licensure comes under local jurisdiction, such as city ordinances.

The American Massage Therapy Association (AMTA) has 4000 members who are listed in a national registry by geographic location (AMTA).

In choosing a massage therapist, there are some important questions to ask:

1. Are they a member of the AMTA or some other professional organization? This indicates that the massage therapist or practitioner has met a standard established by peers, which is usually more stringent than government regulations.
2. Is their practice medical or simply for aesthetics and relaxation? Although massage is always beneficial, a medical practice requires much more training and experience than a practice where the goal is soothing comfort.
3. How long have they been in practice? It takes a minimum of 1 year to begin being proficient as a massage therapist.
4. Do they work with other health professionals? Who? This is an indicator of quality assurance and professionalism.
5. Did their education include anatomy and physiology, business and professional ethics, and whole person assessment? Good schools may or may not be AMTA approved. The longer the course, the more comprehensive the training. If the therapist has had a minimum basic education of 100 hours, ask what additional training he or she has received (e.g., Esalen Swedish massage, Shiatsu, Feldenkrais, Trager®). A practitioner studies for 4 years.
6. Does their technique involve more than the traditional Swedish massage? The chronic pain patient requires an integrated, more gentle approach than traditional Swedish massage.
7. Do they have experience working with chronic pain patients?
8. What is the fee, and how long is the session? Fees range from $25 to $85 per session depending on geographic location and therapist experience. Sessions last from 90 minutes to 2 hours.

CONCLUSION

Massage therapy has much to offer in the management of chronic pain. Patients benefit from stimulation of the cardiovascular system, improved muscle texture and length, reduction of trigger points and muscle spasms, increased energy, deeper sleep, decreased pain, and a heightened sense of well-being, which renews hope.

Other professionals benefit from the amount of focused time the massage therapist spends with the patient in observation and assessment.

Skeptics fear that because massage therapy is at times pleasurable it may become addictive and foster dependence Although this can happen in an already dependent personality, the massage therapist would be quick to point out that the therapy is not always pleasing.

The goals of massage therapy are quite specific. Therapists in a medically oriented practice refer patients to others when the work has reached its maximum restorative effect. At this juncture, people are usually eager to replace therapy sessions with normal life activities.

One side benefit of illness is the learning that comes with it. Throughout their healing journey, people with chronic pain discover many ways to take care of themselves. Having a monthly or quarterly relaxing massage can certainly be one of them.

BIBLIOGRAPHY

AMTA National Office, 1130 W. North Shore Ave., Chicago, IL 60626-4670.

Feldenkrais, M. (1972). *Awareness Through Movement,* Harper and Row, San Francisco.

Montagu, A. (1971). *Touching,* Harper and Row, New York.

Namikoshi, T. (1981). *Shiatsu Therapy, Theory and Practice,* Japan Pub. through Harper and Row, New York.

Pruden, B. (1980). *Myotherapy,* Ballantyne, New York.

Trager, M. (1987). *Trager Mentastics, Movements as a Way to Agelessness,* Station Hill Press, Barrytown, NY.

Travell, J. and Simons, D. (1983). *Myofascial Pain and Dysfunction, The Trigger Point Manual,* Williams & Wilkins, Baltimore.

19 Chiropractic Treatment of Patients with Chronic Pain

Geoffrey Brecher, D.C.

Many chronic pain sufferers consult a chiropractor as a last hope or a last resort after having tried numerous medical and/or surgical approaches without significant help. In some cases, the patient is relieved of long-standing pain after just a few adjustments. There are, however, more complex cases in which the standard chiropractic approach of mobilizing or realigning displaced skeletal joints is not enough, and it is to these cases to which this writing is addressed.

Chiropractic was founded by D.D. Palmer in 1895. Palmer was known as a magnetic healer and used nonmedical, nonsurgical means to restore health to sick individuals. One day, he was able to restore the hearing of a deaf man by adjusting (or realigning) a displaced vertebra in the man's spine. After this initial experience, it was thought that the spinal bones (vertebrae) could, through mechanical, chemical, or mental stresses, become misaligned in relation to other vertebrae above or below the one in question. The displaced vertebra with its surrounding blood vessels, lymph vessels, tendons, ligaments, and muscles could press against one or more of the nerve roots coming out of the spinal cord, or even the spinal cord itself, causing a variety of symptoms including pain and disease.

As the chiropractic field began, it became the chiropractor's task to examine the patient, paying special attention to the spine, to determine which vertebrae were out of position and to reposition them. This was done with the hands.

Today, some doctors of chiropractic also use a variety of instruments for correction. The theory was presented that because part of the nervous system was compromised by the offending vertebrae, the supply of nerve energy (electricity) along the nerve pathway was altered, and the tissues supplied by this pathway would then not function at their full potential, thus setting the stage for disease or malfunction. The chiropractor, by realigning the vertebrae, was able to correct this condition and the patient regained his or her health. Today, we know that the cause of human suffering is not always so simple, and answers still elude even the most experienced chiropractors. Doctors have found that a cooperative effort involving more than one type of therapy offers a promising, broad approach to chronic pain management. I will address this later in more detail.

Today's doctor must learn to recognize when a patient has a chronic pain syndrome. Depending on the severity of the problem, the patient may present with a variety of physical and mental symptoms. Some people suffer mild to moderate chronic pain and use it to retreat from life. Others suffer moderate to severe pain and yet lead an almost normal life.

Many chronic pain patients state that their problem began after one or more accidents. With others, the problem started before or after one or more surgeries. Some have a history that is less spectacular for an initiating event.

Common occurrences among the chronic pain patients, to mention only a few, include:*

1. Pain in numerous, scattered areas or one large area**
2. Muscles that are abnormally tender
3. Tingling, numbness, or burning sensations
4. Tightness and/or stiffness of the muscles
5. Soreness
6. Fatigue
7. Trouble sleeping
8. Depression

The doctor must be careful, however, not to jump to a hasty conclusion or dismiss these patients as psychiatric cases, which many do if they cannot find any "objective" signs. Unfortunately, the standard orthopedic, neurological, and laboratory tests may all be found to be normal. If the orthodox approaches are not working, whether in medicine, chiropractic, or psychology, we must look elsewhere.

When a patient first visits a doctor of chiropractic, he or she will have a health (or rather disease and accident) history taken, receive an examination, and perhaps X-rays will be taken. After analyzing this information, the chiropractor may proceed with his or her treatment and recommendations. The doctor may use his or her hands or an instrument to reposition and mobilize any misaligned spinal or skeletal bones. The doctor may also use heat, cold, ultrasound, electrical muscle stimulation, massage, etc., working also with the patient's muscular system. Specific exercises and/or nutritional recommendations may be made. There are many diverse methods in chiropractic all with the same goal: to remove nerve interference from the body.

The chiropractor deals with the nervous system. This is the first system to develop in our bodies and it controls every other system. Over the years, some chiropractors have come to recognize that relieving pressure on the nerves by realigning the spinal bones gave only partial relief in some of the more complex cases. This initiated clinical research into the role of the bones of the skull, the extremities, and the muscles. Other research has disclosed that sensitivities to certain foods and chemicals initiated and perpetuated nerve irritation. Mechanical and emotional stress was also discovered to cause the same problems.

Addressing and correcting the mechanical problems of the spine is necessary in promoting the health of the patient. However, when a purely mechanical approach is taken (i.e., spinal adjusting), it may be too painful for this type of patient to tolerate or it may not produce stabilization of the spine. In these cases the chiropractor must look to other areas or disciplines for answers.

These more complex cases call for a multispecialty, interdisciplinary approach. In such cases, in addition to the basic chiropractic problem, the patient may have:

1. A biomechanical problem in the feet
2. Cranial faults (abnormalities of the bones of the skull)

---

*Patients may experience some or all of these.
** This may include most of one side of the body.

  3. Food allergies
  4. Metabolic perpetuating factors
  5. Emotional problems

In such cases, unless the multiplicity of associated problems is recognized and addressed by a team of pain management specialists, chiropractic care may have limited value.

The picture of such a team would look like this:*

  1. The chiropractor treats the spinal misalignments and neuromuscular (nerve–muscle) problems.
  2. The medical doctor treats the medical/metabolic aspects.
  3. The psychologist (or psychiatrist) assists the patient with emotional barriers.

Both the doctor and the patient must recognize that in complicated cases, one specialty may not have all the answers.

I will now discuss the particular chiropractic techniques which have been found to be of the most value in treating cases of chronic pain. Note that nutritional therapy in the form of diet and vitamin/mineral supplementation is an important factor which the doctor of chiropractic may or may not choose to use. Since this is covered elsewhere in this book, I will not repeat it here.

Realigning the cranial (skull) bones is most useful in cases of temporomandibular (jaw) disorders and head pain; however it is not limited to just these conditions. The author once had a patient with long-standing hip pain which was relieved by a cranial adjustment. "Cranials" consist of restoring the natural movement of the bones of the skull and face in relation to the craniosacral respiratory mechanism. As we breathe, the bones of our skull move to assist with the circulation of the cerebrospinal fluid which flows through and around our brain and nervous system. One or more of the cranial bones may become fixed and not move normally. This may be caused by trauma, usually from birth through adolescence. Cranial adjustments are performed by chiropractors and osteopaths. The chiropractor will do these adjustments by applying pressure with his finger on specific areas in the patient's mouth. An assistant holds the patient's head to assist with the movement of the cranial bones or to prevent distortion, depending on the adjustment being done.

Another chiropractic technique useful in chronic pain syndromes, which follows very closely the work of Dr. Janet Travell, was developed by Dr. Raymond Nimmo. Dr. Nimmo developed what he called the Receptor-Tonus Technique, in which pressure is applied to the tender, painful muscle or trigger point. He believed that because muscles move bones, the muscle which was too tense would pull on the vertebra to which it was attached, causing a subluxation (spinal misalignment). If, by using pressure, the doctor could begin to get the muscle to relax, the bone would then be free to assume its natural position. He also learned and taught that the trigger point in and of itself could cause pain, muscle weakness, numbness, and tingling. In his procedure, pressure is applied with the doctor's thumb, elbow, fingers, or a small hand-held probe to the painful muscles. This can be uncomfortable, but it is very effective. In severe cases, this technique may be too painful for the patient to tolerate. In such cases, physiotherapies such as ultrasound and electrical muscle stimulation may be helpful.

The most effective technique which this author has found for dealing with chronic pain problems was developed by Dr. William Bennett in the 1920s. It was named Neuro-Vascular

---

* Some or all of the specialists may be needed for a specific case.

Dynamics and deals with the viscerosomatic reflexes of the body. If an organ is not functioning optimally, it sends this information through the nervous system. The information may go directly into the spinal cord, and as a result of this constant nerve signal, that area of the spine can become irritated. The muscles of that area of the spine can become chronically contracted and painful. Subluxations may occur. The chiropractor may adjust that area of the spine, but because the reflex is still active, he or she may adjust that area repeatedly with little or no results. The organ also sends signals through the nervous system to the surface of the body. Dr. Bennett located and mapped these points on the body wall corresponding to each organ. The chiropractor, using these various points, palpates with his or her fingers, searching for increased tension in that area. Sometimes there is pain at these reflex points. The chiropractor gently holds the area with his or her finger. With the other hand contacting a long muscle either in the leg or shoulder area, he or she maintains a stretch reflex. These points are held for a few minutes; then the doctor moves on to the next reflex point. It has been this author's experience that every patient with a chronic pain syndrome has a multitude of these reflexes active.

Chiropractic care is an effective part of dealing with chronic pain problems, especially when used in concert with the other forms of therapy mentioned in this book.

20 Returning to Work

David D. Robinson, Ph.D.

Chronic pain has kept you from working, but you realize that you have to get back to work. You wonder if you can get enough control over your chronic pain to work, and even if you do, you wonder what kind of work you can do, because you cannot go back to your previous job. You worry that no employer will hire you or keep you once they realize that you might not be able to do some parts of the job or that effective pain management takes time. You recognize that you need help in returning to work, but you do not know much about vocational rehabilitation or what kind of help to expect from a rehabilitation counselor.

This chapter is for you. It is meant to acknowledge the difficulties you have and to help you learn how the law protects you and how work can actually help to reduce your pain. It is meant to describe how the process of vocational rehabilitation is designed to operate, how it can get off track, and what you can do to get the vocational rehabilitation services you need and reasonable accommodation to your disability in the workplace. I will describe some best-case/worst-case scenarios and show what you can do in the latter.

You may feel handicapped or disabled. If so, you are not alone. A 1983 report from the Bureau of the Census indicated that about 36 million people — 15% of the population — were handicapped. About 7% of people between 34 and 44 years of age and about 21% of those between 55 and 64 had a work disability (Asch, 1984). The Digest of Data on Persons with Disabilities (1984) uses Social Security Administration data to estimate that 10% of those 18 to 64 years old who participate in the labor force are disabled. A Lou Harris poll found that of the two-thirds of Americans between the ages of 16 and 64 who are not working, two-thirds said they would like to work (ICD Survey, 1986).

The Americans with Disabilities Act (ADA) of 1990 radically changed the return-to-work landscape, as will be explained. Before doing so, it is necessary to define some terms. A handicap represents an obstacle to maximum functioning. "Disability" and "handicap" mean the same thing, but fashion dictates use of "disability" and condemns "handicap." To skim the surface of the employment aspects of ADA in the next few paragraphs requires looking at a number of federal regulations.

Under ADA, a person is considered to have a disability if the person either

1. Has a physical or mental impairment which substantially limits one or more of that person's major life activities (e.g., working, sleeping, sitting, walking, etc.)

2. Has a record of such an impairment (e.g., medical records) or
3. Is regarded as having such an impairment (e.g., "Sam has always been a hopeless alcoholic.")

The law defines physical or mental impairment as any physiological disorder or condition, cosmetic disfigurement, or anatomical loss affecting one or more of several body systems or any mental or psychological disorder.

The definition of the term "impairment" does not include physical characteristics such as eye color, hair color, left-handedness, height, weight, or muscle tone that are within the normal range and are not the result of a physiological disorder. Nor does it include common personality traits such as poor judgment or a quick temper where these are not symptoms of a mental or psychological disorder. Environmental, cultural, or economic disadvantages such as poverty, lack of education, or a prison record are not impairments. The word "Americans" in the title of the act does not imply that the law applies only to American citizens. It applies to all qualified persons with disabilities, regardless of citizenship status or nationality (*Federal Register*, July 26, 1991).

As of July 25, 1994, employers with 15 or more employees are required to avoid discriminating against qualified persons with disabilities in all aspects of employment, including:

> recruitment, advertising, job application procedures, hiring, upgrading, promotion, award of tenure, demotion, transfer, layoff, termination, right of return from layoff, rehiring, rates of pay or any other form of compensation and changes in compensation, job assignments, job classifications, organizational structures, position descriptions, lines of progression, seniority lists, leaves of absence, sick leave, or any other fringe benefits, selection and financial support for training, including apprenticeships, professional meetings, conferences and other related activities, leaves of absence to pursue training, activities sponsored by the employer, including social and recreational programs, and any other term, condition, or privilege of employment (*Federal Register,* July 26, 1991).

A disabled person is qualified if he or she can perform the *essential functions* of the position he or she holds or desires, with or without *reasonable accommodation.* The term essential functions means primary job duties that are intrinsic to the employment position the individual holds or desires. That term does not include the marginal or peripheral functions of the position that are incidental to the performance of primary job functions (*Federal Register*, July 26, 1991). Reasonable accommodations are modifications or adjustments to the job application process, to the work environment, or to the manner in which the job is performed that enable a qualified individual with a disability to be considered for the position the person desires and that do not impose an undue hardship on the business. The rules for undue hardship are strict, and an employer has a heavy burden to demonstrate undue hardship. Certainly, it cannot be a simple as "We can't afford it."

All disabilities, including chronic pain, are genuine barriers to employment. ADA rests on the premise that disability does not mean inability to work. This law focuses on how reasonable accommodation can remove barriers to employment in cases where functional limitation (e.g., pain) interacts with job requirements (Bell, 1993). Consider, for example, an automobile salesman with chronic back pain. The essential functions of this person's job are keeping track of sales leads, generating fresh leads, learning about products and showing them to potential customers, identifying and filling customers' automotive needs, ensuring that all legal documents are properly completed, and helping customers to arrange financing. Marginal aspects of the job include getting the keys out of all the cars in the parking lot and locking them up before going home at night and shoveling snow in winter. Since pain severely limits this particular salesman from getting in and out of a large number of cars to lock them up before going home every night, the employer could obey the law and provide reasonable accommodation by having someone else lock the cars and shovel snow in the winter. The employer could also provide reasonable accommodation by not requiring this salesman to work the usual 70- to 90-hour week, but permitting him to work the hours that he is able to. He was salesman of the month before he was injured, so his expertise would be an asset to the dealership.

If you can perform the essential functions of the job, the law forbids an employer to discriminate against you. It does not mean an employer has to hire you because you are disabled, but it does mean than an employer cannot discriminate against you unless you are unable to perform the essential functions of the job and no reasonable accommodation is possible. If a nondisabled person is better qualified for the job, the employer legitimately can choose that person instead of you.

Workplaces are full of architectural barriers such as doors with stiff closers that are hard to open, doors that swing shut before you can get out of the way, doors pull instead of push to open, windows that are hard to open, jerky elevators, various controls and operating mechanisms that are stiff and hard to work, uncomfortable seating at tables and work surfaces that may be at the wrong height, and steep, long, or narrow stairs. ADA requires employers to make reasonable modifications to the workplace so that persons with disabilities have access to it.

A great many employers are reluctant to hire people with disabilities (*Federal Register,* February 28, 1991), especially people with back or neck problems or with chronic pain due to a work injury. Employers may express interest in your experience until they find that you have a disability. They worry about accidents, liability and worker's compensation insurance expense, work attendance, and your ability to do the job. You need not identify yourself as disabled during the preoffer phase of the application process. The employer must focus his or her questions on your ability to perform the job and may make a job offer contingent upon your passing a preemployment medical examination. During that examination, you may disclose your disability to the doctor, who may discover it anyway. If the doctor has enough information about the job to enable a judgment as to your ability to perform that job, he or she may disqualify you or pass you. If you pass the medical examination, the employer is required to engage in a dialogue with you to identify reasonable accommodations you will need to perform essential functions of the job. Examples of reasonable accommodations for people with chronic pain may include such things as a nearby freezer for ice packs if you use ice to manage your pain; a stand-up desk if you have problems sitting; an electrically powered drafting table that moves up and down and enables you to choose whether to sit or stand; rest breaks as needed; part-time work as needed; an ergonomic chair; job restructuring; part-time or modified work schedule; reassignment to a vacant position; acquisition or modification of equipment or devices; appropriate adjustment or modification of examinations, training materials, or policies; the provision of qualified readers or interpreters, etc. (*Federal Register,* July 26, 1991). In many cases, physical or architectural barriers to effective job performance can be removed at little or no cost. The Job Accommodation Network, a service of the President's Committee on Employment of the Persons with Disabilities, maintains a computer database on such modifications and can provide information about them (toll-free telephone number 1-800-JAN-PCEH). The Network can also put you in touch with the ADA Technical Assistance Centers in your area.

Employment tests (including interviews) must be strictly job related. In other words, the interview and any other tests administered have to focus specifically on what the job requires and assess your ability to perform the essential functions of the position, with or without reasonable accommodation. Otherwise, the tests may be discriminatory and unlawful. If you think that any of the questions on the interview or other test requirements did not address your ability to perform the essential functions of the position in question and you were qualified for the position, you should consult an attorney.

Employers are not the only ones with negative attitudes, stereotypes, and prejudices against persons with disabilities. Many nondisabled people feel uneasy in the presence of people with disabilities. They reject close contact with them and believe that people with disabilities are somehow "different" in character and emotions. They may even believe that disability is punishment for sin or that disability makes a person weak and helpless in all areas of functioning. Many people are unable to focus on other characteristics of persons with disabilities that they would ordinarily use to evaluate each other and to establish normal interpersonal relationships. In the presence of disability, such people may feel a greater sense of their own vulnerability. It is important to be aware of these attitudes so you can do everything possible to avoid giving people reasons to reject you. For example, with regard to the stereotype that individuals who have disabilities are weak and helpless in all areas of functioning, even though you have chronic pain, you should recognize every aspect of you that is powerful and capable. You may have superior know-how in a certain field of work. You may be able to do precision handwork or machine work or work with various other tools. You may be an expert in a process. You may be superb with details. Be conscious of your strengths and apply them to your daily life, including your work. If you draw a blank, you may need vocational testing. If you cannot get testing through your rehabilitation provider, get it from a counselor at your local vocational–technical school. Testing and feedback may be free of charge. If you need reasonable accommodation in the vocational testing process (or in the workplace) (e.g., pain limits you from sitting longer than a half an hour), ask for reasonable accommodation. That might consist of taking part of the test one day and part another day, using a stand-up desk instead of sitting in a chair, etc. It is best to explain your need matter-of-factly, because nondisabled people may fear that they will be unable to maintain a smooth, simple interaction with you (Asch, 1984). If you need to stand, it is better to say up front, "After about 20 minutes, I need to stand for a few minutes and maybe walk a few steps. I'll still be paying attention." Your rehabilitation counselor can help you to identify awkward or unusual behaviors, especially pain behaviors, that may interfere with your relationships with nondisabled people.

WE NEED TO WORK

Work provides a number of important benefits for people. Money is the most obvious, but not necessarily the most important, as long as basic economic needs are met. Work also puts us in contact with other people, which can stimulate us and open up new opportunities for pleasure and satisfaction. It can also provide interesting and challenging activity. Basically, people are motivated to a greater or lesser extent by three things: money and everything it can buy, social interaction, and activity. We all have different preferences for these, and some of us will accept a sacrifice in one or two to maximize a third. For example, you may prefer to work with people but may accept a job without much personal contact to make more money, or you may accept a job that does not pay as well as another job, but you like the work activity and it puts you in contact with people who stimulate you. We humans are problem solvers. Work provides continuing opportunity to solve problems and so has the potential for delivering pleasure and curing our boredom. One of the major causes of job dissatisfaction is that some jobs can be mastered so quickly that they offer no challenge or opportunity for problem solving.

It is important to recognize that boring, low-paying jobs in unsafe or otherwise unpleasant work environments exist and that some owners and managers are unpleasant or exploitative. It is best to stay away from these. However, you need work, so you may accept a job in one of these environments without recognizing what you are getting into and then stay there out of habit or necessity. A person may go to any length to tune out the unpleasantness, including abusing alcohol or drugs. People who have been injured in extremely unpleasant workplaces and whose injuries provide them opportunity to stay home may be psychologically limited from returning to work because of their extreme reluctance to return to such unpleasant circumstances. Just as some workplaces can reinforce work attendance and provide job satisfaction, others can actually serve as punishment to work attendance and provoke such anxiety and dissatisfaction that a person may emphasize reasons to avoid returning to work (Fordyce (1976).

One of the more interesting findings about the relationship between work and chronic pain is that work in a decent environment seems to be good medicine for chronic pain. Pain treatment programs can be designed (1) so that work is part of the treatment program or (2) so the client seeks work *following* treatment. Posttreatment follow-up studies indicate that chronic pain patients who are employed during treatment are much more likely to be working a year or more later than those who do not return to work during treatment (Catchlove and Cohen, 1982; Painter et al., 1980; Tyre and Anderson, 1981). Treatment outcomes of 198 chronic back pain patients in the United States were compared with outcomes of 115 similar patients in New Zealand (Carron et al., 1985). Pretreatment measurements indicated that the U.S. and New Zealand patients were about the same in terms of age, gender mix, length of time since injury, etc. However, on posttreatment follow-up, the New Zealand patients reported much greater improvement than those in the United States and more of them returned to full activity. Factors in the New Zealand system reportedly different from the U.S. system were (1) in New Zealand, worker's compensation is available automatically on a no-fault basis, with no possibility of or need for litigation; (2) vocational rehabilitation is not delayed; (3) patients are directed to return to work, and substantial penalties are imposed if they refuse (if a person cannot find a job in the private sector, the government creates a job); and (4) possible cultural differences regarding how much work a person might be able to do following injury or illness.

When work or simulated work is prescribed as part of a treatment program, the program may be referred to as work hardening. A work-hardening program is designed to get you back into the habit of going to a specific workplace, being on time, and paying attention to the business at hand. Work-hardening programs are often half-day programs. The program day may begin with stretching, followed by a lecture on such topics as care of the back, avoidance of repetitive strain injuries, use and abuse of prescription pain medication, psychosocial barriers to returning to work, and the ins and outs of the worker's compensation system. The purpose of the lecture goes beyond imparting information. It gets you back in the habit of paying attention during a meeting, sitting for a period of time, and perhaps doing something you do not necessarily choose to do. People get out of the habit of doing that when they are off work. After the lecture, there may be some kind of activity designed to increase your tolerance for standing, sitting, bending, pushing, pulling, lifting, or sustained activity of parts of the body that need strengthening, followed by group psychotherapy focusing on return-to-work problem solving, stress management, or other relevant topics.

It is fairly commonly believed in some quarters that chronic pain patients who are receiving worker's compensation or who have litigation pending are less likely to benefit from pain treatment than patients who are not receiving compensation payments or are not litigating. Further, it has been suggested that litigants exaggerate the severity of the pain they experience

— or complain of pain when it is not present — in order to maximize monetary damage awards. The no-fault element in the New Zealand compensation system that eliminates litigation was established with these ideas in mind. A number of published research studies dealing with the relationship between pain and litigation demonstrate a complex relationship among pain, depression, anxiety, litigation, and employment status (Mendelson, 1984; Tait et al., 1990). However, one very simple relationship stands out: being employed is significantly related to positive treatment outcome (Dworkin et al., 1985). When times are hard, when unemployment and the proportion of people receiving food stamps increase and per capita income decreases, disability claim rates increase. Hard times are stressful, and increased stress may make pain problems even more disabling (Volinn et al., 1988).

Research has found that length of time off work because of disability is an important predictor of ability to return to work, but only at older ages. Further, at any age, people who believe that job change is relatively easy have a much better chance of returning to work than those who consider job change extremely difficult or who feel locked into a job (Gallagher et al., 1989).

It seems clear from the evidence that the sooner a person with chronic pain returns to work, the better. Why? One possibility is that when you are solving problems at work or interacting with others, you are not concentrating on pain. You may have found that when you are distracted, you do not notice pain as much. Another possibility is that work provides opportunity for positive stimulation that reduces depression, which may express itself as pain. It is not really necessary to isolate why work is good medicine for chronic pain. The fact that it happens consistently is all we need to know to move in the right direction.

Now let's look at how the process of vocational rehabilitation is designed to work, how it may get off the track, and what you might be able to do to set it right.

VOCATIONAL REHABILITATION AS A PROCESS

Medical treatment for acute injury or illness is a high-technology wonder. As soon as your acute medical problems are solved and your body is ready, you may be moved into a rehabilitation setting, where you may work with occupational and physical therapists, psychologists, and other rehabilitation professionals. As you leave the acute care setting and move into rehabilitation, you move from one world into another. Many rules change. For example, in the acute care setting, things are done *to* you, and your participation and involvement in treatment tend to be somewhat limited. In other words, if you have a broken leg, the doctor sets the leg, puts on a cast, and, barring complications, the leg will heal more or less regardless of what you do. All you have to do is hold still and not sabotage treatment, and when the cast comes off, you have to bear the pain and use it again.

As you move into a rehabilitation mode, you do more for yourself, and less is done *to* you. In rehabilitation, the more involved you are in the process and the more initiative you take, the better, assuming you do not exceed activity limits given by your physician or therapist. It is very important to know that in rehabilitation, nobody is going to fix you, especially in terms of taking away your pain. You have to learn what to do to manage routine pain and pain flare-ups. Effective pain management is very much a matter of acquiring skills. In medical rehabilitation, you get directions from physical and occupational therapists (e.g., do a certain number of repetitions of an exercise or walk a certain number of minutes at a certain rate of speed at a certain incline on a treadmill), and you follow those directions as closely as possible. You cannot wait passively in this situation for someone to fix you. As you progress in rehabilitation, medical treatment offers less and less.

Eventually, your doctor declares that you have reached maximum medical improvement, which means that additional medical care will not do you any more good, and the doctor discharges you. Near the end of treatment, you may get a functional capacity evaluation, which your doctor uses to establish the limits of your physical capabilities and tolerances. Based on this information, your doctor may indicate that you can return to your regular job, with or without restriction. Examples of restrictions may be lifting no more than 20 pounds, sitting no more than 2 hours without a break, and no bending or stooping. Under ADA, preemployment medical examinations do not have to be job related, but if the doctor says you are able to return to a job you do not think you can do or you are unable to return to a job you want to return to, the physician has to base medical opinion on your ability to perform the essential functions of the job, with or without reasonable accommodation. Along with releasing you to return to work, your doctor may give you a disability rating using a standard reference called the AMA rating guide (Engelberg, 1990).

If you are unable to return to your usual occupation, you may need to find another one. One of your priorities should be to determine whether vocational rehabilitation is a benefit under your insurance coverage; if it is not, you can go the office of your state rehabilitation agency. If vocational rehabilitation benefits are covered, your counselor may work for the medical center itself, a private company, a private nonprofit agency, or a state agency. Like medical rehabilitation, vocational rehabilitation is not something done *to* you; again it is something in which you have to participate fully to get anything out of. One of the differences between medical and vocational rehabilitation lies in their methods of reaching objectives. One author put it this way:

> Working with a vocational counselor can be a disappointment for physicians, because the counselor cannot consistently produce the desired result: a job. The patient reaches goals set by the rehabilitation team and leaves the hospital. Vocational rehabilitation is not endowed with advanced technology. It is the newest field in rehabilitation....The vocational counselor usually is only a small part of the adjustment process. Employment usually involves the entire sum of a person's capacities and abilities to adjust to a complex and challenging situation (Walker, 1965).

You have to get very much involved in the rehabilitation process. How does this process work? In the 1970s and 1980s, significant federal legislation brought about increased focus on and public funding for vocational rehabilitation. Some vocational rehabilitation activities are sponsored by private sector enterprises such as insurance companies, self-insured employers, and others. However, dollar for dollar, most vocational rehabilitation is funded by the federal government, and services are actually delivered by state vocational rehabilitation agencies. Federal funds are channeled from the U.S. Department of Health and Human Services through ten regional offices of the federal Rehabilitation Services Administration to the state agencies. The federal regional offices are responsible for overseeing evaluation and work adjustment services, developing service delivery innovations, training, and constructing rehabilitation facilities. In about half the states, two rehabilitation agencies exist: one for individuals with no visual impairments and one for persons who are blind. The rest of the states have just one agency.

Each state agency requires rehabilitation counselors to develop an Individualized Written Rehabilitation Program (IWRP) for each disabled person receiving services. The IWRP considers general and long-term vocational goals and short-term vocational objectives, detailed vocational skills and tasks, and a timetable for task and goal accomplishment. Regardless of whether the rehabilitation counselor works for a state or a private agency, he or she should base the IWRP upon a careful diagnosis of your situation. This basic requirement is supposed to guide your rehabilitation program and ensure a high standard of excellence. One of the purposes of this section is to help you evaluate how well your program meets these standards.

The first step in the vocational rehabilitation process is a preliminary diagnosis to determine eligibility for rehabilitation services. If your rehabilitation services are being funded by an insurance company, this step either may be unnecessary or you may have to hire a lawyer to help you pry these services loose. The second step is a thorough vocational diagnosis that takes place in two stages: medical and socioeconomic/psychological. The third step is treatment. Fourth is termination of services when you complete the program.

Medical diagnosis identifies primary and secondary illness or other conditions and functional limitations as applied to occupations. It should include a medical history and should document how anatomical or pathological conditions affect your ability to function generally and on the job. The weakest part of the medical examination may be the analysis of functional limitations as applied to occupations. The reason for this is that 20,000 different job titles are listed in the fourth edition of the *Dictionary of Occupational Titles*. Most medical doctors are not aware of exactly how your medical condition may affect your ability to work, because they are unlikely to know the functional requirements of your former occupation or any but a few other occupations. Your doctor may be perfectly capable of identifying the extent of your physical and perhaps emotional impairments and can test whether you can or cannot lift a certain amount of weight, can walk a certain distance, or have a certain degree of sensory impairment, but most doctors are unaware of the specific and detailed requirements of most jobs in the labor market. In the best case, an occupational therapist will go with you to your job site to analyze and evaluate the demands of a job for which you may be considered, assess its suitability to your capabilities and tolerances, and identify reasonable accommodations you may need.

However, a busy doctor may release you for return to work without knowing exactly what your job consists of. You have a right to know what job analysis information the doctor is relying upon to evaluate whether you can return to your old job. All other things being equal, it is probably better to return to your old job. But if you do not have the physical or emotional capacity to perform it, you probably need vocational rehabilitation services. The rest of this chapter describes how the evaluation is done, how to recognize a good job on the part of the rehabilitation counselor, how to recognize a bad job, and what to do if you are not satisfied with the service.

After acute and rehabilitative medical and psychological treatment is complete, socioeconomic and further psychological diagnosis should be carried out to evaluate nonphysical abilities and limitations that will affect your rehabilitation plan. Your mental abilities or educational level, vocational interests, and personality might be tested. Your history, attitudes, and motivation will be assessed by interview and in other ways. Your counselor will evaluate your reactions to your disability, whether or not you are having emotional problems related to it, and how it may affect your relations with other people. Psychological evaluation may include paper-and-pencil testing as well as "situational tests" or "work samples." For example, you may be hooked up to various kinds of mechanical apparatus and asked to demonstrate bending, lifting, twisting, pushing, pulling, etc. and may be asked to put things together or take them apart with or without using tools. Situational tests or work samples test your ability to carry out physical activities, assess your level of cooperation and your manner of relating to other people in the environment, your learning speed, and other factors.

Rubin (1978) has characterized the evaluation process for vocational rehabilitation as either short term or long term. Short-term evaluation consists of an intake interview and social history, general medical examination and medical specialty examination (by a neurologist, neurosurgeon, orthopedist, etc.), and a psychological examination (including mental ability, interest, and personality tests). Long-term evaluation consists of all of the above plus work evaluation by means of situational tests and/or work samples. The reason for indicating what is included in short-term and long-term evaluations is to help you to know how to characterize the examination you may get. A short-term examination is a basic minimum. If you do not get at least this basic minimum, you should find out why. On the other hand, if you are fortunate enough to get all the tests involved in the short-term examination, plus situational or work sample testing, do not be impatient or complain. Just hang in there and perform as well as you can.

Computer-assisted systems for matching people to jobs have emerged in recent years. In addition to administering mental ability, interest, and personality tests, your counselor may assess your ability to perform a number of specific job behaviors, such as your ability to read, use numbers, use various kinds of tools, lift certain weights, sit, stand, stoop, bend, reach, work with various kinds of people, etc., and may match these data with a computer database to match your abilities and limitations against the requirements of thousands of jobs listed in the *Dictionary of Occupational Titles* (Botterbusch, 1983) or in some other database (Robinson, 1984). The advantage of a computer-assisted job-matching system is that it can match many more details about your capabilities and limitations with the requirements of a much greater number of jobs than is possible by hand.

Based upon all the information available at a particular time, your counselor may not be able to complete your rehabilitation plan immediately and may indicate the need to extend the evaluation period to a maximum of 18 months (if your rehabilitation services are provided by the state and supported by federal funds). In any case, your rehabilitation plan should be developed *jointly* between you and your counselor, and you should be fully involved in the process. Remember, the vocational rehabilitation plan is not done *to* you; it is done *with* you — and in your behalf.

The treatment phase should involve counseling and guidance, physical and mental restoration, training, and personal adjustment. It should include such prevocational activities as field tours of job sites, rotation through various jobs, and assistance in completing job applications and using public transportation. The plan should call for whatever compensatory skill training (such as Braille if you are visually impaired), speech therapy, gait training, mobility training, and any vocational training you may need (Bitter, 1979) and should identify reasonable accommodations you may need at work.

The goal of the rehabilitation plan is placement in a job that restores you to the highest level of functioning of which you are capable. The job must be commensurate with your abilities, interests, and job potential. This is a very complex set of requirements. People often underrate the difficulty of meeting these requirements (Fishbain et al., 1988).

In the best case, the rehabilitation counselor conducts a comprehensive analysis of your physical and psychological capabilities, prepares an individualized written rehabilitation plan with much involvement by you, and identifies occupations that should enable you to function at your highest level. This involves measuring your capabilities in various ways and identifying various occupations that may fit you. This is the best method of matching you to a job: analyzing your capabilities and limitations as a basis for identifying occupations or jobs that would enable you to function at your highest level. In actual practice, a different, and far less satisfactory, method of job matching may take place. Job openings or training slots may be available and you may be pressured to accept one. By knowing how the process is supposed to work, you should be able to ask intelligent and probing questions as the basis for assigning you to a job or training situation, especially if you have not had mental ability, interest, and personality testing or if you have not been thoroughly involved in the development of your rehabilitation plan.

In the worst case, you may find a very significant difference between the high standards of professionalism found in the medical center and those described above with regard to vocational rehabilitation. A vocational rehabilitation counselor should have a master's degree or some graduate training in that specialty (Athelstan, 1982). Standards of rehabilitation counselor training and preparation vary much more widely than standards in medicine, psychology, occupational therapy, or physical therapy, and therefore quality of job performance among vocational counselors probably varies more than it does among health care professionals. At their best, vocational rehabilitation services can be excellent. But at the low end of quality, a number of problems are evident. Consider a 1974 survey of 378 vocational rehabilitation managers attending a rehabilitation conference (Muthard and Crocker, 1974). The researchers determined that 71% of these managers were employed by state rehabilitation agencies and 29% came from private rehabilitation facilities. Forty-five percent of the state employees indicated that placement and vocational counseling required only on-the-job training and several months of experience. However, employees of rehabilitation facilities said they needed a master's degree — which is a significant difference in opinion between the two groups. The researchers found that counseling and guidance was the largest single activity that counselors performed. The next largest was clerical work. Data recording and reporting was the third most significant activity. The biggest problem the rehabilitation managers claimed was role strain, that is, problems in determining eligibility for services because of changing standards, having a multiplicity of tasks to perform, trying to cope with delays in case processing, and working with unmotivated clients. They also reported lack of knowledge and skills needed to impose their own goals and perceptions on clients, lack of objectivity in their work, and personality conflicts with clients.

We have to be very careful in applying the findings of a 1974 study to situations in other times and places. But Muthard and Crocker's research suggests that tremendous variability exists among rehabilitation managers in their attitudes toward how much training and experience is necessary to do the job and in the kinds of problems rehabilitation counselors face. In places where agencies accept low educational standards, we might expect low standards of rehabilitation counselor selection, job performance evaluation, and pay. In the worst case, rehabilitation counselors have unmanageably large caseloads, are tied up with paperwork, are confused by changes in policies and procedures, and are hard to get along with. Some of them may act more like bullies than therapists. They may be evaluated on the basis of getting clients to return to their old jobs (regardless of how appropriate those jobs might be) or into any job (regardless of the degree to which it may enable their clients to reach their highest level of functioning or may be commensurate with clients' abilities and interests). This is a pretty bleak picture. You need to know about these problems so you can mobilize your resources to improve a bad situation if you are caught in one.

If you are dissatisfied with your program, you should ask questions of your rehabilitation counselor. If you do not get satisfaction at this point, you should complain in writing to your counselor and send a copy of your letter to the director of the agency. If you still do not get satisfaction, complain in writing to the director of the regional office of the Rehabilitation Services Administration and enclose a copy of the letter you wrote to your counselor and the director of the agency, along with copies of their replies, if any. Of course, if your case is not being handled under the state and federal system, your complaint will have to flow through other channels. If you feel as though you are being brushed off, it may be wise to consult an attorney.

SUMMARY AND CONCLUSIONS

You need to get back to work, and you are concerned about your ability to do so and what kind of a job you might be able to do. You need vocational rehabilitation.

Disabled people are protected by law and need that protection because they meet with serious discrimination. Try to minimize your disability in every way you can. Get help to identify any pain behaviors you may exhibit, such as moaning and groaning, grimacing, holding or rubbing the part of your body that hurts, etc., so you do not give people reasons to avoid you.

Get back to work as soon as you can. Work provides a number of important benefits: money, social interaction, and interesting activity. Each of these benefits has a different appeal, and you should try to find a job that enables you to meet your preferences. Returning to work is highly correlated with success in pain treatment; the sooner you return to work, the better.

Most vocational rehabilitation is federally funded, although services are delivered through state rehabilitation agencies. Private sector organizations provide rehabilitation services, too.

In the best case, you will be working with a highly trained, thoroughly capable, professional rehabilitation counselor who will lead you through the process. However, vocational rehabilitation counselors vary considerably in education, training, and experience. In the worst case, you will work with an incompetent or overworked individual and/or an agency in which counselors are undertrained, confused by changing eligibility requirements, buried under a heavy caseload with a lot of paperwork, and where personality conflicts with clients are routine. If you find yourself in that position, you should begin by asking for information. You should ask whether your counselor is formulating an IWRP for you and should say that you know that you should be involved in its preparation. You should ask if you will be taking mental ability, vocational interest, and personality tests and when. If you are directed into a training program or a job on the basis of what appears to be minimal evaluation, you should begin asking questions. If you find that courteous and interested questions on your part are meeting with hostility and/or minimal effort on the part of the counselor, it is time to start a diary and to write letters to your counselor, his or her boss, and the regional office of the Rehabilitation Services Administration or to consult with legal counsel if the system is not responsive. Surely not everyone needs an attorney, but some people definitely do.

Get involved in the process. Cooperate. With the right kind of help, you can find work that is challenging, interesting, and feasible.

BIBLIOGRAPHY

Asch, A. (1984). The experience of disability: a challenge for psychology, *American Psychologist,* 39, 529–536.

Athelstan, G.T. (1982). Vocational assessment and management, in *Krusen's Handbook of Physical Medicine and Rehabilitation,* 3rd ed., Kottke, F.J., Stillwell, G.K., and Lehmann, J.F. (Eds.), W.B. Saunders, Philadelphia.

Bell, C.G. (1993). The Americans with Disability Act and injured workers, *Rehabilitation Psychology,* 38, 103–116.

Bitter, J.A. (1979). *Introduction to Rehabilitation,* C.V. Mosby, St. Louis.

Botterbusch, K.F. (1983). A Comparison of Computerized Job Matching Systems, Materials Development Center, Menomonie Department of Rehabilitation and Manpower Services, University of Wisconsin-Stout; Botterbusch, K.F. (1986). A Comparison of Computerized Job Matching Systems (Revised Edition), Materials Development Center, Stout Vocational Rehabilitation Institute, School of Education and Human Services, University of Wisconsin-Stout.

Carron H., DeGood, D.E., and Tait, R. (1985). A comparison of low back pain patients in the United States and New Zealand: psychosocial and economic factors affecting severity of disability, *Pain*, 21, 77–89.

Catchlove, R. and Cohen, K. (1982). Effects of a directive return to work approach in the treatment of workman's compensation patients with chronic pain, *Pain*, 14, 181–191.

Digest of Data on Persons with Disabilities, Congressional Research Service, June 1984.

Dworkin, R.H., Handlin, D.S., Richlin, D.M., Brand, L., and Vannucci, C. (1985). Unraveling the effects of compensation, litigation and employment on treatment response in chronic pain, *Pain*, 23, 49–59.

Engelberg, A.L. (1990). *Guides to the Evaluation of Permanent Impairment*, 3rd ed. rev., American Medical Association, Chicago.

Federal Register (February 28, 1991). Part VI, Equal Employment Opportunity Commission, 29 CFR Part 1630, Equal Employment Opportunity for Individuals with Disabilities; Notice of Proposed Rulemaking.

Federal Register (July 26, 1991). Part V, Equal Employment Opportunity Commission, 29 CFR Part 1630, Equal Employment Opportunity for Individuals with Disabilities; Final Rule.

Fishbain, D.A., Goldberg, M., Labbe, E., Steele, R., and Rosomoff, H. (1988). Compensation and non-compensation chronic pain patients compared for DSM-III operational diagnoses, *Pain*, 32, 197–206.

Fordyce, W.E. (1976). *Behavioral Methods for Chronic Pain and Illness*, C.V. Mosby, St. Louis.

Gael, S. (1988). *The Job Analysis Handbook for Business Industry and Government*, John Wiley & Sons, New York.

Gallagher, R.M., Rauh, V., Haugh, L.D., Milhous, R., Callas, P.W., Langelier, R., McClallen, J.M., and Frymoyer, J. (1989). Determinants of return-to-work among low back pain patients, *Pain*, 39, 55–67.

ICD Survey of Disabled Americans, Bringing Disabled Americans into Mainstream, A Nationwide Survey of the 1,000 Disabled People, International Center for the Disabled and Lou Harris and Associates, 1986.

Mendelson, G. (1984). Compensation, pain complaints and psychological disturbance, *Pain*, 20, 169–177.

Muthard, J.E. and Crocker. L.M. (1974). Knowledge Utilization Resources and Practices of Vocational Rehabilitation Managers, Regional Rehabilitation Research Institute, College of Health-Related Professions, University of Florida, Gainesville.

Painter, J.R., Seres, J.L., and Newman, R.I. (1980). Assessing benefits of the pain center: why some patients regress, *Pain*, 8, 101–113.

Robinson, D.D. (1984). A flowchart of a computerized system for identifying alternative occupations for rehabilitation clients, in Pain, Supplement 2, Fourth World Congress on Pain of the International Association for the Study of Pain, Seattle, August 31–September 5, p. 644; Robinson, D.D. and Mecham, R.C. (1990). Occupations potentially appropriate for persons with low back pain, in Sixth World Congress on Pain of the International Association for the Study of Pain, Adelaide, S. Australia, April 5.

Rubin, S.E. (1978). *Foundations of the Vocational Rehabilitation Process*, University Park Press, Baltimore.

Tait, R.C., Chibnall, J.T., and Richardson, W.D. (1990). Litigation and employment status: effects on patients with chronic pain, *Pain*, 43, 37–46.

Tyre, T.E. and Anderson, D.L. (1981). Inpatient management of the chronic pain patient: a one-year follow-up study, *Journal of Family Practice*, 12, 819–827.

U.S. Department of Labor Employment Standards Administration (1979). Disabilities by major ranking involving Section 503 complaint cases.

Volinn, E., Lai, D., McKinney, S., and Loeser, J.D. (1988). When back pain becomes disabling: a regional analysis, *Pain*, 33, 33–39.

Walker, R.A. (1965). Vocational assessment and management, in *Handbook of Physical Medicine and Rehabilitation*, 2nd ed., Krusen, F.H., Kottke, F.J., and Ellwood, P.M. (Eds.), W.B. Saunders, Philadelphia, pp. 178–192.

Section V

Medication Management in the Treatment of Patients with Chronic Pain

21 Medications That May Be Useful in the Management of Patients with Chronic Intractable Pain

Michael S. Margoles, M.D., Ph.D.

INTRODUCTION

History and Introductory Remarks

Much has been written about prescribing medications for patients with cancer pain, acute pain, and postoperative pain. Relatively little has been written about prescribing medications for people with chronic nonmalignant pain.

The field of pain therapy began in 1975 and is still in its infancy. Pain problems have been treated since the beginning of time, but the real medical–scientific attack on the problem began recently. As frontiers are pushed ahead, there are many areas in which new approaches to old problems are being developed. The chapters in the section on medication are addressed to the millions of Americans who suffer the agony of day-to-day chronic (more than 6 months) mild to severe pain in one or more areas of the body; pain that results from work injuries, bending injuries, lifting injuries, and auto accidents (whiplash); and pain that begins for no apparent reason. This misunderstood, forsaken, and harassed group of chronic intractable pain patients is usually dealt a "lean cut" when it comes to obtaining adequate medications from the medical profession and from many state medical boards.

The judicious use of medication can be thought of as "first aid" for the management of a chronic intractable pain problem. While never an end in itself, it can be a substantial means to providing help to facilitate return to work, sleep normalization, etc.

The listing of various medicines in the chapters in this section on medication is far from exhaustive. The reader is referred to the drug package inserts, the *Physician's Drug Reference* (PDR), *Drug Facts and Comparisons, The Medical Drug Reference,* and the many other texts and software specifically devoted to detailed presentation of diversified medications.

Course of Disease in Chronic Intractable Pain

Many professionals and patients do not understand that some chronic intractable pain problems become worse with the passage of time. Two of the most common chronic intractable pain problems that can become worse with time are fibromyalgia and myofascial pain syndrome. Many chronic pain patients relate a history of progressive increase of pain and/or pain distribution and a decreased ability to physically function with the passage of time. This downhill course is most frequently related by patients with 3 or more years of symptoms and pain that involves numerous body areas. The problem with some of these persons is that the basic underlying disease process has not been understood and/or adequately treated. A careful, thorough history taken from the person should serve as an indicator of progressive disease. All too frequently, however, the patient goes from doctor to doctor looking for pain relief, and the total history of symptoms and events is not fully explored. A few additional progressive pain problems that could be helped with opioids or opioid-containing analgesics are rheumatoid arthritis, osteoarthritis, ankylosing spondylitis, lupus, arachnoiditis, reflex sympathetic dystrophy syndrome, and countless others.

Many medications help the pain for a while, but they seem to lose their potency over time. This is usually not due to tolerance to the medication(s), but rather is often an indicator that the underlying disease is becoming progressively worse. At that point, there is a need for further physical examination, consultation, and testing. If these approaches prove negative for disease, then more adequate medication needs to be considered for control of pain symptoms.

Good Days and Bad

Most chronic intractable pain problems follow a variable course. There may be days to weeks of relatively low levels of pain and physical dysfunction, and at those times the need for medications is decreased. However, without proper treatment of the underlying disease problem, there is a progression toward more "bad days" with the passage of time. The cautious person adapts to this problem by "giving up" and progressively stops all activities that provoke the pain. This may lead to loss of job and employment productivity, decreased or no sexual activity, decreased social activity, rejection by friends who don't understand, and sometimes divorce and/or suicide.

Complex Problems

Chronic intractable pain and its related discomforts and disabilities can present some of the most complex problems that are seen in medicine. The use of medications as pharmaceutical adjuncts to the overall treatment program represents only a small part of the total patient treatment program. However, this aspect of the treatment of chronic intractable pain, if properly administered, can have a significant salutary effect on the patient and on his or her response to the rest of the treatment program. All too frequently, pharmaceutical support becomes one of the primary struggling grounds between doctor and patient.

Polypharmacy

Poly means many, and *pharmacy* means a pharmaceutical or drug. Some patients will insist on *polypharmacy* (many drugs) in an attempt to find the right combination(s) of drugs that will satisfy their faith in medication to "do the trick" in treating their problems. Some patients may be on tranquilizers, sedatives, muscle relaxers, sleeping pills, analgesics, and antidepressants or mood elevators all at the same time or over a period of time. Their history of drugs used for pain relief reads like a physician's drug reference book. Sometimes as many as 50–60 different prescription medications are tried over a period of 5 years. They do not realize that *medications are to be used as a means to an end and never an end in themselves.* Problems also arise from some patients' continued attempt to find the right drug or combination of drugs that helps them the most.

Some physicians may use a polypharmacy approach to treat all the symptoms that a chronic intractable pain patient presents. Whereas there are specific drugs manufactured for certain diseases, such as insulin for diabetics, there are still no drugs that are specific for the treatment of most types of chronic intractable pain. Therefore, the components of the chronic intractable pain problem, listed below, may each have to be treated with a separate medication or a separate approach for each part of the problem. For example:

Symptom	*Drug or treatment*
Pain	Analgesic, nerve block
Muscle spasm	Muscle relaxer, biofeedback
Stiffness	Anti-inflammatory drug, physical therapy
Burning	Analgesic, tricyclic antidepressant, Inderal®
Numbness	Nerve block or surgery
Depression	Antidepressant, psychotherapy, thyroid, Cortef, estrogen, testosterone
Sleep problem	Sleeping pill, tranquilizer, analgesic, antidepressant, behavior management, estrogen, progesterone
Gut irritation	Antacid or gastric acid secretion blocker
Allergies	Antihistamine

Dosage Range

There is no standard dose of medication suitable for all patients. Drug companies recommend a dosage range for the doctor to follow when he or she prescribes medication. Doctors are expected to stay within the recommended dosage range, but they also have the privilege of giving medication doses that are outside (more than or less than) the recommended dosage range if needed to help provide the desired clinical result. Using doses of medication above the maximum recommended dosing requires careful selection of medication and careful monitoring of the patient. Respect for the medication and the doctor prescribing the medication are vital to a successful doctor–patient relationship.

The amount of medication a patient may need is predicated on a number of factors, including severity of symptoms, present activity level, and goals. For example, a low back pain patient working an 8-hour-a-day manual labor job may require more analgesic medication than a similar individual (one with the exact same back pain problem) who stays home all day. Absorption of a medication may vary from person to person. The best way to establish the proper dose of almost any medication is by blood tests to make sure there is enough of the medication in the bloodstream.

MEDICATIONS: GENERAL STATEMENTS AND SPECIFIC MEDICATIONS

Acute Model

Current teaching about the medication management of pain symptoms has been derived from what is called the "acute model." This applies to pain that is of short duration, usually 30 days or less, and originates from an accident or surgery. This type of pain is usually expected to last no more than 3–6 weeks.

Patient Self-Medicates and Then Sees the Doctor

Much of the chronic mild to moderate pain, with its day-to-day variations in intensity, is treated by the use of over-the-counter medications such as aspirin, Excedrin®, Anacin 3®, Tylenol®, Nuprin®, Advil®, and others. Patients who see a physician for the treatment of a chronic intractable pain problem have usually tried a number of these products.

The Doctor and Medications for Chronic Intractable Pain

The chronic intractable pain patient model is emerging in the medical literature as a complex, ongoing mixture of problems. We are trying and testing medications to find which ones work best for specific pain problems. We physicians lack understanding of exactly what chronic intractable pain is and what causes it. We have theories and opinions. We lack understanding of exactly what each drug has to specifically offer chronic intractable pain patients.

In general, the need for and use of analgesic medication that is more effective than over-the-counter products the patient may already be taking depends on:

1. The cause and severity of the pain problem
2. The patient's desire to use analgesics to relieve some of his or her pain symptoms
3. The willingness of the physician to prescribe appropriate and adequate doses of analgesics

Medications That May Disagree with the Patient

Not all medications are tolerated well by chronic intractable pain patients. One reason is that the person's physiology is compromised. This promotes intolerance to nonsteroidal anti-inflammatory drugs such as aspirin and similar preparations. Some drugs contain nightshades (substances derived from potato, tomato, pepper, or eggplant). The patient taking such a drug might have a nightshade reaction such as a headache, upset stomach, pain flare-up, etc. An example of such a drug is K-Lyte, a fizzy potassium supplement. After experiencing a headache from taking it, a patient showed me where the term "natural flavoring" appeared on the label. Natural flavoring may contain pepper or other nightshade substances.

Drug Representatives

America is a drug-oriented society. Many companies produce pills for many purposes. We use medications to help us cope and function and to rid our bodies of disease.

Drug companies send out marketing representatives who call on doctors at their offices and conferences. They might be seen as a friendly group of "lobbyists" for the pharmaceutical companies. Their goal is to sell the busy physician on using the latest products. These door-to-door sales are backed up by fancy ads in numerous medical and lay public magazines that come the doctor's way throughout the month.

This is where all the doctor's "samples" come from. They are an inducement to try out the new medication in preference to many of the old medications that may still work well.

Generic versus Brand Name Products

Predictable Potency

Brand name medications have "predictable potency," which means that the medication, as originally formulated, will work over and over again, producing the same results in a given type of situation. Brand name medications go through rigorous development and testing procedures before they are approved by the Food and Drug Administration.

Generic medications are those which are made as less costly alternatives to name brand products. A generic medication does not have to pass the same number of stringent criteria that the original brand name product had to. Therefore it can be sold for less money. Generic medications have the same pharmaceutical name and contents as brand name products, but frequently the formulation or production may be slightly different. For example, the way that a product is made or how it is put into pill or capsule form may make it perform slightly differently than the brand name product. A generic product may perform well for a number of patients, but other patients will not get the full potency effect from it. I prefer to think of generics as "carbon copies" of the original. They are not quite as "sharp" as the original.

The Story of Mrs. Jones

A number of factors that influence a person's tolerance to pain and pain medications are outside the individual's domain of control. These may be related to drugs:

1. There is a relative tolerance between drugs.
   a. A pain patient may be "tolerant" to high doses of ingested Darvon® or hydrocodone (Vicodin®, etc.) but be very intolerant to low doses of oral morphine. Morphine is much more potent than Darvon® or hydrocodone.
   b. Some generic analgesic medications are less potent than the brand name medications they imitate.
2. Some patients have a genetic problem that prevents them from getting relief at anything but high doses of opioids or other medications.

For most individuals who need to use medication for a short period of time, a generic may perform as well as a brand name product. However, individuals with chronic intractable pain need predictable and continuous pain relief. Their way of living and earning a living may depend on obtaining predictable pain relief from a medication. Their need for analgesic medication may go on for years. Generic drugs may impair physical performance by providing less than optimal pain control as compared to brand name products.

The following is a hypothetical example, with a factitious individual history, to illustrate the generic versus brand name dilemma. The scenario has occurred with a number of my patients during my 21 years as a pain management specialist.

Brand Name Pain Killer

Pain-ender (fictitious name)
Chemical name: 5-Hydroxy-salicyl-hydrocodone-acetaminophen
Generic name: Hydrocodone and acetaminophen (H&A)

Mrs. Jones is a 35-year-old housewife and executive secretary. Three years ago, she was involved in an auto accident, and since then has had frequent low back and leg pain. The pain interfered with her sleep and her ability to do all her secretarial duties. She was off work for 3 weeks after the accident. When she returned to work, she could work only 6 hours most days. A few days out of the week she had to go home after 4 hours at the office. Her ability to do routine housework was very limited. Vacuuming became torture. The family had to frequently pitch in and help her. As of a year ago, she could work only 4 hours per day and missed 2 days of work every 2 weeks. She never looked all that bad, but nonetheless she was "loosing ground."

She sought help from numerous of the best physicians, but the various therapies were not helping. Eight months ago, she consulted Dr. Vasquez, a physician who was a board-certified pain management specialist. After careful evaluation, he put her on Pain-ender for pain control. She found that if she took six tablets on a time-contingent (by the clock) schedule on her "bad days" and four time-contingent pain tablets on her "good days," it gave her 30–50% pain relief. With the use of the medication, she could work 8 hours a day and do half of her usual housework. She was less irritable and more pleasant to be around. Mrs. Jones' life was back to feeling somewhat normal for the first 3 months after starting the medication.

One day, the pharmacist gave her hydrocodone and acetaminophen (H&A), a generic "equivalent" to Pain-ender. After the second day on H&A, she noted that she could not work the whole day. After 6 hours at work, her back began to act up and she had to go home. Household chores provoked more pain than usual. She increased the dosing of the H&A to eight tablets per day, but the increase in pain relief was minimal. For a time, Dr. Vasquez thought she was developing a tolerance to the drug and possibly abusing it or perhaps had become a drug seeker. Mrs. Jones thought her pain was getting worse. After a month of this dilemma, Dr. Vasquez prescribed Pain-ender and specified that the pharmacist use the brand name product and no generic. After 2 days back on Pain-ender, Mrs. Jones was back to work full time, back to her usual housework (the work she could do while taking four to six Pain-ender tablets per day), and was more pleasant to be around. After that, she obtained the same predictable relief as long as she stayed with Pain-ender.

This type of problem with the use of generics affects relatively few patients. However, those it does affect adversely should be given special consideration for the use of brand name medicine only. Had Dr. Vasquez not put Mrs. Jones back on Pain-ender, he would have been faced with a seemingly runaway pain problem that might have generated a need for magnetic resonance imaging (MRI) (20% produce false-positive results) and back surgery that would have failed. The MRI, surgery, and related expenses would have cost a minimum of $50,000. A lifetime supply of Pain-ender medication would likely not cost that much.

Other Problems Related to Generics

Generics are less expensive imitations of brand name medications. One way to cut costs in manufacturing the generic is to use less expensive ingredients. For instance, manufacturers of generics will use "starch" or "modified food starch" as one of the ingredients in a tablet. Those terms usually refer to potato starch, the cheapest type of starch. Cornstarch is the more expensive type of starch used by pharmaceutical manufacturers and is usually identified as "cornstarch" when it is used. The difference between the two is usually minimal unless you happen to have nightshade syndrome (potato, tomato, pepper, and eggplant). If you have adverse reactions to pills that contain the cheaper type of starch, it is probably the potato starch to which you are reacting.

Consider the case of Patrick P. He had a clinically proven case of nightshade sensitivity and had been given a prescription for Vicodin®. The pharmacist filled it with a generic. Patrick stated the medication worked well compared to the Easprin he had taken before (he was found to have colitis and bleeding ulcers after a year and a half on three Easprin tablets per day) When he took enough generic Vicodin® to get good pain relief, he was hung over the next day. The hangover bothered him and discouraged him from using the medication more than occasionally. This prevented him from returning to active work because of the inability of the medication to give predictable pain relief without significant side effects of tiredness and hangover. Switching him to brand name Vicodin® solved that problem and provided better and more predictable pain relief, so that he could better participate in his rehabilitation program.

Goals of Medication Usage

Chronic intractable pain patients may have to be on one medication or a combination of medications for a number of years. The question of greatest concern is which medications can be given to the patient for long periods of time with the least amount of risk or harm to the patient. Use of analgesic medications for chronic intractable pain patients, as part of the treatment program, can be helpful in accomplishing the following goals:

1. Reduce pain symptoms
2. Improve physical functioning (mobility)
3. Improve sleep that is disturbed by pain and other factors
4. Improve socialization by reducing pain and discomfort
5. Improve work function and decrease absenteeism due to pain-related disability
6. Decrease anxiety, tension, and depression related to the pain problem

A drug may relieve some of the pain that a patient has simply because it relieves some of the tension and anxiety associated with the pain. This is true of the tranquilizers, muscle relaxers, and medications used for sleep. In some cases, a tranquilizer, antidepressant, or muscle relaxer is all the medication a patient will need for control of his or her pain problem. In a similar fashion, many of the opioids and opioid-containing analgesics reduce the anxiety produced by the pain problem by decreasing the pain intensity. This is a characteristic of opioid medications that often is not appreciated in contemplating their use.

The Symptom/Cause "Travel" Model

The main idea here is that you can get to your destination goals quicker with fast-acting medication that controls your pain symptoms. Using opioids and/or opioid-containing analgesics to treat the symptoms of chronic intractable pain can be likened to travel. The "goal" of the "travel" is to be pain free and back to life as usual. We can liken this to a trip to England. There are two ways to arrive there from California. One way is to fly direct from San Francisco or Los Angeles to Washington, D.C. and take the Concord from there to England. The trip takes about 10 hours. The other way is by land and sea. You take the train from San Francisco or Los Angeles to New York. That takes about 3 days. You next travel by ship to England, a journey of more than 2 weeks. In the first instance, you arrive at the "goal" destination about a month ahead of the land/sea travel route. There is time to get a head start on goal-oriented activities, shopping, finding a place to live, getting a job, and starting to work. The person can get back to an active exercise program and "plug into" an active social life. In other words, time lost from usual routine and activities is minimized. The land/ sea route represents the hard and lengthy work that has to be done to treat the cause of the pain problem and get rid of the cause. Both the air/flight and the land/sea models deserve vital consideration in the rehabilitation of a patient with chronic intractable pain. The fast and straight route (use of specific medications to treat the problematic symptom of the pain problem) can get the patient back into the swing of things with the least amount of lost time from his or her usual environment. The long route deals with the cause(s) of the chronic intractable pain problem and attempts to rid the patient of them so that there is hopefully no long-term need for opioids.

These two "trips" can be likened to the two major aspects of treatment necessary in the management of a patient with moderate to severe chronic intractable pain. The air travel model shows what can be accomplished when the *symptoms* are treated, and the land/sea model addresses the more lengthy process of treating the *cause* of the chronic intractable pain problem. Rehabilitation of some chronic intractable pain patients requires that both trips be accomplished simultaneously.

Dosing Schedules for Medications

As Needed

Many medications for chronic intractable pain patients are given on an as-needed or "prn" dosing schedule. This is acceptable for acute pain problems, *but it causes the chronic intractable pain patient to react to his or her pain.* By that I mean that when the pain or related symptom (irritability, tingling, insomnia, pressure, anxiety, tension, tightness, tiredness, fatigue, gut symptoms, depression, cramping, burning, muscle twitching, feeling cold) reaches a certain severity, the patient reacts to it by taking a pain pill. It forces the patient to recognize the pain and related symptom and makes him or her concentrate on it while trying to take something to relieve the it.

Time Contingent and Schedule Contingent

Time contingent and schedule contingent mean that medication is taken by the clock and/or by the schedule, not according to what symptom the patient is experiencing or how intense it may be. Medication is taken around the clock at regular intervals, and on a schedule(s), to suppress a certain amount of pain and related problems on a regular schedule and/or an around-the-clock basis.

For example, you may have chronic insomnia associated with your pain problem. You have to be to work by 8:30 a.m. each morning from Monday to Friday. You may need to sleep 8 hours, from 10:30 p.m. to 6:30 a.m. That 8 hours of rest is crucial for your body to wind down and repair itself. The doctor has prescribed 40 mg of Prozac® and has told you to take it 1 hour before you want to be asleep. You note that the medication takes 1½ hours to get you to sleep. You check with the doctor and you both agree that on work nights your scheduled dose of Prozac® is 40 mg to be taken at 9:00 p.m. The doctor tells you that the scheduled dose of bedtime Prozac® can be 1–2 hours later (10:00–11:00 p.m.).

Initial and Final Dosing Schedules

The schedule below can be used for time-contingent medication dosing. The goal is for the patient to find, within prescribed limits, some continuous pain relief without troublesome side effects. The tablets may be broken up into smaller parts (less than one tablet) if the patient proves to be too sensitive to the one-tablet dose.

Time-Contingent Pain Medication Schedule

Do not use this time-contingent technique without first showing it to and discussing it with your doctor. Begin with one-half tablet every 6 hours. If no significant pain control is obtained, take one-half tablet every 4 hours. If no significant pain control, take one-half tablet every 3 hours. If no significant pain control, take one tablet every 6 hours. If no significant pain control, take one tablet every 4 hours. If no significant pain control, take one tablet every 3 hours. If this dosing does not work, consult your physician for further instructions. Do not use a pill cutter or other device to cut a time-release tablet in half. You may interfere with the time-release mechanism if you do so.

Do not take pain medications more often than at 3-hour intervals unless told to do so by your physician.

The above schedule is reversed when the medication is no longer needed as frequently or when the patient's tolerance for the medication begins to decline. It can then be used to taper the patient off of the medication.

If you are awake at night, when it comes time to take your next dose of medication, take it. If you are asleep at that time, do not wake yourself up to take that dose.

When you are taking your medication by the clock, you do not react to it. You work to suppress some of it by finding the best time interval and dosage strength for taking it regularly. Once you arrive at the most effective time interval and dose, you stay at that dose until you and your therapist agree to change it. Using this approach, you remove *some* of your pain from the problem so that you can begin to respond appropriately to matters other than your pain. By working to suppress some of your pain with the medications, you can then turn your attention to more important matters, such as family, friends, work, and the other aspects of your pain rehabilitation problem.

You need to ask your doctor if he or she would be willing to let you try this method of taking your medication. Without your doctor's permission you would be prescribing for yourself. That would be illegal and could be grounds for a physician to dismiss you from his or her practice because directions were not followed.

Dosing Curves

Figure 21.1 shows the blood level of drug versus the percent of pain relief. The drug depicted represents one of the routinely used nontime-release analgesic medications such as Darvocet-N® 100, Talwin®, Tylenol® with codeine, aspirin with codeine, Vicodin®, Percodan®, morphine, etc. All of these have a relatively short half-life of about 3-6 hours, which means that about 50% of the medication is gone from the blood in 3–6 hours. The curve shows that the pain relief reaches about 40% in mild to moderate pain at about 1–2 hours after the medication is taken by mouth. By the time 3–4 hours has gone by, the blood level is going down and the pain relief is half, down to 20% of what it was when the blood level was maximum. The blood level then goes down slowly from there, and so does the pain relief.

When to Dose (Timing)

To maintain effective pain relief in the treatment of a chronic intractable pain condition, whether of malignant or nonmalignant origin, a number of things must be done. It is best to

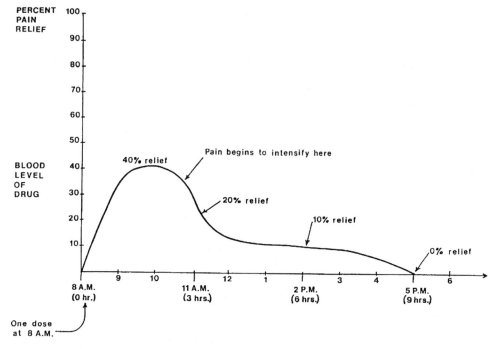

FIGURE 21.1   Dosing by drug half-life. For this graph, assume that the pain is of mild to moderate intensity. Assume that half of the drug clears out of the blood in 3 hours.

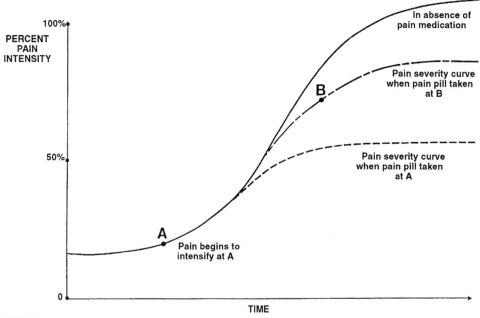

FIGURE 21.2   Pain spike.

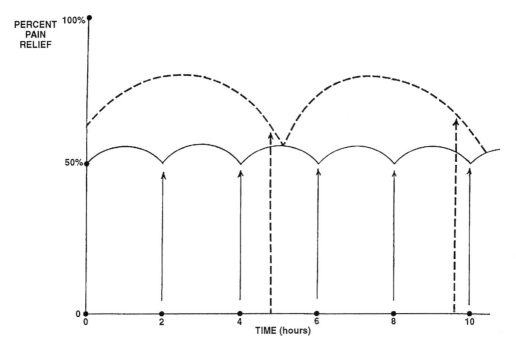

FIGURE 21.3   Frequency of analgesic dosing for a drug with a half-life of 3–4 hours: good versus bad days. (—) Frequency of dosing on days when pain is severe ("bad days"). (---) Frequency of dosing on days when pain is mild ("good days").

take your pain medication when the pain begins to intensify, rather than taking a pill when the pain is at a peak. Figure 21.2 shows a pain spike beginning to occur. In the absence of any medication, it escalates up to sometimes unbearable pain. If the pain medication is taken at "B," there is slight modification of the intensity. However, if enough medication is taken at "A," there is significant modification of the pain flare-up.

Frequency of Dosing: Good Days versus Bad

On the days your pain is more intense ("bad days"), your need for pain medication goes up. Therefore, on "bad days," dosing should be more frequent. This is shown on the lower curve of Figure 21.3. On days when the pain is less problematic ("good days"), you will be able to get the same amount of pain relief with less frequent dosing of your pain medication. This is shown on the upper curve.

Proper Use of Dosage Strengths

Some pain patients cannot tolerate a whole tablet of any pain-relieving medication. This is common in some women. Therefore, when using a time-contingent schedule for taking your medications, you may need to use only half-strength doses. This is shown on the lower curve of Figure 21.4. If your tolerance for a medication is low, you may run into the problem expressed on the upper curve: You begin to take the medication on a time-contingent basis, and before long you become dizzy, light-headed, and tired. In that event, cut the tablet in half, or if a capsule, pour half of it out. After a pause of 4–8 hours, begin dosing on the schedule

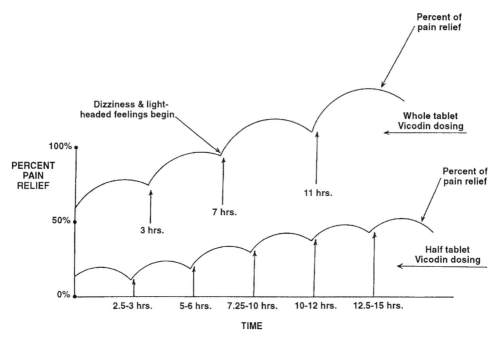

FIGURE 21.4   Proper use of dosage strengths: time-contingent schedule.

shown in the lower curve. Do not cut sustained-release tablets in half. Always inform your physician of any adverse effects of medication, even if the adverse effects are overcome by dose cutting.

Appreciate That in Some Conditions Pain Worsens with Time

A number of pain conditions, if untreated, become worse with the passage of time. This occurs in the more severe and progressive cases of chronic myofascial pain syndrome, fibromyalgia, certain types of cancer, and other conditions. Over time, the pain and dysfunction related to pain become worse and more severe. Therefore, as shown in Figure 21.5, over time it appears as though you are developing a tolerance to your pain medications, but in actuality the pain problem is worsening and there is a relatively increased need for more analgesic medication to adequately control the pain symptoms.

> There is more suffering from taking too little analgesic medication
> than from taking too much.
>
> —The author (1989)

Analgesic Frequency Dosing

Two of the many factors affecting the frequency of dosing of opioids and/or opioid-containing analgesics are potency of the medication and the patient's pain level. An analgesic that is weaker than the patient's pain may have to be taken frequently to get some pain relief (i.e., every 3 hours). An analgesic that is stronger than the pain will be taken less frequently to achieve the same pain relief (i.e., every 4–8 hours).

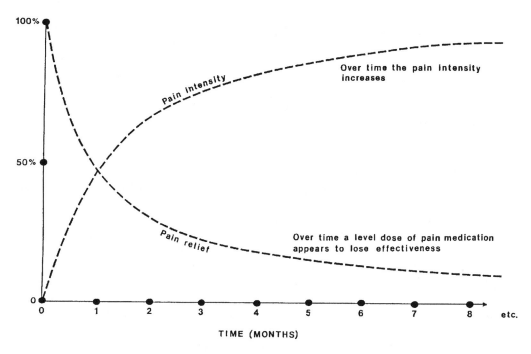

FIGURE 21.5   Pain medication may appear to lose effectiveness over time. In reality, the pain is becoming progressively stronger.

TABLES OF SIDE EFFECTS

A table of some of the more important adverse effects is provided for each category of drugs listed below.

Adverse effects are split into two subgroups: (1) toxic effects and (2) side effects. In any given patient, only one or a few of the symptoms may occur as a manifestation of toxicity or side effect to that drug.

I have not seen a patient manifest all the side effects or toxic reactions listed for a given medication. If you think you are having a problem with toxic or side effects to a prescribed medication, call your physician to discuss the problem.

ANALGESICS: NONNARCOTIC

On the issue of analgesics, it must be kept in mind that the patient may have to stay on pain-relieving medication for a number of years. The search for appropriate medication should focus on those which cause the least harm or potential harm with long-term administration. I generally tend to favor older medications, those that have been around for a while, because we know how they have worked out. Also, the older medications are usually ones that have survived because of little tendency to cause problems.

Nonsteroidal Anti-Inflammatory Drugs

These are drugs that treat pain from inflammation associated with heat, redness, and swelling of tissues and/or joints. They have no cortisone (steroid) in them; the name "nonsteroidal" is used to specify that fact. Nonsteroidal anti-inflammatory drugs (NSAIDs) are a group of weak analgesics. These medications provide pain relief by reducing inflammation and swelling in tissues, as well as a direct analgesic effect. See the table below for some members of this group. One author stated that it was his opinion "…that it has yet to be conclusively proved that the nonsteroidal drugs offer any major advantage over aspirin" (Aranoff, 1985). The most frequently used member of this group is aspirin. "Today, the drug of initial choice for the early treatment of chronic intractable pain remains aspirin" (Aranoff, 1985). There are people who cannot tolerate aspirin or aspirin-like drugs (Motrin®, Naprosyn®, Lodine®, Rufen®, and others) for a variety of reasons. For them, acetaminophen (Tylenol®) is a substitute. Although acetaminophen has the same analgesic strength as aspirin, it does not have the anti-inflammatory properties. This reduces its usefulness somewhat. Zomax® and Oraflex® are NSAIDs that have been removed from the pharmacies by the Food and Drug Administration because of a number of deaths associated with their use. Phenacetin, which is the "P" in APC, is no longer used as a combination ingredient in many preparations because it was found to produce severe kidney damage after long-term use when combined with a number of other ingredients. The NSAIDs are beneficial in short-term use for pain problems of a mild degree that are associated with acute sprain/strain or inflammation of tissues or joints. Each year, about two or three new NSAIDs appear on pharmacists' shelves, yet these drugs have not been dramatically useful in the treatment of chronic intractable pain other than that related to some forms of inflammatory arthritis such as rheumatoid arthritis. Osteoarthritis may or may not have an inflammatory component, and therefore, if no inflammation is present, it may not respond to an NSAID.

The risks and costs of medication and medication-related side effects from using an NSAID may be higher than using Darvon®, codeine, or other opioids (Rose, 1992). These medications may be useful in the treatment of some of the problems associated with chronic intractable pain problems, including morning stiffness, stiffness and soreness of muscles that occur after sports or other exertional activities, menstrual and premenstrual cramping, and common headaches.

To ease some morning stiffness, the NSAID is taken at bedtime. To reduce some of the discomfort that comes from sports or rehabilitation exercises, one tablet is taken 1 hour before the activity. The most effective choice is aspirin. If plain aspirin upsets the stomach, Ecotrin®, which is coated and dissolves farther down in the digestive tract, can be taken instead. These drugs should always be taken with some food to avoid irritation of the gut. While aspirin has to be given every 4 hours to keep the blood levels of it up, some of the newer NSAIDs have to be taken only once per day; examples are Naprosyn® and Dolobid®. Feldene® has to be taken only once per day.

Recently, we began using 50 mg/ml of sodium thiosalicylate as an injectable anti-inflammatory, with potency similar to that of intravenous colchicine injection. This is injectable salicylate. It is an old medication and is available under a number of names. The advantages of this medication are

1. Well tolerated by many patients
2. Potent NSAID
3. Can be injected at any routine injection site in the body
4. Patients can be taught to self-administer this medication
5. Low incidence of irritation of the gut

Because information on this product may be difficult to obtain, package insert material is provided below.

NO-DOLO®; SODIUM THIOSALICYLATE INJECTION

FOR INTRAMUSCULAR USE

DESCRIPTION: Sodium Thiosalicylate Injection (an analgesic, antipyretic agent) is a sterile solution manufactured from Thiosalicylic Add with the aid of Sodium Bicarbonate (30 ml vial) or Sodium Hydroxide (2 ml ampule) for intramuscular administration. Each ml contains 50 mg Sodium Thiosalicylate in Water for injection with 2% Benzyl Alcohol as preservative.

CLINICAL PHARMACOLOGY: In common with the various salicylate compounds thiosalicylate exerts analgesic and antipyretic effects. In antipyretic drugs, the ability to lower temperature Is most readily seen In febrile patients, while normal temperatures do not show much change, action being primarily upon hypothalamic nuclei. The selective central depressant action of salicylates produces analgesia without any apparent cortical effects.

Given Intramuscularly thiosalicylate Is readily absorbed and appreciable amounts detected in the blood within 1½ hour. Salicylates are rapidly distributed through the body tissues. Metabolic changes appear to be made In the kidney and while approximately 50 percent of the salicylate is excreted in 24 hours, some traces are found In urine for periods up 48 hours.

INDICATIONS AND USAGE: Palliative relief of muscular pains, acute gout, arthritis, rheumatic fever, and muscular skeletal disturbance

CONTRAINDICATIONS: Hemophilia, bleeding ulcers, and hemorrhage states are absolute contraindications. Hypersensitivity to salicylates is not an absolute contraindication, but a sensitivity test with 0.05 or 0.1 ml of Sodium Thiosalicylate injection should be made before continuing therapy.

Note: This product contains benzyl alcohol. Benzyl alcohol has been associated with a fatal "Gasping Syndrome" in premature infants and infants of low birth weight.

Contraindicated in those persons who have shown hypersensitivity to any component of this preparation.

WARNING: Salicylates have been reported to be associated with the development of Reye's Syndrome In children and teenagers with chickenpox, influenza and influenza-like infections. Since sodium thiosalicylate is structurally and pharmacological related to the salicylates and appears to share the toxic potentials of the salicylates, Sodium Thiosalicylate Injection is not recommended for use In children and teenagers with chicken pox, influenza and influenza-like infection.

PRECAUTIONS: Febrile children suffering dehydration appear quite prone to salicylate intoxication. Exercise caution with patients suffering oral diseases.

Pregnancy And Lactation: Safe use of sodium thiosalicylate during pregnancy or lactation has not been established.

ADVERSE REACTIONS: Large continued doses of salicylate may produce dizziness, tinnitus, headache, lassitude, profuse sweating, thirst, mental contusion, tremor, delirium and coma, as well as skin eruptions. Disturbances of acid-base and electrolytic balances have also been observed Hemorrhagic disturbances from prolonged larger doses of salicylates are not uncommon. Prescribe sodium bicarbonate per os concurrent with thiosalicylate. Long term usage indicates administration of vitamin K.

DOSAGE AND ADMINISTRATION: It Is advisable to administer this product intramuscularly in order to obviate the usual problems associated with intravenous administration.

In the symptomatic treatment of rheumatic fever, the usual adult IM dosage is 100–150 mg every 4–8 hours for 3 days, followed by 100 mg twice daily until the patient Is asymptomatic.

In the symptomatic treatment of acute gout, the usual adult IM dosage is 100 mg every 3–4 hours for two days, followed by 100 mg once daily until the patient is asymptomatic.

The usual adult dosage for the symptomatic treatment of muscular pain and musculoskeletal disorders is 50–100 mg once daily or once every other day.

Parenteral drug products should be inspected visually for particulate matter and discoloration prior to administration, whenever the solution and container permit.

HOW SUPPLIED: Sodium Thiosalicylate injection, 50 mg/ml, is available in 30 ml multiple dose vials.

Store at 15–30 degrees C (59–86 degrees F).

A slight precipitate may form due to oxidation. If the precipitate does not redissolve when the container is shaken well, the injection should not be used.

CAUTION: Federal law prohibits dispensing without prescription.

Distributed by: CLINT PHARMACEUTICALS, INC., NASHVILLE, TN 37120; 1-800-677-5022

With prolonged use, the NSAID group of medications may lose their effectiveness in many chronic intractable pain patients. Since they work mainly in tissues outside of the central nervous system (brain and spinal cord) that are inflamed, they cannot relieve any of the anxiety produced by pain. These drugs can be excellent for the treatment of arthritis problems, but only when true arthritis exists.

Severe pain due to myofascial pain syndrome (MPS) is usually sustained by the nervous system. Therefore an NSAID will be of little use in controlling the pain of MPS, except in the earliest of cases. If use of an analgesic is called for in the treatment of a patient with MPS, I have found this type of pain responds best to an opioid and opioid-containing analgesic. I have found the same to be true of the severe cases of fibromyalgia that I treat.

Many chronic intractable pain patients are told they have "arthritis," but frequently there is a lack of convincing clinical, blood test, and X-ray findings to back up the diagnosis. The presence of "degenerative changes" in X-rays of the back and neck, along with pain in the same area, does not validate the diagnosis of "arthritis" and does not justify the use of these drugs. If true arthritis is present, a short course of therapy with up to as many as three members of this group of medications is warranted to assess the patient's response to this class of medication.

The X-ray or MRI appearance of degenerative joint disease in the cervical, thoracic, or lumbar spine plus pain in the same area does not mean cause and effect. In fact, short of a fresh compression fracture or metastatic cancer, seen on X-ray or MRI, it is very difficult to say exactly what is causing a pain in the cervical, thoracic, or lumbar spine. MPS is the most common cause of pain in these areas.

Each of the three medications to be used should be chosen from a different one of the chemical classes listed below (e.g., Trilisate®, Indocin®, and Motrin® can be used and evaluated, but Nalfon®, Ansaid®, and Orudis® should not be used in the same patient). However, if there is no convincing pain relief and no overall improvement in the physical functioning of the patient within 3 weeks after beginning the medication, it should be stopped in preference to the use of more potent analgesics (e.g., Vicodin®, Tylenol® + codeine, Percocet®, Percodan®, morphine, Dilaudid®, etc.) for purposes of pain symptom control.

The persistent reliance on "just one more" NSAID is creating unnecessary false hope for both patient and physician and often delays definitive treatment of disabling pain symptoms.

Table of Drugs

Chemical class	Brand name	Generic name	Dose (mg)	Frequency (hours)
Acetylated carboxylic acid	Various	Aspirin	325–1000	4–6
Nonacetylated carboxylic acid	Trilisate®	Choline magnesium trisalicylate	750–1000	12–24
	Dolobid®	Diflunisal	250–500	8–12
	Disalcid™	Salsalate	1000–1500	8–12
Acetic acids	Voltaren®	Diclofenac	50	6–8
	Indocin®	Indomethacin	25–50	8–12
	Clinoril®	Sulindac	150–200	6–8
	Tolectin®	Tolmetin	200–800	6–8
Proprionic acids	Nalfon®	Fenoprofen	200	4–6
	Ansaid®	Flubioprofen	50–100	8
	Motrin®	Ibuprofen	200–800	4–8
	Orudis®	Ketaprophen	25–75	6–12
	Toradol®	Ketorolac	30–60 i.m.	Immediately
	Toradol®	Ketorolac	15–30 i.m.	6
	Naproxyn®	Naproxen	250–500	12
	Anaprox®	Naproxyn sodium	275–550	12
Fenamic acids	Ponstel®	Mefenamic acid	250	6
	Meclomen®	Meclofenamate	50–100	4–6
Enolic acids	Feldene®	Piroxicam	10–20	12–24
Nonacidic compounds	Ralefen®	Nabumetone	500–1000	24

Side Effects

With prolonged use, the incidence of side effects from NSAIDs, such as gastric irritation and bleeding, outright ulcer formation, pancreatitis, thinning of the blood with nosebleeds and easy bruising, liver damage, and kidney damage, tends to increase and therefore limits their usefulness (Brezin, 1979; Curry, 1982; Gary, 1980; Kimberly et al., 1978; Physicians' Drug Alert, 1986). Many deaths each year in the United States are directly attributed to the use of NSAIDs. The NSAIDs can also cause damage to the brain and/or spinal cord through aseptic meningitis and can produce a psychosis, dermatologic problems, hypersensitivity, in some can cause severe sickness on taking the drug, and in a very rare case can cause death. In contrast, the use of narcotics long term in a chronic intractable pain patient does not carry any of this risk. The only long-term risks associated with opioids are respiratory distress and constipation. For a more detailed discussion of the materials in the sections below, refer to *Drug Facts and Comparisons,* a text or set of loose-leaf texts with subjects of interest in the comparison of various current medications.

NSAIDs can become "dangerous drugs" when used long term in a patient with chronic intractable pain. Some of the organ damage may be irreversible or only reversible with long periods of treatment. The NSAID should be stopped at the first sign of gastrointestinal irritation or other organ compromise and the patient converted to a stronger analgesic such as Vicodin®, Percocet®, etc. If the physician is not comfortable with converting the patient to an opioid or opioid-containing analgesic, a specialist familiar with the use of these medications should be called in to manage the patient.

Colchicine

Intravenous colchicine for neck or back disc pain problems is the closest to a "miracle" drug one can find for those problems. It is effective and has a low incidence of side effects. Despite the fact that it has been associated with the treatment of gout for the past 1500 years, it is nothing more than a very potent NSAID.

Colchicine dates back to ancient Roman times and has been used with encouraging success in the treatment of patients with acute and chronic disc pain problems in the neck, low back, and leg (Rask, 1980). Colchicine is administered intravenously in the initial phase of treatment and then by mouth for a period of time. This medication has been proven effective in chronic pain patients using a double-blind study technique (Meek et al., 1984). The drug is effective for some chronic intractable pain patients with low back pain and sciatica, especially if irritation of a disc is suspected. The most common side effect is diarrhea. Some of the other advantages of colchicine are that it is "old" (used in the treatment of inflammations for almost 4000 years), it is inexpensive (usually costs one-fourth to one-sixth the amount that you pay for some of the more modern anti-inflammatory drugs), and it is "good" (low incidence of side effects and can be used for long periods of time without unnecessarily irritating the gut). In patients with a disc-related pain problem of the back or neck who have not been operated upon, the chances of successful help using the colchicine protocol of Rask for chronic intractable pain is 90%, and in the operated patient there is a 67% chance of successful response to the same treatment program. For further information and details about the treatment protocol, contact the American Academy of Neurological and Orthopaedic Surgeons at 2300 S. Rancho Drive, Suite 202, Las Vegas, NV 89102.

Cortisone (Steroids)

There are many cortisone (steroid) preparations available. These medications are pure anti-inflammatory medicines and work to relieve the pain and swelling of tissues and joints that are reddened, hot, swollen, and painful. As a secondary effect, they act as powerful antidepressants, thereby providing the patient with extra ability to cope with the painful situation.

Some fibromyalgia and MPS patients complain of excessive and troublesome tiredness. In these patients, it is wise to obtain an 8:00 a.m. and 4:00 p.m. serum cortisol blood levels. Additional testing for ACTH levels is also warranted to complete the testing. These patients will not generally show abnormal dexamethasone suppression testing. If the a.m. or p.m. levels are in the lower part of the normal range, it is wise to give the patient a test dose of Cortef, in the range of 10–25 mg/day. If a true cortisol problem exists, the patient will obtain an antidepressant effect from the Cortef and his or her energy level will come up.

The injection of a steroid plus local anesthetic into the epidural space (the space between the spinal cord and the bony canal the cord lies in) or facet joints (the major stabilizing joints of the back) of the spine may provide excellent relief of back or neck pain in some chronic pain patients. This can be repeated every other month. If the patient gets a significant energy boost from the epidural, it is wise to suspect there may be a cortisol insufficiency.

In using doses of Cortef of 10–20 mg/day in 50 patients over the last 5 years, there has only been one case of confirmed case of Cushing's disease (excess effect from taking Cortef) and one case of steroid psychosis.

Cortisone medications, whether by mouth or by injection, can cause unwanted side effects. Refer to *Drug Facts and Comparisons* for a more detailed discussion of some of the reactions and problems that may be associated with use of this group of medications. Although the various cortisone-type drugs can be very helpful, their use should not be undertaken casually.

MOOD ELEVATORS, ANTIDEPRESSANTS, AND PSYCHOSTIMULANTS

A psychostimulant is a medication with primary action of stimulation of the central nervous system.

Medications Whose Main Use Is the Correction of Depression and Asthenia

Depression is the most common emotional problem in patients with chronic pain syndromes (Aranoff, 1985). Despite this, depression is often hidden and not always recognized, especially by the family and professionals. The factors responsible for depression that occurs in chronic pain patients are still not known. *Pain tolerance is lowered* in association with long-continued pain and *inadequate sleep* (Sternbach, 1984). Once the cycle of *pain–insomnia–depression* is established, it becomes self-perpetuating and requires the active intervention (Aranoff, 1985) of a support team and often medication.

It is important to realize there may be two types of depression encountered in chronic pain patients. One is *endogenous* or situational depression. The other is based on *anxiety* or anxiousness. When anxiously depressed patients are treated with one of the common antidepressants, such as Elavil®, desipramine, Prozac®, Paxil®, or similar medications, they become overtly anxious and feel "hyped-up," can't settle down, and get palpitations. This may seem to be a paradoxical effect of the medication, but it is not. This group of patients does better on tranquilizer medications. The first group mentioned does better on routine antidepressants. In anxiously depressed patients, the paradoxical effect occurs, causing the patient to become excited and anxious after being on the medication initially or for a while. When this occurs, the pain problem begins to flare up.

A group of drugs that has proved to be very helpful in the treatment of the pain–insomnia–depression cycle and in the rehabilitation of chronic pain patients is the antidepressants (Foley, 1985; Savitz, 1985). They are useful in the treatment of some chronic noncancer pain patients who experience depression, irritability, and difficulty sleeping.

Commonly used antidepressants are listed in the table of drugs that follows. These medications are designed to reduce depression by altering or changing a person's mood or attitude. They usually take 1–2 weeks before any significant mood elevation is noticeable.

Amitriptyline, also known as Elavil®, is frequently used and can sometimes provide pain relief at a low dosage. Sometimes antidepressants seem to work with narcotic or narcotic-containing pain medication, causing improved pain relief.

Despite the widespread use of this class of drugs in the treatment of chronic pain patients, no clinical studies have demonstrated consistently good results with a significant number of pain patients (Pilowsky, 1982; Large, 1980; Foley, 1985). Also, there is little conclusive evidence to support the use of one of the antidepressants over any others in this class of drugs (Monks and Mersky, 1984).

The usefulness of the antidepressant medications is limited by the side effects listed below. As the dosage of the drug is slowly increased, the incidence of side effects increases. At lower doses, they are valuable adjuncts for normalizing sleep. However, at the higher doses, which are usually in the recommended therapeutic range, patients may complain of feeling hung over in the morning.

Only some of the antidepressants (those with high anticholinergic effects) cause constipation. A suggested measure to counteract that undesirable side effect is to use DSS, an over-the-counter medication that holds water in the bowel. Powdered vitamin C (ascorbic acid) or sodium ascorbate at a dose of 1 teaspoon in 10–18 ounces of water or juice per day can act as a mild laxative.

It is important to realize that antidepressants treat symptoms. Many chronic pain patients are depressed as a reaction to their pain problem and the limitations imposed by the disability associated with the pain problem. Drugs will not treat underlying conflicts, family problems, or lack of motivation to return to work. "Therefore, in most cases, chronic pain coexisting with depression must be treated multidimensionally with agents such as the antidepressants and a variety of other medical, psychotherapeutic, and social interventions" (Aranoff and Evans, 1985).

Dosing in chronic pain patient is different than for patients who have classic depressions. Chronic pain patients should begin on the lowest dose of the tricyclic antidepressants being considered (usually 10 mg) and progress up by 10 mg more daily dosing at 3- to 4-day intervals. The correct dose is the one that restores the normal sleep patterns, elevates some of the mood problem, and corrects some of the pain problem.

Although many chronic pain patients will respond to mood elevator or antidepressant medications, many of them are plagued more by asthenia (ICD code 780.7) than endogenous depression. In some cases, this is the major complaint, with pain symptoms being of secondary consideration. Asthenia has two components, weakness and fatigue (Plum, 1992). "*Weakness* is arbitrarily defined as reduced muscle power compared to the person's norm" (Plum, 1992). "*Fatigue*, as employed in medical terms, describes a reduction in performance due to an experienced deterioration in capacity" (Plum, 1992).

Situational depression is also very common in cases of pain that go onto chronicity. The situational depression is based mostly on inability to physically perform usual employment and recreational activities due to pain and inability to enjoy life and friends, etc. because of physical dysfunction secondary to pain.

In the overall rehabilitation of a chronic pain patient, there frequently comes a time when no further progress of recovery can be made until the asthenia is addressed. Asthenia and related symptoms can come from a number of sources. Listed below are some of the more common sources that I have noted in my 21 years as a pain management specialist.

- Low-grade anemia
- Less than optimal potassium (see Chapter 10 for explanation of less than optimal)
- Toxicity from excessive amounts of Tylenol®
- Excessive intake of antidepressants
- Excessive intake of muscle relaxers or tranquilizers
- Excessive intake of opioids or opioid-containing analgesics
- Less than optimal estrogen or progesterone intake
- Excessive intake of progesterone
- Insufficiency (or deficiency) of B vitamins
- Low thyroid levels
- Excessive intake of nightshade foods (potatoes, tomatoes, pepper, or eggplant)
- Inadequate sleep
- Cortisol insufficiency
- Magnesium insufficiency
- Inadequately treated pain symptoms
- Other

Basically, every factor listed above can be diagnosed and treated except "other." Many of my patients feel better (more energy, more endurance, etc.) after a number of the above-indicated factors are corrected, but they may still be plagued with enough residual asthenia symptoms to warrant additional treatment considerations. I have noted that Cylert®, phentermine-containing medications, Ritalin®, and Dexedrine® are four choices that may be of help in trying to remedy the asthenia problem.

The medications indicated below are usually thought of for the treatment of narcolepsy, attention deficit disorder, and appetite control. The fact is that they are all stimulants of one type or another. Some chronic pain patients need a stimulant medication to relieve asthenia so they can become productive people either at home or at work. If you read the material for each medication carefully, you will see, usually under "unlabeled" uses, that these medications may have a role in treating this condition.

Numerous of the more severe/seriously involved of the chronic pain patients will have gained 20–30 pounds in the first 5 years that follow the onset of their pain problem. Most all of the psychostimulants are appetite suppressants. While that is not my primary recommendation for the use of these medications, weight loss may be facilitated by the use of these medications.

The psychostimulants can also be likened in their actions to antidepressants. Many of the tricyclic antidepressants (TCAs) and selective serotonin reuptake inhibitors (SSRIs) have little or no effect on many of the seriously/severely afflicted chronic pain patients (for example, see grades 3 and 4 MPS in Chapter 10). In cases where the TCAs or SSRIs are of no significant help for asthenia, use of one of the psychostimulants should be considered.

Care must be emphasized in the use of the psychostimulants. A small dose of medication may be helpful, but a larger dose may irritate muscles (spasms, charley horse, etc.) and become counterproductive to overall rehabilitation and recovery.

With respect to phentermine, pemoline, methylphenidate, and amphetamines, the possibility of abuse potential exists. Regarding the occurrence of dependence in chronic pain patients, each case must be judged on an individual basis. A patient can be dependent on a medication without being addicted to it and without abusing the medication.

Table of Medications and Dosing

Referred to *Drug Facts and Comparisons* for a more detailed discussion of some of the dosing and problems that may be associated with the use of this group of medications.

Note that all doses given are for adults. No dosing for children is given.

Chemical class	Brand name	Generic name	Dose (mg)	Frequency
Tricyclic antidepressants	Elavil®	Amitriptyline	10–300	Once or multiple
	Endep®			
	Aventyl® pulvules	Nortryptyline	25	3–4 times
	Pamelor®			
	Tofranil®	Imipramine	25–200	3 times
	Adapin®	Doxepin		
	Sinequan®		75–300	Divide to 3 doses
	Surmontil®	Trimipramine maleate	75–200	Divided doses
	Asendin®	Amoxapine	50–300	2–3 times per day

Chemical class	Brand name	Generic name	Dose (mg)	Frequency
	Norpramin® Pertofrane®	Desipramine	50–300	Once or divided doses
	Vivactil®	Protriptyline	5–60	3–4 doses
	Anafranil®	Clomipramine	25–250	Divided doses with meals
	Ludiomil®	Maprotiline	25–225	Once or divided doses
Quadracyclic antidepressants	Desyrel®	Trazodone	50–400	Once or multiple
Selective serotonin reuptake inhibitors	Zoloft®	Sertraline	50–200	Once[a]
	Paxil®	Paroxetine	20–50	Once[a]
	Prozac®	Fluoxitine	20–80	Once or twice
	Luvox®	Fluvoxamine	50–30	Once or twice
Psychostimulant	Cylert®	Pemoline	18.75–112.5	Once in a.m.
Anorexiants– psychostimulants	Fastin®	Phentermine	8	3 times/day
	Obephen®	Phentermine	15	Twice
	Phentrol®	Phentermine	15	Twice
	Zantryl®	Phentermine	15	Twice
	Adipex-P®	Phentermine	15	Twice
	Ionamin®	Phentermine	15	Twice
	Didrex®	Benzphetamine	25–50	1–3 times/day
	Bontril PDM®	Phenmetrazine	35	2–3 times/day
	Dital® [b]	Phenmetrazine	105	Once
	Tenuate®	Diethylpropion	25	3 times/day
	Tenuate Dospan® [b]	Diethylpropion	75	Once
	Mazanor®	Mannzidol	1	3 times/day
	Pondimin®	Fenfluramine	20	3 times/day
	Phenoxine®	Phenylpropanolamine	25	3 times
	Dexatrim® Premeal	Phenylpropanolamine	25	3 times
	Acutrim® 16 hour	Phenylpropanolamine	75	Once
		Methylphenidate	5	2–3 times daily
			10	2–3 times daily
	Ritalin®	Methylphenidate	10	2–3 times daily
	Ritalin-SR® [c]	Methylphenidate	20	Once
Psychostimulants		Dextroamphetamine	5	1–4 per day
	Dexedrine®	Dextroamphetamine	10	1–2 per day
	Dexedrine® spansules[c]	Dextroamphetamine	5	1-4 per day in a.m.
			10	1-2 per day in a.m.

[a] For the SSRIs dose, changes should be done at intervals of at least a week between dosage alterations.

[b] Slow release.

[c] Time release.

Functions

The tricyclics, trazodone, and SSRIs act to stimulate the production of antidepressant substances intrinsic to the nervous system. On the other hand, caffeine, Cylert®, phenylpropanolamine, methylphenidate, and the amphetamines contain chemical substances which act directly on the central nervous system. Methylphenidate is a mild cortical stimulant with central nervous system actions similar to the amphetamines.

Uses and Goals

With the medications in this class of drugs, we may attempt to achieve multiple desirable goals. Some of these goals might be more responsibilities at work, added housework, increased social activity, etc.

No one medication works for all patients. Therefore, when attempting to achieve these goals, a number of medications from this class of drug may be needed to be tried in succession until the desired result is achieved. Only very rarely will as many as two medications from this class be needed to be used simultaneously to achieve the desired result. The medications listed here are merely a partial listing of medications that I have found useful in the chronic intractable pain patients I have treated over the last 22 years. Other medications not listed here are equally as effective.

Only very rarely will as many as two medications from this class be needed to be used simultaneously to achieve the desired result. Thus far, only the use of a TCA, most commonly amitriptyline or desipramine, plus a psychostimulant such as pemoline, phentermine, or amphetamine has been assessed. The additive and synergistic effects have produced enough positive results to warrant the recommendation of combination of these medications in some of the more complex and challenging patients. After each medication is tried individually and found to be partially effective, they are then used together. Each medication is started out at a low but effective dose and elevated slowly at weekly intervals until the desired positive mood and energy effects are noted by the patient, physician, or both. Every other week, medication one, TCA, is elevated. On the in-between weeks, the psychostimulant is elevated. There is reason to believe that this would work well with SSRIs.

These medications are useful for some chronic pain patients as follows: improve asthenia, depression, and alertness; may relieve some of the tiredness that comes from a range of drugs including NSAIDs to opioids, tranquilizers, and muscle relaxers; improves cognitive thinking; improves memory in some patients; improved energy to perform household and work-related duties; improvement in mood allows the patient to tolerate his or her pain; improves interpersonal and social relationships; and improves sleep.

All the psychostimulants mentioned, except Ritalin®, have been used extensively on a small segment of my patients (about 7% of my total patient population [280 patients]). The psychostimulants have been used as part of the overall rehabilitation of my patients for the past 11 years. For the most part, my patients are middle-class Americans, who may or may not be employed. My patients are *motivated* to become improved regardless of the severity of their pain problem and related disability. There have been no documented cases of drug dependence syndrome (DDS) when the World Health Organization criteria listed in Chapter 22 have been used as the "gold standard" by which to make the assessment of DDS to psycho-stimulants.

Potential Problems

Tricyclic Antidepressants

TCAs lower the seizure threshold. The should be used with caution in patients with a history of seizures, urinary retention, urethral or ureteral spasm, or glaucoma and with extreme caution in patients with cardiovascular disorders such as severe coronary heart disease with ECG abnormalities, progressive heart failure, conduction disturbances, angina pectoris, or paroxysmal tachycardia. In high doses, TCAs may produce arrhythmias, sinus tachycardia, and prolong conduction time.

Schizophrenic or paranoid patients may exhibit a worsening of psychosis with TCA therapy, and manic-depressive patients may experience a shift to a hypomanic or manic phase.

They should be used with caution in reduced doses for patients with hepatic and renal impairment.

They may impair mental or physical abilities required for the performance of potentially hazardous tasks.

Sedation and anticholinergic effects are reported most frequently. Tolerance to these effects develops, but side effects may be minimized by starting with a low dose and then gradually increasing the dose. Other effects include:

- Orthostatic hypotension, hypertension, syncope, tachycardia, palpitations, myocardial infarction, arrhythmias
- Bone marrow depression
- Confusion (especially in the elderly), disturbed concentration, hallucinations, disorientation, decrease in memory, feelings of unreality, delusions, anxiety, nervousness, restlessness, agitation, panic, insomnia, nightmares, hypomania, mania, drowsiness, dizziness, weakness, fatigue, headache, depression, sleep disorder, abnormal dreaming, migraine, depersonalization, irritability
- Myoclonus, twitching, paresis, asthenia
- Nasal congestion, excessive appetite, weight gain or loss, increased perspiration, flushing, chills, myalgia, back pain, arthralgia, muscle weakness
- Dry mouth, blurred vision, disturbance of accommodation, increased intraocular pressure, constipation, paralytic ileus, urinary retention, delayed micturition, urinary tract dilation
- Although not indicative of addiction, abrupt cessation after prolonged therapy may produce nausea, headache, vertigo, nightmares, and malaise
- Nausea and vomiting, anorexia, epigastric distress, diarrhea, flatulence, dysphagia, abdominal cramps, pancreatitis, black tongue, dyspepsia, esophagitis, eructation, rarely hepatitis and jaundice, elevation in transaminase, changes in alkaline phosphatase
- Breast enlargement, menstrual irregularity, increased or decreased libido, painful ejaculation, impotence, nocturia, urinary frequency, urinary tract infection, dysuria, vaginitis, breast pain, amenorrhea

Trazodone

- Not recommended for use during the initial recovery phase of myocardial infarction; may be arrhythmogenic in some patients
- Priapism has been reported in patients receiving trazodone; patients with prolonged or inappropriate penile erection should discontinue use immediately and consult a physician

- May produce drowsiness, dizziness, or blurred vision; patients should observe caution while driving or performing other tasks that require alertness, coordination, or dexterity
- Hematuria, delayed urine flow, increased urinary frequency, urinary incontinence/retention
- Decreased appetite, sweating, clamminess, weight gain or loss, malaise, nasal/sinus congestion, increased appetite, apnea, alopecia, edema

Selective Serotonin Reuptake Inhibitors

- Use cautiously in patients with a history of mania. The long elimination half-life of fluoxetine and norfluoxetine means that changes in dose will not be fully reflected in plasma for several weeks, affecting titration to final dose and withdrawal from treatment.
- Nervousness, insomnia, drowsiness, fatigue, asthenia, tremor, increased sweating, dizziness, anxiety (fluoxetine), headache (paroxetine), dry mouth (paroxetine, sertraline), male sexual dysfunction (sertraline); cardiac problems or cold extremities; edema or orthostatic hypotension; abnormal gait, amnesia, apathy, ataxia, convulsions, delusions, depersonalization, emotional lability, euphoria, hallucinations, hostility, incoordination, libido increased, manic reaction, psychosis, vertigo, abnormal EEG, antisocial reaction, depression, myoclonus, paralysis, torticollis, agoraphobia, sleep disorder, abnormal thinking
- Dysphagia, eructation, esophagitis, gastritis, gingivitis, glossitis, abnormal liver function tests, melena, stomatitis, thirst, bloody diarrhea, cholecystitis, cholelithiasis, colitis, duodenal ulcer, enteritis, fecal incontinence, hematemesis, hepatitis, hepatomegaly, hyperchlorhydria, increased salivation, jaundice, liver tenderness, mouth ulceration, salivary gland enlargement, stomach ulcer, tongue discoloration, tongue edema
- Arthritis, bone pain, bursitis, tenosynovitis, twitching, bone necrosis, chondrodystrophy, muscle hemorrhage, myositis, osteoporosis, pathological fracture, rheumatoid arthritis, arthralgia, generalized muscle spasm, tendinous contracture, tenosynovitis, arthrosis, myopathy, pathological fracture, muscle cramps/weakness
- Asthma, epistaxis, hiccups, hyperventilation, pneumonia, apnea, hemoptysis, hypoxia, laryngeal edema, lung edema, lung fibrosis/alveolitis, pleural effusion
- Abnormal ejaculation, amenorrhea, breast pain, cystitis, dysuria, fibrocystic breast, impotence, leukorrhea, menopause, menorrhagia, ovarian disorder, urinary incontinence/retention/urgency, urination impaired, vaginitis, abortion, albuminuria, breast enlargement, dyspareunia, epididymitis, female lactation, hematuria, hypomenorrhea, kidney calculus, metrorrhagia, orchitis, polyuria, pyelonephritis, pyuria, salpingitis, urethral pain, urethritis, urinary tract disorder, urolithiasis, uterine spasm, vaginal hemorrhage
- Cyst, facial edema, hangover effect, jaw pain, malaise, neck pain, neck rigidity, pelvic pain, abdomen enlarged, hypothermia

Caffeine

Caffeine is available in many over-the-counter preparations such as Nodoz®, coffee, and carbonated beverages such as Coca-Cola®, Pepsi®, Mountain Dew®, and others. Small amounts may be of benefit in the management of patients with MPS, but if taken in excess may cause irritability of the muscles and pain.

Pemoline

- Administer with caution to patients with significantly impaired renal function.
- Perform liver function tests prior to and periodically during therapy; discontinue use if abnormalities are revealed and confirmed by follow-up tests; elevated liver enzymes are not rare and appear reversible upon drug discontinuance.
- The similarity of pemoline to other psychostimulants with known dependence liability suggests that psychological or physical dependence might occur.
- Insomnia is a most frequent problem and usually occurs early in therapy prior to optimum therapeutic response; it is often transient or responds to dosage reduction.
- Dyskinetic movements of tongue, lips, face and extremities; abnormal oculomotor function (e.g., nystagmus); convulsive seizures; increased irritability; mild depression; dizziness; headache; drowsiness; hallucinations.
- Weight loss, weight gain, stomach ache or nausea.

Phentermine

Phentermine should not be taken by patients who have advanced arteriosclerosis, symptomatic cardiovascular disease, moderate to severe hypertension, or hyperthyroidism.

These drugs are chemically and pharmacologically related to the amphetamines and have abuse potential.

May produce dizziness, extreme fatigue, and depression after abrupt cessation of prolonged high-dosage therapy; patients should observe caution while driving or performing other tasks requiring alertness (Facts and Comparisons, 1996).

Fenfluramine's central effects are mediated by 5-hydroxytryptamine (5-HT) in the brain stem. A rapid reduction in 5-HT in the brain can lead to depression. This commonly occurs immediately following abrupt withdrawal of fenfluramine; therefore, do not discontinue abruptly (Facts and Comparisons, 1996).

Depression may be provoked while the patient is taking fenfluramine or following abrupt withdrawal, especially in those with a history of mental depression. Control symptoms of depression by reinstituting therapy; follow by gradual withdrawal (Facts and Comparisons, 1996).

- Palpitations, tachycardia, arrhythmias, hypertension or hypotension, fainting, precordial pain, pulmonary hypertension, ECG changes
- Nervousness, restlessness, dizziness, insomnia, weakness or fatigue, malaise, anxiety, tension, euphoria, elevated mood, drowsiness, depression, agitation, tremor, dysarthria, confusion, incoordination, tremor, headache, change in libido
- Dry mouth, unpleasant taste, nausea, vomiting, abdominal discomfort, diarrhea, constipation, stomach pain
- Dysuria, polyuria, urinary frequency, impotence, menstrual upset
- Bone marrow depression, hair loss, ecchymosis, muscle pain, chest pain, excessive sweating, clamminess, chills, flushing, fever, myalgia, gynecomastia

Phenylpropanolamine

This is a sympathomimetic medication commonly used as a decongestant. This product is available in numerous over-the-counter preparations.

- Not to be used in persons having cardiovascular disease, hypertension, hyperthyroidism, kidney disease, diabetes, hypersensitivity or idiosyncrasy to sympathomimetic amines, glaucoma, depression
- Average doses may be strong enough to induce severe hypertensive episodes
- Restlessness, dizziness, insomnia, headache, bizarre behavior, tremor, increased motor activity, agitation, hallucinations

Methylphenidate

Do not use for severe depression of either exogenous or endogenous origin. It may lower the seizure threshold in patients with a history of seizures. Use cautiously in patients with hypertension. Patients with an element of agitation may react adversely. Perform periodic complete blood count and differential and platelet counts during prolonged therapy.

This drug is listed by the Drug Enforcement Agency (DEA) as a schedule 2 medication, which means the abuse potential is considered to be high. Give cautiously to emotionally unstable patients, such as those with a history of DDS or alcoholism. This type of patient may increase dosage on his or her own initiative.

- Skin rash, urticaria, fever, arthralgia, dizziness, headache, dyskinesia, drowsiness, tachycardia, angina, cardiac arrhythmias, palpitations, anorexia, nausea, abdominal pain, weight loss during prolonged therapy, nervousness and insomnia usually controlled by reducing dosage and vomiting the drug in the afternoon or evening

Amphetamines

Amphetamines have a high potential for abuse. Administration for prolonged periods may lead to DDS.

- Use cautiously in patients with hypertension; may cause dizziness; observe caution while driving or performing other tasks that require alertness
- May cause palpitations, tachycardia, and elevation of blood pressure
- Overstimulation, restlessness, dizziness, insomnia, dyskinesia, euphoria, dysphoria, tremor, headache, changes in libido, rarely psychotic episodes at recommended doses
- Dry mouth, unpleasant taste, diarrhea, constipation
- Reversible elevations in serum thyroxine (T_4) levels have occurred with heavy amphetamine use

Refer to *Drug Facts and Comparisons* for a more detailed discussion of some of the reactions and problems that may be associated with the use of this group of medications.

Do not give these medications to patients who have advanced arteriosclerosis, symptomatic cardiovascular disease, moderate to severe hypertension, hyperthyroidism, hypersensitivity or idiosyncrasy to the sympathomimetic amines, glaucoma, or agitated states.

Patient Instructions

General Comments

Do not crush or chew time-release medication.

Selective Serotonin Reuptake Inhibitors

SSIRs may cause dizziness or drowsiness. Patients should be instructed to observe caution while driving or performing tasks that require alertness, coordination, or physical dexterity.

Pemoline

Take daily dose in the morning. If dizziness occurs, use caution when performing tasks that require alertness. Notify physician if insomnia occurs and continues.

Phentermines

May cause insomnia; avoid taking medication late in the day. Weight reduction requires strict adherence to dietary restriction. Do not take more frequently than prescribed. Notify physician if palpitations, nervousness, or dizziness occurs.

Medication may cause dry mouth and constipation; notify physician if these become pronounced.

May produce dizziness or blurred vision; observe caution while driving or performing other tasks that require alertness.

Fenfluramine may cause drowsiness. Avoid concomitant consumption of alcohol. These drugs should generally be taken on an empty stomach; mazindol may be taken with meals to reduce gastrointestinal irritation.

Phenylpropanolamine

Discontinue use if rapid pulse, dizziness, nervousness, insomnia, or palpitations occur.

Methylphenidate

Take last daily dose early in the evening (prior to 6:00 a.m.) to avoid insomnia. May be taken without regard to presence or absence of food in the gut.

May mask symptoms of fatigue. Use caution while driving or performing other tasks that require alertness.

Time-release tablets have a duration of approximately 8 hours and may be used in place of regular tablets when the 8-hour dosage of the time-release tablets corresponds to the titrated 8-hour dosage of the regular tablets.

Amphetamines

Prescribe or dispense sparingly. Take early in the day (especially sustained-release dosage forms) to avoid nighttime insomnia. Do not increase dosage, except on physician's advice. May impair ability to drive or perform other tasks that require alertness. Notify your physician if you have problems with nervousness, restlessness, insomnia, or dizziness.

CENTRALLY ACTING ANTIANXIETY AND SKELETAL MUSCLE RELAXANT AGENTS

There are two types of muscle relaxants. One type works directly on the muscle and its nerve connections. The other works on the central nervous system to calm any abnormal signals that may be going to the muscles. In this section some of the central nervous system agents will be discussed.

Medications Whose Main Use in Chronic Intractable Pain Patients Is to Produce Partial Tranquilization, Relief of Unwanted Anxiety, and Reduction of Muscular Tension

This group of drugs provide an adjunct to rest, physical therapy, and other measures for the relief of discomfort associated with painful muscular conditions. They can be effective in managing muscular spasms in some patients.

In the presence of persistent or repeated episodes of muscular spasms or cramping, the physician must also blood test for less than optimal levels of potassium, calcium, magnesium, and other vital biochemical factors within the internal milieu that directly affects muscle tone and irritability.

By the time a chronic intractable pain patient gets to a pain management specialist, he or she may have been treated with three muscle relaxer/tranquilizers, two hypnotics, four antidepressants, three NSAIDs, and up to three analgesics of the opioid or opioid-containing analgesics class. It is only normal that when the patient requests a medication from the doctor, the patient will frequently ask for the drug that gave the best results in the past. Some doctors consider this evidence of the patient being a drug addict (but it does not fulfill enough criteria to classify the patient as having DDS [see Chapter 22 for the criteria for DDS]). I see this as the patient knowing which drug worked best in the past and requesting that medication from the treating physician.

Table of Medications and Dosing

Note that all doses given are for adults. No dosing for children is given.

Drug	Treatment range (mg/day)[a]	Half-life (hours)[b]	Rapidity of start of medical effect
Alprazolam (Xanax®)	0.75–4	12–15	Mid range
Diazepam (Valium®)	4–40	20–80	Very quick
Lorazepam (Ativan®)	2–4	10–20	Mid range
Oxepam (Serax®)	30–120	5–20	Mid range
Carisopradol (Soma®)	1050–1400[c]	4–6	Quick
Cyclobenzaprine (Flexeril®)	1–2 g 4 times/day	1–3 days	Mid range
Methocarbamol (Robaxin®)	20–40	1–2	Mid range

[a] Oral administration.

[b] The amount of time needed to eliminate one-half of the drug from the body.

[c] A rare chronic intractable pain patient can tolerate up to 2100 mg/day and function with no psychologic or physical impairment.

Chemical class	Brand name	Generic name	Condition	Dose (mg)	Frequency
Benzodiazepines	Serax®	Oxazepam	a	10–15	3–4 times daily
			b	15–30	3–4 times daily

[a] Mild to moderate anxiety, with associated tension, irritability, agitation, or related symptoms of functional origin or secondary to organic disease.

[b] Severe anxiety syndromes, agitation, or anxiety associated with depression.

Chemical class	Brand name	Generic name	Dose (mg)	Frequency
Benzodiazepines	Ativan®	Lorazepam[a]	0.5	In the elderly, use 1–2 mg daily in divided doses
			1	For anxiety, 2–6 mg/day (range 1–6 mg), divided into 2–3 times daily
			2	
	Xanax®	Alprazolam[b]	0.25	For anxiety, start with 0.25–0.5 mg three times per day; maximum total dose of 4 mg/day
			0.5	
			1	
			2	
	Valium®	Diazepam[c]	2	Elderly patients or in the presence of debilitating disease: 2–2.5 mg one or two times daily initially; increase gradually as needed and tolerated
			5	
			10	Adjunct in skeletal muscle spasm; 2–10 mg three or four times daily; management of anxiety disorders and relief of symptoms of anxiety: 15–30 mg/day, depending upon severity of symptoms
Psychostimulants	Soma®[d]	Carisopradol	350	Adults: 350 mg three or four times daily, with the last dose at bedtime; a rare chronic intractable pain patient will be allowed to take up to six tablets per day

[a] When higher dosage is needed, increase the evening dosage before the daytime doses.

[b] For the elderly, use a maximum of 0.25 mg three times per day.

[c] Oral: individualize dosage. Increase dosage cautiously to avoid adverse effects. Management of anxiety disorders and relief of symptoms of anxiety (depending upon severity of symptoms): 2–10 mg two to four times daily (Facts and Comparisons, 1996). A rare chronic intractable pain patient can tolerate up to 100–120 mg of diazepam per day and function normally, without side effects. Whenever oral 5 mg diazepam three times a day would be considered appropriate dosage, one 15-mg sustained-release capsule daily may be used.

[d] It has been my experience that one to three tablets an hour before bedtime can be used as a safe sedative medication with a half-life such that it does not cause hangover in the morning.

[e] Facts and Comparisons, 1996.

Chemical class	Brand name	Generic name	Dose (mg)	Frequency
Centrally acting skeletal muscle relaxant	Flexeril®	Cyclobenzaprine	10	Give 10 mg three times daily (range 20–40 mg daily in divided doses); do not exceed 60 mg/day
	Robaxin®	Methocarbamol	500 750	Initial: give 1.5 g four times daily; maintenance: 1 g four times daily, 750 mg every 4 hours, or 1.5 g three times daily; for the first 48–72 hours, 6 g/day is recommended (for severe conditions, 8 g daily may be administered) and thereafter reduce to approximately 4 g daily[e]

Addiction is in the person, not in the pill.

—The author (1997)

Functions

The relation of pain to the nervous system is a very complex subject that has been the subject of extensive research over the last 20 years. What follows is a summary statement of the research. There are many events that can initiate spinal and cortical excitatory responses. This can occur with trauma, emotional stress, and other stimuli. Cortical excitation, if pronounced, can cause intensification of pain that is extant. This class of medications can cause a reduction of pain through the calming of the spinal and cortical excitatory responses. Each medication has a different mechanism of action and will produce a different clinical effect.

Cyclobenzaprine

Cyclobenzaprine is structurally related to the TCAs. It can relieve skeletal muscle spasm of local origin without interfering with muscle function. It is ineffective in muscle spasm due to central nervous system disease. It acts primarily within the central nervous system at the brain stem. Cyclobenzaprine is well absorbed after oral administration, but there is large intersubject variation in plasma levels (Facts and Comparisons, 1996).

Orphenadrine

Its analgesic properties come from its central actions at the brain stem. It does not directly relax tense skeletal muscles.

Methocarbamol

Mechanism of action may be due to general central nervous system depression. The drug has no direct action on the contractile mechanism of striated muscle, motor endplate, or nerve fiber. It does not directly relax tense skeletal muscles.

Uses and Goals

The goals we are attempting to achieve with medications in this class of drugs may be multiple (i.e., more office work and better social skills). No one medication works for all patients. Therefore, when attempting to achieve these goals, it may be necessary to try a number of medications from this class of drug in succession until the desired result is achieved. Only very rarely will it be necessary to use as many as two medications from this class simultaneously to achieve the desired result. The medications listed here are merely a partial listing of medications that I have found useful in the chronic intractable pain patients I have treated over the last 22 years. Other medications not listed here are equally as effective.

The cry that the benzodiazepines are addictive is just about as intense as that for the opioids or opioid-containing analgesics. As we will see in later parts of the medication sections, under the heading of DDS, addiction is a property of the person and not the pill. There are two types of depression seen in chronic pain patients: (1) that which is due to internal and situational problems and (2) that which is due to anxiety. Those patients with anxiety-related depression respond better to the benzodiazepines or similar antianxiety medication than the medications seen here in the section on mood elevators and antidepressants. Giving a TCA or SSRI antidepressant to an anxiously depressed chronic pain patient could have disastrous consequences. About one-half of my patient population has depression due to anxiety.

The antianxiety agents can also be considered muscle relaxers and vice versa The mechanism of action is the reduction of tension in the muscles. Anxiety produces tension. This can also cause pain in patients with MPS.

This group of drugs causes relaxation of muscles indirectly. It lowers the levels of tension and anxiety by working on the brain. This relaxes the tension in muscles.

These are the drug of choice in chronic intractable pain patients with anxiety problems and panic disorders. However, anxiety is too often inappropriately treated with a benzodiazepine instead of discussion and support. When anxiety is a part of the chronic pain problem, these medications should be used only as adjuncts to a well-planned and well-executed psychotherapy program aimed at the cause(s) of the anxiety problem.

Because they reduce anxiety, the benzodiazapines may provide relief of pains that are related to muscular tension. In some patients, the centrally acting antianxiety agents and skeletal muscle relaxants may enhance pain relief when combined with an analgesic.

The two most commonly used benzodiazepines in my practice are diazepam and alprazolam. Patients will tell the physician which of these worked best in the past. This could be used as a starting guide if the physician is inclined to listen to the patient.

Oxazepam and lorazepam are metabolized to inactive compounds and therefore have relatively short half-lives and durations of activity. Because of their simple one-step inactivation, oxazepam or lorazepam may be preferred in patients with liver disease and in the elderly. Sustained clinical effects require multiple daily doses; significant accumulation does not occur. The other agents with prolonged half-lives may be administered as a single daily dose at bedtime. The elimination half-life of diazepam and desmethyldiazepam is prolonged in obese patients; total metabolic clearance does not change (Facts and Comparisons, 1996). In addition to use as antianxiety agents, some benzodiazepines are also useful as hypnotics, anticonvulsants, and muscle relaxants.

Additionally, diazepam and alprazolan can be used for panic attacks that are seen in some chronic intractable pain patients.

Lorazepam is used for the management of anxiety disorders or for the short-term relief of the symptoms of anxiety or anxiety associated with depressive symptoms. Oral lorazepam appears useful for chronic insomnia. A small percentage of the patients I see derive benefit from 2–4 mg of lorazepam at bedtime for correction of a sleep deficit problem. Lorazepam given sublingually is absorbed more rapidly than after oral administration and compares favorably to intramuscular administration.

Alprazolam is used for the management of anxiety disorders or for the short-term relief of the symptoms of anxiety. Anxiety associated with depression is also responsive. It is also of value in the treatment of panic disorder with or without agoraphobia.

Diazepam is used for the management of anxiety disorders or for the short-term relief of the symptoms of anxiety. It can also be used as an adjunct for the relief of skeletal muscle spasm due to local pathology (e.g., inflammation of muscles or joints) or secondary to trauma. It also has a role in the treatment of spasticity caused by upper motor neuron disorders (e.g., cerebral palsy and paraplegia). It can be of value in the management of panic attacks.

Carisopradol

Carisoprodol is a relative of meprobamate (a tranquilizer medication whose history began almost 50 years ago). It can be used as adjunct for the relief of skeletal muscle spasm due to local pathology (e.g., inflammation of muscles or joints) or secondary to trauma.

Cyclobenzaprine

Cyclobenzaprine can be used as an adjunct to rest and physical therapy for relief of muscle spasm associated with acute painful muscle conditions. A dose of 10–40 mg/day appears to be a useful adjunct in the management of the fibrositis (fibromyalgia) syndrome.

Muscle spasm associated with acute, painful musculoskeletal conditions is generally of short duration. Muscle spasm secondary to overuse of the muscle usually lasts for short periods of time (up to 6 weeks). Cyclobenzaprine can be of value in treatment of muscle pain of up to 6 weeks in duration.

Palpable muscle tightness with associated tenderness that lasts longer than 6 weeks is due to myofascial taut bands. Cyclobenzaprine has been shown to be of value in treating some of the longer lasting cases and some cases of tender and painful myofascial taut bands. Therefore, therapy for longer periods may be appropriate.

Methocarbamol

Methocarbamol can be used as an adjunct to rest, physical therapy, and other measures for the relief of discomfort associated with acute and chronic painful musculoskeletal conditions.

Potential Problems

Refer to *Drug Facts and Comparisons* for a more detailed discussion of some of the reactions and problems that may be associated with the use of this group of medications.

The benzodiazepines contain medications with long half-lives (diazepam) and ones with shorter half-lives (oxepam). Because of the long half-life of diazepam (20–80 hours), a patient might take 5 mg at bedtime for two to four nights and become overly sedated during the daytime hours. On the other hand, some infrequent patients metabolize the medication very quickly and can take 10 mg of diazepam every 4–6 hours without cumulative sedative effects after months to years of taking the medication.

The greater the anxiety and tension level in some chronic intractable pain patients, the greater their tolerance for these medications.

Individual variation among patients calls for careful titration of the medication against the patient's anxiety or pain level.

Benzodiazepines

These agents are not intended for use in patients with a primary depressive disorder or psychosis or in those psychiatric disorders in which anxiety is not a prominent feature.

Dependence. Prolonged use of therapeutic doses can lead to dependence. Withdrawal syndrome has occurred after as little as 4–6 weeks of treatment. It is more likely if drug was short-acting (e.g., alprazolam), taken regularly for >3 months and abruptly discontinued. Higher dosages may not be a factor affecting withdrawal (Facts and Comparisons, 1996)

Renal function impairment. Usual precautions should be observed in the presence of impaired renal or hepatic function to avoid accumulation of these agents. Lorazepam injection is not recommended in these patients. Metabolites of clonazepam are excreted by the kidneys; to avoid excess accumulation, caution should be exercised in patients with impaired renal function. Also, clonazepam is contraindicated in patients with significant liver disease (Facts and Comparisons, 1996).

In those patients in whom depression accompanies anxiety, suicidal tendencies may be present, and protective measures may be required. Dispense the least amount of drug feasible to the patient (Facts and Comparisons, 1996).

Transient mild drowsiness is commonly seen in the first few days of therapy. If persistent, the dosage should be reduced. Other less frequent problems include sedation and sleepiness, depression, lethargy, apathy, fatigue, hypoactivity, lightheadedness, memory impairment, disorientation, restlessness, confusion, crying, sobbing, delirium, headache, slurred speech, syncope, tremor, vertigo, dizziness, euphoria, nervousness, irritability, difficulty in concentration, agitation, inability to perform complex mental functions, unsteadiness, ataxia, incoordination, weakness, constipation, diarrhea, dry mouth, coated tongue, nausea, anorexia, change in appetite, vomiting, difficulty in swallowing, increased salivation, gastritis, incontinence, changes in libido, urinary retention, bradycardia, tachycardia, cardiovascular collapse, hypertension, hypotension, palpitations, edema, diplopia, nystagmus, urticaria, pruritus, hair loss, hirsutism, ankle and facial edema, diaphoresis, paresthesias, hepatic dysfunction (including hepatitis and jaundice), leukopenia, anemia, lymphadenopathy, and elevations of LDH, alkaline phosphatase, ALT, and AST.

Oxazepam

Oxazepam is be used for the management of anxiety disorders or for the short-term relief of the symptoms of anxiety. Anxiety associated with depression is also responsive to oxazepam, as is anxiety, tension, agitation, and irritability in older patients (Facts and Comparisons, 1996).

Lorazepam

Information about lorazepam is found here in numerous areas relating to the benzodiazepines.

Alprazolam

Information about alprazolam is found here in numerous areas relating to the benzodiazepines.

Diazepam

Information about diazepam is found here in numerous areas relating to the benzodiazepines.

Carisoprodol

"In clinical use, psychological dependence and abuse have been rare, and there have been no reports of significant abstinence signs. Nevertheless, use the drug with caution in addiction-prone individuals" (Facts and Comparisons, 1996).

Carisoprodol should be administered cautiously to patients with compromised liver or kidney function. It may cause impairment of physical and mental faculties required for the performance of potentially hazardous tasks. Chronic intractable pain patients should use caution while driving or performing other tasks that require alertness, coordination, or physical dexterity.

Bothersome symptoms may manifest as dizziness, drowsiness, vertigo, ataxia, tremor, agitation, irritability, headache, depressive reactions, syncope, insomnia, tachycardia, postural hypotension, facial flushing, nausea, vomiting, hiccoughs, and epigastric distress.

Cyclobenzaprine

Because of its anticholinergic action, cyclobenzaprine should be used with caution in patients with a history of urinary retention, angle-closure glaucoma, and increased intraocular pressure. It may impair mental or physical abilities required for performance of hazardous tasks; patients should observe caution while driving or performing other tasks that require alertness, coordination, and physical dexterity (Facts and Comparisons, 1996).

Other adverse reactions are as follows:

- Tachycardia, syncope, arrhythmias, vasodilation, palpitations, hypotension, edema, hypertension, myocardial infarction, heart block, stroke, drowsiness (39%), dizziness (11%), fatigue, tiredness, asthenia, blurred vision, headache, nervousness (1–3%), convulsions, ataxia, vertigo, dysarthria, paresthesia, tremors, hypertonia, malaise, tinnitus, diplopia, decreased or increased libido, abnormal gait, delusions, peripheral neuropathy, Bell's palsy, alteration in EEG patterns (Facts and Comparisons, 1996)
- Confusion, disorientation, insomnia, depressed mood, abnormal sensations, anxiety, agitation, abnormal thinking and dreaming, hallucinations, excitement, dry mouth, nausea, constipation, dyspepsia, unpleasant taste, vomiting, anorexia, diarrhea, gastrointestinal pain, gastritis, thirst, flatulence, paralytic ileus, tongue discoloration, stomatitis, parotid swelling (Facts and Comparisons, 1996)
- Urinary frequency or retention, impaired urination, dilation of urinary tract, impotence, testicular swelling, gynecomastia, breast enlargement, galactorrhea
- Abnormal liver function, hepatitis, jaundice, cholestasis, sweating, skin rash, urticaria, pruritus, photosensitization, alopecia, muscle twitching, local weakness, myalgia, bone marrow depression, leukopenia, eosinophilia, thrombocytopenia, elevation and lowering of blood sugar levels, weight gain or loss

Methocarbamol

Adverse reactions include lightheadedness, dizziness, drowsiness, nausea, urticaria, pruritus, rash, conjunctivitis with nasal congestion, blurred vision, headache, and fever (Facts and Comparisons, 1996).

Patient Instruction

Benzodiazepines

The following material applies to the benzodiazepines as a group: "May cause drowsiness; avoid driving or other tasks requiring alertness. May be taken with food or water if stomach upset occurs. Patients on long-term or high dosage therapy may experience withdrawal symptoms on abrupt cessation of therapy; do not discontinue therapy abruptly or change dosage except on advice of physician" (Facts and Comparisons, 1996).

Carisopradol

Carisopradol may be taken with food or meals if gastrointestinal upset occurs. It may cause drowsiness or dizziness. Patients should observe caution while driving or performing other tasks that require alertness, coordination, or physical dexterity. Alcohol and other central nervous system depressants should be avoided. If dizziness (postural hypotension) occurs, sudden changes in posture should be avoided and caution should be exercised when climbing stairs, etc. (Facts and Comparisons, 1996).

Cyclobenzaprine

Cyclobenzaprine may cause drowsiness, dizziness, or blurred vision. Patients should observe caution while driving or performing other tasks that require alertness, coordination, or physical dexterity. Alcohol and other central nervous system depressants should be avoided. It may cause dry mouth (Facts and Comparisons, 1996).

Methocarbamol

Methocarbamol may cause drowsiness, dizziness, or lightheadedness. Patients should observe caution while driving or performing other tasks that require alertness, coordination, or physical dexterity. Urine may darken to brown, black, or green. The patient's physician should be notified if skin rash, itching, fever, or nasal congestion occurs (Facts and Comparisons, 1996).

SEDATIVES AND HYPNOTICS (SLEEPING MEDICATIONS)

Medications Whose Main Purpose Is the Correction of the Sleep Disorder Which Comes with Some Chronic Intractable Pain

As one of my patients put it, "Without a good night's sleep, you're shot!" She is a 57-year-old business executive who fell backwards onto the office floor in 1977. She has had MPS and fibromyalgia pain in almost her whole body since that time. She lives in constant pain. She takes Vicodin® during the day for pain control. She uses MS Contin® at bedtime for pain control and to facilitate her sleep, which is disturbed by her pain. Simply easing enough of the pain helps her sleep fairly comfortably at night.

The sleep disorders common to chronic pain patients include:

1. Insomnia (abnormal inability to sleep)
2. Difficulty falling asleep
3. Frequent awakenings
4. Early morning awakenings
5. Arising in the morning feeling tired and unrested

6. Feeling exhausted
7. Feeling drained of energy
8. Difficulty staying asleep

If the patient's sleep is impaired because of pain, numbness, and tingling and/or twitching of the muscles, one of the medications listed in the table below can be used. It will usually suppress some of the bothersome nighttime symptoms and produce a more restful sleep. If pain is the only problem that causes sleep problems, an adequate dose of a proper analgesic at bedtime may facilitate better sleep.

Table of Medications and Dosing

Note that all doses given are for adults. No dosing for children is given.

Generic name	Brand name	Usual adult oral dose (mg)	Rapidity of start of medical effect	Half-life (hours)
Flurazepam	Dalmane®	15–30	Mid range	47–100
Temazepam	Restoril®	15–30	Slow	9.5–12.4
Triazolam	Halcion®	0.125–0.5	Mid range	1.5–5.5
Diazepam	Valium®	4–40	Mid range	20–80
Zolpidem tartrate	Ambien®	5–10	Quick	2.5
Chlorpromazine	Thorazine®	10–80[a]	Slow	10–20

[a] According to work in the practice of Michael S. Margoles, M.D., Ph.D.

Functions

Benzodiazepines generally decrease sleep latency and decrease the number of awakenings and the time spent in stage 0 (awake stage). Flurazepam, quazepam, and temazepam decrease stage 1 (descending drowsiness). Stage 2 (unequivocal sleep) is increased by all benzodiazepines, and most benzodiazepines shorten stages 3 and 4 (slow wave sleep). Temazepam has prolonged stage 3 and shortened stage 4 in neurotic patients or patients with depression. All but flurazepam prolong REM latency. REM sleep is usually shortened, but with temazepam or low-dose flurazepam, this may not be the case. The result of benzodiazepine administration is an increase in total sleep time (Facts and Comparisons, 1996).

Uses and Goals

The goals we are attempting to achieve with medications in this class of drugs may be multiple (i.e., more restful sleep, decrease overall pain, improve ability to work, better social skills, etc.). No one medication works for all patients. Therefore, when attempting to achieve these goals, a number of medications from this class of drug may need to be tried in succession until the desired result is achieved. The medications listed here are merely a partial listing of medications that I have found useful in the chronic intractable pain patients I have treated over the last 22 years. Other medications not listed here are equally as effective.

Some of the more severely afflicted chronic intractable pain patients suffer disturbed sleep because of nocturnal myoclonus, a bothersome twitching of the lower extremities. The problem may be bad enough that the spouse with the disease repeatedly kicks the unaffected spouse. The condition usually responds well to Klonopin® (clonazepam), a membrane stabilizer (anticonvulsant) medication that both blocks the nocturnal myoclonus and produces sedation.

Insomnia is characterized by difficulty in falling asleep, frequent nocturnal awakenings, or early morning awakening. Medication can be used for recurring insomnia or poor sleeping habits and in acute or chronic medical situations that require restful sleep. Insomnia is often transient and intermittent; therefore, prolonged administration is generally not recommended.

Because insomnia may be a symptom of other disorders, consider the possibility that the complaint may be related to a condition for which there is more specific treatment. "Specific treatment" might consist of psychotherapy plus an antidepressant. Recurrent waking may be due to pressure on active and hyperirritable myofascial trigger points. For example, an active myofascial trigger point in the gluteus minimus muscle may produce tenderness at the greater trochanter on one side. When the patient rolls to that side and brings pressure to bear on the trochanter, the pain wakes the patient up. This can happen repeatedly throughout the night. Simply and skillfully injecting the gluteus minimus myofascial trigger point will rid the patient of that problem.

In my practice, I have used Dalmane®, Restoril®, and Valium® for 5–10 years in a small group of patients without significant side effects. There is no one benzodiazepine that is best for chronic intractable pain patients.

Halcion is not recommended for this group of patients. It is too short acting for chronic intractable pain patients. These patients usually have difficulty going to sleep and staying asleep. A medication like Halcion® will help the first part of the problem, but not the second (difficulty staying asleep).

Minor versus Major Sedatives/Hypnotics

Some major tranquilizers need to be used as a sedative/hypnotic medication for some patients. The designations minor and major are arbitrary ones that I developed for use in my office, based on the following characteristics. The minor medications are used in patients with "minor" pain problems, and the major medications are used in patients with "major" sleep and pain problems.

Some of the following differences between minor and major pain problems help to distinguish which patients should be considered for the major medications to aid in restoring sleep patterns toward normal:

Item	Minor	Major
Area of pain	Limited	Broad and multifocal
Overall disability secondary to pain	Mild	Moderate to severe
Hyperirritability of the tissues	None	Frequent and diffuse
Adequate response to benzodiazepine, Soma®, Ambien®, etc.	Produces adequate sleep	Very little correction of abnormal sleep

An analgesic can act as a sedative because of sedative side effects it may have at higher doses. However, sedative medications, in most cases, cannot act as an analgesic because they have no analgesic properties.

Chlorpromazine HCl

Many of the most painful patients cannot get to sleep or stay asleep. This is when a medication like chlorpromazine may be effective.

I began to evaluate the benefits of using chlorpromazine (Thorazine®) about 3 years ago. I had found that a portion of my severely afflicted chronic pain patients could not get a restful night's sleep despite the use of a potent analgesic and one of the more commonly used sedative–hypnotic medications (Dalmane®, Restoril®, etc.). I discovered that most of this group of patients responded well to the use of a potent analgesic (1 hour before retiring) and chlorpromazine at 20–80 mg taken 2–3 hours before bedtime.

This medication is a major tranquilizer. In doses of 100–1000 mg/day, the medication is used as an antipsychotic drug. In doses of 10–50 mg by mouth or by injection, it is used in the treatment of nausea or vomiting.

Potential Problems

Refer to *Drug Facts and Comparisons* for a more detailed discussion of some of the reactions and problems that may be associated with the use of this group of medications.

Benzodiazepines

In general, the warnings, precautions, and adverse reactions are the same for this group of benzodiazepines as for the centrally acting antianxiety and skeletal muscle relaxant agents. Refer to *Drug Facts and Comparisons* for discussion of the medications that are covered here but not covered elsewhere in this book.

Zolpidem Tartrate

This drug has not been used extensively in my program because it does not seem to work any more effectively than other of the minor medications that aid sleep. Refer to *Drug Facts and Comparisons* for more extensive discussion of this medication.

Chlorpromazine HCl

Tardive dyskinesia, a syndrome that consists of potentially irreversible, involuntary dyskinetic movements, may develop in patients treated with major tranquilizer drugs.

The syndrome can develop, although much less commonly, after relatively brief treatment periods at low doses. There is no known treatment for established cases of tardive dyskinesia, although it may remit, partially or completely, if major tranquilizers are withdrawn.

If signs and symptoms of tardive dyskinesia appear, discontinuation of use of the drug should be considered (Facts and Comparisons, 1996).

Drowsiness may occur during the first or second week, after which it generally disappears. If troublesome, the dosage should be lowered. Patients should be cautioned against performing activities that require alertness (e.g., operating vehicles or machinery). The medication should be used cautiously in depressed patients and patients in an agitated state with depression (particularly if a suicidal tendency is recognized).

Lethargy and decreased sensation of thirst due to central inhibition may lead to dehydration, hemoconcentration, and reduced pulmonary ventilation. If the above signs appear, especially in the elderly, remedial therapy should be instituted promptly. Use with caution in respiratory impairment due to acute pulmonary infections or chronic respiratory disorders.

Use with caution in patients with cardiovascular disease, mitral insufficiency, seizure disorders, renal function impairment, impairment of liver function, and patients with a history of glaucoma. Jaundice may occur during the second to fourth week after therapy is begun. Refer to *Drug Facts and Comparisons,* 1996 for a more in-depth discussion of the above material.

Patient Instruction (Patient Information)

Because some patients exposed chronically to major tranquilizers will develop tardive dyskinesia, all patients for whom chronic use is contemplated should be informed about this risk, if possible.

Nonprescription Sleep Aids

There are many over-the-counter products that can work well in the early stages of any chronic pain problem where sleep begins to become disturbed. These include Benadryl® and many others.

MEMBRANE STABILIZERS (ANTICONVULSANTS)

A membrane stabilizer is a medication whose primary action is to decrease abnormal signaling coming from the central nervous system.

Medications Whose Main Purpose is to Correct Abnormal Signaling from Numerous Cells in the Body

Emphasis here is on nerve or brain tissue.

Tables of Medications and Dosing

Note that all doses given are for adults. No dosing for children is given.

Chemical class	Brand name	Generic name	Dose (mg)	Frequency
Membrane stabilizer	Dilantin®	Phenytoin sodium[a]	30	100–300 mg/day
			50	100–300 mg/day
			100	100–300 mg/day
			125	100–300 mg/day
	Klonopin®	Clonazepam[b]	0.5	Adults: Begin dosing not to
			1	exceed 1.5 mg/day in three
			2	divided doses; increase in increments of 0.5–1 mg every 3 days until desired effect is achieved
	Depakene®	Valproic acid	Tablet 250	Dosing suggested here is
			Syrup 250	adjunctive therapy for migraine headaches, as well
		Divalproex	125[c]	as neuropathic pain and
			500[c]	related abnormal signals; begin 125 mg at bedtime; if

[a] Clinically effective serum levels are usually in the range of 10–20 µg/ml.

[b] For the patient with nocturnal myoclonus, either the spouse says there is less kicking or the patient reports less awakening due to kicking activity (kicking will cause less jumps and jerks during sleep).

[c] Time-release tablets.

Chemical class	Brand name	Generic name	Dose (mg)	Frequency
				no response after 2 weeks, graduate dosing to 250 mg at bedtime; if no response, stop the medication
	Neurotontin®	Gabapentin	100-mg caps 300-mg caps 400-mg caps	Effective dose is 900–1800 mg/day in divided doses three times per day; titration to an effective dose can take place rapidly, giving 300 mg on day 1, 300 mg twice per day on day 2, and 300 mg three times per day on day 3; however, many of the chronic intractable pain patients are sensitive to dosage escalation that is too rapid, and this applies to any medication intended for use in this group of patients; I therefore start the patient at 100 mg three times per day; every other day the dosing is increased by 100 mg until a maximum of 1800 mg/day is achieved; if no positive results are obtained, taper the patient off the medication by decreasing 100 mg every day

Functions

The primary site of action of the hydantoins appears to be the motor cortex, where the spread of abnormal electrical activity is inhibited. Possibly by promoting sodium efflux from neurons, hydantoins tend to stabilize the threshold against hyperexcitability caused by excessive stimulation or environmental changes capable of reducing membrane sodium gradient.

Uses and Goals

These medications are used primarily for the treatment of seizures and related disorders. They have also found use for the treatment of neuropathic symptoms of pain, burning, bothersome tingling, and a number of other strange or perverted sensations. One of the medications, clonazepam, has been found of use in the treatment of nocturnal myoclonus.

The goals we are attempting to achieve with medications in this class of drugs may be multiple (i.e., more office work, better social skills, etc.). No one medication works for all patients. Therefore, when attempting to achieve these goals, it may be necessary to try a number of medications from this class in succession until the desired result is achieved. The medications listed here are merely a partial listing of medications that I have found useful in the chronic intractable pain patients I have treated over the last 22 years. Other medications not listed here are equally as effective.

It should be noted that neuropathic pain and related abnormal signals may come from two source locations. There may be direct signals from local peripheral nerve degeneration. In this instance, the signals are going to the brain from abnormal, degenerated tissue at the site where the symptom is felt. Alternatively, a diseased focus in the sensory cortex of the brain may be projecting (referring) abnormal signals to the periphery (the area of the body where the neuropathic pain and related abnormal signals are felt). In the most severe and complex cases, both types of signaling will be present.

The majority of the patients in my practice are men and women who have failed in numerous other pain programs. In general, they are the severely afflicted chronic intractable pain patients. This type of patient is discussed in Chapter 10 on MPS in the sections on grade 3 and grade 4 patients. This group of pain patients comes with multifocal pain in numerous body areas, including headaches of the tension or migraine type in about 50%. The multifocal pain is either pure MPS in origin or a mixture of MPS, fibromyalgia, and neuropathic pain. In general, these patients do not respond well to membrane stabilizer medications. In this group, the benzodiazepines work well in about 50% as an antianxiety medication. Clonazepam has been found to be of some help in the management of some patients with nocturnal myoclonus. Valproic acid has been a helpful preventative medication in about 30% of the migraine headache patients.

Gabapentin, a recently released membrane stabilizer, has been attempted on 20 of my patients, but has not shown significant results. In one of my patients, the gabapentin made the pain more tolerable, but did not cut back on the 875 mg of MS Contin® per day that it takes to keep her gainfully employed.

About 12 years ago, this group of patients was treated with hydantoins with no significant help.

Clonazepam

- Periodic leg movements during sleep (nocturnal myoclonus) (0.5–2 mg per night)
- Neuralgias (deafferentation pain syndromes) (2–4 mg/day)

Potential Problems

Refer to *Drug Facts and Comparisons* for a more detailed discussion of some of the reactions and problems that may be associated with the use of this group of medications.

Hydantoins

Conversion of hydantoins occurs in the liver; elderly patients or those with impaired liver function or severe illness may show early signs of toxicity. The drug should be discontinued if hepatic dysfunction occurs. Blood counts and urinalyses should be performed when therapy is begun and at monthly intervals for several months thereafter. Blood dyscrasias have occurred. If lymph node enlargement occurs, attempt to substitute another anticonvulsant drug or drug combination. Osteomalacia has been associated with phenytoin therapy. Adverse effects include ataxia, dysarthria, slurred speech, mental confusion, dizziness, insomnia, transient nervousness, motor twitchings, diplopia, fatigue, irritability, drowsiness, depression, numbness, tremor, headache. Toxic hepatitis and liver damage may occur.

Benzodiazepines

For more complete information, refer to the information on benzodiazepines in the section on centrally acting antianxiety and skeletal muscle relaxant agents.

Valproic Acid

Significantly reduced plasma protein binding has occurred in renal insufficiency, cirrhosis, and acute viral hepatitis. Discontinue immediately in the presence of significant hepatic dysfunction, suspected or apparent. Thrombocytopenia, inhibition of the secondary phase of platelet aggregation, and abnormal coagulation parameters have occurred. The most common initial side effects are nausea, vomiting, and indigestion, usually transient and rarely requiring discontinuation of therapy. Diarrhea, abdominal cramps, constipation, anorexia with weight loss, and increased appetite with weight gain may occur. Sedation, tremor, ataxia, headache, "spots before eyes," dysarthria, dizziness, incoordination, emotional upset, depression, psychosis, aggression, hyperactivity, behavioral deterioration, transient hair loss, skin rash, petechiae, photosensitivity, generalized pruritis, altered bleeding time, thrombocytopenia, bruising, hematoma formation, frank hemorrhage, relative lymphocytosis, leukopenia, eosinophilia, anemia, bone marrow suppression, bone marrow toxicity suggestive of a myelodysplastic syndrome, and minor elevations of AST, ALT, and LDH are frequent and appear to be dose-related. Occasionally, increases in serum bilirubin and abnormal changes in other liver function tests occur. Severe hepatotoxicity and death may occur. Irregular menses, abnormal thyroid function tests, parotid gland swelling, and breast enlargement may also occur, as may edema of extremities and weakness.

Gabapentin

Adverse effects include somnolence, dizziness, ataxia, fatigue, nystagmus, nausea or vomiting, headache, fever, abdominal pain, diarrhea, convulsions, confusion, insomnia, emotional lability, rash, acne, asthenia, malaise, facial edema, allergy, generalized edema, weight decrease, chill, strange feelings, lassitude, alcohol intolerance, hangover effect, hypertension, hypotension, angina pectoris, peripheral vascular disorder, palpitation, tachycardia, migraine, murmur, atrial fibrillation, heart failure, thrombophlebitis, myocardial infarction, cerebrovascular accident, pulmonary thrombosis, ventricular extrasystoles, bradycardia, premature atrial contraction, pericardial rub, heart block, pulmonary embolus, hyperlipidemia, hypercholesterolemia, pericardial effusion, pericarditis, anorexia, flatulence, gingivitis, glossitis, gum hemorrhage, thirst, stomatitis, increased salivation, gastroenteritis, hemorrhoids, bloody stools, fecal incontinence, hepatomegaly, dysphagia, eructation, pancreatitis, peptic ulcer, colitis, blisters in mouth, tooth discoloration, perleche, salivary gland enlarged, lip hemorrhage, esophagitis, hiatal hernia, ematemesis, proctitis, irritable bowel syndrome, rectal hemorrhage, esophageal spasm, hyperthyroid, hypothyroid, goiter, hypoestrogen, ovarian failure, epididymitis, swollen testicle, cushingoid appearance, bruises (resulting from physical trauma), anemia, thrombocytopenia, lymphadenopathy, white blood cell count increased, lymphocytosis, arthralgia, tendinitis, arthritis, joint stiffness/swelling, positive Romberg test, costochondritis, osteoporosis, bursitis, vertigo, hyperkinesia, paresthesia, abnormalities of the deep tendon reflexes, syncope, abnormal dreaming, aphasia, hypesthesia, dysesthesia, paresis, cerebellar dysfunction, positive Babinski sign, decreased position sense, apathy, hallucination, depersonalization, euphoria, feeling high, fine motor control disorder, meningismus, alopecia, eczema, dry skin, increased sweating, urticaria, hematuria, dysuria, urination frequency, cystitis, urinary retention/incontinence, vaginal hemorrhage, amenorrhea, dysmenorrhea, menorrhagia, kidney pain, leukorrhea, genital pruritus, nocturia, abnormal vision, eye pain, photophobia, bilateral or unilateral ptosis, eye hemorrhage, hearing loss, earache, tinnitus, inner ear infection, otitis, taste loss, unusual taste, eye twitching, ear fullness, eye itching, abnormal accommodation, sensitivity to noise, eye focusing problem, watery eyes, retinopathy, glaucoma, iritis, corneal disorders, lacrimal dysfunction, degenerative eye changes, retinal degeneration, miosis, chorioretinitis, strabismus, eustachian tube dysfunction, labyrinthitis, otitis externa, and odd smell.

Patient Instruction

Phenytoin

This medication should be taken with food to reduce gastrointestinal irritation. Patients should maintain good oral hygiene (regular brushing and flossing) while taking phenytoin and inform their dentist of medication usage.

It can cause drowsiness, dizziness, or blurred vision; alcohol may intensify these effects. Patients should use caution while driving or performing other tasks that require alertness, coordination, or physical dexterity and notify their physicians if drowsiness, slurred speech, or impaired coordination (ataxia) occurs.

Valproic Acid

If gastrointestinal upset occurs, valproic acid should be taken with food. Tablets or capsules should not be chewed. They should be swallowed whole to avoid irritation of the mouth and throat. Valproic acid may cause drowsiness; patients should observe caution while driving or performing other tasks that require alertness, coordination, or physical dexterity. It should be taken at bedtime to minimize effects of central nervous system depression (Facts and Comparisons, 1996).

Gabapentin

Gabapentin should be taken only as prescribed. Patients should be advised that gabapentin may cause dizziness, somnolence, and other symptoms and signs of central nervous system depression. Accordingly, patients should be advised to neither drive a car nor operate other complex machinery until they have gained sufficient experience on gabapentin to gauge whether or not it affects their mental or motor performance adversely (Facts and Comparisons, 1996).

ANTICONSTIPATION MEDICATIONS

Constipation can be a factor in the pain syndrome itself or can be a side effect of medication. Medications known to produce constipation are the TCAs (amitriptyline, desipramine, etc.) and some of the opioid and opioid-containing analgesics. The general approach to this problem is easily remedied by putting more fiber in the diet (fruits and vegetables). For some, this has no effect. In a number of cases, gentle laxatives such as Senokot® and Senokot S® (a natural plant laxative) can be of value. In some of the more resistant cases, milk of magnesia taken regularly throughout the day can be of value. With some of the stronger analgesics, such as methadone and morphine, constipation can be a serious problem. A combination of Senokot® and milk of magnesia may be of better benefit here. Small doses of each can be taken throughout the day. For the more problematic constipation, herb teas may be of great value. One is "Dieters' Green Tea" and the other is "Super Slimming Tea." Both of the teas can be purchased in Japanese markets and health food stores. Lactulose can be of great benefit in the last cases mentioned.

BIBLIOGRAPHY

Aranoff, G. (1985). Psychological aspects of nonmalignant chronic pain: a new nosology, in *Evaluation and Treatment of Chronic Pain,* Aranoff, G. (Ed.), Urban and Swarzenberg, Baltimore, pp. 471–484.

Aranoff, G. and Evans, W. (1985). Pharmacological management of chronic pain, in *Evaluation and Treatment of Chronic Pain,* Aranoff, G. (Ed.), Urban and Swarzenberg, Baltimore, pp. 435–449.

Brezin, J. et. al. (1979). Reversible kidney failure and nephrotic syndrome associated with nonsteroidal antiinflammatory drugs, *New England Journal of Medicine,* 301, 1271–1273.

Curry, R. (1982). Acute renal failure after acetaminophen (Tylenol) ingestion, *Journal of the American Medical Association,* 247, 1012–1014.

Facts and Comparisons (1996). *Drug Facts and Comparisons,* Wolters Kluwer, St. Louis.

Facts and Comparisons (1996a). *Drug Facts and Comparisons,* Wolters Kluwer, St. Louis, pp. 1245–1251

Foley, K. (1985). Adjuvant analgesic drugs in cancer pain management, in *Evaluation and Treatment of Chronic Pain,* Aranoff, G. (Ed.), Urban and Swarzenberg, Baltimore, pp. 425–433.

Gary, N. et. al. (1980). Indomethacin (Indocin)-related acute renal failure, *American Journal of Medicine,* 69, 135–136.

Kimberly, R. et. al. (1978). Reduction of renal (kidney) function by newer nonsteroidal anti-inflammatory drugs, *American Journal of Medicine,* 64, 804–807.

Large, R. (1980). The psychiatrist and the chronic pain patient: 172 anecdotes, *Pain,* 9, 253–263.

Meek, J., Guidice, V., and Enrick, N. (1984). Colchicine highly effective in disc disorders: results of a double blind study, *Journal of Neurological and Orthopaedic Medicine and Surgery,* 5, 213–220.

Monks, R. and Mersky, H. (1984). Psychotropic drugs, in *Textbook of Pain,* Wall, P. and Melzack, R. (Eds.), Churchill Livingston, New York, pp. 526–537.

Rask, M. (1980). Colchicine use in 500 patients with disc disease, *Journal of Neurological and Orthopaedic Medicine and Surgery,* 1, 1–18.

Rose, H. (1992). Personal communication.

Savitz, D. (1985). Medical evaluation of the chronic pain patient, in *Evaluation and Treatment of Chronic Pain,* Aranoff, G. (Ed.), Urban and Swarzenberg, Baltimore, pp. 47–49.

Sternbach, R. (1984). Acute versus chronic pain, in *Textbook of Pain,* Wall, P. and Melzack, R. (Eds.), Churchill Livingston, New York, pp. 174–175.

22 When I Control the Pain, I Control My Life: Opioids and Opioid-Containing Analgesic Medication in the Management of Chronic Intractable Pain

Michael S. Margoles, M.D., Ph.D.

INTRODUCTORY REMARKS ABOUT THE USE OF OPIOIDS OR OPIOID-CONTAINING ANALGESICS

In general, in patient circles and medical circles, the ignorance surrounding the use of opioids or opioid-containing analgesics is appalling. The war against illicit drug use frequently strikes home when a physician prescribing legitimate medication is apprehended and prosecuted for allegedly prescribing too much opioid pain-relieving medication for a motivated patient who was using the medication to make a living and provide for his or her family.

There is a legitimate and an illegitimate use of "narcotics" in the United States. In many instances, those of us in the medical profession and regulatory bodies appear not to know how to accurately differentiate between the two scenarios.

In general, there is a trend toward treating chronic intractable pain patients with any medication other than opioids or opioid-containing analgesics. The latest fad in that direction is Neurontin®. Whereas Neurontin® may be a good anticonvulsant, it has not been indicated in the treatment of any type of painful condition (Facts and Comparisons, 1996).

We are also faced with the constant pressure to "taper" patients off of opioid analgesics that may be helping in their overall rehabilitation, because there is a fear of "addiction" on long-term use of the opioids or opioid-containing analgesics in the treatment of chronic intractable pain. My 21 years of pain management practice and the medical literature state that "addiction" with long-term use of opioids or opioid-containing analgesics for the long-term treatment of chronic intractable pain patients is not a significant problem.

1-57444-103-5/99/$0.00+$.50
© 1999 by CRC Press LLC

Patients are reluctant to take the opioids or opioid-containing analgesics because they fear addiction. Doctors hesitate to prescribe the opioids or opioid-containing analgesics for fear of lengthy and expensive prosecution by their licensing board. Some pharmacists will not stock certain of these medications for the same reasons relating to unnecessary exposure to possible prosecution.

The mention of these medications usually strikes fear in the hearts of patients, medical boards, hospital boards, and doctors alike. The use of opioids ("narcotics") is bathed in mysticism and confusion both in the patient community and in the professional community.

Before embarking upon the medications and how they are used, some concise definitions and understandings are necessary. The terms "addicted," "habituated," and "hooked" have no reliable meaning any more because everyone has a "definition" or "understanding," but none is quite complete.

In 1980, the World Health Organization (WHO) gave a practical and applicable definition of drug-related problems when it coined the term drug dependence syndrome (DDS). The definition is detailed but not boringly long; it is concise and precise. It presents the syndrome of "addiction" as having multiple abnormal personality characteristics.

Unless a person has 80% or more of the criteria for DDS, he or she is not addicted. There are a few exceptions to the rule, which will be presented.

ADDICTION AND THE DRUG DEPENDENCE SYNDROME

Chronic pain patients use narcotics to live.
Drug addicts live to use narcotics.

Some Introductory Remarks

Every case of "chemical dependency" is not a case of DDS and is not a case for detoxification ("detox"). In some clinical cases, dependence on a potentially addicting drug, if carried out with the proper supervision, can be of benefit to the patient.

Drug Dependence Syndrome Does Not Equal
Chemical Dependency Does Not Equal Addiction

The following is a tentative statement that has not been qualified by extensive clinical study. However, it is based on the author's 5 years of experience with a drug addict population in Harlem, New York, and 21 years of prescribing controlled substances to chronic intractable pain patients: To qualify for a diagnosis of DDS, the patient/person has to have at least 80% of the profile characteristics listed below.

Drug Dependence Syndrome and Addiction

The terms addiction, dependence, tolerance, drug abuse, hooked, dependent, and habituated are commonly used in a confusing fashion by lay, medical, and regulatory persons. These terms have been replaced by the WHO with "drug dependence syndrome." DDS relates to a syndrome that is not bound by the old ways of thinking and avoids the dualism inherent in the use of terms such as psychological dependence and physical dependence.

DDS is a socio–psycho–biological syndrome manifested by a behavioral pattern in which the use of a given psychoactive drug (or class of drugs) is given *sharply higher priority over other behaviors which once had significantly greater value.* A key descriptive element is the priority given to drug seeking over other behaviors (Edwards, 1980). The emphasis in defining DDS is a ***change*** *in usual and acceptable behavior patterns to unusual and unacceptable behaviors.*

Characterization of Drug Dependence Syndrome

DDS is a characteristic of the patient, not a characteristic of the drug. At the core of the person with DDS is a profound alteration of personality manifested by being consumed by an overwhelming involvement (compulsive behavior) with the controlled substances upon which he or she is dependent. The drug literally becomes the person's whole way of life. The person sleeps, eats, and lives for the controlled substances. He or she favors socially unacceptable behavior such as stealing, lying, prostitution, and/or misappropriating funds to obtain and use controlled substances. People will lie, cheat, and steal for drugs. The controlled substances they seek become a substitute for reality. There may be significant disruption of family and interpersonal relationships. They are usually not well kept and have poor dental hygiene. There is a strong tendency to relapse (recidivism) to consuming controlled substances after they have been "detoxed" (appropriately withdrawn from the drug). The person with DDS takes a psychoactive substance ("drug"), in a compulsive and repetitive habit or ritualistic manner, for a "high" or euphoric effect, despite physical, psychological, or social harm. Because tolerance to euphoria develops quickly, there is a need for progressive escalation of the drug dosing. During the euphoric state, morals and ethics may be compromised in ways not acceptable before the drug took effect. It becomes easier to commit crimes and behave in other unacceptable ways.

Drug-Seeking Behavior

Drug-seeking behavior is manifested by:

- Hoarding or selling medication(s) a person is dependent on
- An intense desire for controlled substances and overwhelming concern about their continued availability
- Evidence of compulsive controlled substance use which is manifested as unsanctioned dose escalation, continued dosing despite significant side effects, use of the drug to treat symptoms not targeted by the therapy, or unapproved use during periods of no symptoms
- Manipulation of the treating physician or medical system for the purposes of obtaining additional controlled substances
- Altering prescriptions to obtain controlled substances
- Acquisition of controlled substances from nonmedical sources
- Unapproved use of other drugs (particularly alcohol)
- Consulting numerous therapists concurrently (physician, dentist, podiatrist, etc.) to obtain prescriptions for controlled substances; this usually occurs at multiple pharmacies
- Numerous excuses to get more controlled substances

Unsanctioned Use of a Controlled Substance

Unsanctioned use of a controlled substance is manifested by:

- Consuming another person's medications
- Taking more of a controlled substance than is prescribed

- Dissolving and injecting, by any route, controlled substances that are meant for oral administration
- A patient giving his or her controlled substances to a spouse, relative, or friend
- Not taking a controlled substance according to the written or oral directions of a therapist or pharmacist
- A patient repeatedly (more than once) fails to call the prescribing therapist to clarify questions about the use of a controlled substance
- Unauthorized escalation of the ingestion of a controlled substance

Establishing Drug Dependence Syndrome

Although DDS can theoretically be established by review of records, the preferred method is by interview and physical examination. The interview and physical examination should be conducted by a specialist familiar with DDS patients. If the medication is being used for pain control in a chronic pain patient, a physician familiar with various chronic pain conditions, including myofascial pain syndrome, should physically evaluate the patient. This helps to authenticate the presence of disease as the reason for taking the controlled substance.

The "Con"

This section addresses some of the personality alterations seen in persons with DDS, persons with abnormal drug-seeking behavior, or illicit drug-oriented persons. The "con" is the drug-seeking person. Con also refers to the game(s) of stories the drug seeker plays to obtain drugs. Persons with DDS characteristically "con" their "mark" (the physician or person who is the source of the con's drug[s] or drug money) for drugs or money to obtain drugs.

In obtaining drugs, there is usually a basic con going on (going down), with the mark unaware of its occurrence. I call this the "basic continuing." There is a pattern that cons the sympathy of the mark. The con frequently uses the "Oh, poor little old me" approach with the mark to obtain sympathy. This is especially true when women con a male physician with seductive behavior. The mark is usually a person who demonstrates a desire to help the impoverished and/or suffering persons. The con may appear downtrodden and oppressed.

The mark is manipulated with lexicon or "jive-talk." If you are perceptive or cognizant, you can feel the "torque" when the con is moving in on you. The appeal is to your sympathies and "soft spots." Cons make you feel sorry for them and their predicament. They have a "needy" appearance. They sound needy. One of the classic remarks is, "Okay, Doc, I'll stop using this medication, but can you prescribe it just one more time for me, and then no more." Next week, the person is back for more with a new con.

The con that comes with drug addicts and drug-seeking behavior is typified as follows:

- Bold and affrontive in a bad way, not a proud way
- Stark
- Without conscience
- Without humility
- Desperate
- Urgent (pressures the mark to forget usual policy and procedural steps in ordering or dispensing the drug)
- Selfish
- Self-centered
- Takes advantage of the mark

- Dishonest
- Clandestine
- Surreptitious
- Secondary gain
- Deception
- Plotting in a decisive way against the mark
- Strong denial

Denial of Personal Problems

The person with DDS denies the negative effect of the drug on his or her life. He or she express no worries or concerns about becoming or being a person with DDS. Normal persons, not used to taking this type of medication, are almost constantly plagued by this type of worry.

Examples of Nondrug Dependence Syndrome Drug Use

If a patient depends on a narcotic and/or narcotic-containing analgesic to promote employment and provide for his or her family, this is not DDS. If an individual uses a narcotic and/or narcotic-containing analgesic to relieve pain and/or the anxiety associated with pain (depends on the medication for a physical and/or psychologic reason), this is not DDS.

Chronic pain patients are goal oriented, whereas DDS patients are drug oriented.

Behaviors Embodied in Drug Dependence Syndrome ("Addiction")

Behaviors embodied in DDS ("addiction") include:

- Personality alterations around obtaining the drug:
  - Abstinence syndrome after drug abruptly stopped
  - Family is disrupted due to personality alterations related to drug use
  - Hygiene may be poor, especially dental
  - Manipulation of family members and friends
  - Priority is given to drug-seeking behavior
  - Rapid dose escalation
  - Stealing, lying, denial of drug problem, compromised morals, prostitution
  - Taking drugs for euphoria or desire for a "rush"
- Drug-seeking behavior:
  - Acquisition from nonmedical sources
  - Altered prescriptions
  - Hoarding and/or selling drugs
  - Ignoring negative impact and influences of the drug
  - Manipulation of the physician to get more drug
  - Multiple excuses to get more drug
  - Multiple therapists and multiple pharmacies
  - Strong desire for the drug for other than medical use
  - Use of additional drugs, most commonly alcohol
- Unsanctioned use:
  - Consuming another person's medications
  - Giving medication to others

- Injecting oral medication
- Unsanctioned dose escalation
- Using the drug for unapproved indications

Closing Comments

H. Wesley Clark, M.D. offered the following observation: "The chronic pain patient, although at risk for addiction, must not be considered addicted simply because of the long term use of psychoactive substances, physical dependence and/or tolerance to the medications" (Clark, 1988)

The following sources were used in preparation of the material in this section: Clark (1988), Edwards (1981), and Portenoy (1990).

PAIN SEVERITY

There is a tendency to trivialize chronic intractable pain patients. It is a put-down based on ignorance on both the family/public side and the professional side. This occurs because the patient is frequently not showing much in the way of reaction to the pain.

Some doctors will not pay much attention unless the patient is visibly oozing blood or has a known painful condition that can be documented with technology, such as an EKG for a heart attack, etc. My own personal experience points up the fact that most physicians are poorly trained in the physical examination and diagnosis of patients with chronic pain. This does not mean that chronic intractable pain is any less painful than a heart attack or broken bone.

I believe we need to look at the works written for myofascial pain syndrome (MPS) by Janet G. Travell, M.D. and David G. Simons, M.D. (Travell and Simons, 1983). By the time they wrote their first book on the subject of MPS, Dr. Travell had been in medical practice for about 53 years, and Dr. Simons had been in practice for about 35 years. Both were professors at well-known universities. Here is what they said about pain severity in MPS: "Severity. The severity of symptoms from myofascial trigger points ranges from painless restriction of motion due to latent myofascial trigger points so common in the aged, to agonizing incapacitating pain caused by very active myofascial trigger points. The potential severity of this common malady is illustrated by one housewife who, while bending over cooking, activated a quadratus lumborum myofascial trigger point that felled her to the floor and caused pain so severe that she was unable to reach up and turn the stove off to prevent a pot from burning through its bottom."

"Patients who have had other kinds of severe pain, such as that due to a heart attack, broken bones, or renal colic, say that the myofascial pain from trigger points can be just as severe. Despite their painfulness, myofascial trigger points are not directly life threatening, but their painfulness can devastate the quality of life" (Travell and Simons, 1983). Some of the chronic intractable pain patients have this degree of pain constantly and in an ongoing fashion for years.

We can also look at pain severity in reverse, noting what type of medication it takes to control the pain. Some of the grade 3 and grade 4 MPS patients (see Chapter 10) have pain severe enough to call for 20–30 4-mg Percodan® or Dilaudid® tablets per day to bring about 50% pain control. An occasional patient needs 75- to 100-µg/hour Duragesic® patches and 4-mg Dilaudid® tablets at 20–30 tablets per day. A rare patient in this group needs 50–100 mg of injectable Dilaudid® per day plus 75- to 100-µg/hour Duragesic® patches or similar medication combination for years.

TOLERANCE

Introduction

Tolerance for opioids and/or opioid-containing analgesics is a complex topic. Many variables affect it. It varies with factors related directly and indirectly to the individual and his or her pain problem.

Tolerance, as it relates to persons with DDS (referring to the true "drug addict"), is markedly different from "tolerance" seen in chronic pain individuals who use opioids and/or opioid-containing analgesics for gainful and productive purposes.

Concepts embodied in the term "tolerance" can be confusing and elusive. On the one hand, it pertains to escalation of the consumption of an opioid drug. On the other hand, it pertains to ill-defined concepts relating to both the legal and illegal use of numerous medications classified as controlled substances.

A controlled substance is any medication or substance that is "scheduled" (rated), according to abuse liability, by the U.S. Department of Justice. These substances can only be prescribed by practitioners that are licensed to practice in fields of medicine, dentistry, and podiatry. Actual controlled substance prescribing privileges are granted by issuance of a special numbered certificate issued by the Department of Justice.

Some examples of schedule III medications are Tylenol® and codeine, Fiorinal® with codeine, and Vicodin®. Some examples of schedule II medications are morphine, Percodan®, Dilaudid®, and Demerol®.

The severity of chronic nonmalignant pain can be agonizing and incapacitating (Travell and Simons, 1983). As the severity of the pain goes up, the need for (tolerance for, ability to tolerate) more pain-relieving medication usually goes up.

Confusion exists in the use and understanding of the term tolerance. One person's *euphoria* (a feeling or elation or well-being) may be another person's *dysphoria* (an emotional state marked by anxiety, depression, and restlessness). Dysphoria is the abnormal or unpleasant state of mind (agitation, anguish, feeling of bodily discomfort or abnormal tiredness, haziness of thinking) that comes from taking relatively too much of a drug in a person who takes it for pain-relieving purposes. For example, in a person taking an opioid and/or opioid-containing analgesic for a painful condition, if the pain-producing disease is lessened or completely alleviated, the patient experiences or begins to experience dysphoria. The individual then decreases the drug intake or stops it altogether because of increasing dysphasia while on the medication.

Tolerance, with respect to opioids and/or opioid-containing analgesics, means that certain side effects of the drug generally lessen with the passage of time. Some of the effects are euphoria, respiratory depression, tiredness, dizziness, dysphoria, insomnia, disorientation, drowsiness, nausea, vomiting, diarrhea, dry mouth, constipation, itching, and rash.

Another way to think of tolerance for opioids and opioid-containing analgesics is as a container that can hold a substance. When a person's container is full, pain relief is optimal. However, every individual has a different sized container, and nobody has yet figured out how to tell how big each individual's container is and when an individual's container may be full, other than by report of the individual. The "size" (tolerance for opioids and/or opioid-containing analgesics) of the container may change noticeably with the numerous variables mentioned throughout this section on tolerance. For example, the individual who experiences mild constant pain from an ongoing headache may need one nonopioid pain tablet per day to obtain adequate pain relief. This same person may need two pain tablets per day if the intensity of the pain doubles or the area of pain involvement increases as the pain spreads into the neck and shoulders.

Another individual with similar initial pain may obtain no pain relief from the nonopioid medication used above, but will obtain pain relief from an opioid-containing pain tablet. The individual who needs more medication for pain relief is mistakenly said to have a high tolerance for the analgesic. In contrast, people who obtain pain relief with only small amounts of pain-relieving medication are said to have a low tolerance. The use of the terms high and low tolerance is relative and is not backed up by scientific studies.

Dynamic Change

Some chronic nonmalignant pain problems become worse with the passage of time (Margoles, 1983). Chronic pain individuals may report progressive increase of pain severity, pain distribution, emotional problems, pain-related physical dysfunction, and progressive disability over time. This progressive physical and emotional dysfunction may be related to pain severity or the underlying disease that is causing the pain.

In general, the greater the level of pain and the more constant it is, the greater may be the tolerance for higher quantities and potencies of pain-relieving medications to control it. For example, consider similarities with a kitchen fire. If a fire starts on the kitchen stove, and you catch it early, you can put it out with a towel or glass of water. However, if you wait until the whole kitchen begins to burn, it will take much more water and additional fire-fighting equipment to control it.

As the disease progresses back toward normal and the severity of the pain diminishes, the tolerance for analgesic medication goes down and the medication may cause the individual to feel tired, sleepy, or groggy, all of which can be manifestations of mild toxicity to opioids and/or opioid-containing analgesics. If that happens, it is a signal to begin tapering back on the medication.

Factors Affecting Tolerance

Each person with chronic pain who takes pain-relieving medication has an individual tolerance for medications. This means that one is able to take into his or her body a certain amount (dosage) of a medication and not have ill effects from it. Tolerance addresses an individual's ability to take, accept, and metabolize a medication. One authority recently stated, "A variety of opioid analgesics now available are able to relieve severe pain in most individuals but the doses required for some individuals may render others breathless" (Mather, 1990).

Analgesia is another effect that lessens with time. There is no reason why any receptor-activated effect (primary and side effects) would not lessen with time, due to tolerance (Supernaw, 1992).

Tolerance, when used with respect to the body's ability to accept opioids and/or opioid-containing analgesics, is a relative term and may vary according to the following factors.

Individual Factors

- Age of individual
- Severity of pain
- Degree of physical dysfunction caused by pain
- Degree of emotional and cognitive dysfunction produced by the pain
- Ability to absorb the medication from the gut

- Ability of the liver to activate the medication
- Number of surgeries
- Surgical status (preop versus postop)
- Family dynamics
- Employment status
- Menstrual cycle
- Individual motivation
- Length of time on the medication
- Coping abilities
- Work status
- Depression
- Tension
- Stress level
- Anxiety level
- Height and weight of the patient
- Rehabilitation status
- Individual's goals
- Marital status and, if married, status of marriage
- Spouse status
- Maturity of the individual
- Individual's support system
- Individual's compliance
- Individual's nutritional status (Margoles, 1990, in press)
- Past drug usage patterns (Portenoy, 1990)
- Degree of physical functioning that the medication allows

Physician Factors

- Doctor's bias
- Doctor's politics
- Degree of patient's suffering
- Pressure from the doctor's licensing board
- The physician's knowledge of pain and pain-producing pathology
- Physician peer pressure
- Physician knowledge of the pharmacokinetics of the medicine being prescribed
- Doctor's compassion

Climate and Natural Phenomena

After an earthquake, tornado, or other natural disaster, the tolerance for analgesic medication is likely to go up. The reason is that persons are frequently thrown about during such events, and when this happens, they may be unable to completely protect their painful areas from reinjury or strain. Natural disasters are also accompanied by increased emotional distress. Distress due to this and other causes tenses painful muscles and can make them hurt more.

Emotional stress alone is known to cause intensification of pain signals related to numerous different types of pain. Most noteworthy in this area is MPS. Cold climate can also increase pain in MPS patients and other conditions.

Brand Name Analgesic versus Generic

Other factors outside an individual's domain of control also influence a person's tolerance to pain and pain medications. These may be related to drugs and different types of drug manufacturing.

A pain patient may be "tolerant" to high doses of ingested codeine or hydrocodone but be very intolerant to low doses of oral morphine. This tolerance is relative to the potencies of the schedule III medications versus the schedule II medications.

Some generic analgesic medications are less potent than the brand name medications they imitate. Some generic products will perform well for a number of individuals, but other individuals will not get the full potency effect. For most individuals who will need to use the medication for short periods of time, a generic may perform as well as a brand name product. However, chronic pain patients with constant (intractable) pain need predictable and continuous pain relief. Their way of living and earning a living may depend on obtaining predictable pain relief from a medication. Their need for analgesic medication may go on for years. Generic drugs may impair physical performance by providing less than optimal pain control as compared to the brand name product.

The following is a hypothetical example, with a fictitious individual history and a fictitious drug, to illustrate the generic versus brand name dilemma. The scenario has occurred in a number of my patients during my 21 years as a pain management specialist.

Brand name: Pain-ender
Generic name: Hydrocodone and acetaminophen (H&A) (generic for Vicodin®)

Mrs. Jones is a 35-year-old housewife and executive secretary. Three years ago, she was involved in an auto accident and since then has had frequent low back and leg pain. The pain interfered with her sleep and her ability to do her secretarial duties. She was off work for 3 weeks after the accident. When she returned to work, she could work only 6 hours most days. A few days out of the week she had to go home after 4 hours at the office. Her ability to do routine housework was very limited. Vacuuming became torture. The family had to frequently pitch in and help her. As of a year ago, she could work only 4 hours per day and missed 2 days of work every 2 weeks. She never looked all that bad, but nonetheless she was "loosing ground."

She sought help from numerous of the best physicians, but the various therapies were not helping. Eight months ago, she consulted Dr. Smith, a physician who was a board-certified pain management specialist. After careful evaluation, he put her on Pain-ender for pain control. She found that if she took six tablets on a time-contingent schedule on her "bad days" and four time-contingent pain tablets on her "good days," it gave her 30–40% pain relief. With the use of the medication, she could work 8 hours per day and do half of her usual housework. She was less irritable and more pleasant to be around.

Mrs. Jones was back to feeling somewhat normal for the first 6 months after starting the medication. One day, the pharmacist gave her hydrocodone and acetaminophen (H&A), a generic "equivalent" to Pain-ender. After the second day on H&A, she noted that she could not work the whole day. After 6 hours at work, her back began to act up and she had to go home. Household chores provoked more pain than usual. She increased the dosing of the H&A to eight tablets per day, but the increase in pain relief was minimal. For a time, Dr. Smith thought she was developing a tolerance to the drug, and possibly abusing it, or perhaps had become a drug seeker. Mrs. Jones thought her pain was getting worse. After a month of this dilemma, Dr. Smith prescribed Pain-ender and specified that the pharmacist use the brand name product and not the generic. After 2 days back on Pain-ender, Mrs. Jones was back to work full time, back to her usual housework, and was more pleasant to be around. After that, she obtained the same predictable relief as long as she stayed with the Pain-ender.

Self-Imposed Limits

Individuals may electively decide to limit their intake of a controlled substance. One of my patients wrote:

> There are three reasons why I would never abuse the analgesics he (Dr. Margoles) prescribes for me:
>
> 1. I am a computer programmer who plies his trade solely by the clarity of his mind. If I take too much (medication) I can't concentrate (because of dysphoria). If I take too little I can't concentrate (because of pain).
> 2. I have a precisely regulated allotment for a specific length of time. If I take too much on any one day, I know that I have a regular torrent of pain waiting for me in just a short time. One experience of that is sufficient.
> 3. I would never do anything that might jeopardize Dr. Margoles or add to his burden in any way. This is the most compelling reason of all.

Tolerance Types

Medication-related tolerance is present when, after exposure to a drug, higher and higher amounts of the drug are required to produce a given response (Edwards, 1981). Tolerance to effects of a drug will develop at different rates to opioids and/or opioid-containing analgesics. The fastest tolerance with respect to opioids and/or opioid-containing analgesics develops to their euphoria-producing effects. For that reason, drug addicts have to take ever-increasing doses of drugs to get the same "high." One of the slowest types of tolerance is that related to the pain-relieving effects of the medication. Patients of mine have remained on stable dosing of schedule II and schedule III analgesics for years. However, if the disease process changes over time for the worse, the need for pain medication will go up. The tendency to produce respiratory depressant problems will decrease over time, and usually quickly, if the medication dosing is kept at level dosing. The tendency to constipation will remain level, and problematic, in a number of patients, but many become tolerant to the constipating effects of opioids.

Metabolic Tolerance

This relates to the increase in the capacity to metabolize a drug. It can be induced by the substance itself or by some other agent or capacity (Edwards, 1981).

In this situation, the pain remains constant, but the consumption of drug increases over time. The basis is that the drug induces its own accelerated metabolic breakdown, and hence there is a need to consume more drug to produce the same analgesic or euphorigenic effect.

Therefore, the more drug consumed, the faster the body metabolizes it up to a certain point, and the greater the demand for oral consumption of the drug. This routinely happens during the first 1–3 months after initiating treatment with most opioids and/or opioid-containing analgesics and is a reflection of initial controlled substances gradient.

Genetic Tolerance

This refers to the few chronic pain patients who have a natural ability to accommodate rather (and sometimes surprising) high doses of controlled substances (Minkus, 1991). When they take in the medication, not enough of it is converted to a form that the body can use for pain relief. These patients may have fewer pain-related receptors that respond (with pain relief) when properly stimulated by medication (Supernaw, 1992).

Apparent Tolerance

In this situation, the rise and fall of pain severity and drug consumption go up or down together. Increased pain severity causes increased need for analgesic medications. Decreasing pain severity lowers the need for analgesic medications. In this instance, if the individual continues at the same analgesic dosing, dysphoria and negative tolerance set in as the analgesic overpowers the dwindling pain symptoms.

Many medications help the pain for a while, but they seem to lose their potency over time. In chronic pain patients, this is generally not due to tolerance to the medication(s), but is often a reflection of the underlying disease becoming worse. At that point in the treatment and evaluation of the patient, there may be a need for further examination, consultation, and testing. If these approaches prove negative for operative or specific treatable disease, more adequate medication needs to be given for the control of pain symptoms.

Good Days and Bad

Most chronic pain follows a variable course. There may be days to weeks of mild pain during which the need for analgesic medication is decreased. However, in some cases, without proper treatment of the underlying disease process there is a progression toward more "bad days" over time. The cautious individual (or one denied access to adequate analgesics) adapts to this problem by giving up and progressively cutting back or stopping all activities that provoke the pain. This may lead to the loss of employment and decreased social and sexual activity (see Figure 21.3). On the days that the pain is more intense ("bad days"), the tolerance for pain medication goes up and dosing will be more frequent. This is shown on the lower curve. On days when the pain is less problematic ("good days"), the individual will be able to get the same amount of pain relief with less frequent dosing of pain medication. This is shown on the lower curve.

Dynamic Tolerance Related to Premenstrual Syndrome

Many chronic pain individuals are women in the menstrual years. These women may have had mild low back pain related to their premenstrual syndrome (PMS) before a traumatic event initiates a chronic headache, neck ache, or backache. After the onset of the chronic pain problem, each month, in addition to the usual PMS, they may have a cyclical moderate to severe flare-up of the posttraumatic headache, neck ache, or backache during the time of PMS. During this period of 7–10 days, the tolerance for pain medications usually goes up. It returns to usual consumption levels after the PMS passes.

Anticipated Tolerance

Anticipated tolerance relates to stereotypical thinking This is a guessing game, played by physicians, that may leave a deserving individual "high and dry" when there is a genuine need for analgesic medication in excess of the doctor's expectations (Angel, 1982).

I see this most frequently in women of medium build who have severe pain. D.S., a 37-year-old woman, was in severe pain for 10 years while under my care. In the last 2 years, she took a static dosing of eight Percodan® tablets per day to work 8–10 hours per day and take care of her activities of daily living. The medication was used to control pain in her head, neck, left shoulder, arm, wrist, hand, elbow, upper and lower back, and the entire left lower extremity. The pain resulted from a series of five automobile accidents. The fifth automobile accident ruptured a disc in her neck. She had a cervical disc removal and fusion 2 years ago, and this relieved 30% of her neck and arm pain. She is 5 feet 4 inches tall and weighs 123 pounds.

Recently, she was in the hospital recovering from a myelogram that was used to evaluate her severe postoperative persistent low back and leg pain. She was to be discharged by the neurosurgeon who performed her myelogram. He recommended Vicodin® (one tablet is about one-half the strength of Percodan®) every 4 hours for pain control while at home. She said, "Do you mean two every 4 hours?" He said, "Oh no, that will leave you breathless."

He anticipated that such opioid dosing might cause an overdose, but did not reckon with the fact she could tolerate eight Percodan® tablets per day without ill effects before going into the hospital for the myelogram.

Also, when he said to take the medicine every 4 hours, he anticipated a maximum of six tablets per day. When she said 2 every 4 hours, he assumed she might try to take a maximum of 12 tablets per day. Many chronic pain individuals, if told they can take a maximum of two tablets every 4 hours, will not go over six to eight tablets per day.

Medication Usage During Periods of Changing Tolerance

When individuals regularly experience apparent increased tolerance, due to the numerous factors mentioned above, physicians can prescribe a spectrum of analgesics to combat the symptoms as they vary (only a few of the possible medications that can be used for each type of symptom are shown in the table below):

Symptom	Drug or treatment
Mild pain	Nonsteroidal anti-inflammatory drugs Muscle relaxer Tylenol® and codeine #3
Moderate pain	Vicodin® Percocet®, Percodan® Tylenol® with codeine #4 Lorcet 10® Fiorinal® Darvon®
Intense pain	Oxycodone Demerol® tablets Methadone tablets
Severe pain	Morphine tablets Dilaudid® tablets Demerol® injection Duragesic® patches Injectable morphine sulfate or Dilaudid®

PREVAILING SCHOOLS OF THOUGHT AND ATTITUDES IN THE USE OF OPIOIDS OR OPIOID-CONTAINING ANALGESICS IN VARIOUS TYPES OF CHRONIC INTRACTABLE PAIN MANAGEMENT

Introduction

We are prone to confusion because there are no current standards to cover the subject of opioid usage in patients with nonmalignant intractable pain.

Chronic Opioid Usage: Two Points of View

At present, the medical field is extremely polarized as to how opioids are used and for what indications they are used. Guidelines have been published for use of opioids in acute traumatic pain and postsurgical pain, but relatively few guidelines are yet available for chronic intractable pain. Therefore, there are two prevalent views on usage of opioids or opioid-containing analgesics in the treatment of patients with chronic intractable pain:

1. The medications are being used to maintain an addiction.
2. The medications are being used to alleviate pain and promote normal function.

Some therapists refuse to use opioids or opioid-containing analgesics for other than pain due to:

- Cancer, but only for pain due to cancer that involves the bones by way of metastasis
- Surgery, immediately after an operation and for up to 3 weeks after the surgery
- Severe injuries with broken bones, but only for up to 6 weeks after the injury

Some therapists may fear the use of opioids or opioid-containing analgesics. This may occur in the form of threat of a medical board or Drug Enforcement Agency investigation. There may be fear of a malpractice case for using the medications outside of "community standards." It is the fear of these adverse events occurring (there is even risk of the doctor losing his or her license to practice medicine) that prevents many therapists from prescribing opioids or opioid-containing analgesics for their patients.

Some clinicians claim that the use of opioids or opioid-containing analgesics is counterproductive in noncancer and nonsurgical patients. Considerations for use of these medications are swept aside, claiming that they promote "pain games," "addiction," or the patient will become "hooked."

Some therapists do not believe that patients can handle the responsibility of using opioids or opioid-containing analgesics.

There are those who routinely use opioids or opioid-containing analgesics. These therapists who do not attach danger to the use of the medications in the management of their patients. The use of opioids or opioid-containing analgesics is just another part of the routine therapy that is considered in the management of patients with pain of diverse etiologies. In this situation, the clinician tailors the therapeutic program to meet the patient's needs. If the patient's pain goes beyond what the nonsteroidal anti-inflammatory drugs or schedule III (Tylenol and codeine®, Vicodin®, etc.) medications can do, he or she then moves right into the use of the schedule II (morphine sulfate, Dilaudid®, Levo-Dromoran®) medications.

In this case, the therapist is knowledgeable about the side effects and addiction liability of the opioids or opioid-containing analgesics and feels comfortable with their usage.

His or her doctor–patient rapport is good, and both doctor and patient understand the potential hazards of using this type of medication.

Appropriate practice of medicine is followed, and the therapist monitors the patient for addiction, DDS, and abuse problems. The medications are used to promote all the goals indicated in the section on criteria for use of opioids or opioid-containing analgesics. The therapist considers the risks and benefits of using the opioids or opioid-containing analgesics and decides that the benefits outweigh the risks.

Some clinicians feel very uncomfortable about giving opioids or opioid-containing analgesics to any of their patients for any reason.

Confusion Among Therapists and Setting Unreal Standards

"Chronic pain syndrome"* is usually presented as a clinical problem with subjective pain complaints, but has no organic basis. This is routinely considered an emotional problem, and the conclusion is that opioids are not given for emotional problems.

This group of patients is further characterized as having pain that lasts longer than 3 months which has failed to respond to "conventional treatment" and usually results in analgesic addiction, muscle atrophy, depression, vocational maladjustment, and financial problems.

The chronic pain syndrome patient group is further accused of having nonanatomical pain distribution (e.g., pain in areas it should not be in) and symptom magnification. Symptom magnification means that the patient is exaggerating what little seems to be there.

There are times when those relating the shortcomings of patients with "chronic pain syndrome" sound like a religions order bent on making sure these patients are misunderstood and mistreated worldwide.

After reviewing many of the histories and physicals performed by these therapists, it is my opinion that (1) they do not do adequate evaluations of the chronic pain patients they see and (2) they do not know how to interpret what they do find on the patients evaluated.

Centralist versus Peripheralist

There are two basic but arbitrary divisions in the pain field: centralist and peripheralist. The centralist believes that all chronic pain is merely a memory in the brain's pain receptor area and that all the tissue injury responsible for production of the original pain problem is gone by about 6–12 weeks after the injury occurred. Some of the centralists tell their patients that their current perception of pain is nothing more than a "track" on the brain. In essence, they are telling the chronic pain patient that the whole problem is basically an emotional or tension-related disorder.

A centralist can also be referred to as a pure behaviorist. His or her approach to the patient with chronic pain is to solely use behavior modification techniques, pacing, and cognitive restructuring to create a mode of adaptation to the pain for the patient. Theoretically, this blunts the patient's perception of pain and suffering.

From Marie J.:

> It was Dr. Mk. who kept gently prodding me to see Dr. Mg. Before my first visit with Dr. Mg., I was afraid that he would tell me what all the other doctors had told me: "It's all in your head." I was in a lot of pain, had very little energy, and getting worse

---

* A nonspecific name commonly given to patients who have actual cases of fibromyalgia or MPS.

with every passing day, and no one could figure out why, so all that was left was "It's all in your head."

The pure peripheralist believes that all chronic pain is caused by damaged tissue that is chronically deranged, such as the effects of postoperative scarring that appears to be causing ongoing pain after an operation or internal scarring of muscles that may follow an automobile accident. The primary modes of therapy are built on thinking that all components of the pain are due to tissue damage. Therapy may be medication, injections of muscles, or surgery. There is also a strong reliance on diagnostic procedures such as X-ray, EMG, MRI and CT scans, and myelograms.

Ultimately, the decision to give (administer) adequate doses of pain-relieving medication to a chronic pain patient will depend, to an extent, on whether a pain therapist physician is a centralist or peripheralist.

The centralist may tend to avoid surgery at all costs, and the peripheralist may perform surgery more than is needed. There are numerous other examples that can be cited. It is difficult to reconcile the dichotomy against the fact that we know very little about the cause for most types of chronic intractable pain. The knowledgeable pain management specialist can achieve a balanced thinking that incorporates material from both points of view. When a therapist is swayed too much in either direction, his or her thinking ultimately works to the disadvantage of the patient. This may cause problems in the delivery of medical care.

It is my observation that the centralist physicians may not be well trained in comprehensive clinical physical examination of patients with chronic pain. This impairs their ability to establish the presence of organic pathology as a contributor to the ongoing pain.

CRITERIA FOR WHEN TO USE AN OPIOID OR OPIOID-CONTAINING ANALGESIC IN THE TREATMENT OF PATIENTS WITH CHRONIC INTRACTABLE NONMALIGNANT PAIN

The following criteria have been developed at my pain center:

1. The patient is unable to obtain adequate relief of pain symptoms after:
   a. Tylenol® or aspirin + codeine or Vicodin® in adequate time-contingent doses. Depending on the patient's liver status, up to ten tablets per day can be given for either of these two drugs.
   b. Talwin® or other agonist–antagonist medication such as Stadol®, etc.
   c. Three different (from differing chemical groups) nonsteroidal anti-inflammatory drugs.
   d. Use of an antidepressant.
2. The patient gives a history of significant allergic response or intolerance to the drugs mentioned above.
   a. The therapist may need to verify this by doing a review of records or calling other physicians who have treated the patient.
3. The patient is unable to perform a significant number of the routine activities of daily living and/or employment because of marked handicap due to the pain brought on by these activities.
4. The patient is clearly able to report the dysfunction caused by the pain (i.e., can't paint, can't drive a car, can't go to work, can't cook a meal, etc.).
5. Duration of pain symptoms is not crucial.

6. Pain severity is moderate to severe, and this is determined by proper good faith, history, review of records, review of symptom chart, review of visual analogue scale, and comprehensive pain-oriented physical examination.

7. The patient agrees that the opioid analgesic will be used to become more active (productive) at home and/or at work.

8. The patient demonstrates to the therapist a desire to get well. This may be difficult to assess. Review of records from other offices can help here.

9. The patient demonstrates to the therapist a desire to follow therapeutic directives (the doctor's directions and advice).

10. No other therapy is indicated for the patient, such as surgery for a ruptured disc or a cancerous lesion. However, if a pain problem has a definite cause, and surgery is planned, analgesics can be given to aid in relief until the surgery is performed. Once a cancerous lesion is established as a source of chronic pain, the pain symptoms can be treated with opioids.

11. No other known illnesses will be masked or aggravated by the use of opioid analgesics.

12. The patient understands the abuse potential of the medication.

13. To "buy time" for the surgeon. Sometimes the patient looks like a possible surgical candidate. However, there is need for more time for evaluation and observation before booking the surgical date. The patient is frequently anxious and very distressed. Patients like this become irritable and begin to insist that the surgical procedure get under way soon. Use of enough strong analgesic can block up to 50% of the pain. This can relieve the stress on the surgeon, the referring doctor, the patient, and the patient's family.

14. Discretion, maturity, wisdom, and experience of the patient must be assessed. Individuals who demonstrate ability to use medication properly, with no tendency to abuse or inappropriate escalation of the dosing, may be kept on this type of medication indefinitely if needed.

15. To restore near normal physical and/or emotional function.

REQUIREMENTS FOR ADMINISTERING OPIOIDS AND/OR OPIOID-CONTAINING ANALGESICS TO PATIENTS WITH CHRONIC INTRACTABLE PAIN (SUPERNAW, 1991)

1. The therapist has to understand what chronic pain is.

2. The therapist has to understand what DDS is.

3. The therapist has to understand the pharmacokinetics and differential absorption of opioids and/or opioid-containing analgesics and how they can vary from race to race and person to person.

4. The therapist has to understand that nonsteroidal anti-inflammatory drugs and acetaminophen are potentially dangerous drugs for long-term administration (greater than 6 weeks) in chronic intractable pain patients and have limited use in this patient population.

5. The therapist should consider opioid analgesics only when one or more of the following conditions exists: (a) there has been demonstrated analgesic treatment failure using nonopioid analgesic(s), (b) the pain is significantly more debilitating than moderate pain, and/or (c) the patient has a history of adequate response to opioid therapy.

6. The therapist must understand the nature of opioid agonist, partial agonist, antagonist, and antagonist/agonist mechanisms.

7. The therapist must be aware of any respiratory problems the patient has prior to prescribing any opioid analgesic. Some severe respiratory diseases may preclude the use of opioids and opioid-containing analgesics or may call for special precautions and patient monitoring when these medications are administered.

8. The therapist must be able to evaluate and to manage the adverse drug reactions associated with opioid analgesics.

OPIOIDS AND/OR OPIOID-CONTAINING ANALGESICS

Introduction

In my 21 years as an orthopedic surgeon and pain management specialist, I have made the following observation:

> There is more suffering from taking too *little* pain medication
> than from taking too much.

Part of the practice of medicine is to provide relief of pain and suffering when a definite disease condition cannot be cured or remedied by other means. That is as important a part of medicine as surgically removing a gall bladder when it is diseased or performing orthopedic surgery to relieve problems of a diseased hip by doing a total joint replacement. It is just as important in inoperable cases (cases for which there is no relevant surgery or multiply operated failed back or neck surgeries) to find some way to make painfully dysfunctional patients functional.

Some people have to lie on the floor because their pain prevents them from laying in a bed. Some people cannot get out into the world because their pain and dysfunction related to pain are so great.

If we can get these people up and functioning, even with dependence on an analgesic, it is my experience and my opinion that it is better to have the drug dependence than to promote unnecessary atrophy and disuse of muscles and bones and isolation. "Dependence" is not a dirty word when it pertains to using appropriate doses of opioids to return a chronic intractable pain patient to gainful employment or to gardening, housework, hiking, enjoying life, etc.

Opioids or opioid-containing analgesics are the most effective class of analgesic pain relievers. They can relieve pain that is mild to severe in quality and intensity, depending on which medication is chosen. In the treatment of chronic noncancer pain, the use of the more potent opioid analgesics, on a long-term basis, is currently one of the most controversial topics in the field of medicine and pain management.

A great deal of mysticism, taboo, and ignorance continues to surround the use of these "forbidden" medications. It seems that the only time people can get morphine or Dilaudid® is when they are about to die of a painful cancer or in the immediate period following a surgical procedure. Even then, there seems to be a tendency to undermedicate cancer and postoperative patients.

When severe pain strikes, whether severe migraine headache, severe back spasm, or severe leg pain, a trip to the emergency room may get you a shot of Demerol®. However, if you are one of the "regulars" on the emergency roster, you may have to wait 1–3 hours and then be accused of being a drug seeker or other type of humiliation. Following that, you may be sent home after a Toradol® (nonsteroidal anti-inflammatory drug) injection, which does next to nothing for your pain.

The opioids are analgesics (pain relievers or "pain killers"). They can also relieve the anxiety that comes with pain (Foley, 1985). They can be used both to control pain symptoms and to aid the patient in increasing physical activity level. Their potencies range from weak to strong.

Opioids are also referred to as "controlled substances" because the Drug Enforcement Agency controls the dispensing of them by designating which have the highest and lowest potential for abuse.

Controlled substances, including opioids and/or opioid-containing analgesics, can be a formidable adjunct in the pain individual's overall rehabilitation program. Two factors prevent many physicians from prescribing adequate amounts of controlled substances: (1) fear of arrest or sanction by the medical board for allegedly overprescribing opioids and (2) history taking and physical examinations that are inadequate to reveal the patient's pain severity.

Many chronic pain patients are not interested in taking opioids and/or opioid-containing analgesics for their pain symptoms. In order to consider the use of such medications, they have to be properly approached and introduced to the subject. The clinician must make it worthwhile for them to consider taking the medication. If the physician does not appeal to the fact that the medications can make them more mobile, slow the onset of osteoporosis, and possibly promote an earlier return to work and many other activities, many patients will not even consider the use of the medication.

Regarding the monthly outlay of money for her opioids and/or opioid-containing analgesics, Louise T. said, "I'd rather spend my money on something more fun than paying my pharmacy bill."

Most of the analgesics of the opioid and opioid-containing type can cause sedation and drowsiness if the dosing is above the intensity or severity of the pain. For this reason, when this class of medications is chosen for treatment of pain symptoms, treatment should be started with the least sedating members of the group and progress to those that are stronger and more sedating.

A clinician who has proper understanding of chronic pain, pain-relieving medications, and concepts related to tolerance can enhance the overall management of the individuals he or she treats. Using opioids and opioid-containing analgesics for physical functional gain or gainful employment is different than using them for "recreational" purposes. Not all physicians feel comfortable or capable in prescribing opioids.

The judicious use of analgesic medication can be thought of as "first aid" for the management of a chronic intractable pain problem. While never an end in itself, it can be a substantial means to an end such as return to work, sleep normalization, etc.

In a recent publication, two authors stated: "The treatment of patients with intractable (stubborn, obstinate) pain of non-malignant origin with opioids is not recommended. However, if other treatment avenues have been excluded or exhausted, then it would seem unethical to withhold from these patients the pain relief provided by opioids" (Glynn and Mather, 1982). "It may also be unethical to withhold pain relief from these patients while they are in the process of being worked up" (evaluated) (Rose, 1992).

When we choose to give a narcotic(s) to a chronic intractable pain patient to control pain symptoms and/or increase physical activity level, we're not promoting addiction, we are preventing suicide.

—The author (1997)

Recently, a major drug company reported that when morphine is used by some patients with chronic pain, they "noted a lack of increasing tolerance to morphine dosages and saw no evidence of addiction despite the fact that each patient was allowed to titrate (take as much medication as needed) their dosage to suit his analgesic (pain relieving) needs" (Lilly, 1980).

Opioids are the most effective of all the analgesics for producing pain relief, even in chronic pain patients (Houde, 1974; Foley, 1986). This group of medications, depending on the drug chosen, can treat pain symptoms that are mild to severe in degree. *This group of drugs has the highest record for safety and the lowest record of adverse side effects on long-term use* (Gilman et al., 1980; Margoles, 1984; Porter and Jick, 1980). Opioid analgesic medications are associated with a low risk of "addiction" when they are used for the treatment of legitimate medical problems (Gilman et al., 1980; Medical Board of California, 1991).

Whereas the pain-relieving potency of nonsteroidal anti-inflammatory drugs and the lower potency opioid-containing analgesics (Vicodin®, Tylenol with codeine®, etc.) levels off with increasing dosage ("ceiling effect"), most of the stronger analgesics in the opioid family (Drug Enforcement Agency classification of "schedule II") do not lose their potency for relieving pain as the dosage is increased (no ceiling effect) (Gilman et al., 1980). Pain relief is usually obtained in a linear fashion (e.g., as more drug is taken, more pain relief is obtained) (Boas et al., 1985). The exceptions to this linear rule are codeine, Talwin®, Stadol®, and Buprenex®.

The opioids should be viewed as another one of the options available in the treatment of chronic pain patients and should not be viewed as a treatment that should be avoided at all costs. The proper way to administer opioids for analgesic purposes is to give enough to enable the patient to function in most of his or her usual activities of daily living.

In addition to relieving pain, many of the opioid analgesics relieve anxiety. These two attributes of potent pain relievers make them suitable for chronic pain patients who have pain plus a great deal of anxiety associated with their pain.

It can roughly be stated that Percodan®, morphine sulfate, and other schedule II analgesics are to some chronic intractable pain patients what gas is to a car. It helps the patient get from point A to point B.

> No patient should ever wish for death because of his physician's reluctance to use adequate amounts of effective opioids. Such patients, while they may be physically dependent, are not considered "addicts" even though they may need large doses on a regular basis...
>
> —Jaffe (1980)

Medical Opinion on Opioid Effect

It has been said that when a patient takes an opioid or opioid-containing analgesic such as codeine, Percodan®, Demerol®, Vicodin®, etc., the body's own pain killer, endorphin, is suppressed, and this allegedly causes increased pain and an increased need for pain medication to control the increased pain. Such conclusions have not been supported by valid medical research and can only be viewed as speculation, theory, or opinion. My observations over the past 21 years seem to show the following. Patient given opioids and opioid-containing analgesics soon discovers they can do more physically. They will push to the limit of what the pain medication will relieve. They then decide that they want to do more and can accomplish this only with the help of more or stronger doses of pain medication. The illusion is that the patient has developed a "tolerance" to the original pain-relieving medication, but that generally is not the case. A very small percentage of real pain patients (less than 1%) are drug abusers or drug seekers and will escalate the dosing of pain medication for reasons as yet unknown.

In my experience with chronic pain patients, what small "highs" they obtain from opioid analgesics: (1) wear off fast (Gilman et al., 1980; Margoles, 1984) and (2) are usually not to the patient's liking (Margoles, 1984). One patient stated that she took her pain medications strictly for "survival." "Chronic pain patients who are in a lot of pain generally feel down. When they take the medication, they feel "great" (Rose, 1992).

> Chronic pain patients use narcotics to live; *drug addicts* live to use narcotics.
>
> —Margoles (1989)

The Doctor and the Administrative Law System

Even though the laws on prescribing opioids or opioid-containing analgesics (Intractable Pain Act) may have changed in your state, you may find your doctor resistant to prescribing opioids or opioid-containing analgesics for your pain problem.

Before we go further, I am convinced you need to know some of the dynamics behind the prescribing of opioids or opioid-containing analgesics and what each professional faces before he or she writes a prescription for a schedule 2 medication. Drug Enforcement Agency (DEA) designation of a medication as a schedule 2 labels the medication as having a strong tendency to addiction or abuse. A few of the many medications in this group are morphine or Dexedrine®. Most doctors have 20–25 years of schooling (including the primary grades) before they get into practice. They apply for a license in the state(s) in which they wish to practice and are granted the right to be licensed by the state, if they pass specific testing for the licensing and have proof of proper training. They also apply to the DEA to obtain a certificate to prescribe opioids and other potentially abusable drugs. The DEA certificate is issued only if proper information is provided supporting the fact that the individual is a competent licensed physician with no related legal problems. In California, and some other states, there is an extra step. A practitioner who wants to prescribe schedule 2 medications needs to obtain "triplicate" blanks from the California Department of Justice; 56% of physicians in California do not use triplicates, presumably because it puts them under added surveillance from a state regulatory agency.

The medical board in any state is there for many purposes, one of which is to ensure that the consumer of medical services obtains high-quality, competent, consciences medical care. In California, persons having difficulties with physicians can file an anonymous or nonanonymous complaint with the Medical Board of California by calling a toll-free number. All complaints are investigated. Not all complaints are based in provable fact. In the 1980s, one of my pain management competitors filed an unfounded anonymous complaint against me with my medical board. This was not the first time he used a complaint with the Medical Board of California to try to put me out of business.

Unfortunately, the manner in which physicians are treated after complaints are lodged against them leaves many physicians in shock. They are like "sitting ducks," with no real protection once an investigative process has begun against them. A doctor coming under investigation and prosecution for allegedly overprescribing or misusing opioids or opioid-containing analgesics has little guarantees under present law in most states, and the same is true for the patients he or she is allegedly overprescribing to. California has the Intractable Pain Act of 1990, which offers California doctors some protection. There is no insurance that covers a doctor being investigated by a medical board. There is no access to public defenders to cover such a mishap. Malpractice insurance does not pertain here. The doctor has to pay for his or her own defense, which can cost $50,000 to $150,000 or more.

In California, doctors are prosecuted under "administrative law." That means you are guilty until proven innocent. Any decision made by a judge at any level (administrative, superior, appellate, etc.) is not binding and can be overturned by the licensing board. There is no trial by jury or trial by peers. If the case is sent for review by an "expert," it is reviewed by one "expert" who may or may not be as advanced in his or her thinking as the doctor accused of overprescribing. The accused physician does not get to face his or her accuser. That means an anonymous complaint can put a doctor out of business. The accusation becomes fact, regardless of what it is based on. Lastly, a doctor who loses a case against the Medical Board of California has to pay all court costs for the state of California as well as his or her own court costs.

Given all this, what doctor would want to prescribe opioids or opioid-containing analgesics for anything but the most severe cancer pain?

Other factors are fear of prosecution, scare tactics, and smear tactics by the medical boards. The person filing the complaint has nothing to worry about. If a patient makes a mistake in judgment while using opioids, the doctor is held liable for it. The whole process is more like persecution than prosecution. Doctors going through this process are treated like "dirt," no matter what their record looked like before. The basis of an investigation may be unclear. If you cannot be firmly investigated on one type of charge (i.e., addicting a patient to pain medication), the medical records will be reviewed until something can be found to charge the doctor with and, at minimum, put him or her on probation.

The whole process is humiliating, embarrassing, demeaning, and degrading to the professional on trial. Doctors have been known to commit suicide during or after this type of investigation.

If there are any patients in question, the state will not interview them and will not call them in to participate in the hearings. "Experts" used by the state in such a process may not be expert enough to pass judgment on the situation in question.

Other Opinions About Opioids

For some individuals, opioids and/or opioid-containing analgesics are the most "definitive" treatment that can be offered for pain management. Consider the case of Mary E. She was a 54-year-old housewife and mother of three grown children. Her husband had a good job and was a good provider. Because her three back surgeries had failed to relieve her severe back and leg pain, she and her husband enjoyed little or no social life. Many days, she had too much pain to walk any farther than to the mailbox. At times, episodes of burning in the legs were severe. Sometimes severe cramps would grab her calves or thighs and keep her awake all night. She frequently awoke in the morning feeling exhausted. Shopping was painful. When she could make the beds, she had to do so on her knees. Her back pain prevented her from picking up her wonderful grandchildren, whom she loved very dearly. Along with the pain came disability. At one time, she had been a very active person. She enjoyed shopping, going to baseball games, and many other activities. It had been 3 years since her last surgery. Doctors had nothing encouraging to say. She began to teach her husband to cook and provide for himself so she could end her life and stop being a burden to him and a misery to herself. Consider the options still open to Mary to restore her to an active and meaningful life:

- *Surgery.* The chance of success of a fourth operation on her back was 0%. That included percutaneous (through the skin) stimulation with an electrode implanted into the back and a host of other possible cutting and fusing procedures.

- *Physical therapy.* The chance of success with any known machine, technique, program, or device was 0%.
- *Transcutaneous electrical nerve stimulator (TENS).* The chance of success with any known TENS unit was 0%.
- *Chiropractic treatments.* In the hands of a good soft tissue chiropractor, the chance of successful resolution of some of her pain and dysfunction was 20–30%. The anticipated amount of pain relief would be 20–30%.
- *Biofeedback and/or relaxation training.* The chance of successfully controlling more than 10% of her pain with this technique is 0%.
- *Behavior modification.* Mary was a bright and positive person. She was optimistic and outgoing. She accepted and tolerated her pain as well as could be expected. However, I felt she could benefit from more of this therapy. The therapy was administered in my office. The chance of successfully modifying Mary's pain with behavior modification was 0%. The chance of successfully modifying Mary's attitude about her pain using behavior modification was 100%.
- *Inpatient pain management with "detox" and rehabilitation.* Mary was not on much medication when she came to my outpatient program. She took a couple of Darvocet® every day and only when the pain was at its worst. She said she was not "hooked" on the medication. She said she would stop using the medications for about 2–3 days every month because she was afraid she would get "addicted" if she took them too much. She denied any withdrawal symptoms during the couple of days she would be off the Darvocet®. I was not impressed that she had a drug problem that required detoxification (withdrawal from the medication). Her attitude toward her pain and dysfunction was one of reality. Her reasons for considering suicide were not groundless. We then considered the costs and realities of an inpatient program. Depending on where she would go, the costs would be $20,000 to $35,000 for 6 weeks of treatment. The chance of her obtaining any results was 30%. The chance of her losing her gains in the months that followed that program was 80%.
- *Medication treatment.* With the implementation of a program in which Mary was taught time-contingent, flexible controlled substance dosing using opioids and/or opioid-containing analgesics, her chance of successful control of her pain and pain related dysfunction is 100%. The anticipated amount of continuous relief was 30–50%.
- *Use of Elavil® and other antidepressants.* The chance of successful control of her pain is 20%. The amount of anticipated pain relief would be 20–30%. The chances of the Elavil® by itself producing a more restful sleep is 30–40%. Combining Elavil® or another antidepressant with an opioid or opioid-containing analgesic enhanced the chance of producing a more restful sleep to 60–70%.

Table of Drugs: Opioid and Opioid-Containing Analgesics

Chemical class	Brand name	Generic name	Dose (mg)[a]	Frequency[b]
Opioid	Demerol® tablets	Meperidine	qs	q2–4 hours
	Demerol® injection			q2–4 hours
	Dilaudid®	Hydromorphone	qs	q2–4 hours*
	Dilaudid® suppositories	Hydromorphone		q2–4 hours*

Chemical class	Brand name	Generic name	Dose (mg)[a]	Frequency[b]
	Demerol® injection			q2–4 hours
	Dilaudid®	Hydromorphone	qs	q2–4 hours*
	Dilaudid® suppositories	Hydromorphone		q2–4 hours*
	Dilaudid® injection, 2 mg/ml	Hydromorphone	qs	q2–4 hours*
	Dilaudid injection, high potency, 10 mg/ml	Hydromorphone	qs	q2–4 hours*
	Dolophine® tablets	Methadone	qs	q4, 6, 8, or 12 hours
	Dolophine® injection	Methadone		q4, 6, 8, or 12 hours
	Levo-Dromoran®	Levorphanol	qs	q6 hours
	Morphine tablets	Korphine	qs	q2–4 hours*
	Morphine suppositories	Morphine		q2–4 hours*
	Morphine injectable	Morphine	qs	q2–4 hours*
	Oramorph®	Controlled-release morphine	qs	q8–12 hours
	MS Contin®	Controlled-release morphine	qs	q8–12 hours
	Duragesic®	Fentanyl patch	qs	q3 days
	Percodan®	Oyxcodone + aspirin	Up to 10 per day	q2–4 hours
	Percocet®	Oxycodone + acetaminophen	Up to 10 per day	q2–4 hours
	Oxycontin®	Time-release oxycodone	qs	q12 hours
	Roxicodone®	Oxycodone	qs	q2–4 hours*
Opioid containing	DHC	Dihydrocodeine	Up to 6–8 per day	q2–4 hours
	Darvon®	Propoxephyne	Up to 8 per day	q2–4 hours
	Tylenol + codeine #4® (60 mg codeine)	Acetaminophen + codeine (60 mg)	Up to 10 per day	
	Vicodin®	Hydrocodone 5 mg + acetaminophen	Up to 10 per day	q2–4 hours
	Lorcet 10/650®	Acetaminophen + 10 mg hydrocodone	Up to 8 per day	q2–4 hours
	Vicodin ES®	Acetaminophen + 7.5 mg hydrocodone	Up to 8 per day	q2–4 hours

[a] qs means the patient should consume a quantity of medication sufficient to relieve 30–50% of the pain symptoms.

[b] q3–4 hours = every 3–4 hours, q12 = every 12 hours, etc.

Dosing Frequency

All dosing is done at the frequency indicated in the right-hand column of the table above. There are rare occasions when the pain level soars and the analgesic medication appears to not work when given at 2- to 4-hour intervals. There are at least three choices of therapeutic approach at this point: (1) switch to a more potent analgesic, (2) use more medication, or (3) dose every hour. Every-hour dosing can be accomplished with medications marked with an asterisk in the table above.

Formula Thinking

Formula thinking is used by some regulatory bodies (people) in the review of a patient's consumption or a physician's prescription of opioids and opioid-containing analgesics. This allegedly picks up overprescribing or overconsuming of opioid analgesics.

Formula thinking takes the number of pills consumed per day, week, month, or year and arbitrarily defines the count to mean the patient has an addiction problem if the number of pills consumed per day, month, or year passes a certain theoretical "normal" number. A formula-type equation would read as follows:

$$\frac{\text{Number of pills}}{\text{Time interval}} \neq \text{Does not equal addiction}$$

The actual calculation is as follows:

$$\frac{\text{Patient takes 180 tablets per month}}{\text{30 days per month}} = 6 \text{ pills per day} \neq \text{Does not equal addiction}$$

Factors not considered in "formula thinking" are as follows:

1. Age of patient
2. Severity of pain
3. Number of failed surgeries
4. Surgical status (preop versus postop)
5. Relevant diagnoses that relate to pain
6. Family dynamics
7. Tolerance for analgesic medications
8. Blood levels of the medication in questions
9. Employment history
10. Present employment
11. Patient motivation
12. Rehabilitation status
13. Patient's goals
14. Marital status
15. Spouse status
16. Primary gain
17. Secondary gain
18. Tertiary gain
19. Emotional status
20. Competency of the prescribing physician to handle the prescribed medications adequately
21. Help from local pharmacists
22. Size and competency of the doctor's office staff
23. Doctor's bias
24. Doctor's politics

25. Degree of patient suffering
26. Degree of physical functioning that the medications allow
27. Maturity of the patient
28. Patient's support system
29. Progressive tolerance
30. Negative tolerance
31. Patient compliance
32. Patient's nutritional status
33. Pressure from the doctor's licensing board
34. Past drug usage patterns, if available
35. Degree of anxiety
36. Skill of the doctor's office staff in the surveillance of patients on medications
37. The physician's knowledge of pain and pain-producing pathology
38. Physician peer pressure
39. Physician knowledge of the pharmacokinetics of the medicine being prescribed
40. Financial factors
41. Doctor's compassion
42. Various "fudge factors" (Kentucky windage, etc.)
43. Adequacy of absorption and liver metabolism
44. Degree of physical disability the pain produces

At present, there are no "normal" patients, and there are no normal numbers to use with this formula. There is no absolute number of pills taken per day that establishes the diagnosis of DDS ("addiction").

For example, Richard has a severe low back pain problem. He takes ten 15-mg morphine pain tablets per day and gets 40% pain relief. Donald has a similar pain problem and takes 20 15-mg morphine pain tablets per day to obtain 35–40% pain relief. Is Donald "addicted" compared to Richard? The answer is no. Donald has a genetic processing problem that calls for more morphine to be utilized to obtain the same amount of pain relief that Richard gets. Donald may depend (is more "dependent") on more medication for similar pain relief to Richard.

This example demonstrates the concept of individual variation. Faculties and functions of the human body can vary significantly from one human to another. A simple example of this concept would be that Richard feels full after eating one small piece of pie (one-sixth of a pie) and Donald feels full after eating a larger piece (one-fourth of a pie).

A chronic intractable pain patient taking 100–200 mg methadone or morphine sulfate per day for pain control is not a drug addict. The total amount of opioid or opioid-containing analgesics per day does not establish whether or not a patient is a drug addict.

Advantages of Opioids and/or Opioid-Containing Analgesics for Some Chronic Pain Patients

Analgesic. Medications in this group are analgesics that act on the brain's pain center.

Muscle relaxer. Opioids may relax muscles that are tight due to tension caused by pain.

Tranquilizer. These medications can provide tranquilizer effects for patients who are tense and tight due to the effects of pain

Sleeping medication. For those who cannot sleep due to pain, the pain relief produced by the opioid analgesics can give a better night's sleep than a regular sleeping pill. (Sleeping pills are usually tranquilizers of one sort or another. They sedate and make you tired. None of them are analgesics.) Taken in high enough doses, the opioids will also produce a tired sensation which can induce sleep in some patients. At times, it is best to add a tranquilizing medication to the opioid to supply both the sedation and pain relief.

Mood elevator. Depression frequently accompanies chronic pain and is a result of the chronic pain and its activity-restricting effects on persons who at one time were very active. If the opioid is strong enough to relieve pain and allow restoration of activity level, the person will experience some improvement in mood. He or she will feel lighter and less burdened by the pain. Some patients will interpret this as a high, but it is merely a return to normal (Rose, 1992).

Combined with anti-inflammatory drugs. If an anti-inflammatory drug is combined with an opioid (i.e., aspirin + oxycodone = Percodan® aspirin + codeine, aspirin + morphine, etc.), the following are noted (a word of caution: some chronic pain patients are intolerant to nonsteroidal anti-inflammatory drugs and should not be treated with them):

- Enhanced pain relief
- Decreased stiffness
- Decrease in some swollen joints

"It should also be noted that some patients are intolerant to opioids (severe gastrointestinal complications and severe nausea)" (Supernaw, 1992).

Slow or reverse atrophy of muscles. Chronic pain is frequently accompanied by weakening of the muscles due to disuse. If the patient is not up and doing activities from day to day, the muscles all over the body begin to waste. The prudent but aggressive use of opioids and/or opioid-containing analgesics promotes return toward normal activity level and decrease of muscle atrophy. The use of opioids can also promote getting in shape for more aggressive physical therapy programs.

Put an end to "doctor shopping" (Rose, 1992). Chronic pain patients may "shop" from doctor to doctor looking for pain relief. During this phase of their recovery, they may be labeled as "drug addicts." In most cases, once a patient finds a physician willing to supply the relief he or she need, the patient no longer has to "shop" and can expend energy on improving physical and emotional functioning and quality of life. Pseudoaddiction is patients who doctor shop and doctor hop and are constantly seeking to get medicine to relieve their pain. This is not true addiction or drug-seeking behavior; this is pain-relief-seeking behavior (Rose, 1992).

Promote earlier return to work. If the medication is not being used to mask the pain of a malignant process such as a tumor in a bone that might break with too much activity, and if the cause of the pain is known but only partially treatable (i.e., severe MPS or severe primary fibromyalgia syndrome [fibromyalgia, fibrositis] or similar pain-producing disease), opioids and/or opioid-containing analgesics can be used to return the patient to work. Earlier return to work can be accomplished with these medications compared to most other methods of therapy. Implementation of this class of medications, with blood testing to assure adequate blood levels of analgesic, gives more predictable analgesia than any other form of treatment in most cases of chronic intractable pain. On the other hand, reliance solely on analgesics to effect a return to work should not be promoted in a patient with chronic pain.

Promote rehabilitation efforts. These medications can be used to promote better compliance in physical rehabilitation programs. Some aspects of physical rehabilitation can be brutal, painful, and trying. This may occur in routine physical therapy, a back school program, sports rehabilitation, and some phases of myotherapy, rolfing, and chiropractic work. With suitable medication to combat troublesome flare-ups related to the rehabilitation efforts, the pain patient is more apt to tackle bothersome aspects of the overall rehabilitation program. The medication represents "incentive" to accomplish the more problematic parts of the recovery program.

Aid in flushing out troublesome myofascial trigger points. Opioids and opioid-containing analgesics can be used to increase overall activity level through pain suppression. Some of the more important myofascial trigger points will only become well defined at a higher physical activity level. Once activated, through increased activity level, the important myofascial trigger points can be properly defined and dealt with.

Promote patient compliance during myofascial trigger point injections. Some of the more severely involved MPS patients have extremely irritable trigger points (posttraumatic hyperirritability syndrome). Injection of the more irritable trigger points can be extremely irritating and exceedingly painful. When this occurs, patients become reluctant to have repeat myofascial trigger point injections if the pain and soreness are sufficiently discouraging with each trigger point injection session. If this becomes a problem, MPS patients can be premedicated with an intramuscular injectable opioid, such as morphine sulfate or Dilaudid®, 10–20 minutes before the trigger point is injected. This stops a lot of the irritation that occurs when the trigger point is properly needled.

Promote return to normalcy. The "right" amount of opioid or opioid-containing analgesic medication reestablishes sleep to restful and restorative, allows the patient to return to almost all job and home duties, causes the minimum number of side effects (e.g., constipation and nausea), reduces much of the anxiety caused by pain, and allows enough up time to minimize atrophy or wasting of muscles.

Can act as an "energizer." This effect is found most commonly with Vicodin®, Lorcet-10® (and other hydrocodone-containing analgesics), and Dilaudid® pills or injection. The mechanism of action here is not understood. These medication do not work as an energizer in all patients. In 20–30% of patients in my practice who are taking the mentioned medications, if the pain is stronger than the capability of the opioid or opioid-containing analgesics being used, the energizing effect will not usually be seen. In some cases, this is a bothersome side effect, causing insomnia and other problems associated with increased energy. If the pain medication gives good pain control but causes anxiety (too much energized feeling), a muscle relaxer or tranquilizer can be added to resolve the undesired side effect of anxiousness.

Diane's Story

Diane was a 44-year-old female barber. Her back pain problem started with a slip-and-fall injury at a large department store. Over the ensuing 5 years, she had two unsuccessful back surgeries. She had been to a number of pain clinics where the emphasis was on coping techniques and learning to live with the pain. She had complied well with the therapy that was given, but was unable to physically function despite the good intentions of her therapeutic team.

In March 1992, after her first 8 hours of evaluation by a well-trained and competent pain management specialist, she wrote him the following letter:

...You can't imagine how appreciative I am to have finally found such a great doctor. I know you've reviewed my records and have an idea of what I've gone through, but there's a lot more to it that isn't written into records. This has been the absolute worst thing that has ever happened to me. I have faced several obstacles in my life that would have crushed most people, but this by far is the hardest one to overcome. I look back and wonder how I've survived it for this long. There were so many times I wanted to give up. I tried everything I thought would help me, but nothing worked. By the time I came to you I didn't have much hope left. Dr. Kcabon told my attorney and I that I refused to "adapt to my disability." He was right about that. I will never adapt to it. Adapting is another word for quitting in my book. Had I "adapted" and given up the search for a doctor that could help me I would have never found you. I have changed since my first visit to your office. My friends and family can see the difference in me. The difference is that I now have hope. I went to every doctor, physical therapist, pain clinic, etc. that I thought could help the pain, but nothing worked. I couldn't even get two doctors to agree on a diagnosis let alone the treatment. When their treatments did not work, the failure became me. I was "overreacting to the pain," "I had a low pain threshold," I was having "a bad reaction to the pain," etc., etc. I was accused of being a drug addict, neurotic and oversensitive.

The drug addict accusation has been the hardest one to handle. I hate stigma that is automatically given to people who need narcotics for pain. You are made to feel weak because you can't "tough out" the pain. Once when I was paying for my office call, I said to the receptionist, "I think the doctor made a mistake. He gave me 100 Lortab® last month and this time he gave me only 60." She said, "The doctor is cutting down on prescribing these pills, because everybody wants them." I did not say anything back to her, but I thought to myself, "Wants them? What about patients like me that *need* them for a legitimate reason?" Throughout this entire ordeal I have argued with everyone over the "drug addict" issue. I have had to defend myself to everyone, even my own attorneys. I understand it to some degree. Here is Dr. Kcabon (especially) telling them that their client is addicted to the pain medicine. He's the doctor and supposed to know that thing when he sees it and who am I? I'm not only a lay person, but I'm the one taking the narcotics. It's like being sane in a mental ward or innocent in prison. Who's going to believe you over the authority figure? Everyone seems to forget that I've asked every single doctor if there was any other treatment for this pain that could replace the Lortab®. I tried everything they suggested no matter how painful it was, like epidurals, surgeries, anything. When I ran out of things to try, their only suggestion was to get off of the pain medicine. They had no suggestions as to how I was to handle the pain; they just wanted me off of the pills. One time Dr. Kcabon told my attorney that I had tried to get pain medicine from his patients. I couldn't believe my ears, nor did I know why he would say such a thing. Nevertheless I had to go through the stress of defending myself for months. It was important for me to not "let it go." I felt that if my credibility was gone, I'd be sunk. I only knew one of Dr. Kcabon's patients and that was a girl in a wheelchair, from my church. I don't even know if she takes pain pills, which is beside the point. The point is that I couldn't believe that anyone would think I would take someone else's pain medicine. If there's anyone that knows how much a person in pain needs their pain medicine, it's me. I would never do that to anyone. I felt so hurt that I had to address such a viscous accusation. This made me so angry and hurt that I didn't go back to Dr. Kcabon again. He was my only source of pain medicine, but I didn't care. I wasn't about to sacrifice my last ounce of self-respect by going back to him. I went out and got another doctor the next day. I had wanted a different doctor for a long time. This was the push I needed. Dr. Kcabon is a very temperamental person, especially for a pain doctor.

Every time Chuck and I left his office we were angry or I was crying. He would cut off my pain medicine whenever he felt like it or cancel my refills. He would literally scream at me if I told him that four Lortab® a day wasn't enough to help the pain. One time it was two days before my refill was due to be filled. I had taken two extra pills and I was out of medicine. Chuck called his office to tell him that I was out of medicine and in a lot of pain. His office told us to go to the ER at Harwick. We went and when we returned we called his office to tell them what was done for me. The ER doctor gave me a very small prescription of Lortab®, just enough to make it through the weekend, and a shot of Demerol®. We went in to see Dr. Kcabon on Monday. He screamed at me so bad that I cried. He felt like we were trying to pull a "fast one" on him, even though we called his office and they told us to go to the ER and we told them what was prescribed there. There were many times that Kcabon got upset with us and I knew when he got mad that my medicine would be canceled. It caused constant stress. Kcabon wasn't the only doctor to treat me like this, but he was the worst. Many times I've been told by doctors, "You have a back pain problem and now you have a drug problem too." If I thought I had a drug problem, which I don't, I would chose the drug problem over 24 hours of pain forever. It is my opinion that no sensible person would want to be a "drug addict," but no sensible person wants to suffer every minute of every day either. It boils down to taking the medicine or living with pain that beats the tar out of you. What choice is there?

There is nothing in a person's life that prepares them for chronic pain. By the time you're my age you usually know what acute pain is, but it always goes away. I think that is why this is so disappointing and frustrating. It changes your entire life. You aren't fun any more, you aren't as sympathetic to other people's minor problems, you're hateful and come close to losing your faith in God and everything. The people you love the most seem to end up paying for your misery. It seems like your life is spent in doctors' offices and you never get better. I compared it to cancer, because it reminds me of my mom when she had cancer. The doctors cut on you and cut on you, but you still don't get better. The bad thing about chronic pain is that you don't *get to* die. Dying isn't even a privilege for us. I am sure that no chronic pain patient wants to die, they just want the pain to go away. I know that's what I want. I, for once in my life, have a lot to look forward to. I have a man that I love and want to marry, which means so much to me. I have many close friends that I love. I want my life back the way it was, full of life. I used to be thought of as the "life of the party." Now I'm just a drag to be around. My entire life is consumed with doctors and lawyers. Oftentimes I feel that this case shouldn't be one of personal injury, but wrongful death. No matter how much money I wind up with, it will never make up for the 5 years of suffering.

I know it's hard for such a caring doctor like you to think that other doctors aren't the same way, but believe me they aren't. I have had a couple of doctors that were nice, but they were few and far between. I haven't felt like any of them were on my side, until you. It means a lot to be able to have a good relationship with your doctor and feel like the two of you are a team. It's important to feel as though you can be honest and you won't be reprimanded for your honesty.

As of 5/27/93 the patient had made fair progress. Although numerous therapies were being employed in her management, she was asked to comment on (make a list of) the benefits of taking 350–400 mg of oral morphine tablets per day.

...The improvement is pretty basic to explain. I simply have less pain when I take the morphine, and when I don't take it my pain is unbearable. Without pain medication to control this pain, my life is not worth living.

I explained that I would do this list as soon as I finished the letter for my attorney. I explained I had been so busy that I couldn't see straight. I explained how bad this typewriter was (is) hurting my back. I explained to you that I am so stressed from having too much to do that I could run away somewhere and never come back. I have ironing stacked a mile high and I haven't even been able to do my nails, which I always kept up before. The medicine helps me but only so far. I still can't be up 8 hours a day getting things done. It helps a great deal and makes my life livable, but it isn't a cure-all. The more I have to lay down, the more I get behind. That means that the times I feel good, I have to go like hell to accomplish what other people accomplish in their normal length of day. If I get behind by one thing a day, in 6 years you are really behind. My life doesn't stop because I feel bad and don't have the money to hire everything done like some people.

Medication is the only thing in the world that helps chronic pain people have the strength of go on living:

This pain is not the kind of pain that you can just grit your teeth and bear it. That pain medicine is no less important to us than another person's insulin. When our pain medicine is threatened it just makes you realize how your life is out of your control. Our sanity hangs on those pills, because this pain can literally make you nuts. I am not suicidal in the least, but take away the only thing that takes the pain away and it's a different story.

During the course of 1993, Diane took a level dosing (no escalation of the dose during the year) of 350–400 mg of morphine tablets per day. She took nontime-release morphine because she could not afford the more expensive time-release morphine. Here is what she said in response to my request to tell me what advantages the morphine provided her compared to not having the medication available to her:

I can walk for longer distance: sometimes an hour or a little longer.
I recovered a chair: it took me 4 days working a couple hours every day.
I can sit for slightly longer but it's still the hardest thing I do.
I go shopping more now than I did before.
I am doing more flower arrangements and crafts in general.
I spent almost a whole day sightseeing with Chuck's sister. I felt real bad when I got home, but I did it.
I can ride in the car for longer distances.
I can go out to eat more than before and I can sit for longer after eating.
I can do more housework than before. I still can't vacuum without paying for it dearly.
The morphine does nothing permanent as far as curing my pain. The pain is right back to severe as ever when the dose wears off and my abilities diminish to almost zero. I also still have many days where nothing helps, not even the morphine. If I overdo, the pain overrides the morphine too.

Sandra's Story (Written 12/15/90)

When I was hit by a car while riding my bike to the health spa in 1974 (at age 24), I was sure that the fact that I worked out daily, took my vitamins, and generally tried to live a healthy lifestyle would protect me from problems with healing that the doctor in the emergency room to which I was taken warned me about. But I continued to hurt...

I followed the advice of several chiropractors, and I continued to exercise when I was able to. I had been told that I had a "hairline fracture" of the bones somewhere in the back of the pelvis, but since I had never been hospitalized following my accident, I thought that the fact that I took calcium–magnesium supplements would heal any injury to my bones and the muscular exercising I did would strengthen my abdominals and my spine. I continued to hurt, but I was young and strong…

In early February 1979, I was in the crash landing of a small plane near Palmdale, CA. We were all able to leave the scene without assistance, but my back and right hip really hurt, and the pain worsened over the next few days. I tried heat and stretching, but when those did nothing, I sought the help of a chiropractor again. Unfortunately, his manipulations did nothing, but when he X-rayed my back, he noticed what he called "bone spurs" and he set me up for a course of treatment. When I got home from the first session with him, I stooped down to get something from the bottom drawer of my dresser and I was unable to straighten up. The pain was sharp and excruciating. I called my family physician, who saw me right away, but only said that it would take about 2 weeks for the pain to go away. He just said I was getting old (she was age 27 then). He told me to use a heating pad for 20 minutes at a time every hour and to stay in bed. At the end of the 2 weeks, during which time he had also given me Talwin® for pain relief and to relax me, the pain was still the same as when I first called him. I was anxious to get back to work, so he recommended that I see a specialist, as he (my family physician) did not want to continue to treat what was becoming a chronic condition. He said there were advances being made in the treatment of back pain, and he had recently spoken with a doctor who he thought could help me. Dr. Michael Margoles is the doctor my family physician sent me to. I was in some of the worst pain I had ever felt and called for an appointment right away…

Dr. Margoles examined me thoroughly at my first visit and explained the concept of trigger points to me, followed by an example involving some muscles in my upper back that had bothered me off and on, especially after writing a lot or driving my car. I was pleased to find that such a simple-seeming injection could make such a big difference. Unfortunately, the same kind of trigger point injections did not relieve the pain in my lower back, right leg, ankle, and foot. In June of 1979, Dr. Margoles gave me an epidural injection that relieved all of the back, leg, and foot pain almost miraculously. I was able to stop taking any and all medications, which had included, up to the epidural, aspirin and Talwin®.

My husband and I had been considering starting a family, but my back and leg pain had precluded the thought of carrying a pregnancy. Following the epidural procedure, however, I was feeling so well I became pregnant as soon as I could, in July 1979, a little over a month after the epidural. I had a comfortable pregnancy, continuing my work as a photolithographic lead inspector and trainer on second shift up until just before my term in April 1980. I walked 3–5 miles a day throughout my pregnancy, and following my daughter's birth, I continued to walk daily, with her in a front or back carrier, for at least 3 miles a day, in complete comfort. I returned to work 3 months afterward, still on second shift, and was promoted to lead step-and-repeat photolithographer within the year. I continued to have no pain…

On March 11, 1982, I was working in the clean room of the production area I was supervising as lead person, when I entered the camera chamber to extract raw materials for an operator I was training. The door into the chamber of this type of camera has a positive air flow, to keep any microcontaminants out of the process of exposing photoresist. As I opened the door, I caught my wedding ring in the door seal, and as the door was forced open by the positive air flow, I was pulled back, even as

I was continuing a forward motion. The clean room shoe coverings I was wearing began to slip, and I was pivoted into the operating camera equipment. I pulled myself away as hard as I could, in order to prevent damage and costly downtime to the machine if I had run into it. I consequently torqued my spine in all the pulling and twisting and immediately felt a sharp, searing pain from the back of my waist, down my right leg. As I was the responsible person on duty, still responsible for seeing to the shutdown procedures with just a trainee to assist me, I was unable to go to the Industrial Clinic to which my company subscribed, as I would have if it had been an employee working under me. I thought the pain would go away, was just pulled muscles. I cried all the way home, however, because my right foot and leg hurt so badly, and I know it affected my driving because I was pulled over not far from home by the California Highway Patrol for driving erratically (speeding up and slowing down). When I explained what my problem was, I fortunately did not get a ticket, but I did become even more concerned about my ability to do the things I usually had to do on a daily basis (grocery shopping the next day, driving to work at a job I enjoyed, getting my daughter to her play group, etc.). I didn't know what else to do, so when I got home, I took a hot bath, a shot of brandy (to ease the pain), an aspirin, and went to bed with the heating pad, just like I had when my back had hurt before.

The next day, I was unable to sit to drive, but I went to work. From there, I finally couldn't stand it any more and asked my supervisor to let me go to the Industrial Clinic. Once there, I was seen by a doctor, prescribed Parafon Forte®, and set up for a course of ultrasonic treatments. These treatments were horribly painful, but I tolerated them as long as I could, thinking that there must be pain involved in the healing process and, although I hate to admit it, the technician giving me the treatments was a young, good-looking man whom I didn't want to embarrass by crying from the pain, so I hid my face during treatments, until he was out of the room. Finally, about 2 weeks later, I wasn't getting any better. I, in fact, felt increasing pain, interfering with sleep, as well as my usual daily activities. I could no longer pick up my not yet 2-year-old child, and I worried about making mistakes at work because I couldn't concentrate. While driving to the clinic for treatment, the pain suddenly began stabbing and shooting down my leg, from the back of my waist down. When I reached the clinic, I burst into tears because it hurt so bad, and I finally asked the technician doing the ultrasound if I should feel so much pain during treatment (I had had ultrasound during my pregnancy to determine due date, and I had felt no pain at all). He was shocked that I hurt during treatment and showed me on my forearm, which didn't hurt, how the treatment should feel. It didn't hurt my arm at all, I told him, but it made the pain in my back and leg much more intense. He apologized and told me I should not have any more treatment with ultrasound; it sounded to him like a pinched nerve.

They called my husband to come for me at the clinic, and when I got home, I called the personnel office at work to inform them I wanted to see my own doctor, even though the time limit for treatment at the clinic had not expired.

I called Dr. Margoles because he had helped me before. I thought an epidural would fix me right up, since it had helped so much last time. Dr. Margoles asked if the medication I was taking eased the pain, and I had to admit it didn't. I wanted to go back to work, so he prescribed Percodan®, which finally eased the pain, so I was able to return to work, first for 4 hours a day, and finally I was able to go back to 8 hours and 10 hours when it was required.

I underwent another epidural, this time performed by another physician I was sent to by Dr. Margoles. The result of this procedure was totally unlike the previous, and I was wracked with a tremendous flare-up of pain for several weeks after. I continued to take the only medication that allowed me to keep working.

While taking Percodan® in carefully monitored doses, I continued to work and received promotions. I worked as a supervisor for 2 years, and in 1984 I moved into the electron-beam photolithographic lab at the company at which I worked. I remained on second shift, and as the equipment involved in this process was relatively new at the time, I often was at the lab with field service personnel until three or four in the morning when the machines were down and required test programs run. I maintained my working hours, I believe, only because the Percodan® I was taking allowed me to work relatively free of pain. I never felt "dopey" or fuzzy while taking the medication, and Dr. Margoles warned me not to exceed the doses he prescribed. Occasionally, I would reduce the amount of medication I took, on my own, whenever I had free time or a period of time when I was not working during holidays, so that I would reduce the chances of developing a tolerance for the pain medication. I didn't want to take more than I had to so as to reduce the pain to a "livable" level. Meanwhile, Dr. Margoles and I tried several other medications to move away from narcotics. None of them worked satisfactorily. I tried all of the tricyclics, with allergic-type reactions to all I tried. I took Klonopin® for about 6 months, but I finally realized it was making me very depressed, so I stopped taking it. Between the insurance company and Dr. Margoles' referrals, I have seen several doctors, none of whom had been able to reduce my pain without medication. Long-term physical therapy did little to reduce my pain either.

Every time I walk on uneven ground, I experience pain that I can only equate to biting down on hardtack with a rotten tooth. I have been in a car that has had to slam on the brakes to avoid a collision, and the subsequent pain I experienced is what I imagine it must feel like to get shot. The pain is always in the same places, and it wakes me up often. I was hospitalized in traction in 1985 following one such incident. I felt a little better following traction, but not significantly. I am thankful to be able to continue working, but I know I am only able to do so because I am easing the pain with medication.

In 1985, I quit working for the company I had worked for since 1977, hoping that taking some time off would help me to reduce the pain by reducing the daily stresses that accompany a two-income family and raising a small child while living in the fast lane career-wise. Both my husband and I agreed that his continued promotions in sales and marketing would cover us financially. However, my pain did not abate, and it became inviting to go back to work when a business acquaintance called to ask for my expertise in setting up a new custom photolithographic company. I agreed to work only part-time, so that I could continue my plan of stress reduction, but within 6 months, the production manager was fired, and I was asked to take his place. Reluctantly, I agreed. I soon grew to love the power and freedom that came from setting up the shop the way I thought it should be, and soon I was working directly with the customers, functioning as the customer service manager, as well as continuing as the production manager. I promoted a promising employee into a supervisory position to assist me, and soon I found myself driving a territory from San Carlos to Los Gatos, working with the engineers with whom we did business to alter existing microcircuitry in ways most production shops were unwilling to handle. I loved the challenge, and I enjoyed working with my boss, my crew, and the customers I directly worked with. The driving, however, was increasingly painful, even in the automatic LeSabre station wagon I bought in 1986. By this time, however, I had no choice, I felt.

I quit working again in 1988, when my family moved into a bigger house that required more of my time to manage. I hated to move out of the work force, particularly since I enjoyed my work so much, but I still thought that if I was able to have more time, my pain would be more manageable. The physical therapist I was seeing at the time agreed that I needed more time to do the exercises she recommended. And I felt I needed more time to get to work with my daughter, a dancer and gymnast who not only needed me to drive her to lessons and competitions but needed my help in achieving her scholastic goals. It seemed that no matter who I had as her day-care provider after school, even when it was provided by off-duty teachers on campus, she still was not able to complete her homework. I was able to provide the discipline only when I was able to get home before 6:00 p.m., which was becoming less and less frequent, so I quit to provide the necessary framework for her to complete her tasks in a timely fashion and get the grades, finally, that I knew she was capable of attaining, with little or no pressure. I am proud to say that, entering middle school, she has been an A student since I have been able to be at home with her every day after school. Her study habits have improved 100%, as has our relationship, now that I am available to her and not exhausted by long hours.

I continued to require pain medication, and Percodan® was working well for me until I had a myelogram at the suggestion of Dr. Gest in 1989. I was not expecting any repercussions from the procedure, since I was informed that the dye used now is far more easily absorbed and flushed from the body than the dies used in past years. I had heard it was a painful procedure with the old dye, but I was not afraid having the myelogram done with the new dye, especially as I was highly medicated when I was sent in for the procedure. I was, therefore, shocked when the needle was inserted and I felt a blazing, burning, and stabbing pain from the point where the needle, I think, was inserted all the way down my right leg and into my toes. I couldn't help but cry. Dr. Gest said, "You shouldn't be feeling a thing!" and then he told me I had scar tissue pressing at the L4–L5 space, and there was nothing that could be done about it. I didn't see him again in the hospital, but when I asked the nurses, who brought me the pain medication he prescribed (Demerol®), they told me that no one performed operations to remove scar tissue in the back because the risk of cutting into the muscles was too great to go in after tissue that, unlike a ruptured disc, was not going to go anywhere. I accepted that, but what I could not accept was the pain flaring up, uncontrollably, and only relieved by the Demerol® injection in the hospital, where I stayed overnight. The next day, no amount of Percodan® relieved the pain, so I called Dr. Margoles. I was afraid to be taking so many pills, with no result. He told me that the next higher medication to try was morphine and that he recommended the injectable form. My husband picked up the prescription and the medication, and I was finally able to get some relief. Since then, I have tried the nontime-release pill form of morphine, and MS Contin® (time-release morphine sulfate), but it seldom if ever works by itself. By the time I take enough pills to relieve the pain, I have made myself sick to my stomach. The pills do work however in conjunction with the injectable morphine.

In December of 1989, Dr. Margoles prescribed a new antidepressant medication suggested by a doctor he sent me to for consultation at a major university. The medication, Prozac®, was not used for depression, per se, but, as I understand it, antidepressant medications have successfully treated chronic pain in some cases. I took it in ever-increasing doses for 6 months, during which time I remember feeling nothing at all emotionally, not even happiness or pleasure when it would have been appropriate, but I still had the pain. Dr. Margoles also had me try methadone, to replace the morphine, but that medicine made me feel really fuzzy and incapable of driving, which the injectable morphine does not. I have to drive my daughter to lessons on a daily basis, so I was afraid to continue the methadone by itself or in conjunction with other medications.

Last February, a friend who works for the high school district in which I live suggested that I should take the AB65 test to become an instructional aide. I had worked with handicapped children in high school and college, so I thought this might be something I would enjoy doing and, as my friend pointed out, the hours would still get me home when my daughter needed me, and the hours were not as long as I had previously done. I wanted to take the test then, but was unable to do so until it was administered in September 1990, as my daughter was home sick at the time the test was given in February. I was a little anxious, as I had not been tested, except in daily life, for my skills in math or English, although I had always been a good student, in both high school and college. Unfortunately, I also was in a great deal of pain on the day I was tested, from a fall at home earlier in the week. (The numbness in my right leg sometimes causes me to fall when my leg "gives out" on me unexpectedly.) However, I arrived at the appointed test time, took the test, and awaited my test results in the mail, as I had been told they would arrive before I could apply for a job. The next day, however, the district personnel office called me, asking if I would be interested in temporary work. The woman who called said they were very impressed with my test scores and that of the 50 or 60 applicants, mine were the only perfect scores. I was relieved and gratified. I felt that I had done well on the test, but knowing my scores were "impressive" gave me the added confidence I needed to undertake a job unlike any I had done for over 20 years. I agreed to take the position also because the fact that it was temporary gave me an "out" if I didn't like the work or if my pain made it impossible for me to continue beyond the contracted time period of 3 months.

That time period is almost up now, and I know I love working with special education kids, and I will be applying for the job permanently. My supervisor is anxious to hire me on a permanent basis as well, he tells me, and my co-workers say I am not only doing a great job, but I often do more than my share. They all know about my pain problem and that I have to take medication, but they are unaware of the type of medication I take, and it obviously does not interfere with my ability to do my work. In fact, I don't think I could be at work without medication. The 14-mile drive to school, the long walks between classes, and my work assisting wheelchair-bound students between classes whenever necessary would be impossible without the help that medication affords me. So far, I have had two incidents of extreme pain flare-up that would have necessitated my leaving work and possibly my husband leaving work to drive me home, but the morphine injection has eased the pain enough to allow me to attend classes to take notes for students who are mainstreamed but unable to physically write for themselves, and without my doing this, the students I work with would not be able to work in the main student body or get the passing grades that will graduate them as productive members of society. I feel a deep sense of responsibility to the students with whom I work, and I want to continue this work.

I have tried, over the past years, physical therapy of various types, antidepressant medications, exercises prescribed by several therapists as well as those available in the popular press for "backache," the TENS unit, I have the best mattress that money can buy, all the special pillows that are supposed to help back pain, and I have a supportive family who do what they can to help me. Nothing relieves my pain except narcotic pain medications. I want to continue working, and I want to be able to love my husband and raise my child to be a strong, productive member of our world, and I do not think I can do these things when I am in constant, unmitigated pain that robs me of my sleep, prevents me from concentrating on life around me, and makes me feel sick and unhappy to be alive and sentient. With the medications I am presently taking, and only with them, I can reduce my pain to a livable level that allows me to function and participate in my family and the society to which I would like to contribute and to which I feel I am making daily contribution.

As of 1997, Sandra has been on a level dosing of morphine sulfate injection at an average of 300 mg/day since 1993. In 1993, injectable Dilaudid-HP® (about eight times as powerful as morphine sulfate injection) was tried, but it did not help as much as the morphine sulfate injection. At rare times, when her pain flares up from a twist or fall, I allow her to take extra morphine sulfate injection for 3–5 days. She is also on a complete program for MPS management. The myofascial trigger point injections are supplying more pain relief with the passage of time. Other than the morphine sulfate injection, there is no other treatment for her postmyelogram arachnoiditis.

OPIOID (NARCOTIC) AGONIST ANALGESICS

Medications Whose Main Use Is the Relief of Pain and the Suffering Related to the Pain Experience

No patient should ever wish for death because of his physician's reluctance to use adequate amounts of effective opioids. Such patients, while they may be physically dependent, are not considered "addicts" even though they may need large doses on a regular basis...

—Jaffee and Martin (1980)

The table below gives common brand names and the corresponding generic name:

Brand name	Generic
	Codeine
Duragesic®	Fentanyl
Vicodin® and others	Hydrocodone
Dilaudid®	Hydromorphone
Levo-Dromoran®	Levorphanol
Demerol®	Meperidine
Dolophine®	Methadone
MS Contin®, Oramorph®, and others	Morphine
Percodan®, Percocet®	Oxycodone
Numorphan®	Oxymorphone
Darvon®	Propoxyphene

Introduction

This section contains the classic descriptions of opioids (agonists, narcotics). Subjects covered include uses, functions, potential problems, and patient instructions for narcotics as a group. The opioid agonists are the most powerful analgesics (ones that can be used to partially or totally control any type of pain). When used properly, the incidence of side effects is minimal. The main bothersome side effects of the opioid agonists are constipation and tiredness (sedation). When patients are properly supervised and guided, these medications can be used for years without complications.

Review of the potential problems section of this material may seem frightening. However, if proper principles of dosing are adhered to, the incidence of serious side effects will be minimal compared to long-term use of Tylenol® or nonsteroidal anti-inflammatory drugs (NSAIDs). Serious side effects from NSAIDs include necrosis of liver, kidney damage, sterile meningitis, and ulcers with perforation of the gut. Refer to the section on NSAIDs in the part of Chapter 21 that deals with the these substances.

Functions

Agonists

Narcotic analgesics are classified as agonists, mixed agonist–antagonists, or partial agonists by their activity at opioid receptors in the body. An agonist is a drug that acts in the same fashion as the natural opium derivatives such as morphine or codeine; semisynthetic derivatives such as hydromorphone, oxymorphone, and oxycodone; and synthetic derivatives such as meperidine, levorphanol, and methadone.

Mixed Agonist–Antagonists

Mixed agonist-antagonist drugs (e.g., nalbuphine [Nubain®] and pentazocine [Talwin®]) have agonist activity at some receptors and antagonist (acting to defeat the results of an agonist) activity at other receptors. Also included are the partial agonists (e.g., butorphanol [Stadol®], buprenorphine [Buprenex®]). While these medications may be tolerated by some of the mildly painful chronic pain patients, there may be significant side effects, plus lack of adequate pain control in the more severely involved chronic pain patients. All of these preparations are available by injection. Butorphenol is available in nose spray, and pentazocine is available in tablet form. Because of their partial antagonist activity, none of these drugs should be administered to a patient who is actively taking agonists of any type. Before starting a person dependent on agonists on an agonist–antagonist medication, the patient should be tapered off the agonist(s) and be free of the medication for 24–48 hours. Then the agonist–antagonist medication can be started.

Of note is the lingering effects of some agonist–antagonist medications. For example, one of my patients was on Buprenex® for about a month. She then stopped that medication and went back to her agonist, Dilaudid® tablets and injections. She stated that the Dilaudid® felt relatively ineffective for the first 24 hours of taking the medication, but 24 hours after stopping the Buprenex®, the Dilaudid® began to provide the pain relief she was used to.

Characteristics of Opioid (Agonist) Analgesics

Generic name	Brand name	Type of pain relieved[a]	Start of effects (minutes)	Duration of action (hours)	Equal doses oral (mg)[b]
Codeine	None	Mi–Mo	10–30	4–6	200
Fentanyl	Duragesic®	Se	7–8	1–2	
Hydrocodone	Vicodin® [c]	Mi–Mo	15–45	4–8	60
Hydromorphone	Dilaudid®	Mo–Se–In[d]	15–30	4–5	7.5
Levorphanol	Levo-Dromoran®	Mo–Se	30–90	6–8	4
Meperidine	Demerol®	Mo–Se	10–45	2–4	300
Methadone	Dolophine®	M–Se	30–60	4–6	20
Morphine	MS Contin® [e]	Mo–Se–In[d]	15–60	3–7	60
Oxycodone	Percodan® [f]	Mo	15–30	4–6	30
Propoxyphene napsylate	Darvon®	Mi–Mo			
	Darvocet®		30–60	4–6	200

[a] Mi = mild, Mo = moderate, Se = severe, In = intolerable.

[b] Morphine is the standard used here.

[c] Others include Anexia®, Anexia 7.5®, Lortab®, and Lorcet 10®, among others.

[d] Only the injectable works for intolerable pain.

[e] Morphine I R® (immediate release), Oramorph SR-30®.

[f] Percocet®, Endocet®.

Uses and Goals

These medications are used for relief of moderate to severe pain. Some agents are also used for their anticoughing and antidiarrheal effects.

Methadone, in addition to being an excellent analgesic medication, is also used in the detoxification ("detox") of persons addicted to narcotics. It seems that methadone is a narcotic with low addiction potential.

When using rectal morphine suppositories (RMS), take note of the following. There are two bases that can be used as a foundation for the manufacturing of RMS. One melts at a lower body temperature. Most of the more severely painful chronic intractable pain patients run basal temperatures around 98 degrees Fahrenheit. Therefore, the product made by Upsher-Smith is the correct RMS to be used for these patients, because it melts at lower body temperatures. If other brands are used, pain relief will be short (10–20 minutes), and the suppository will come out only partially dissolved.

Potential Problems

The opioids may have a variety of problematic pharmacological effects. The most common unwanted effects are tiredness and constipation. When medication dosing is used strictly for pain relief, these effects are rarely seen. If the dosing of opioid medication exceeds the patient's needs, the unwanted effects will usually, but not always, be seen. Also, given a steady intake of opioid, if the patient's pain problem is reduced in intensity, the incidence of unwanted effects may increase.

It is noteworthy that some chronic intractable pain patients have reported that the use of injectable morphine and injectable Dilaudid® has been associated with much less incidence of constipation than the use of oral morphine or Dilaudid®.

Respiration may be depressed because the breathing center becomes less sensitive to carbon dioxide. Tolerance to this potential problem area develops rapidly when opioids are taken continuously; then depression of respiration becomes less and less of a problem.

Effects on the heart and circulatory system are manifested by feeling dizzy when getting up from sitting or lying down, as well as a sensation of feeling dizzy and/or faint or fainting.

Edema can be a problem in the management of a small number chronic intractable pain patients when methadone, Duragesic®, and morphine sulfate are used. If this occurs, a mild diuretic such as Maxide® can be helpful. Maxide® is a potassium-sparing diuretic, and this feature is desirable in patients with MPS. Rare chronic intractable pain patients will need up to 60 mg of Lasix® per day to manage the edema problem.

The urinary or gastrointestinal systems may manifest problems by retention of urine or inability to pass urine or fecal matter. Constipation may manifest as being mild to severe. Constipation can become a real problem. Proper attention to bowel hygiene, with use of anticonstipation medications such as Senokot® tablets, some of the herb teas, or small doses of milk of magnesia products, may be warranted.

All opioids and opioid-containing analgesics are metabolized in the liver and excreted primarily in the urine. Meperidine is metabolized to normeperidine, a breakdown product with significant pharmacologic activity. It is significant that as normeperidine accumulates, it can actually make a pain problem worse. I believe that infrequent use (every 3–4 days) of meperidine may be of benefit to the patient, but frequent use may make the pain symptoms worse.

Other potential effects include euphoria, dysphoria, apathy, mental confusion, nausea* and vomiting, delirium, insomnia, increased energy, agitation, anxiety, fear, hallucinations, night-

---

* It is important to know that patients with certain pain conditions such as migraine headache and some of the more severely painful cases of MPS may become nauseated for reasons related to pain severity, and not related to opioid intake, when their pain becomes severe.

mares, vivid dreams, disorientation, drowsiness, sedation, lethargy, impairment of mental and physical performance, skeletal or uncoordinated movements, coma, mood changes, weakness, headache, mental cloudiness, blurred vision, visual disturbances, double vision, constriction of pupils, tremor, convulsions, toxic psychosis, depression, and increased intracranial pressure.

Kidney and liver malfunction may cause prolonged duration of action and cumulative effect. Smaller doses may be necessary. Other effects include ureteral spasm and spasm of vesical sphincters, urinary retention or hesitancy, and reduced libido or potency.

Facial flushing, chills, faintness, peripheral circulatory collapse, tachycardia, bradycardia, arrhythmia, palpitations, chest wall rigidity, hypertension, hypotension, feeling faint when getting up from lying down or sitting, fainting, and phlebitis following intravenous injection have also been reported.

Opioids may obscure diagnosis or clinical course in acute abdominal or acute chest conditions.

Use caution in elderly and debilitated patients and in those suffering from conditions accompanied by hypoxia or hypercapnia when even moderate therapeutic doses may dangerously decrease pulmonary ventilation. Exercise caution in patients sensitive to central nervous system (brain) depressants and those with decreased respiratory reserve (e.g., emphysema, severe thoracic kyphosis, etc.), prostatic hypertrophy, urethral stricture, gall bladder disease, and recent gastrointestinal or genitourinary surgery.

Observe closely patients with known seizure disorders for morphine-induced seizure activity.

Additional Unwanted Effects of Opioids

Some qualifying remarks are necessary with respect to using these medications in patients who have moderate to severe intractable pain, not related to cancer, and who have fibromyalgia, MPS, reflex sympathetic dystrophy syndrome, arachnoiditis, or similar-pain producing disorders.

Symptom	Comments
Euphoria	Some patients have stated that the presence of pain is like carrying around extra weight. It drags a person down. The absence of pain in some persons is characterized as feeling more energetic and more able to do things. This could be mistaken for euphoria.
Insomnia	Many of these patients have sleep disorders that began before the use of opioids or opioid-containing analgesics. Pain reduction by using an opioid may actually promote a better night's sleep.
Anxiety	Pain and all the psychological stress it brings can cause anxiety. Two opioids, hydrocodone and hydromorphone, can cause anxiety by themselves, and this is a characteristic of these two drugs independent of their pain-relieving qualities.
Nightmares	Present in about 15% of my patient population.
Drowsiness, sedation, lethargy	Many of the chronic pain patients who require opioids or opioid-containing analgesics are already plagued by chronic fatigue, drowsiness, sedation, or lethargy. If the patient notes that these symptoms are made worse by using opioids or opioid-containing analgesics, then the analgesic must be suspected as contributing to the problem.

Symptom	Comments
Impairment of mental acuity	Many of the chronic pain patients are plagued by decreased mental acuity. This may be based on the fact that moderate to severe pain can be very distracting. If acuity is further diminished with addition of opioids or opioid-containing analgesics, medication cutbacks should be considered. On the other hand, distraction and loss of acuity caused by pain may be improved by the use of an opioid which lessens the pain.
Impairment of physical performance	This is commonly part of fibromyalgia, reflex sympathetic dystrophy syndrome, arachnoiditis, and severe MPS. In general, the proper use of opioids enhances overall physical performance.
Mood changes	This is commonly part of fibromyalgia and severe MPS. Opioids may cause minimal additional problems here.
Mental cloudiness	This is commonly part of fibromyalgia, severe MPS, reflex sympathetic dystrophy syndrome, or arachnoiditis. Opioids may cause minimal additional problems here. May be a sign that too much opioid is being used.
Constriction of pupils	Seen in a very small percentage of these patients with fibromyalgia and severe MPS.
Depression	This is commonly part of fibromyalgia, severe MPS, and reflex sympathetic dystrophy syndrome. Opioids may cause minimal additional problems here.
Visual disturbances	May be a sign that too much opioid is being used.

Contraindications

Do not give these medications to patients who have a history of abnormal sensitivity to opioids, acute bronchial asthma, upper airway obstruction, acute alcoholism, increased intracranial pressure, or head injury.

Patient Instruction

These medications may cause drowsiness, dizziness, or blurring of vision. Patients should exercise caution while driving or performing other tasks that require alertness and should avoid alcohol or other central nervous system depressants while taking these medications. Patients should notify their physician if nausea, vomiting, or constipation becomes prominent. If gastrointestinal upset occurs, these agents may be taken with food or antacid. The patient's physician should be notified if shortness of breath or difficulty in breathing occurs.

For a more comprehensive review of the above subject matter, including the opioid (narcotic) pain-relieving medications, refer to *Drug Facts and Comparisons,* 1996 or a later issue.

Opioid analgesics have abuse potential. Only a very small percentage of the patients who receive opioids for medical reasons develop DDS ("addiction") upon repeated usage of these medications (Porter and Jick, 1980).

In 1994, the Medical Board of California addressed these issues by stating: "Physical dependence and tolerance are normal physiological consequences of extended opioid therapy and are not the same as addiction...Patients with chronic pain should not be considered addicts or habituates merely because they are being treated with opioids" (Medical Board of California, 1994).

Abstinence Syndrome (Withdrawal)

Some genuine addicts and a number of chronic pain patients can go off of relatively large doses of opioids with few or no withdrawal symptoms.

In patients who demonstrate withdrawal symptoms, the severity is related to the degree of dependence, the abruptness of withdrawal of the medication, and the drug being used. Usually, the shorter the duration of the drug, the more dramatic the withdrawal response. Generally, withdrawal symptoms develop at the time the next dose would ordinarily be given. For morphine, the symptoms gradually increase in intensity, reach a maximum in 36–72 hours, and subside over 5–10 days. In contrast, methadone withdrawal is slower in onset, and the patient may not recover for 6–7 weeks. Meperidene withdrawal often runs its course within 4–5 days. Hydrocodone (Vicodin®, Lorcet 10®, Anexia®, etc.) peaks at 48–72 hours.

Withdrawal caused by narcotic antagonists (Narcan®, Nubain®, etc.) is manifested by onset of symptoms within minutes and maximum intensity within 30 minutes.

Symptoms of Withdrawal Regardless of Cause

Early	Intermediate	Late
2–4 hours after effects of last dose have ended	Up to 10–12 hours after effects of last dose have ended	24–36 hours after effects of last dose have ended
Yawning	Mydriasis	Muscle spasm
Tearing of eyes	Hair standing on end	Nausea
Clear discharge from nose	(gooseflesh)	Diarrhea
"Yen sleep"	Flushing	Vomiting
Sweating	Fast heartbeat	Abdominal and leg pains
	Twitching	Abdominal and muscle cramps
	Tremor	Hot and cold flashes
	Restlessness	Insomnia
	Irritability	Intestinal spasm
	Anxiety	Coryza
	Loss of appetite	Repetitive sneezing
		Increase in body temperature, blood pressure, respiratory rate, and heart rate
		Spontaneous orgasm
		Chills
		Bone and muscle pain in back and extremities

Tapering Intake of Medication

Should you desire to taper off a potentially addicting medication, a recommended 17-day schedule of tapering is as follows:

- On day 1, cut original dose by 20% of original amount.
- On day 5, cut the day 1 amount by 20% of the original amount.
- On day 9, cut the day 5 amount by 20% of the original amount.
- On day 13, cut the day 9 amount by 20% of the original amount.
- On day 17, discontinue substance or medication.

For example:

Original daily dose	30	25	20	18	16	10	8
Day 1	24	20	16	14	13	8	6
Day 5	18	15	12	10	10	6	4
Day 9	12	10	8	6	7	4	2
Day 13	6	5	4	2	3	2	1
Day 17	0	0	0	0	0	0	0

IMPORTANT POINTS ABOUT SUGGESTED DOSING SCHEDULES FOR TAKING OPIOIDS AND/OR OPIOID-CONTAINING ANALGESICS

General Principles of Medication Dosing and Rationale

Dosing regimens recommended here are to be considered as a starting point. Each person's needs must be met by tailoring the analgesic(s) to meet the specific situation. This also applies to recommended dosages for opioids or opioid-containing analgesics in the *Physician's Desk Reference, Drug Facts and Comparisons,* and similar references. While the recommended doses for most analgesic medication are adequate for most patients, in some cases the recommended doses of analgesics can only be considered a starting point.

All opioids or opioid-containing analgesics are safe to use in an outpatient setting. Patients need to be thoroughly screened for their ability to manage the medication in a trustworthy fashion.

Unfortunately, there are very few physicians who understand what chronic pain is, its changing nature, its variations in intensity, its causes, the fact that pain is not the only symptom that accompanies the patient, its ups and downs, various tolerance-related issues, how and why it disturbs sleep patterns, its effects on mood and thinking, its effects on cognitive functioning, and how to perform meaningful history taking and physical examinations of patients with chronic pain.

The reality of pain control is that the body is not making enough normal pain killer (endorphin) or it is being made adequately but is not being transported to the site in the body where it is needed. Therefore, the person in pain wants to put enough pain-relieving medication into his or her body to make up for what it is not presently making.

Those who become skillful at proper analgesic dosing will be able to adjust the medication dosing for some of the normal ups and downs (variations of pain intensity). For example, if you are going to be driving your car for half an hour and know this will predictably aggravate your back pain, you can compensate for this by taking a little extra medication. You may get a job working 2–4 hours per day, but vibration and sounds at the job site aggravate your headache and/or backache and make you miserable. If you know how to stage your medication dosing going into the job, you can block some of the pain and discomfort.

It is easier to block pain when it is on the rise than to try to block it at the top of a peak (spike). Once a pain problem has gone to a severe spike, in some of the more severe cases, the only medication that will subdue it is an injectable opioid such as Demerol®, morphine sulfate, or Dilaudid®.

While dosing a pain problem* throughout the day, if a pain flare-up occurs, the patient may have need to aggressively apply extra pain medication to reduce the intensity. The patient

---

* Using your pain medication to keep the pain at a tolerable level.

needs to obtain prior permission* for the medication increase. The usual formula I give is as follows: the analgesic medication is increased 25–50% for no more than 3–5 days. If the flare-up continues for more than 5 days, the patient needs to be seen in the office of the doctor for further evaluation as to what is causing the pain flare-up.

Taking the medication on a regular basis (i.e., time contingent or schedule contingent), instead of just when in pain, allows better control of flare-ups when they occur.

For those who take pills for pain control, on days when the pain spikes up and faster control is needed, crushing the pain pill between two spoons and taking the powder will allow the medication to work in about one-half the usual time.

For patients with constant pain but whose levels of activity and pain intensity vary quite a bit, a spectrum of analgesic medications may have to be prescribed. For example, when the pain is

Very mild	NSAID, Tylenol®, or aspirin
Mild	Darvon®
Moderate	Tylenol #4®
Moderately severe	Percodan®
Severe	Morphine, Dilaudid®, methadone, injectable morphine sulfate, etc.

Analgesic pain-relieving medication must be used in an aggressive fashion. It is a weapon to be used against your pain problem. Think of it like pouring water on a fire. You keep pouring the water on the fire until it is under good control or is out. The pain-relieving medication *gives you control* of your pain problem. You now have a weapon to go after your pain in the same way you would rub out grime in a shower with suitable cleanser or use hot soapy water to wipe away dirt from a window.

Common concerns about addiction to this type of medication are more fancy and fear than fact and reality. The term addiction has become a "junkie" or "wastebasket" term without meaningful definition. Most people think that addicted means "hooked." You get on the drug and then you can't get off. In reality, the reason you can't get off is because the pain relief is so great that you cannot function without the medication that relieves your pain. You get off the medication and your pain starts hurting badly and you cannot go to work anymore. That is not "hooked"; that is a normal dependency and is promoted by medical practitioners and medical licensing boards, so the patient can get back to normal functioning activity.

Material quoted here will be anecdotal and based on the author's 21 years of pain management experience. No double-blind or double-blind crossover studies using potent analgesics (schedule II) in severe chronic intractable pain patients have been carried out by this author. I am aware of no such studies in the present medical literature. The reason for this lack of such studies is not clear.

Studies in the medical literature using schedule III analgesics versus placebo have been equivocal. I believe the results of these studies could have been better than equivocal if a potent schedule II medication had been attempted against a placebo.

Medication Dosing for the Treatment of Chronic Intractable Pain Patients

The examples given below represent only a fraction of the medications and strategies that may be employable in the management of intractable pain.

---

* The doctor and patient have a preexisting agreement that if the need arises to increase the analgesic medication, the patient will notify the physician by telephone or leave a message.

Anexia® with 7.5 mg of Hydrocodone + Acetaminophen (A Medication for Moderate Intensity Pain)

This medication is 1.5 times as strong as Vicodin®, Lorcet®, or Anexia D®. It gives pain-relieving effects for 3–4 hours, and if the pain is moderately severe, pain control may last for only 1–2 hours. If you "overshoot the mark" with pain medication of this type, it will make you feel a little dizzy and tired. If you "undershoot the mark," you will not have pain control (20% relief for 30 minutes by using one tablet). This medication is not the weakest and is not the strongest. The table for matching pain intensity with analgesic medication later in this chapter indicates that if you have a pain that is at 7–8 intensity and you have a medication that is of class 2 analgesic potency, you may get only a minimal amount of pain relief using the class 2 medication.

Short-Acting Medications

The idea with this and other short-acting (half-life of 3–4 hours or less; half-life is the time it takes for half of the medication to disappear from the bloodstream) medication is to take advantage of the half-life of the medication. If the half-life of the medication is only 3–4 hours, then take it every 3–4 hours to get consistent pain relief. If you take it every 4 hours but are not getting much pain relief after the third hour, take the medication every 3 hours. Sometimes taking a whole tablet every 3 hours will "knock you out," but taking one-half tablet every 3 hours will not do this and may provide some good steady pain relief.

Cheryl's Story: Short-Acting Medications and Fear of Addiction — "Life without Movement Is Not Worth Living"

Cheryl is a 49-year-old housewife who has been a patient in my practice for the last 12 years. Her pain problem began after two automobile accidents. Over time, the pain progressed to involve all four extremities and the torso, neck, back, and head. In addition to the body pain, she was plagued by disabling migraine headaches.

About the only predictable help for her disabling intractable pain problem came from the medication she mentions. A good deal of the time during our visits over the last 5 years has been spent trying to convince her to take adequate amounts of analgesic medication. She had genuine fears of becoming "addicted" to the medication or developing a dependency or tolerance to it with the passage of time. This method of treatment has been pursued to allow her to function better while more definitive therapy is being developed to help patients such as Cheryl who have severe pain and the related physical incapacity caused by it. Of late, she seemed to understand what I have been trying to accomplish with the judicious use of strong analgesics in patients with her type of chronic, severe, multifocal MPS (this type of patient is frequently mistaken for severe cases of fibromyalgia). I recently asked her to give me a short statement about the benefits of the medication:

> Pain is nature's way to inform the body to stop action that is causing harm. We have so many labels to put "pain" into levels that are acceptable to the society we live in. There is acute, chronic, tolerable, mild, and the one that has become my long companion: myofascial.
>
> It has taken over my life: days, nights, hours, minutes, and the very seconds of every moment. I have spent years in physical therapy. I have spent a fortune in medical bills and drugs. I have been struck, stabbed, pushed, pulled, iced, heated, X-rayed, and MRI'd until I feel like I have a degree in the medical field.

Nothing had given me the relief from the pain or the ability to do even the minor things of daily living that most people take for granted, until I began to take a very small white tablet the size of a baby aspirin. It was morphine.

Morphine tablets have given me back a part of my life that had been taken away by the never-ending pain. Since I began taking the medication in adequate amounts, I can brush my hair, get dressed to some degree without assistance, do some very light household chores, and look forward to each and every day. Without the morphine tablets I would suffer so much I could only pray that God would take me because life without movement is not living.

At my recommendation, her consumption of 30-mg morphine sulfate tablets went from 272 mg/day in 1995 to 427 mg/day in 1997.

Stay Ahead of Your Pain

The overall goal is to use your pain medication to stay ahead of your pain symptoms. Many times, chronic pain patients are given pain medication and told to take it when they hurt. The reality is many chronic pain patients hurt all the time! Therefore, it is a good idea to develop a consistent attack on your pain to provide ongoing relief, to accomplish as many of your daily tasks as possible. Take a steady dose of pain medication throughout the whole day to get yourself up and moving.

Who Gets Pain-Relieving Medications?

Some patients, if given sufficient pain relief, return to the fast-paced life that may have burned them out and caused the pain problem in the first place. This use of analgesic pain medication may be detrimental to the patient's overall recovery. The physician must make his or her choices on a case-by-case basis. These decisions are very difficult to make.

The physician must be ready to take a patient off analgesic medication if he or she feels the medication is being used by the patient for overachieving or self-abuse. These patients must be taught pacing skills.

Patients to be given potent analgesics must be properly assessed and selected. This is done by taking a thorough history, performing an adequate physical examination, and arriving at a proper diagnosis to support the use of analgesic medication (analgesic medication can be as weak as Darvocet® or as strong as Dilaudid®).

Tylenol® Problems

A word of caution about Anexia 7.5® or other similar medications: Regular daily ingestion of more than 3.2 g of acetaminophen (Tylenol®) is not recommended. Anexia 7.5® has 500 mg of acetaminophen per tablet. Therefore, intake should not be in excess of five tablets per day. There are circumstances in which higher amounts of Tylenol® can be consumed, but the patient must be closely followed by the physician and by laboratory testing to assess for liver/kidney damage or clinical toxicity (Rose, 1996).

Individual Variation

Although the occurrence of the problem to be mentioned is not common, it happens frequently enough to warrant mention. With opioids, as with other medications, patients may have bothersome adverse reactions to a number of the stronger analgesics, necessitating a switch to another member of that family of medications. A clinical case of one of my patients will be used to demonstrate this problem. Patient R.S. was 38 years old when she first consulted me for pain in her right shoulder, low back, right lateral hip, right posterior, and anterior thigh, plus medial and lateral right knee pain.

Medication	Adverse reaction
Dilaudid®, 4-mg tablets	Nightmares Listless Crying
Percodan®	Hurts gut
Morphine, 10-mg tablets	Nightmares Thrashing about in bed Feelings of generalized malaise
MS Contin®, 15-mg tablets	Nightmares Thrashing about in bed Feelings of generalized malaise
Methadone	Nightmares Thrashing about in bed Feelings of generalized malaise

R.S. has done well since she was switched to Levo-Dromoran® and Roxicodone® in September 1996.

Similarly, patient J.S. was plagued with gut cramping and nausea when she attempted to take morphine sulfate tablets for her back and arm pain problem. Although low-dose methadone (20–30 mg/day), combined with Lorcet 10® tablets (six to eight tablets per day), gave rather good pain control, pushing up the bedtime dose irritated her gut. This prevented her from increasing the dose of methadone when pain flare-ups occurred.

Opioid versus Opioid-Containing Analgesics: Morphine Sulfate Oral Solution Dosing (A Short-Acting Medication for Strong Pain)

With Anexia®, Vicodin®, Tylenol #3®, Percocet® and Percodan®, the therapist is limited in quantity to prescribe because aspirin (in Percodan®) and Tylenol® (in Percocet®, Vicodin®, and many others) can be toxic to organs of the body in sufficiently high dose. However, when the narcotic alone, oxycodone (from Percocet® and Percodan®), morphine, Dilaudid®, or fentanyl, is used, the only significant side effects to worry about are sedation and constipation.

"High Tolerance"

A small subset (about 9%) of patients I have seen have a relatively high tolerance for opioids. These patients can tolerate 300–600 mg or more of morphine, 20–60 mg of oral Dilaudid®, 100–300 mg of injectable Dilaudid®, 200 mg of oral methadone (Dolophine®), and up to 570 milligram of injectable Dolophine per day with no long-term (up to 5 years in some cases) ill effects.

Precaution on Tapering

Never stop taking any of the medications mentioned in this chapter abruptly. Before tapering off, consult your physician for a tapering schedule or use the one included in this chapter.

Rudy E.

Rudy E. was injured at work a number of years before he saw me. He presented with sciatic-type pain in the right hip and leg. His pain was moderate to severe and prevented him from working.

During one of his major flare-ups, it was determined that 10–12 7.5-mg Anexia® tablets per day could not control the pain adequately. There was concern for the amount of acetaminophen (Tylenol®) consumed per day in his Anexia®. He was therefore switched to methadone (a pure opioid and pure agonist) instead of an opioid-containing opioid. He did well on the methadone. With the use of methadone, he was able to return to work.

At times, he had problems with severe breakthrough pain. For those periods, he needed a potent short-acting opioid. Morphine sulfate was chosen. Morphine sulfate oral solution comes in a number of strengths. The one chosen for Rudy was 10 mg/5 ml (5 ml = 1 teaspoon) or 10 mg per teaspoon. Directions for Rudy E. were as follows: Begin ½ cc (1 mg) every half hour to 2 hours for medium flare-up pain. If of no help, add ½ cc more to each dose, to a maximum of 2 teaspoons (10 cc or 20 mg) every 2–4 hours. The morphine sulfate oral solution can be added to any liquid to cut down on the bitter taste. This medication goes to work quickly (10–15 minutes) and gives pain-relieving effects for up to 3–4 hours. However, if the pain is very severe, the pain-relieving effects may last for only 1–2 hours.

Benefits of Long-Acting or Controlled Time-Release Opioids

The following medications are included in this group of long-acting analgesics:

Chemical class	Brand name	Generic name	Dose (mg)	Frequency
Opioid	Dolophine®	Methadone	qs	q4, 6, 8, or 12 hours
	Levo-Dromoran®	Levorphanol	qs	q6 hours
	Oramorph®	Controlled-release morphine	qs	q8–12 hours
	MS Contin®	Controlled-release morphine	qs	q8–12 hours
	Duragesic®	Fentanyl patch	qs	q3 days
	Oxycontin®	Time-release oxycodone	qs	q12 hours

Note: q = every; qs = quantity sufficient = take enough to relieve sufficient amounts of pain.

These medications are either naturally long acting (e.g., methadone or Levo-Dromoran®) or are formulated to be time release (e.g., MS Contin®, Oxycontin®, etc.). The usual benefit is decreased need for frequent dosing. These medications can usually be taken every 8–12 hours. They are also useful for controlling pain through the hours of sleep at night.

Instructions: Morphine Sulfate Time-Release Tablets for the Treatment of Intractable Pain

This consists of MS Contin®, Oramorph®, or similar tablets. Time-release morphine comes in 15-, 30-, 60-, 100-, and 200-mg strengths.

The example below uses 15-mg tablets. In reality, this medication progression can be used with any of the time-release opioid analgesics. For example, when patients gets to day 13, they are taking four MS Contin® 15-mg tablets per day. Four of the 15-mg tablets equal 60 mg. Therefore, patients are taking 60 mg twice per day.

Day 1   15 mg in the morning or at night
Day 2   Same

Day 3	15 mg bid (12 hours apart) (two tablets)
Day 4	Same
Day 5	Two 15-mg tablets in the morning and one tablet 12 hours later (total of three tablets)
Day 6	Same
Day 7	Two 15-mg tablets bid (12 hours apart) (total of total tablets)
Day 8	Same
Day 9	Three 15-mg tablets in the morning and two 15-mg tablets 12 hours later (total of five tablets)
Day 10	Same
Day 11	Three tablets bid (total of six tablets)
Day 12	Four tablets in the morning and three tablets 12 hours later (total of seven tablets)
Day 13	Four tablets bid[a] (12 hours apart) (total of eight tablets)
Day 14	etc.

Note: bid = twice per day.

[a] Day 13 dose could also be one 60-mg tablet every 12 hours.

A small number of patients need these tablets every 8 hours, and an even smaller number of patients do well when they are taken every 6 hours.

Dosage increases should be stopped if tiredness sets in, thinking becomes clouded, or nausea and vomiting develop. As you gradually increase your dose of MS Contin® (or similar drugs), begin to taper down on your consumption of Anexia®, Percocet®, Vicodin®, etc. Do not stop the MS Contin®, etc. medication abruptly. First, call your physician for directions. In the worst-case scenario, if you need to taper the medication but have no professional to help reverse the order of the MS Contin®, start at day 13 and begin to taper yourself down, right down to day 1 dosing, and then stop use of the medication.

Instruction Sheet: Methadone (Dolophine®) When Used to Control Intractable Pain

This medication is most commonly available in 10-mg tablets. The usual stigma associated with this excellent analgesic is that methadone, the generic, has been associated with detoxification of drug addicts for many years. Therefore, any person using the medication may be assumed to be a drug addict. For patients with chronic intractable pain, methadone is an inexpensive and very effective analgesic, providing pain relief that compares very favorably with orally administered morphine or Dilaudid®. It is generally tolerated well by a great number of chronic pain patients. In most cases of intractable pain, the medication is long acting (up to 12 hours or more) and is ideal as an analgesic that will work throughout the night. In many patients, the medication can be taken on an every 12-hour basis. A shorter acting opioid, such as Dilaudid® or nontime-release morphine sulfate, can be used for breakthrough pain, if needed, during the 12 hours between doses. A small number of patients can tolerate this medication on an every 6- or 8-hour basis with good pain control and no compromise of cognition or problems with tiredness.

Methadone is 85% absorbed on oral administration (Foley, 1986), which in some instances makes it almost as powerful by mouth as by injection.

If the patient gets too much sedation on dosing every 12 hours, convert to one dose, usually at bedtime, to get the benefits of all night long pain control and relief of some of the morning pain and stiffness.

The following is a dosing schedule for 10-mg methadone tablets or 10-mg Dolophine® tablets to begin use in a progressive fashion.

Day 1	5 mg (half a tablet) (morning or evening)
Day 2	Same
Day 3	5 mg bid (12 hours apart) (total of half of a 10-mg tablet twice per day)
Day 4	Same
Day 5	10 mg in the morning and 5 mg 12 hours later
Day 6	Same
Day 7	10 mg bid (12 hours apart) (total of two 10-mg tablets)
Day 8	Same
Day 9	15 mg (one and a half tablets) in the morning and 10 mg 12 hours later (total of two 10-mg tablets)
Day 10	Same
Day 11	20 mg bid (12 hours apart) (total of four 10-mg tablets)
Day 12	30 mg in the morning and 20 mg 12 hours later (total of five 10-mg tablets)
Day 13	30 mg bid (12 hours apart) (total of six 10-mg tablets)

Note: bid = twice per day.

Next, continue to slowly increase the dosing until a good therapeutic effect is achieved or is stopped by a side effect.

Stop dosage increases if tiredness sets in, thinking becomes clouded, or nausea and vomiting develop. As you gradually increase your dose of methadone, begin to taper down on your consumption of the medication it is replacing. The 17-day taper schedule can be used to taper the drug the methadone is replacing, but the taper schedule for the medication that the methadone is replacing can usually be cut in half (see below). "Original daily dose" refers to the daily dose of the medication methadone will replace. Look across the top of the table to find the number of pills or cc's of medication taken daily, and use the tapering schedule below it to taper off the medication as your methadone intake goes up. This table is approximate, and the tapering process should be supervised by a physician.

Original daily dose	30	25	20	18	16	10	8	4
Day 1	24	20	16	14	13	8	6	3
Day 3	18	15	12	10	10	6	4	2
Day 5	12	10	8	6	7	4	2	1
Day 7	6	5	4	2	3	2	1	0
Day 10	0	0	0	0	0	0	0	

Changing the Dosage and Type of Analgesic Medication

Usual Progression

Going directly from a mild to strong analgesic (such as Vicodin® to Duragesic® patches) may result in death of the patient. Dosing analgesics upward, as the pain dictates or as the pain escalates, must be done stepwise.

Most chronic pain patients will get relief of pain and return of reasonably normal function with three to four Vicodin® tablets (or similar medication) per day.

A Small Group of Patients Need More

A small number of patients (9% of the population in my entire practice) on opioids or opioid-containing analgesics will require strong analgesics to control their pain and/or get them back to near normal function.

Over the past 21 years of my pain practice, I have noted that a small group of patients, those with the more severe chronic and intractable pain, have been found to need higher intakes of opioids and opioid-containing analgesics or stronger analgesics to get adequate pain relief. Within this small group of patients, I have encountered some who can tolerate extremely high intakes of opioids or opioid-containing analgesics. This high tolerance is due to a genetic problem that relates to decreased opioid receptor site sensitivity or inability to convert adequate amounts of the drug to useful medications within the body. One percent of my entire population has benefited from the use of injectable analgesics.

Stewart's story, presented in Chapter 26, illustrates the use of injectable analgesic for maintenance of gainful employment.

Strategy for Moving to Stronger Medications

Oxycodone is the active opioid ingredient in Percodan® and Percocet®. It can also be ordered as a separate 5-mg tablet.

If a patient has 30% pain relief on six oxycodone tablets per day but a blood level of oxycodone is 20 ng/ml (normal range = 17–36 ng/ml), move up to eight to ten tablets per day to get more pain relief. The patient is to reassess the pain severity and intensity on a daily basis. If the patient indicates 50% relief and the blood testing registers 28 ng/ml, this should be an acceptable clinical situation. Unfortunately, there are many clinical combinations of patient and drug that do not work out this well.

If the blood level is 47 ng/ml, pain relief is 30% or less, and function has not improved much with the use of 10–14 oxycodone tablets per day, there is a need to move up to a stronger pain-relieving medication (provides a stronger quality of pain relief) such as morphine, methadone, or Dilaudid®.

MATCHING PAIN INTENSITY WITH ANALGESIC MEDICATION

Pain intensity scale	Classification of analgesic potency	Approximate matching analgesic medication
10– • • • • • • • • •	Class 4 analgesic	**Fentanyl injection** **Duragesic® patches** **Dilaudid® injection (hydromorphone)** **Morphine injection** **Dilaudid® suppository** **Rectal morphine suppository** **Dilaudid® tablets** **MS Contin® tablets (time-release morphine)** **Oramorph® tablets (time-release morphine)** **Demerol® injection**
7.5– • • • • • •	Class 3 analgesic	**Morphine tablets, immediate release** **Morphine tablets** **Methadone tablets (Dolophine®)** Demerol® tablets, Stadol® injection, Buprenex® injection Percodan®, Nubain® injection, Talwin® injection Oxycodone (Roxicodone®) Oxycontin® (time-release oxycodone)

Pain intensity scale	Classification of analgesic potency	Approximate matching analgesic medication
5.0– • • • • • • • • • •	Class 2 analgesic	Percocet® (oxycodone + acetaminophen), Stadol® nasal Lorcet 10® (hydrocodone 10 mg + acetaminophen) Anexia 7.5® (hydrocodone 7.5 mg + acetaminophen) Tylenol + codeine #4®, Talwin® Aspirin + codeine #4 Vicodin® (hydrocodone + acetaminophen) Ultram® Tylenol + codeine #3® Fiorinal® Fioricet® (butalbital) Darvon®, Darvocet®, and Darvocet-N® 100 (propoxyphene)
2.5– • • 0	Class 1 analgesic	NSAIDsa Tylenol®

Note: Medications that appear in bold type will usually not demonstrate ceiling effects for severe intractable pain (see Figure 22.1). All the other medications (below) demonstrate ceiling effects for severe pain.

a These include, but are not limited to, acetaminophen, Advil®, Anaprox®, Ansaid®, Butazoladin®, Clinoril®, Disalcid®, Dolobid®, Feldene®, ibuprofen, Indocin®, Lodine®, Meclomen®, Medipren®, Motrin®, Nalfon®, Naprosyn®, Orudis®, Rufen®, Tolectin®, Toradol®, Trilasate®, Tylenol®, Voltaren®, and others.

In the preceding table, class 4 pain is the worst (graded 7.5–10 in intensity) and class 1 pain is the least bothersome (graded 0–2.5 in intensity). This table indicates some of the many ways to proceed when attempting to control pain symptoms. First the NSAIDs are used, then the weak analgesics such as Darvon®, Fioricet®, etc. Next, as one attempts to provide enhanced pain control, the intermediate analgesics (Tylenol with codeine #3®, Ultram®, Vicodin®, etc.) and moderate strength analgesics (Lorcet 10®, Percodan®, etc.) are utilized. If these fail to provide control of pain, the strong (morphine, methadone) and very strong (Dilaudid®, Duragesic®, etc.) analgesics are brought into the treatment program.

General Considerations in Analgesic Dosing Principles

In general, the farther down the scale one goes (from 10 toward 0 in pain intensity), the higher incidence of undesirable side effects on long-term usage. This is usually due to the acetaminophen (Tylenol®) or aspirin that is combined with the medication. The most bothersome complications from the stronger narcotics are constipation and, less frequently, tiredness. The side effects from extended (2 months or more) use of the NSAIDs may be kidney failure, sterile brain abscess, gastritis or ulcers of the gut, liver problems, and more. Proper use of all these medications dictates that the physician start with the lowest potency medications, such as the NSAIDs, and slowly progress upward in potency until the patient is functioning at near normal (prepain) levels of activity.

In some cases, combinations of these medications must be used. For instance, a patient may use MS Contin® every 12 hours and nontime-release morphine every 3–4 hours for breakthrough pain. Levo-Dromoran® may be combined with Naprosyn®. In very severely afflicted

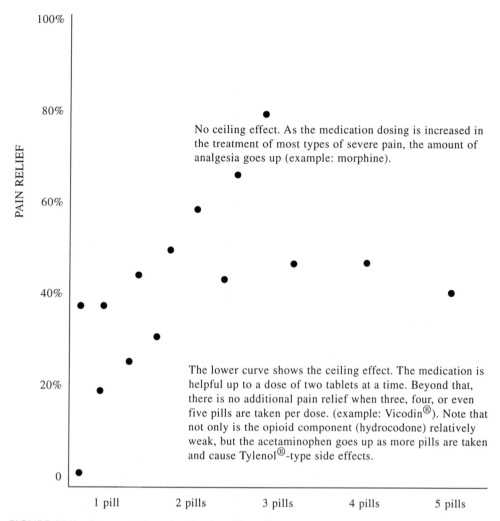

FIGURE 22.1 Demonstration of analgesic ceiling effects.

patients, Duragesic® patches (give level pain relief for 2.5 days or more) may need to be combined with high-potency Dilaudid® injections (for severe breakthrough pain), etc.

Motrin® may be found to be a good drug in the treatment of a patient, but chronic administration of the drug is questioned because of the known side effects. In that case, enough Vicodin® can be added to accomplish what at least one-half of the Motrin® is doing, and the Motrin® dose can be reduced. This may be true for other opioid/NSAID combinations. Cutting the NSAID dose in half greatly reduces the probability of significant side effects on long-term administration.

Insights

Keep the following in mind: What one person considers grade 10 pain, another person might consider level 6 or 7. Likewise, for the use of medications, one person's level 10 pain will respond well to oxycodone or Lorcet 10®, but another person's level 10 pain will respond only to injectable Dilaudid®. These are true clinical findings. Each patient must be respected for assessment of his or her pain and dysfunction related to pain. The clinician must decide which "10" will respond to the Lorcet® and which will respond to the injectable Dilaudid®. This is part of what makes pain management a complex endeavor.

HOW TO DECIDE WHETHER TO USE AN ANALGESIC, AND HOW TO GET OPTIMAL PAIN RELIEF FOR A PAINFUL CONDITION

Suggested Progressive Medication Dosing: Steps and Stages

If the situation calls for an analgesic medication, there are numerous steps and stages that must be followed. Before prescribing any analgesic medication for a patient in pain, the physician is legally obligated to perform a "good faith" medical examination. The history and physical examination sections of the good faith medical examination must be comprehensive enough to provide the physician (and possibly an independent medical reviewer) sufficient data on which to base his or her decision to use an analgesic medication.

Obviously, the criteria and complexity for giving Motrin® are not as strict and demanding as those for deciding to use Percodan® or morphine tablets.

Clinical Examples

Listed below are a few types of commonly encountered patients that may present in a general medical practice and a few that might be encountered in a pain management practice. For each case, a very brief summary of the pain intensity, CPT code (evaluation and management complexity), and type of analgesic medication that may apply is provided. In the examples, if a person with back pain is put onto a class 4 analgesic medication for pain symptom control, the assumption is that the patient has already been through numerous medications from class 1 to 3 analgesics to treat his or her pain.

Note that these cases are of a general nature and are used to demonstrate what class of analgesic(s) might be used to treat a given type of pain. Another assumption here is that a comprehensive good faith medical examination has been done and that all other troublesome diseases (diabetes, liver problems, obstructive pulmonary disease, etc.) are under satisfactory control.

Each type of problem will be summarized in tabular format. The tables will address the significant points of each case scenario. The first table is the prototype from which the others are derived.

Prototype Table of Data to Be Presented

Pain intensity (range = 0–10)	AMA CPT code for new patient (complexity)	Class of pain[a] medication for this case
Tenderness	Localized or spread over broad areas	
Redness	Localized or generalized	
Swelling	Local or generalized	
Impairment of physical function	Grade 1 = minimal; 2 = moderate, can do most of usual work but 50% physically impaired; 3 = severe, cannot perform gainful employment, bed bound at least 30% of each day	
Location of pain		

Approx. expected duration of analgesic medication usage	

a See the table of matching pain intensity with analgesic medication.

The following terms are derived from California Worker's Compensation Board literature: moderate = causes marked handicap in the performance of activities of daily living (ADL); severe = precludes the performance of ADL and/or job duties that bring on the pain.

Acute Ankle Sprain

Pain intensity (range = 0–10)	AMA CPT code for new patient (complexity)	Class of pain medication for this case
2–5	99201-99202	Class: 1–2
Tenderness		Localized
Redness		Localized
Swelling		Localized
Impairment of physical function		Grade 1
Location of pain		Localized
Approx. expected duration of analgesic medication usage		2-6 weeks

Acute Back Sprain/Strain

Pain intensity (range = 0–10)	AMA CPT code for new patient (complexity)	Class of pain medication for this case
3–7	99203	Class: 1–3
Tenderness	Localized to low back, and usually in the area of pain	
Redness	None to localized	
Swelling	None to localized	
Impairment of physical function	Grade 1–2	
Location of pain	Low back to upper buttocks	
Approx. expected duration of analgesic medication usage	2–6 weeks	

Chronic Moderate to Severe Back Pain

Pain intensity (range = 0–10)	AMA CPT code for new patient (complexity)	Class of pain medication for this case
0–8	99205	Class: 2–4
Tenderness	Localized to both sides of buttock, one or both piriformis muscles, and to variable extent up the paraspinal muscles from the sacrum to the upper thoracics involving the iliocostalis lumborum, longissimus thoracis, iliocostalis thoracic, and the multifidus at one or a number of levels	
Redness	Usually none	
Swelling	Usually localized to the sacral area and may be difficult for the examiner to visualize	

Impairment of physical function	Grade 1–3
Location of pain	Usually in the muscles along side the spine, from T8 to the sacral region, and/or in both or one side of the buttock; may have sciatic pain down one leg, and rarely the sciatica affects both legs
Approx. expected duration of analgesic medication usage	3 months to years; possibly the duration of the person's expected life span

Chronic Shoulder Pain

Pain intensity (range = 0–10)	AMA CPT code for new patient (complexity)	Class of pain medication for this case
6–7	99203-99204	Class: 2–3

Tenderness	Localized to shoulder and neck
Redness	Generally not seen unless an infection is present
Swelling	Local or generalized — mild
Impairment of physical function	Grade 2–3
Location of pain	Shoulder: front, back, side, any one area, or all three can be involved
Approx. expected duration of analgesic medication usage	Months to years; if an organic cause for the pain is found and taken care of, use of medication will drop to none at all (class 1–2 or less)

Chronic Moderate to Severe Back and Neck Pain

Pain intensity (range = 0–10)	AMA CPT code for new patient (complexity)	Class of pain medication for this case
3–10	99205 or greater	Class: 2–4

Tenderness	Neck and back, plus paraspinal and extremity involvement; in severe cases of fibromyalgia and MPS, tenderness may be diffuse and widespread; the more severe the involvement, the greater and more pronounced the diffuse tenderness
Redness	Generally not present
Swelling	Mild pretibial edema may be seen in some of the more severe cases; swelling may be due to use of methadone and/or morphine
Impairment of physical function	Grade 2–3; the greater the areas of pain involvement, the greater the amount of physical dysfunction and the greater the need for opioids or opioid-containing analgesics to counteract the physical dysfunction
Location of pain	Neck, back, extremities, paraspinal muscles, hands, feet, torso, or abdomen; one, a number, or all of these areas may be involved
Approx. expected duration of analgesic medication usage	From months to years or for the rest of the patient's expected lifetime

Postoperative Neck Pain ("Failed" Neck Surgery, Aracnoiditis)

Chronic back and neck pain, postoperative neck surgeries that seem to fail, and postoperative low back surgeries that seem to fail all have numerous features in common. Pain severity rating, area of pain involvement, pain intensity, and other factors all begin to look alike as they head into the 2- to 3-year mark after the injury or after the surgery. Therefore, the following tables for postoperative neck and back pain will look very much like that for chronic back and neck pain.

Pain intensity (range = 0–10)	AMA CPT code for new patient (complexity)	Class of pain medication for this case
3–10	99205 or greater	Class: 2–4
Tenderness	Neck and back, plus paraspinal and extremity involvement; in severe cases, fibromyalgia and/or MPS may be present; tenderness may be diffuse and widespread; the more severe the involvement, the greater and more pronounced the diffuse tenderness	
Redness	Generally not present	
Swelling	Mild pretibial edema may be seen in some of the more severe cases; swelling may be due to use of methadone and/or morphine	
Impairment of physical function	Grade 2–3; the greater the areas of pain involvement, the greater the amount of physical dysfunction and the greater the need for opioids or opioid-containing analgesics to counteract the physical dysfunction	
Location of pain	Neck, back, extremities, paraspinal muscles, hands, feet, torso, or abdomen; one, a number, or all of these areas may be involved	
Approx. expected duration of analgesic medication usage	From months to years or for the rest of the patient's expected lifetime	

Postoperative Back Pain ("Failed" Back Surgery, Arachnoiditis)

Pain intensity (range = 0–10)	AMA CPT code for new patient (complexity)	Class of pain medication for this case
3–10	99205 or greater	Class: 2–4
Tenderness	Neck and back, plus paraspinal and extremity involvement; in severe cases, fibromyalgia and/or MPS may complicate the postoperative pain picture; tenderness may be diffuse and widespread; the more severe the involvement, the greater and more pronounced the diffuse tenderness	
Redness	Generally not present	
Swelling	Swelling above the sacrum can be seen by patient and therapist; presacral swelling may reach a moderate degree; mild pretibial edema may be seen in some of the more severe cases and may be solely based on intake of opioids; morphine and methadone are the agents most likely to produce the pretibial edema	

Impairment of physical function	Grade: 2–3; the greater the areas of pain involvement, the greater the amount of physical dysfunction and the greater the need for opioids or opioid-containing analgesics to counteract the physical dysfunction
Location of pain	Neck, back, extremities, paraspinal muscles, hands, feet, torso, or abdomen; one, a number, or all of these areas may be involved; see the figures for grade 4 MPS in Chapter 10
Approx. expected duration of analgesic medication usage	From months to years or for the rest of the patient's expected lifetime

Chronic Multifocal (Multiple Locations of the Body Involved)

Arthritis

Pain intensity (range = 0–10)	AMA CPT code for new patient (complexity)	Class of pain medication for this case
3–6	99202-99204	Class: 1–3
Tenderness	Localized to numerous joints in the upper and/or lower parts of the body	
Redness	Localized to numerous joints in the upper and/or lower parts of the body	
Swelling	Localized to numerous joints in the upper and/or lower parts of the body	
Impairment of physical function	1–3	
Location of pain	Localized to numerous joints in the upper and/or lower parts of the body	
Approx. expected duration of analgesic medication usage	Months to years	

Progressive Disabling Fibromyalgia

Pain intensity (range = 0–10)	AMA CPT code for new patient (complexity)	Class of pain medication for this case
3–10	99205 or greater	Class: 2–4
Tenderness	In the more severe cases, neck and back plus paraspinal and extremity involvement; in severe cases, tenderness may be diffuse and widespread; the more severe the involvement, the greater and more pronounced the diffuse tenderness	
Redness	Generally not present	
Swelling	Mild pretibial edema may be seen in some of the more severe cases and may be solely based on intake of opioids; morphine and methadone are the agents most likely to produce the pretibial edema	
Impairment of physical function	Grade 2–3; in general, the greater the areas of pain involvement, the greater the amount of physical dysfunction and the greater the need for opioids or opioid-containing analgesics to counteract the physical dysfunction	

Location of pain	Neck, back, extremities, paraspinal muscles, hands, feet, torso, or abdomen; one, a number, or all of these areas may be involved progressively
Approx. expected duration of analgesic medication usage	From months to years or for the rest of the patient's expected lifetime

Progressive Myofascial Pain Syndrome (MPS)

Pain intensity (range = 0–10)	AMA CPT code for new patient (complexity)	Class of pain medication for this case
3–10	99205 or greater	Class: 2–4

Tenderness	Progressive neck, back, paraspinal muscle, and extremity involvement; in severe cases, tenderness may be diffuse and widespread; the more severe the involvement, the greater and more pronounced the diffuse tenderness
Redness	Generally not present
Swelling	Mild pretibial edema may be seen in some of the more severe cases and may be solely based on intake of opioids; morphine and methadone are the agents most likely to produce the pretibial edema.
Impairment of physical function	Grade 2–3; the greater the areas of pain involvement, the greater the amount of physical dysfunction and the greater the need for opioids or opioid-containing analgesics to counteract the physical dysfunction
Location of pain	Neck, back, extremities, paraspinal muscles, hands, feet, torso, and/or abdomen; one, a number, or all of these area may be involved
Approx. expected duration of analgesic medication usage	From months to years or for the rest of the patient's expected lifetime

THE NEED TO OBTAIN INDEPENDENT MEDICATION USAGE REVIEW

Many states have now enacted "intractable pain bills" to provide patients better access to schedule 3 and schedule 2 analgesics and to provide some protection to doctors who prescribe these medications for their patients. One of the provisions of these bills, either explicit or implied, is that the physician's use of opioids or opioid-containing analgesics should be reviewed by an independent practitioner, outside of the treating physician's practice, and preferably one who is a specialist in the diagnosis and management of chronic pain. This ensures that the physician's use of opioids meets with acceptable community medical standards.

However, at present there are no absolute standards for the use of schedule 2 opioid analgesics in the management of the pain component in chronic intractable pain patients. This acts as a deterrent to the prescribing of these stronger analgesics for chronic intractable pain patients. In the treatment of chronic intractable pain patients, the directions about medication usage in the *Physician's Desk Reference* and *Drug Facts and Comparisons* are merely a suggested starting point in the use of schedule 2 opioid analgesics.

If the practitioner is involved in a multispecialty practice, it is assumed that the chart will be reviewed by other members of the group, and therefore formal review, using a document such as the one below, is not necessary. If there is any question in this matter, it is best for the practitioner to have his or her patient reviewed by another physician who specializes in the diagnosis and management of chronic pain. I have used the controlled substances review request letter (see below) with over 300 of my patients. It has been reviewed by medical board agents, reviewers for the medical board, and medical board consultants. It seems to satisfy the need for a structured independent controlled substances review. The language for this letter was developed from the November 1985 and June 1991 "California Action Report," a quarterly put out by the Medical Board of California. The sections used dealt with the board recommendations on the use of opioids or opioid-containing analgesics for the treatment of chronic intractable pain patients.

The procedure proceeds as follows:

- The original letter is sent to the consultant.
- A copy is put into the patient's chart.
- A copy is given or sent to the patient, with a note telling the patient to contact the doctor to set up the medication review.
- When the review is done, the consultant fills it out and sends it back to the referring physician.
- Any recommendations from the reviewer must be acted upon by the physician requesting the review.

The following is a sample letter for obtaining independent medication review:

MICHAEL S. MARGOLES, M.D., Ph.D.
177 San Ramon Drive
San Jose, California 95111-3615
(408) 226-0318 FAX (408) 226-0626
Diplomate, American Board of Orthopedic Surgery
Diplomate, American Academy of Pain Management

Date: (date the form was filled out)

To: (name, address, and telephone number of the consultant who will perform the evaluation [consultation])

Re: (name of patient)

Dear Doctor:

My patient is being referred to you for review of usage of controlled substance(s). These medications are one of a number of therapies presently used in (his/her) treatment/management program.

The Medical Board of California recognizes that there is a subset of patients who fall under the category of chronic intractable pain.* These patients may be treated with appropriate modalities, including opiates (MBC Action Letter, June, 1991 and July 1994). Among their recommendations, the board advised periodic independent

---

* As used here, intractable pain means a pain state in which the cause of the pain cannot be removed or otherwise treated. In the generally accepted course of medical practice, no relief or cure of the cause of the pain is possible or none has been found after reasonable efforts to do so. Reasonable efforts include, but are not limited to, evaluation by the attending physician and one or more physicians specializing in the treatment of the area, system, or organ of the body perceived to be the source of pain.

review of the patient and treatment, including controlled substance (opiates, seda-tives, sleeping medication, etc.) usage.

In my opinion, this patient suffers from intractable pain as part of the total clinical problem. I believe the use of controlled substances is providing relief of some of the pain symptoms, relief of some of the dysfunction related to pain, aiding return to a more normal physical activity level, and facilitation of response to other therapies used in the overall pain management program.

My patient's current diagnoses are (put in the diagnosis and ICD number, similar to the following example):

1. Arachnoiditis — 322.2
2. Myofascial pain syndrome, multifocal, severe — 729.1
3. Posttraumatic painful polyneuropathy — 356.4
4. Fibromyalgia — 729.0

The controlled substance(s) currently being used to treat this patient are (put in the substances, similar to the following example):

Medication	Average consumption per day	Starting date of the medication
MS Contin, 60-mg tablet	11 per day	12/13/93
_____	_____	_____
_____	_____	_____

While using the medications, under my care, there has been no evidence of drug dependence syndrome, drug-seeking behavior, or unsanctioned use. Consumption of the above medications has been level, with no unexplained escalation of con-sumption.

Please check all of the following (use the back of this sheet or a separate sheet to explain where requested).

- Do you believe my patient has intractable pain? ☐ yes ☐ no If no, please explain.

- Do you notice any evidence of drug dependence syndrome (see attached sheets for definitions)? ☐ yes ☐ no If yes, please explain.

- Do you feel my patient shows evidence that would indicate the medications were used to obtain euphoria? ☐ yes ☐ no If yes, please explain.

- Do you detect any evidence of an abstinence syndrome? ☐ yes ☐ no If yes, please explain.

- Do you feel the medications are being used to facilitate pain control? ☐ yes ☐ no If no, please explain.

- Do you detect drug-seeking behavior? ☐ yes ☐ no If yes, please explain.

- Do you observe evidence of toxicity to any of the medications? ☐ yes ☐ no If yes, please explain.

- Do you feel any or all of the medication-oriented goals listed below are being achieved? ☐ yes ☐ no If no, please explain your concerns.

Goals: better social and interpersonal function, better physical functioning with respect to activities of daily living and/or employment, improved ability to do household work and chores, enhanced overall independence in physical functioning, and improved ability to interact with friends and/or family members

* Do you feel the medications are appropriate for my patient's needs and goals?
  ☐ yes ☐ no If no, please explain.

* Do you feel there are any additional diagnoses? ☐ yes ☐ no If so, please list them below.

_____

_____

Please answer the above questions and return this letter to my office. Please sign on the line above "signature of reviewer."

If you have further comments, observations, or therapies to recommend, please dictate a note to me or write them on the lines below

_____

_____

_____

_____   _____

Signature of reviewer   Date

Sincerely,

Michael S. Margoles, M.D., Ph.D.

A summary about drug dependence syndrome is attached to present some of the characteristics to be considered for in assessment.

DRUG DEPENDENCE SYNDROME SUMMARY

The old term "addiction" has been replaced by the World Health Organization's phrase "drug dependence syndrome." Drug dependence syndrome is a socio-psycho-biological syndrome manifested by a behavioral pattern in which the use of a given psychoactive drug (or class of drugs) is given sharply higher priority over other behaviors which once had significantly greater value, (i.e., drug use comes to have greater relative value). A key descriptive element is the priority given to drug seeking over other behaviors.

Behaviors embodied in drug dependence syndrome ("addiction") include:

Personality alterations around obtaining the drug
* Abstinence syndrome after drug abruptly stopped
* Family is disrupted due to personality alterations related to drug use
* Hygiene may be poor, especially dental
* Manipulation of family members and friends (by trying to make them feel bad, guilty, or responsible in some way for the mishap that has befallen the individual)
* Priority is given to drug-seeking behavior
* Rapid dose escalation
* Stealing, lying, denial of drug problem, compromised morals, prostitution
* Taking drugs for euphoria; desire for a "rush"

Drug-seeking behavior
- Acquisition from nonmedical sources
- Altered prescriptions
- Hoarding and/or selling drugs
- Ignoring negative impact and influences of the drug
- Manipulation of the physician to get more drug
- Multiple excuses to get more drug
- Multiple therapists and multiple pharmacies
- Strong desire for the drug for other than medical use
- Use of additional drugs, most commonly alcohol

Unsanctioned use
- Consuming another person's medications
- Giving medication to others
- Injecting oral medication
- Unsanctioned dose escalation
- Using the drug for unapproved indications

OPIOID CONTRACTING

The use of opioids in the treatment of chronic intractable pain patients is a complex endeavor. There are many possible complications when opioids are used as part of the overall treatment plan. It is therefore vital that the physician explain the reasons for opioid usage, anticipated side effects and complications, duration of opioid usage, and more at the initial visit(s). The following is a simple contract that can be used to attest to the fact that the physician and patient discussed the use of opioids in detail.

SAMPLE OPIOID CONTRACT

INFORMED CONSENT OF THE PATIENT: I _____
understand   Patient's name
and have been informed of the risks and benefits of the narcotic(s) (opioid[s]) medication that may be used in my treatment. I understand the addiction potential, the
possibility of adverse reactions to the medication, and the possibility of developing
dependency on the medication. I understand the risks and benefits of this/these drug(s)
compared with other treatment methods. I understand that if I fail to obtain medical
and/or medication reviews, laboratory tests, or if I fail to keep up with return visits to
Dr. Margoles' office, I may be tapered off my medication(s) and discharged from Dr.
Margoles' practice with notice being given. I will disclose to Dr. Margoles all other
sources of medication I am receiving.

Patient signature _____   Date _____

Witness signature _____   Date _____

Doctor signature _____   Date _____

BIBLIOGRAPHY

Ajemian, I. (1977). An oral morphine mixture for intractable pain, *Canadian Family Physician,* 23, 1506–1507.

Angel, M. (1982). The quality of mercy, *New England Journal of Medicine,* 306, 98–99.

Aranoff, G. (1985). Psychological aspects of nonmalignant chronic pain: a new nosology, in *Evaluation and Treatment of Chronic Pain,* Aranoff, G. (Ed.), Urban and Swarzenberg, Baltimore, pp. 471–484.

Aranoff, G. and Evans, W. (1985). Pharmacological management of chronic pain, in *Evaluation and Treatment of Chronic Pain,* Aranoff, G. (Ed.), Urban and Swarzenberg, Baltimore, pp. 435–449.

Baker, B. (1981). Personal communication.

Berken G. et. al. (1982). Methadone: an effective agent in managing intractable pain as a symptom of psychotic anger, *Annals of New York Academy of Sciences,* 398, 83–86.

Boas, R., Holford, N., and Villiger, J. (1985). Clinical pharmacology of opiate analgesia, in *Advances in Pain Research and Therapy,* Vol. 9, Fields, H., Dubner, R., and Cervero, F., (Eds.), Raven Press, New York, pp. 695–708.

Boas, R., Holford, N., and Villiger, J. (1985). Opiate choice and drug use, *The Clinical Journal of Pain,* 117–125.

Bonica, J. (1957). Management of myofascial pain syndromes in general practice, *Journal of the American Medical Association,* 164, 732–738.

Bonica, J. (1984). Local anesthesia and regional block, in *Textbook of Pain,* Wall, P. and Melzack, R. (Eds.), Churchill Livingston, New York, pp. 541–557.

Brechner, T., personal communication.

Brezin, J. et. al. (1979). Reversible kidney failure and nephrotic syndrome associated with nonsteroidal antiinflammatory drugs, *New England Journal of Medicine,* 301, 1271–1273.

Brose, W. (1991). Personal communication.

Bruera, E., Brenneis, C., Michaud, M., and MacDonald, R. (1989). Influence of the pain and symptom control team (PSCT) on the patterns of treatment of pain and other symptoms in a cancer center, *Journal of Pain and Symptom Management,* 4, 112–116.

Clark, H.W. (1988). Chronic pain and the chemical dependency specialist, *California Society for the Treatment of Alcoholism and Other Drug Dependencies News,* 15(1), 8.

Cooperman, H. (1979). Lifting the mantle of mystery, *Nursing Mirror,* July 5.

Crook, W. (1986). *The Yeast Connection,* Professional Books, Jackson, TN.

Curry, R. (1982). Acute renal failure after acetaminophen (Tylenol) ingestion, *Journal of the American Medical Association,* 247, 1012–1014.

DSM-III-R (1987). *Psychoactive Substance Abuse Disorders, Diagnostic and Statistical Manual of Mental Disorders,* 3rd ed. rev., American Psychiatric Association, Washington, D.C., pp. 165–172.

Edwards, G. (1981). Nomenclature and classification of drug and alcohol-related problems: a WHO memorandum, *Bulletin of the World Health Organization,* 59, 225–242.

Facts and Comparisons (1996). *Drug Facts and Comparisons,* Wolters Kluwer, St. Louis.

Facts and Comparisons (1996a). *Drug Facts and Comparisons,* Wolters Kluwer, St. Louis, pp. 1245–1251

Foley, K. (1985). Adjuvant analgesic drugs in cancer pain management, in *Evaluation and Treatment of Chronic Pain,* Aranoff, G. (Ed.), Urban and Swarzenberg, Baltimore, pp. 425–433.

Foley, K. (1986). Personal communication.

Foley, K. and Portenoy, R. (1986). Chronic use of opioid analgesics in non-malignant pain: report of 38 cases, *Pain,* 25, 171–186

Fordyce, W. (1976). *Behavioral Methods for Chronic Pain and Illness,* C.V. Mosby, St. Louis, p. 212.

Gary, N. et. al. (1980). Indomethacin (Indocin)-related acute renal failure, *American Journal of Medicine,* 69, 135–136.

Gilman, A., Goodman, L., and Gilman, A. (1980). *Goodman and Gilman's The Pharmacological Basis of Therapeutics,* 6th ed., Macmillan, New York, pp. 494–583.

Glynn, C and Mather, L. (1982). Clinical pharmacokinetics applied to patients with intractable pain: studies with Pithidine (Demerol), *Pain,* 13, 237–238.

Graham, J. (1985). Headache, in *Evaluation and Treatment of Chronic Pain,* Aranoff, G. (Ed.), Urban and Swarzenberg, Baltimore, p. 112.

Havsy, H. (1984). Colchicine use in 110 patients with disc disease, *Journal of Neurological and Orthopaedic Medicine and Surgery,* 5, 221–224.

Houde, R. (1974). The use and misuse of narcotics in the treatment of chronic pain, in *Advances in Neurology: An International Symposium on Pain,* Bonica, J. (Ed.), Raven Press, New York, pp. 527–538.

Jaffe, J. (1980). Opioid analgesics and antagonists, in *The Pharmacological Basis of Therapeutics,* Goodman, L. and Gilman, A. (Eds.), Macmillan, New York, pp. 494–534.

Jaffe, J. (1980). Drug addiction and drug abuse, in *The Pharmacological Basis of Therapeutics,* Goodman, L. and Gilman, A. (Eds.), Macmillan, New York, pp. 535–579.

Jaffe, J. and Martin, W. (1980). in *Goodman and Gilman's The Pharmaceutical Basic of Therapeutics,* 6th ed., Macmillan, New York, p. 512.

Kimberly, R. et. al. (1978). Reduction of renal (kidney) function by newer nonsteroidal anti-inflammatory drugs, *American Journal of Medicine,* 64, 804–807.

Large, R. (1980). The psychiatrist and the chronic pain patient: 172 anecdotes, *Pain,* 9, 253–263.

Lilly (1980). Eli Lilly Pharmaceutical Company, personal communication.

Margoles, M. (1983). The stress neuromyelopathic pain syndrome, *The Journal of Neurological and Orthopaedic Surgery,* 4, 317–322.

Margoles, M. (1983). The pain chart: spatial properties of pain, in *Pain Measurement and Assessment,* Melzack, R. (Ed.), Raven Press, New York, pp. 214–225.

Margoles, M. (1984). Opioid usage survey of the members of the American Pain Society, unpublished data.

Margoles, M. (1990). Myofascial pain syndrome: clinical evaluation and management of patients, in *Innovations in Pain Management: A Practical Guide for Clinicians,* Vol. 1, Weiner, R. (Ed.), Paul Deutsch Press, Florida, 15-3–15-63.

Margoles, M. (in press). Vitamins by injection in the treatment of patients with chronic pain, *Journal of Neurological and Orthopedic Medicine and Surgery.*

Margoles, M. and Margoles, M. (1984). The use of narcotic analgesics in the treatment of chronic orthopedic pain patients (COPP) — an informal and retrospective study of 95 patients, *Pain,* Supplement 2, S31.

Mather, L. (1990). Pharmacokinetics and pharmacodynamic profiles of opioid analgesics: a sameness amongst equals? *Pain,* 43, 3.

Medical Board of California (1991). Action Report.

Medical Board of California (1994). Prescribing Controlled Substances for (Intractable) Pain, pp. 4–5.

Meek, J., Guidice, V., and Enrick, N. (1984). Colchicine highly effective in disc disorders: results of a double blind study, *Journal of Neurological and Orthopaedic Medicine and Surgery,* 5, 213–220.

Monks, R. and Mersky, H. (1984). Psychotropic drugs, in *Textbook of Pain,* Wall, P. and Melzack, R. (Eds.), Churchill Livingston, New York, pp. 526–537.

Physicians' Desk Reference (1986). Medical Economics Company, Inc., Oradell, NJ.

Physician's Drug Alert (1986). Piroxicam (Feldene)-Induced Pancreatitis, August, p. 58.

Pilowsky, I. et. al. (1982). A controlled study of amitriptyline (Elavil) in the treatment of chronic pain, *Pain,* 14, 169–179.

Porter, J. and Jick, H. (1980). Addiction rare in patients treated with narcotics, *New England Journal of Medicine,* 302, 123.

Portenoy R.K. (1989). Opioid therapy, in *Interdisciplinary Rehabilitation of Low Back Pain,* Tollison, D. and Kriegel, M. (Eds.), Williams and Wilkins, Baltimore, 1989, pp. 137–157.

Portenoy, R.K. (1990). Chronic opioid therapy in nonmalignant pain, *Journal of Pain and Symptom Management,* 5 (Suppl.), S46–S62.

Rask, M. (1980). Colchicine use in 500 patients with disc disease, *Journal of Neurological and Orthopaedic Medicine and Surgery,* 1, 1–18.

Raskin, N. (1987). Personal communication.

Rose, H. (1992). Personal communication.

Rose, H. (1996). Acetaminophen and hydrocodone levels in chronic pain patients, *American Journal of Pain Management,* 6(1), 17–20.

Sacramento Medical Society (1990). *The Painful Dilemma — The Use of Narcotics for the Treatment of Chronic Pain,* Sacramento Medical Society, Sacramento, CA.

Savitz, D. (1985). Medical evaluation of the chronic pain patient, in *Evaluation and Treatment of Chronic Pain,* Aranoff, G. (Ed.), Urban and Swarzenberg, Baltimore, pp. 47–49.

SB 1802 (1990). State of California "Intractable Pain" Bill, approved September 30.

Simons, D.G. and Travell, J.G (1984). Myofascial pain syndromes, in *Textbook of Pain,* Wall, P. and Melzack, R. (Eds.), Churchill Livingston, New York, pp. 263–276.

Sternbach, R. (1974). *Pain Patients Traits and Treatment,* Academic Press, New York, pp. 64–65.

Sternbach, R. (1984). Acute versus chronic pain, in *Textbook of Pain,* Wall, P. and Melzack, R. (Eds.), Churchill Livingston, New York, pp. 174–175.

Stimmel, B. (1985). Pain analgesia and addiction: an approach to the pharmacologic management of pain, *The Clinical Journal of Pain,* 1, 14–22.

Supernaw, R. (1991). Personal communication.

Supernaw, R. (1992). Personal communication.

Travell, J.G. and Simons, D.G. (1983). *Myofascial Pain and Dysfunction: The Trigger Point Manual,* Williams and Wilkins, Baltimore.

Washburn, T. (1984). Personal communication.

Wilkinson, H. (1982). *The Failed Back,* Harper and Row, Philadelphia, p. 173.

Zimmerman, J. (1980). Senior Special Investigator, Board of Medical Quality Assurance, personal communication.

23 Sally's Story: Opioid Usage Over a Number of Years in a Chronic Pain Patient

Michael S. Margoles, M.D., Ph.D.

ATTEMPTING TO RETURN TO NORMAL LIFESTYLE AND APPARENT TOLERANCE TO PAIN-RELIEVING MEDICATION

By the time we become adults, most of us have decided on a lifestyle to pursue. When pain strikes, we may be at any of the many stages of our chosen life pursuits. Suddenly, if the pain is severe enough, we may have to give up our job, caring for our children or parents, mowing the lawn, training horses, gardening, and myriad other activities we used to take for granted. If our pain problem is only of a minor nature, such as persistent bursitis of the shoulder, we may only have to give up our weekly racquetball game and nothing else for the rest of our lives.

Let's consider the case of Sally (age 36), who is an executive buyer for a large department store chain. As an executive buyer she made a reputation for being reliable, hard working, honest, sincere, forthright, and one of the most effective and efficient employees in the 56-year history of her company. She and her daughters cared for a 2000-square-foot two-level house. Richard, her husband (age 38), took care of the quarter-acre of property which also includes her garden For the 5 years preceding the onset of her pain problem, her annual salary averaged $77,000. Her two teenage daughters are Tina (age 14) and Tonya (age 16). Sally became afflicted with a commonly occurring progressive, disabling soft tissue pain problem that was a combination of myofascial pain syndrome (MPS) and fibromyalgia syndrome. However, her MPS component was a variation of MPS called posttraumatic hyperirritability syndrome, a condition that relates to a small number of the overall MPS population. It is a severe and disabling cause of soft tissue chronic pain problems. It is described in Appendix 3 of this chapter and can be found in Chapter 10 under the descriptions of grade 3 and 4 patients.

Sally is not just a person with a pain problem; she is a person with a quality of life issue who has a pain problem. The life was intended; the pain was not.

At this point in the 21-year-old field of pain management, we have to face the fact that although thousands of therapists have begun to devote their efforts to pain management, we have not yet arrived at definitive therapy for many pain sufferers. Research is accelerating in this area, and many answers will be forthcoming in the next 10–20 years. Sally has a devastating and viscous pain problem that is destroying her life and her livelihood, not to mention her savings and other important issues. Some therapy is needed to bridge the gap for Sally, so she can remain physically, physiologically, and emotionally stable while she waits for those 10–20 years to pass.

We have to face the fact that routine therapy for fibromyalgia is nonsteroidal anti-inflammatory drugs (NSAIDs) and antidepressants. Some tender point injections may be carried out. The standard therapy for MPS is stretch and spray, NSAIDs, correction of perpetuating factors , mild analgesics, and myofascial trigger point injections. Some of these therapies are generally inadequate for patients who have the very severe progressive and/or disabling varieties of these diseases. Although treatment of perpetuating factors for MPS is vital and mandatory, few clinicians pursue these (see Chapter 10 for a discussion of perpetuating factors).

Severe and Progressive Pain

When I talk about severe and progressive chronic fibromyalgia or MPS pain, I am not talking about a pain that is relieved with two Bayer® aspirin and a tender/trigger point injection, meditation, or some stretch exercises. I am talking about a pain that will not respond to anything — headache, backache, neck ache, or any ache that will not or has not positively, definitively, and unquestionably responded to anything and/or anybody who has tried to do something for you or it.

Let's take a good hard look at "pain" medications, because these may be one of the most important methods of pain symptom control that could get Sally into the next decade or two, still intact and ready to reap the benefits of the final, definitive solution to her pain problem and accompanying disability. This may be the best means of pain symptom control that promotes compliance with other aspects of the pain management program.

Some professionals think that giving opioids to a chronic pain patient is fraught with dangers, the worst being addiction. They feel that opioids are to be avoided at all costs. This statement about opioids is similar to saying that everyone who owns a Corvette, Camaro, or Mustang is a speed demon, out looking for a thrill or a drag race. Following the same logic, one could say that everyone in a bar is an alcoholic.

Promoting Progressive Physical Rehabilitation

In my 21 years of experience with use of opioids in a chronic pain practice, I have noted there are many chronic pain patients who can use opioids with maturity and in a way that promotes their physical rehabilitation and return toward normal living.

I believe that given enough pain relief, many moderately to severely afflicted chronic pain patients could become fairly well self-rehabilitated (a savings of millions of dollars in rehabilitation costs). If their disease process has been allowed to progress to noticeable muscle atrophy, some form of structured physical rehabilitation program will be needed for their overall rehabilitation.

Sally's Symptom Chart

Sally's symptom chart (December 1992) related the following:

- Moderately severe pain
- Numbness, burning, and weakness of the right arm, leg, and right side of the back from the shoulder to the lower part of the buttock
- Cramping of muscles in the back of both thighs and calves
- Muscular twitching that was periodic in her right arm and leg and in the left eyelid
- Light pain, numbness, and tingling in the left arm and leg
- A tightness in the back of her neck that was more problematic on the right side
- Occasional right-sided headaches that tended to become problematic during the PMS part of her cycle
- Sharp, shooting pains of short duration between her shoulder blades from T3 to T7

Sally rated her pain at 8.9 on a scale of 0 (no pain) to 10 (excruciating, the worst ever). After seeing numerous doctors and pursuing numerous therapies, she came upon a specialist in pain management who had been trained according to the principles of medication management in the table of matching pain intensity with analgic medication provided in Chapter 22 and other rational medication-prescribing practices. (The farther down on the intensity scale one goes [from 10 toward 0], the higher incidence of undesirable side effects on long-term usage of the indicated medications. The main complications from the stronger narcotics are tiredness and constipation. The side effects from using the NSAIDs for too long are kidney failure, sterile brain abscess, ulcers of the gut, and liver problems, among others. Proper use of these medications dictates that the physician start with the lowest potency medications, such as the NSAIDs, and slowly progress upward until the patient is functioning at near normal [prepain] levels of activity. In some cases, combinations of these medications must be used. For instance, a patient may use MS Contin® and nontime-release morphine during the day. Levo-Dromoran® may be combined with Naprosyn®. In very severely afflicted patients, Duragesic® patches may need to be combined with high-potency Dilaudid® injections.)

The approach that each doctor used in treating Sally was similar. Each doctor noted that Sally had much treatment over the previous seven years. Sally's previous doctor had drawn the line at four Vicodin® tablets per day, stating she would become "addicted" if she took more than that.

Sally's Problems

By the time Sally saw the doctor:

- She had progressive pain and dysfunction for 3 years.
- She had become bedridden most of the time.
- She did not go out and socialize with friends.
- She had fatigue.
- She could no longer garden.
- She had great difficulty getting to the grocery store or post office.
- Her husband and children did most of the cooking and cleaning.
- She had given up horseback riding.
- Because of the severity of her neck and back pain, she could read her favorite novels for no more than 10 minutes a day.
- She had been gaining weight because of her lack of ability to exercise and keep up her usual activity level (she gained of 30 pounds in 12 months time). This was an embarrassment to her. Her wonderful figure was fading into someone she did not recognize in the mirror. Her clothes went up two sizes.

- She had noted weakness in her right arm and leg.
- She could sit or stand for no more than 30 minutes before needing to lay down.
- Her sleep was repeatedly interrupted by pain in her right arm and leg and spasms in her back. There was no comfortable sleeping position. She had tried numerous cervical pillows, numerous mattresses, and multiple pillows without much help. Some nights she would go to sleep sitting in the recliner because she could not lay flat on the bed.
- Driving her automobile had become very tiring and painful when she drove for more than 20 minutes.
- Her marriage had become stressful.
- Her back, hip, and leg pain was so bad that she had decreased love-making with her husband to 20% of what it was before the back pain started. When she spreads her legs for love making, she gets sharp jabs of pain in her mid buttock that are more problematic on the right side.
- She had become more irritable.
- She had very limited involvement with her daughters. This was the time in their lives when they needed to learn many of the routine household responsibilities.
- She constantly had to fight back depression due to all the emotional damage caused by her pain problem.
- She was too tired to put on makeup.
- Mornings were terrible. She literally rolled out bed and fell onto her knees. She then put one hand on the dresser and one hand on the bed. With a lot of groaning, she slowly got up, bent over, and got into the semi-erect posture. She had to immediately start walking or spasms set into her back and the back of her thighs. She had to walk at least 10 minutes to get to the vertical or near vertical position. This took a great deal of energy and left her fatigued.
- Exposure to vibration, such as that from a passing truck, aggravated her pain.
- Emotional stress, such as anger, or being frightened aggravated her pain.
- If her body was suddenly jarred, such as bumping into someone or getting hit by a shopping cart, her pain might flare up for weeks.
- Physical activity for more than 20 minutes could make her pain flare up for up to 2–3 days or more.
- She noted a marked change in her handwriting (she was right-handed).
- When the pain was at its worst, she noted a marked change in her voice.

A Well-Motivated Patient's Activity Level Will Generally Ascend to the Highest Level Allowed by the Doctor and/or by the Medications Prescribed for Pain Control

In the area of drug usage, it has been my experience that the euphoria of the drug addict is interpreted as dysphasia (anguish, agitation, disquiet, restlessness, malaise) when it happens to a chronic pain patient. However, the properly selected patient will not demonstrate euphoric-type behavior. Unlike street addicts who experience euphoria from drugs like heroin, pain patients get no highs from their opioid pills, shots, patches, or suppositories. They just get varying degrees of pain relief. Chronic pain patients willfully avoid getting a "buzz" from the medication. This abnormal feeling is counterproductive to them and their goals. Drug addicts use narcotics and other illicit drugs to "check out"; a chronic pain patient could use opioids or opioid-containing analgesics to "check in" (to become a productive member of society).

Apparent Tolerance

In the well-motivated chronic pain patient, the ability to accommodate higher intake of opioid analgesics usually reflects the effects of increased physical activity level ("apparent tolerance") and is not a true physiological tolerance that reflects greater body processing of the drug.

Sally began treatment with Dr. Smith in December 1992. After extensive evaluation, he began her medication treatment with three Lorcet 10® tablets (equivalent to six Vicodin®) per day. With that amount of analgesic medication, Sally could cook one meal. She related this with glee to her physician, Dr. Smith. He was impressed that she was on her way to getting well. This went on for a few weeks.

However, she had been bedridden for so long that many of her muscles had become weak, although visible atrophy was minimal (atrophy occurs on both sides and is difficult to detect). She knew there was atrophy by what she knew of herself.

Being an industrious person, she attempted to clean some windows and do a little shopping. Her atrophied muscles would only carry her so far and then she got tired. Her muscles became stiff and sore as she attempted to increase her physical activity level. Her increased activity activated latent infraspinatus and scalene anterior myofascial trigger points in the right shoulder and neck (see Chapter 10). These were injected with 0.5% procaine with 35% success in relieving the right shoulder pain, but she continued to have a generalized elevated pain level. She needed more pain control for her activity-related pain flare-up so she could continue to rehabilitate herself.

She appealed to Dr. Smith, who, after some hesitation allowed her to go to four to six Lorcet 10® tablets per day. With six Lorcet 10® tablets per day, Sally could shop for and cook two meals per day, still with pain. She reported this to Dr. Smith, and he documented that in her chart. She told him that the pain had been bothersome in the right neck, shoulder, elbow, and thumb, plus index finger. After study of the myofascial trigger point charts (Chapter 10), it was obvious that she has scalene and infraspinatus muscle trigger points. After proper palpation of the neck muscles, Dr. Smith injected the right scalene anterior muscle right behind the sternocleidomastoid muscle. When the infraspinatus muscle was injected, she felt a horrible shocking, lightening sensation go down her right arm and into her thumb. When the right scalene muscle was injected, she felt a pronounced deep ache radiating into the shoulder, down the arm, and into the hand. The local twitch response from the injections was severe with each muscle injected. Her body jerked involuntarily and noticeably during each injection procedure. The right arm felt sore and "dead." It took about 5 days for the pain and soreness to wear off, and the net effect of the myofascial trigger point injection was, at most, very small. The experience was not to her liking.

During each of the visits in which a myofascial trigger point injection was to be done, Dr. Smith listened to Sally and most times drew a pain chart to document what he heard her say and confirmed it with her by showing her the symptom chart (see the glossary at the end of this chapter for a definition of myofascial terms). He then determined where the myofascial trigger point(s) would most likely be. The muscle was approached and the taut band sought out. Within the taut band, palpation was performed until spot tenderness (the myofascial trigger point) was found. When the spot tenderness was found, a number of effects would be noted. Sally might demonstrate a jump sign. In determining which myofascial trigger point to inject, Dr. Smith preferred to elicit a pain recognition response in which Sally would tell him that his palpation of the myofascial trigger point was triggering at least some of the pain or other symptoms of which she was complaining. When he actually injected the myofascial trigger point, he knew that if a local twitch response was elicited, the likelihood of a successful outcome was good. However, over the years, he had many patients in whom the local twitch response was not elicited during a myofascial trigger point injection, but the outcome was good because he followed the above principles to find the most likely myofascial trigger point to inject. (Depending on the expected tenderness and local twitch response, premedication with some injectable tranquilizer [such as Valium®] or an opioid [such as morphine, Dilaudid®, or similar medication] might be used to suppress the very pronounced local twitch responses that come from the most active myofascial trigger points. The massive, sometimes total body, twitch responses that occur with injection of the very active myofascial trigger points could cause rebound pain in any or many places of the body. This is a most unpleasant experience for the patient.) Each myofascial trigger point injection was followed by stretch and spray and then warming of the area of stretch and spray.

Overall, Sally was thrilled. She could see some light at the end of the tunnel. There was hope! With the increase in her pain-relieving medication, she then proceeded to more time out of bed, a bit of gardening, and a longer trip to the grocery store per week. Her atrophied muscles could only carry her so far and then she got tired. Her muscles become stiff and sore as she attempted to increase her physical activity level. Her increased activity activated a few more latent trigger points, this time in her left low back and left buttock. When Dr. Smith suggested myofascial trigger point injections, she was willing to undergo the procedures, but became very apprehensive because of the awful pain during the last injections. Dr. Smith perceived her apprehension. He suggested some medication to sedate her to make the procedure more tolerable. His nurse drew up 10 mg of morphine, 25 mg of Phenergan® and $1/2$ cc of 2% Xylocaine® and injected into the upper right buttock. Before the injection was given, Dr. Smith told the nurse to inject deeply into the fatty area but not into the muscle. He pointed out to the nurse that unnecessary injections into myofascial muscles could cause postinjection pain, soreness, and stiffness that might last days to weeks. A misdirected therapeutic (medication-containing) injection could possibly activate a latent myofascial trigger point, causing short or long periods of pain and/or disability.

Twenty minutes later, he injected Sally's right iliocostalis lumborum, at the first lumbar level. Within 30 minutes, she had 30% pain relief in the lower right buttock, but she still had an elevated general pain level. She needed additional pain control for her activity-related pain flare-up so she could continue to rehabilitate herself (routine physical therapy or routine chiropractic care at this point would possibly still cause her pain to flare up too much at this point). Pain had become bothersome at night and interfered with her sleep. Dr. Smith taught her the benefits of taking a long-acting, inexpensive pain-relieving medication, methadone. Sally was now in her fourth month of treatment.

Sally was to start at one 10-mg methadone tablet one hour before bedtime. Every other night she was to increase by one-half additional tablet until her sleep and morning stiffness improved. (Methadone, Oxycontin®, Oramorph®, or MS Contin® taken at bedtime in some cases can reduce morning stiffness related to fibromyalgia or MPS. These medications can also reduce nighttime pain that keeps the patient awake.)

Three weeks later, Sally reported that her nighttime pain was markedly reduced when she took two methadone tablets before going to sleep. Mornings were less problematic. She stated that in the mornings, she used to wake up feeling as though she was coated with a stiffening resin all over her body. With the use of the methadone, this problem was cut in half. However, she said she had trouble getting to sleep. She was therefore told to combine one to two Soma 350® (a muscle relaxer that can be used to induce sleep) tablets with her bedtime methadone. After a few nights of improved sleep, she felt well enough to invite her friend Betty to lunch. She has not seen Betty in over 6 months. They had stayed in touch by phone. After lunch, Sally went home and did a lot of gardening. The pain flare-ups caused a major setback for 6 weeks. Dr. Smith understood that an MPS patient should only flare up for a few days. He ordered a panel of blood tests and found that she had a low blood count with accompanying low iron level. Her blood potassium level was at the bottom of the normal range. Her B12 level was at the lowest quarter of the normal range, and her folic acid level was in the middle of the range. Her estrogen and testosterone levels were very low. All these levels were considered to be less than optimal for the myofascial component of her pain problem. Dr. Smith corrected this by giving her the oral B-complex program listed below. He supplemented this with self-administered quarter-strength B-complex shots every other day. He prescribed 10 meq of time-release potassium, at two tablets twice per day. She was given supplements of microcrystalline estrogen, microcrystalline testosterone, and natural progesterone. After 5 weeks on the above program, she began to feel almost like a new person.

Oral Vitamin Direction Sheet, B-Vitamin Injections

Oral Vitamin Directions Sheet

Bronson product	#[b]	Week 1	Week 2	Week 3	Week 4	Thereafter
			Number of items to take per day[a]			
B complex with C and E	4	1	2	3	4	4
Mineral insurance formula	12	1	2	3	3	3
Folic acid, 800-µg tablets	97	1	1	2	2	2
Vitamin C, time release, 1000 mg	78	1	2	2	2	2

	Full	Half	Quarter
B-complex injection syringe #1			
Dexpanthenol, 250 mg/ml (B5)	1 cc	$\frac{1}{2}$ cc	$\frac{2}{10}$ cc
2% lidocaine (Xylocaine)	$\frac{1}{2}$ cc	$\frac{1}{2}$ cc	$\frac{2}{10}$ cc
B-Complex 100 (mixed B-complex)	1 cc	$\frac{1}{2}$ cc	$\frac{2}{10}$ cc
Riboflavin, 50 mg/ml (B2)	$\frac{1}{2}$ cc	$\frac{1}{2}$ cc	$\frac{2}{10}$ cc
B-complex injection syringe #2			
Dexpanthenol, 250 mg/ml (B5)	$1\frac{1}{2}$ cc	$\frac{1}{2}$ cc	$\frac{2}{10}$ cc
Folic acid, 5 or 10 mg/ml (Bc)	$\frac{1}{2}$ cc	$\frac{1}{2}$ cc	$\frac{2}{10}$ cc
Hydroxcobalamin, 1000 µg/ml (B12)	$\frac{1}{2}$ cc	$\frac{1}{2}$ cc	$\frac{2}{10}$ cc

___X___ Use alternate injection program: Inject a #1, skip a day, inject a #2, skip a day, inject a #1, skip a day, inject a #2, etc.

[a] When more than one per day is indicated, it is best to split the dose and take one dose in the morning and one in the evening. If three doses are indicated, take them before breakfast, lunch, and dinner. If four or more are indicated, break up the dosing any way you like.

[b] This is the unique number assigned to each Bronson product. For instance, #4 is assigned to nontime-release B complex with C and E. If you call Bronson and say you want a 250-tablet bottle of product #4, they know it is nontime-release B complex with C and E. Bronson can be reached at 800-610-4848.

Sally's activity level continued to increase, and so did the pain. Dr. Smith converted the daytime medication from Lorcet 10® to one to two 5-mg oxycodone tablets every 4–6 hours for better pain control.

At about 7 months after he began treating Sally, Dr. Smith repeated most of his extensive original physical examination of her (7/14/93). He found there was still absence of a number of the deep tendon reflexes in her upper extremities. In the lower extremities, the knee jerks were normal and the ankle reflexes were diminished on both sides. There was decreased pinprick sensation testing in a number of the dermatomes of the upper and lower extremities.

The pinwheel was standardized at C4 on both sides. He next used a goniometer to measure the passive hypertension of the left index finger metacarpophalangeal joint. It measured 90 degrees, which meant she should be rather flexible. He used a goniometer to measure the range of motion of the neck and shoulders. There was slight but definite improvement He checked the trapezius, sternocleidomastoid, pectoralis major, and latissimus dorsi muscles. Taut bands and tenderness were noted in all these muscles, but the incidence of jump sign was down by 30%, a sign of good progress. Muscle testing of a number of the shoulder muscles showed a small but definite improvement. Straight leg raising was positive at 35 degrees on the right and 45 degrees on the left. She complained of tight hamstring muscles on both sides and pain radiating down the side of the leg on the right (this is not a sciatic distribution). Dropping her hip and leg over the side of the table on the right showed a flexion contractor of 25 degrees on the right. When this was repeated on the left, the hip extended to neutral and then she complained of pain in the low back. Muscle testing the ankle dorsiflexors showed minimal weakness on both sides. Muscle testing the extensor of the great toe showed moderate weakness on both sides. After she stood up, he checked the level of the pelvis from behind. She was noted to be 0.4 inches shorter on the right side. When the range of motion of her lumbar spine was tested, she missed touching her toes by 19 inches because of pain in the buttock and low back. She could extend to 10 degrees. She could laterally bend 15 degrees bilaterally. When asked to perform a deep knee bend, she could do range of motion of 45% of normal. Her balance was about 50% of expected and her strength was 50% of expected. She complained of pain in her rectus femoris muscles and patellas on both sides.

The short left leg was corrected with a series of lifts under the left heel: 2 mm was used for 2 weeks, 4 mm for 2 weeks, 7 mm for 2 weeks, and finally a 1-cm lift permanently. On the follow-up visits, she indicated that the lifts were helping.

Dr. Smith left town for 4 weeks to attend a medical conference and take a vacation. His partner, Dr. Jones, took over for him. Sally saw Dr. Jones for a routine appointment (that she would have had with Dr. Smith). After reviewing her chart, Dr. Jones took very little relevant history and performed no physical examination. Nonetheless, he looked at her and said, "By now you've become a drug addict." Upon hearing this, she was shocked and broke into tears. She tried to explain what the medication had done for her, but he was not moved by her statements.

He noticed she was heavier than when she was seen last year. She had gained 30 pounds. He inquired about her eating habits. She said she did not eat much. She asked if he had any answers for her. He said, "Just stop eating!" She thought to herself, "I'm down to three low-fat Ensure® and smaller portions than I used to eat in the past. What Dr. Jones is saying just doesn't make sense."

She told him that when she tried to do many of her usual activities, her activity would be blocked by bothersome pain flare-ups (caused by one or more of the many myofascial trigger points she had). With respect to many of the activities that were important to her, he said, "Just don't do that."

Dr. Jones told her that her pain was related to depression and put her on 20 mg of Prozac® daily. He told her she had to get hold of herself and lick this pain. He told her, "No pain, no gain." He recommended that she sign up for a pain management class at Good Standards Hospital. She told him that she went through the program a year ago. He told her that she did not understand the value of the program and told her to take a similar program at Good Intention Hospital. She knows from conversations with other pain patients that the program at Good Intention is the same as the one at Good Standards.

Dr. Jones tapered her off the oxycodone, methadone, and Soma®. Within the week, she found that she could no longer garden, shop, or go out with friends due to the return of the pain (that was blocked by the analgesics). She felt shattered, hopeless, and terrified. She was depressed because the light at the end of the tunnel had gone out. She was again relegated to being bed-bound most of the time. Although the Prozac® lifted her mood a bit, it did nothing for the pain. It was now 8 months since her treatment with Dr. Smith began.

However, Sally did find that correcting the perpetuating factors, plus the couple of myofascial trigger point injections, had left her with an overall 15–20% pain relief. It was not enough to be too active, but she found that she could cook an occasional meal. She could go to the store with the use of her disabled parking sticker. Her husband loaded and unloaded the cart as she pushed it. Most of the time she used an electric cart that she could ride in the store. This convenience was supplied by the store.

At the end of 4 weeks, Dr. Smith returned. At her next visit with him, she explained what had happened. He apologized for not having told Dr. Jones what to do in his absence. He assured her that her chart would be structured in a way to avoid that in the future.

Dr. Smith put Sally back on the methadone, Soma 350®, and oxycodone. Because of the physical setback from being disabled for almost a month, it took her 13 days to get back to the activity level she was at just before Dr. Smith left town. It was now 9.5 months since her treatment with Dr. Smith began.

Strain Right Shoulder, Lunch with Betty, Fatigue, Dexedrine®

Sally went back to her gardening. There was joy in the work and a sense of accomplishment. She was excited about what she had done. She took a photo of her garden and showed it to Dr. Smith at her next visit. This labor of love in the garden had activated an additional myofascial trigger point in her lower right buttock and had caused a "strain" in her right shoulder.

She was having lunch with her friend Betty on a weekly basis. This was a real treat for Sally because she had begun to feel very socially isolated since the onset of her pain problem. She was now out of bed much more consistently from day to day.

Fatigue was becoming bothersome at this time. She reported it to Dr. Smith. Over the next 8 weeks, she was tried on Paxil®, Zoloft®, Elavil®, Norpramin®, phentermine, Ritalin®, Cylert®, and finally 6-mg time-release Dexedrine® capsules. It was found that taking four of the Dexedrine® capsules in the morning would give her enough of an energy boost to accomplish more of her usual activities of daily living.

It was now early December 1993. She was able to do most of the cooking. She had been able to prepare about half of the Thanksgiving dinner. Last year at that time, the most Sally could muster up was enough energy to go out to a restaurant with her two daughters and husband to celebrate the holiday. After dinner, she had to return to bed because the pain and fatigue had become more pronounced. December 1993 was joyful because she was heading back toward the mainstream of life.

In December 1993, Sally, Tina, and Tonya cooked a wonderful Christmas dinner for the family and six friends. As the prayer was given before the meal, Sally's heart was filled with overwhelming thankfulness to the Lord for restoration of her life. Tears of gratitude and happiness streamed down her cheeks. Her current therapy program had provided 40% overall pain relief, better stamina, and improved physical function.

When dinner was finished and all the guests were relaxing with conversation and gifts, Sally and her daughters served desserts and ice cream. At one point, Sally got up to serve more dessert and her right hip momentarily gave out. She had to grab hold of Richard to keep from falling. That hip had been progressively problematic since 2 months after the hip and leg began to hurt.

The next morning (12/26/93), after finishing her shower, she twisted to her right as she stepped over the shower ledge. When her right foot touched the floor, she felt a sharp muscle spasm in her right hip. At that same instant, her right hip gave away. As she came crashing toward the floor, she hit the wooden clothes hamper with her right side (at the lower rib cage level). As she continued to fall, her back was sharply twisted and she let out a loud scream. She wound up on the linoleum floor, on her right side, and in excruciating pain. Because her chest and back muscles were in acute spasm, she could barely catch her breath. Tonya was the first to arrive. She was terrified at her mother's distress. She didn't know what to do. Sally told her to call Dr. Smith and tell him what had happened. Dr. Smith said to have Sally brought to the emergency room. Richard had not left for work yet. He helped her over to the bed to lie down for a moment. She had him bring her an oxycodone tablet, a Soma 350® tablet, and some water. The medication was of no help. Tonya and Richard got her into some loose clothing. A brassiere was out of the question because of the location of the pain.

With Tonya on one side and Richard on the other, Sally was slowly taken down the stairs to the car. Each step caused jerking and horrible pain. Luckily, the reclining seats in the car made the trip to the hospital more bearable. Upon arrival at the emergency room, she was transferred to a stretcher and logged in. X-rays were taken of her ribs and spine. The ribs were normal, but she had the appearance of a small compression fracture at the eighth thoracic vertebrae. It was difficult to tell if the fracture was old or new. After Dr. Smith evaluated her, he told her to go home and rest for the next 1–2 weeks. He told her to double the bedtime methadone and increase the daytime oxycodone by 25–50% until the flare-up subsided. She was to see him at the office a week later.

When Sally saw Dr. Smith a week later, her rib and upper back pain was clearing. However, she had severe pain radiating down the right in a sciatic distribution. Her ankle and foot were weak. She was dragging the right leg and had marked difficulty walking on it. She had taken to using a cane because weight bearing on the right was so painful. Dr. Smith reassured her and gave her a prescription for Motrin®.

When seen a week later (1/8/94), the painful leg problem had not changed. Pain was causing marked distress. He told her to stop the daytime oxycodone and started her on one to four 2-mg Dilaudid® every 3–4 hours as needed.

When seen a week later (1/15/94), she said the Dilaudid® provided better pain control than the oxycodone, but the leg had begun painful spasms and numbness down the side. At times, it was difficult to control the leg.

When Dr. Smith evaluated her, the ankle reflex was absent on the right side. He suspected that she might have ruptured a disc during the fall. He referred Sally to a neurosurgeon, Dr. Worthington, and an orthopedic surgeon, Dr. Swartz, for surgical evaluation. A lumbar MRI and discogram were performed. The findings showed small to moderate disc bulges at L4–L5 and L5–S1. The surgeons were not convinced that surgery was needed at the time, but indicated that the situation could get worse over time. They recommended an epidural steroid injection.

For unknown reasons, the insurance carrier paid for the neurosurgeon consult but not the orthopedic surgeon. The answer given was that one consultant was enough. Dr. Smith attempted to explain the need for the two different specialists. However, the insurance company sent back a standard form letter stating that only one of the two consultants was authorized by her insurance plan. By now, 14 months of treatment had gone by.

Dr. Mosby, an anesthesiologist, was called to do the epidural (2/15/94). He met Sally in the emergency room. Dr. Mosby was an elderly man. He was kind and took as much time as Sally needed to understand the procedure and the expected results. He asked her a number of questions in order to determine the correct level to inject at. Her vital signs were taken.

She put on a gown and lay on her right side. The special table she was on was tilted up to allow the epidural injection components to run down the nerves on her right side. The doctor had her slowly bend as far as she comfortably could, bending her head toward her knees. He then numbed the skin at the L4–5 area and waited a few minutes for the anesthetic to work. He then used a specially prepared tray and assistance from a nurse to draw up Marcain® and Depomedrol® into a syringe. He attached a 22-gauge 3.5-inch spinal needle to a glass syringe. The plunger was pulled back to the 5-cc mark. He inserted the needle into her right L4–5 region and began to direct the needle toward the ligaments that stretched between the two lumbar levels. Soon he felt an inaudible "pop" as the needle went through the ligamentum flavum. The needle came to rest on the undersurface of the ligament. He pushed the plunger and noted that he could easily inject 4 cc of air into the epidural space. At about the time of the "pop," Sally felt sharp pain shooting down her right leg. She tensed a bit. Dr. Mosby reassured her that the medication would soon be in and the pain would be numbed. She relaxed as best as she could. Richard was there holding her hand. Dr. Mosby switched to the medication-containing syringe and injected it into the epidural space. Within minutes, she began to feel a numbing sensation in the areas where she had hurt so terribly. Dr. Mosby told her to go home, take some pain medication, if needed, and rest for the following 24 hours.

On the way back home, Sally noted that the pain relief was substantial. She breathed a sigh of relief. By the next day (2/19/94), she felt that the epidural injection gave her 50% relief of the pain in her right leg. The relief lasted $2\frac{1}{2}$ weeks. During that time, she was able to get back to gardening, housework, teaching her daughters matters relating to household responsibilities, and some shopping. After $2\frac{1}{2}$ weeks (3/1/94), the pain and dysfunction slowly returned to the right leg. Ten days later (3/11/94), the radiating pain was strong and beyond what her methadone and Dilaudid® could control.

One week later, she saw Dr. Smith. He noted the limp and the use of the cane. The grimacing on her face with each step told him she was back to the preepidural pain level.

Dr. Mosby was called again to do a repeat epidural. She was scheduled for a repeat epidural a week later (3/25/94). He met her at the emergency room and the same procedure was performed. This time he ordered premedication with 15 mg morphine sulfate, 50 mg Phenergan®, and 1 cc of 2% Xylocaine® (to reduce the effects of the pain and discomfort from the procedure). After questioning her, he felt that the right L5–S1 interspace was the proper level to treat. The procedure was carried out and the patient sent home.

By a week postinjection (4/1/94), Sally had experienced no relief from the epidural injection. Pain and physical dysfunction related to pain were back. She was showing signs of a drop foot on the right and had begun to drag the leg again. Twenty milligram of methadone plus up to 32 2-mg tablets of Dilaudid® per day were not providing adequate pain control. (This represented a substantial dose of pain medication. In most nonpain patients, one or two of the Dilaudid® tablets would be enough to knock them out for a number of hours.)

One week later (4/8/94), she was referred back to Dr. Worthington for further surgical evaluation. He recommended use of a myelogram to further define the findings on the MRI. Two days later (4/10/94), Dr. Worthington performed the myelogram in the X-ray department. He was aware of the fact that patients such as Sally could experience pain flare-up and headaches during and after the procedure. Forty-five minutes before the procedure, he had the nurse give Sally two injections. One contained 4 mg of Dilaudid® plus 1 cc of 2% Xylocaine®. The other shot contained 50 mg of Phenergan® plus $\frac{1}{2}$ cc of 2% Xylocaine®. He instructed the nurse to inject deep into the fat and not the muscle. He told her to use the smallest gauge needle, a 27-gauge $1\frac{1}{4}$-inch needle. The medication was very helpful in reducing the amount of pain and discomfort associated with the myelogram.

He used water-soluble dye for the myelogram. Routine myelography views and CT scan views were taken during the procedure. The myelogram showed an extruded disc fragment (ruptured disc) in the space between the L4 and L5 disc spaces. It was obvious that the fragment had ruptured at the L4–5 level and then began to travel downward. It appeared to be resting against the L5 nerve root. The cause of her enhanced right leg pain had been found.

Dr. Worthington advised Sally and Richard to have the fragment taken out as soon as possible, because it was causing inflammation of the tissues in the canal, especially the L5 nerve root, and pressure on that nerve root. After discussing the matter with Dr. Smith, Richard and Sally decided to go ahead with the operation. Dr. Smith and Dr. Worthington conferred before the operation. Dr. Smith gave Dr. Worthington a summary of the pain medications Sally was presently taking and a profile of her doctor–patient relationship with him. Dr. Smith advised Dr. Worthington that if 64 mg of oral Dilaudid® was not controlling her pain before the operation, compensation for that needed to be made in the postoperative pain medication.

Sally was scheduled for surgery on April 20. Dr. Swartz was the assistant. At the time of the operation, after doing a standard posterior lumbar approach, once they got through the ligamentum flavum it was noted that the L5 nerve root was being pinched, inflamed, and irritated by a large disc fragment. After the free fragment had been removed, the surgeons went to the disc space and located and removed a number of additional free fragments that had not extruded yet. Because of the pressure on the nerve, it looked blanched. Once the disc fragment was removed, the nerve returned to its normal healthy color.

Two hours after the procedure, Sally awoke in the recovery room. She immediately noted that the cramping, spasms, and sharp pain were gone from the right leg. She could move it without agonizing pain. She was elated.

She had and I.V. in her left arm with a patient-controlled analgesia machine. Dr. Worthington had instructed the nurses to set the machine to deliver up to as much as 5 mg of Dilaudid® per hour if she needed that much. He told the staff what Dr. Smith and he had discussed preoperatively. After reviewing her usage and needs for opioid analgesics, they determined that Sally had a natural resistance to opioids ("high tolerance"). Therefore, she needed to be given more than most patients. All the medical personnel involved in her care knew that the proposed dosing regimen would probably kill most people. However, they knew that Dr. Smith and Dr. Worthington were capable and credible physicians. Nonetheless, Sally's vital signs were monitored more closely than usual during the first 24 hours postoperatively.

Sally averaged 3–4 mg of Dilaudid® per hour for the first 28 hours, 1–2 mg/hour for the subsequent 18 hours, 1 mg/hour for the next 10 hours, and then was switched to oral 2-mg Dilaudid® tablets at a prescription of up to three to four tablets every 2 hours as needed for pain control.

Dr. Worthington wrote an order that Richard could give Sally her vitamin shots while in the hospital. Dr. Smith had instructed Richard and Sally to begin the full-strength shots daily, starting 4 days before the surgery. They were told to stay at that dose until 10 days after the surgery and then taper back to the usual (half-strength doses every other day) dose. Sally was up and about in record time. By 36 hours postoperatively, she was walking, with minimal assist from Richard, and not dragging the right leg. At that time, the spasms and cramping were rapidly going away from her right leg.

The medical staff on the floor where she was staying was amazed at the speed of her recovery. They were also amazed at her pattern of Dilaudid® usage and how quickly she went from intravenous to oral pain medication so quickly. She was discharged in the morning on 4/24/94.

By 2 weeks from the time of the surgery (5/10/94), she could walk on the leg again. The leg dragging had stopped. The disc-related pain was gone, and all that remained was the myofascial and fibromyalgia pain that was troublesome before the injury that had ruptured the disc in her back.

By 1 month postoperatively, all surgically related pain was gone. She was left with most of the pain problem described on her symptom chart of December 1992.

Dr. Smith continued her on the 2-mg Dilaudid® tablets at one to four tablets every 3–4 hours as needed for daytime pain control, 20 mg methadone at bedtime, and Soma 350® for bedtime sedation as needed.

During her visit of 5/27/94 Dr. Smith, taught her about using her Dilaudid® tablets on a time-contingent basis. That meant taking the medication by the clock and not according to how bad her pain felt. Sally was apprehensive about taking pain medication period, because she felt that she might really become addicted or "hooked." Relatives had been pressuring her to consider something other than the pain medication for control of her pain. Dr. Smith told her that he could appreciate her dilemma.

He stated that taking the medication on a time-contingent basis would result in the least amount of addiction because it stopped the patient from reacting to the pain. He also stated that patients like her (with a family, executive position, children, supportive husband) were the least likely to become addicted to an opioid analgesic medication.

To initiate the time-contingent dosing, he told her to get a wristwatch with an alarm or one with an alarm countdown timer. He recommended she look into buying a Casio Databank® watch. She was to start the medication at two 2-mg Dilaudid® tablets every 4 hours. The idea was to suppress as much of the pain as possible before it became intense or problematic. She was to report back in a week to get further directions from Dr. Smith about the time-contingent medication.

Her next visit was on 6/6/94. She said she had bought the watch he requested. It was not too feminine, but was functional. She said the pain relief would last about 3 hours, and then the pain would begin to peak in intensity during the third to fourth hour. She was continuing on all the vitamins (oral and injectable), minerals, and hormones that had been prescribed for her. Dr. Smith told her to change the dosing to two tablets every 3 hours.

She returned on 6/20/94. She told Dr. Smith that pain control was good with the two 2-mg Dilaudid® tablets every 3 hours. Her up time was about 60% of the day, and she could cook most meals. She had better interaction with her husband and her daughters. With the help of a disability parking sticker, she could do much of the shopping with some help from Richard or her daughters. She was meeting with Betty and their friend Marge for lunch three days out of the month. She could do some household chores, but using the vacuum cleaner and reaching (e.g., to the second shelf or higher in a cupboard) provoked too much pain in her back. When asked to point to the problem pain area, she used her right index finger to point backward, just under the shoulder blade, at the latissimus dorsi muscle. He had her scheduled to have it injected.

Sally came in on 6/30/94. Ruth, the nurse, drew up 4 mg Dilaudid® plus ½ cc of 2% Xylocaine® In a second syringe she drew up 25 mg Phenergan® plus ½ cc of 2% Xylocaine®. The medications were injected into the left buttock, making sure to inject into the deep fat and not the muscle. Sally removed her clothes from the waist up and put on a gown. Ruth put her into the prone position. Dr. Smith came in 15 minutes later. With his left hand, he picked up a wad of latissimus dorsi muscle just to the outside (lateral side) of the scapula. He began rolling the taut band between his index finger and thumb until he found a prominent tender spot (myofascial trigger point. He kept pressure on that area for about 25 seconds. At that point, Sally said she could feel some faint pain along the inside of her right arm and a very faint discomfort into the low back in some of the areas that hurt when she tried to do household chores. Ruth handed Dr. Smith a 5-cc syringe, with a 25-gauge 2-inch needle, containing 3 cc of 0.25% Marcaine®. He inserted the needle and began running it slowly in and out of the muscle in a circular fashion, just piercing the fascia and slightly beneath the fascia to the muscle of the latissimus dorsi. The needle never came out all the way, but was merely brought up near the skin surface, and then redirected to a different part of the muscle. During this procedure, the muscle twitched visibly as each active myofascial trigger point was inactivated. There were eight local twitch responses and six accompanying jump signs. Most of the jump signs were minor to moderate in strength, but two of them caused a massive downward pull of her shoulder. One took her completely by surprise, as a flash of accompanying pain hit her low back and shoulder at the same time. When this happened, she let out a scream.

When seen on 7/14/94, Sally told Dr. Smith that injection to the latissimus dorsi muscle had decreased some of the tingling in her right arm, had loosened some of the tightness in her back and buttock, and she was beginning to regain some more strength in her right arm and hand. There was less tendency to drop things she was holding in her right hand.

Over the next 4 months, and at 2-week intervals, using the same premedication, additional myofascial trigger point injections were carried out. The specific muscles injected were right and left sternocleidomastoid muscles (both sternal and clavicular parts of the muscle) for her headache problem; right and left trapezius 3, 2, and 1 for upper back and headache pain; right and left iliocostalis thoracis at thoracic levels 4, 5, 7, 8, 9, 10, and 11 for tightness and pain in the back and chest; right and left longissimus thoracis at thoracic levels 4, 5, 7, 9, 10, and 11 for tightness and pain in the back; and right scalene anterior, middle scalene, and scalene posterior for pain and numbness in the right upper extremity and also for carpal tunnel syndrome symptoms that she had been having in her right wrist. The right gluteus medius 1, 2, and 3 plus the right gluteus minimus anterior and posterior were injected for weakness in the right hip. The right rectus femoris, vastus intermedius, and both vastus medialis myofascial trigger points were injected for pain and weakness in the right knee. All these injections were completed by 11/14/94. Each series of injections produced positive results.

On her visit of 12/26/94, Sally informed Dr. Smith that the intensive course of myofascial trigger point injections had produced an overall 50% relief of her continuing pain problems, including the carpal tunnel syndrome. This relief began a week after the series was completed. She experienced good relief of the pain and weakness in her right arm and leg. Her sitting, standing, and walking tolerances were increased. Driving a car was easier. The stress in her marriage was easing up. Because her activity level was up, she was burning more calories and slowly losing weight. Love making with Richard was becoming less painful, less problematic, and more pleasurable. She could read her favorite novels for up to 25 or 30 minutes instead of 10. Before her pain problem began, she could read her favorite books for up to 90 minutes. She was excited about all the improvements.

She had begun a low-impact aerobics class and had signed up for the back school program at her local YMCA. Dr. Smith also suggested behavioral therapy to combat the grieving associated with her devastating pain problem. He sent her to Dr. Foreman for the behavioral therapy and stressed additional needs for pacing skills, since Sally had a past history of overdoing it in the days before her pain problem.

Dr. Smith reviewed her intake of pain medication. She was still taking 20 mg of methadone at bedtime and eight time-contingent 2-mg Dilaudid® tablets per day. He knew this was characteristic of other patients with the same problem, but decided to challenge her medication intake to ascertain whether or not her answer would be valid. He wanted to know why staying at the same opioid pain-relieving medication dosing was important to her.

Sally proceeded to give him an analysis of why the pain medication dosing remained unchanged. The basic premise was that after all the preceding treatments had produced 50% pain relief, she decided to push for more activity and more return to being the active type of person she was before the pain problem began. When she increased her activity level, she felt additional pain from latent myofascial trigger points becoming active in her mid and lower back. As the latent myofascial trigger points became active, her pain level increased. Therefore, her need for analgesic medication remained the same, but she was then at a markedly increased activity level compared to December 1992, when she stared with Dr. Smith. Dr. Smith was well aware of this phenomenon in well-motivated patients, and he felt her reasons for staying at the present level of pain medication intake were adequate.

On the more tangible side, she told Dr. Smith that before coming to see him, she really avoided going to bed with Richard, in case he was in an amorous mood. The reason for this "was because after making love, Richard would roll over and go to sleep, while she went from bed to couch to chair to floor because of pain." She said, "I love Richard dearly, but even a deep kiss gets me nervous possibly that later we would make love." Also she said, "It takes the way I feel about my femininity to a new low. Since I now have proper medication to take, I know we can make love and I know that after, I have no pain and can cuddle and bring even more closeness into our relationship. The one big advantage is I feel like a whole woman once again."

In early January 1995, she reported to Dr. Smith that the two K-Tabs® (750 mg of potassium each) at twice per day had relieved a significant amount of the cramping in both of her legs. However, when her activity level escalated, she was still plagued by leg cramps that interfered with some of the more aggressive activities, such as brisk swimming and fast, brisk walking for more than one to two blocks. Dr. Smith repeated the blood analysis for potassium. The result now was 4.4 meq/liter. This was about a mid-range reading. He therefore increased the potassium intake to five K-Tabs® per day. She was blood tested again a week later. The retest showed her to be slightly short of the top of the normal range. More importantly, the leg cramping due to swimming and brisk walking was improving. She was kept at a dose of two K-Tab® tablets three times per day after that.

During the Christmas season and in early January 1995, she went off her vitamin injections because she became too busy with all the preparations for the holidays. A month later, on 1/30/95, when she saw Dr. Smith for a follow-up evaluation, she complained of tiredness during the previous 3 weeks and feeling run down. She felt that her pain medication was losing its effectiveness. The first question he asked was, "When did you take your last vitamin shot?" Suddenly she remembered what she had done and was embarrassed to tell him she had not had a vitamin shot in about a month. He told her those complaints could be due to a number of medical problems, including being off the vitamin injections. He suggested the first treatment to try was to go back on the vitamin injections and check back with him in 3–4 weeks. She finished the visit by telling him that she had remained on the oral vitamin program. He told her that in some of the chronic pain patients, including her, a malabsorption problem prevented complete absorption of a number of the B vitamins. The B-vitamin injections guaranteed that her body was getting some of the most important B vitamins and in adequate amounts. He concluded by telling her that some doctors refer to the injection program as giving the patient an "expensive urine." It was his opinion that it was better to have an "expensive urine" than to have an expensive chronic pain problem.

When Sally came back on 2/27/95, she told Dr. Smith that he had been right about the vitamin shots. After 6 days of being back on them, she could feel the improvement in her energy and the effectiveness of her pain medication.

On her visit of 6/26/95, additional history was taken by Dr. Smith. Sally said that 50% of her chronic pain problem was either resolved or under control. Her leg cramps were 25% of what they were previously. Pain medications consisted of two time-contingent 2-mg Dilaudid® tablets every 4 hours, 10–20 mg of methadone at bedtime, and one Soma® at bedtime as needed. Occasionally she took one Soma 350® during the day for muscle spasms. Sixty-five percent of her fatigue was gone. With the help of her daughters and a disability parking sticker, she was able to do all the shopping and meal preparation. She could read her favorite novels for up to an hour. She had lost 25 of the 30 pounds she had gained after the pain problem began. The analgesic medication had been helpful in that it facilitated keeping her activity level up. Seventy percent of the weakness in her right arm and leg was either resolved or under control. She could sit, stand, or walk for up to an hour. She could drive an automobile for up to an hour before pain became problematic. The stress was 90% gone from her marriage. Making love was more pleasurable and spontaneous. The Dilaudid® did not interfere with her ability to have an orgasm.

A comprehensive physical reexamination was carried out at that visit. The results were compared to those of the original physical examination.

Dr. Smith had found the absence of the biceps and brachioradialis deep tendon reflexes on both sides; the return of the biceps reflexes showed an improvement. In the lower extremities, the knee jerks were normal and the ankle reflexes were normal on both sides. There was not much decrease in pinprick sensation when testing the dermatomes of the upper and lower extremities. He next used a goniometer to measure the passive hypertension of the left index finger metacarpophalangeal joint. It measured 80 degrees, which meant she should be rather flexible. He used a goniometer to measure the range of motion of the neck and shoulders. There was definite improvement of an additional 25% in the range of motion of the areas tested. He checked the trapezius, sternocleidomastoid, pectoralis major, and latissimus dorsi muscles. Taut bands and tenderness were noted in all these muscles, but the incidence of jump sign was down by 50%, a sign of good progress. When the right latissimus dorsi myofascial trigger point was compressed, she complained of pain radiating down the inside (side closest to the body) in the upper and lower right arm. (Even though this muscle had been previously injected, his finding would indicate additional myofascial trigger point[s] in the latissimus dorsi muscle.) Muscle testing of a number of the shoulder muscles showed improvement. Straight leg raising was positive at 65 degrees on the right and 70 degrees on the left. She complained of tight hamstring muscles on both sides and pain radiating down the side of the leg on the right (this was not a sciatic distribution). Dropping her hip and leg over the side of the table on the right showed a flexion contractor of 25 degrees on the right. When this was repeated on the left, the hip extended to neutral and then she complained of pain in the low back.

Muscle strength testing of the hip abductors (gluteus minimus, normal = 5/5 rating) revealed weakness secondary to myofascial trigger point on the right. Strength was rated at 4B/5 (the "B" stands for breakaway weakness). This means the hip was weak and gave way during the manual muscle testing. Strength of the left hip was mildly weak compared to what was expected. Muscle testing the ankle dorsiflexors showed minimal weakness on both sides. Muscle testing the extensor of the great toe showed moderate weakness on both sides. After she stood up, he checked the level of the pelvis from behind. She was noted to be 0.4 inches (1 cm) shorter on the right side. She had been wearing her 1-cm lift in the right heel to compensate for the leg length problem. When the range of motion of her lumbar spine was tested, she missed touching her toes by 7 inches because of pain in the buttock and low back. She could extend to 18 degrees. She could laterally bend 20 degrees bilaterally. When asked to perform a deep knee bend, she could do range of motion of 55% of normal. Her balance was about 65% of expected, and her strength was 70% of expected. She complained of pain in her rectus femoris muscles and patellas on both sides.

Toward the end of the physical examination, she was placed in the prone (on her belly) position on the exam table to palpate muscles along the spine on both sides. The iliocostalis thoracis and longissimus thoracis muscles were palpated from T1 to T12 on both sides. The longissimus thoracis revealed taut bands and tenderness on both sides at T4, T6, T10, and T11. Jump signs occurred when the muscle was palpated at T6 and T11 on the right and at T10–11 on the left. When pressure was applied to the right T11 myofascial trigger point, Sally complained of pain radiating up the back to her right shoulder and down the back and into her right leg. Examination of the iliocostalis thoracis showed tenderness at T3, 4, 5, 6, 8, 9, 10, and T11. When the iliocostalis thoracis myofascial trigger points at T6, 8, 9, and T11 were palpated, the tenderness response was extreme, with the patient demonstrating marked jump signs. The referral of pain from all of these was pronounced and reported in right shoulder blade, right side of the chest, right side of the upper and lower abdomen, right low back, sacroiliac joint, right buttock, and down the outside and back of the right leg to the foot.

The net result of the history and physical examination data showed that Sally was making progress in a positive direction. She continued to slowly progress in a positive direction from June 1995 to August of the same year.

On 9/3/95, she got up in the middle of the night to go to the bathroom. The room was very dark. As she got out of bed, she tripped over a suitcase that Tonya had left by the bedside. She lost her balance and began to fall. She grabbed the dresser drawer with her right hand and arm to break the fall. When this happened, she acutely twisted her right ankle, leg, buttock, and low back. The pain in her back and down her leg was excruciating. She let out a loud scream. Everybody woke up and went to see what was happening. The agony was so severe that she wet herself because she was paralyzed by the pain. Richard placed a call to Dr. Smith, who luckily was able to speak to him. Dr. Smith recommended Sally increase the dose of Dilaudid® to a maximum of three to four of the 2-mg tablets as often as every 2 hours to try to control the severe pain. Dr. Smith said to call the office in the morning and ask Ginger, his secretary, for an appointment. Sally called the next morning. Ginger told Sally there was only a short visit available the following day. She scheduled Sally for that visit and a regular visit a week later on 9/12/95.

When Sally saw Dr. Smith on 9/5/95, he noted that she was in marked to severe distress, even though she was on the increased dosing with the Dilaudid® tablets, and was walking with the use of crutches. She was not putting any weight on the right leg. He noted an ace bandage around her right knee. He inquired about the use of the bandage. She told him it was to treat some swelling that had started in the knee after the fall. It was obvious to him that the increased dosing of Dilaudid® tablets was having little effect on her current pain flare-up.

He took off the ace bandage and inspected the knee. He found it to be moderately swollen. It was very tender to the touch. Minimal movement of the knee by Dr. Smith caused a severe pain reaction, as evidenced by grimacing and shock-like reactions to her body. Because the pain was obviously severe, he decided to put her on Dilaudid® injection, to be administered by Sally to herself. He told her that the principles of drawing up the injection were the same as for the vitamin shots. The injectable Dilaudid® was 2 mg/ml. He also told her to stay on her oral Dilaudid®, which he boosted to 4-mg tablets. He recommended one to two of the 4-mg tablets every 3–4 hours. If she had breakthrough pain that was beyond what the oral Dilaudid® could control, she was to give herself from ½ to 2 mm of the Dilaudid® injection at no more than every 4 hours. He also told her to switch to the full-dose vitamin shots and to take them daily: a #1 shot on one day, a #2 shot the next, a #1 shot the next day, and so on. Dr. Smith told Ginger to schedule Sally to meet him at 11:00 a.m. at the emergency room on Saturday, 9/9/95, to have her knee aspirated. After returning home that day, Sally installed a couple of night-lights in the master bedroom and master bathroom.

On Saturday, she and Richard met Dr. Smith at the emergency room . She told him she was averaging 1½–2 ml per injection (3–4 mg) during the day and took about three to four injections per day. She was placed on a gurney and the ace bandage was taken off. The troublesome swelling was still evident. He drew up 4 ml of injectable Dilaudid® (8 mg) and injected her with it. After 30 minutes, she was feeling much less pain. He opened a sterile aspiration tray and, after preparation of the skin, used an approach from the lateral (outside) aspect of the knee), with an 18-gauge needle, to remove bloody fluid. About 30 ml of blood-tinged fluid was removed.

After the fluid was removed, he was able to perform an evaluation of the knee. His conclusion, after the examination, was that she probably sprained a ligament in the knee, with a partial tear of it. He did not think she had a torn meniscus. He wrapped the leg from mid-calf to mid-thigh with cast padding. Next he applied an ace bandage over that and then put the leg into an immobilizing knee splint. He said she would need about 3–6 weeks for the ligament tear to heal. He told her to continue her present medication program. She said her sleep was disrupted by pain. He prescribed 10-mg Elavil® tablets and told her to take two to eight tablets before retiring.

Sally next saw Dr. Smith on 9/12/95. She told him the Dilaudid® injection was being used mainly for the severe pain in her back and buttocks. The injectable Dilaudid®, combined with the stronger tablets, was giving her an average of 50% overall pain relief. Putting her leg in a splint was aggravating the back pain. He assured her the splint would be off as soon as possible. He told her to begin light weight bearing on the right foot with the assist of the crutches. He sent her to physical therapy to begin exercises in the splint. She told him the Elavil® was of no help for sleep. He prescribed 10-mg Sinequan® tablets and told her to follow the same dosage schedule as for the Elavil®.

Sally called the office on 9/19/95 and told Ginger to tell Dr. Smith that the Sinequan® was not helping. Dr. Smith phoned in a prescription for 20-mg Prozac®, with directions to take one to three capsules at bedtime.

Prozac® did not help. During the next few weeks, Dr. Smith tried her on Zoloft® at 100 mg at bedtime, Paxil®, and Luvox®, all without help.

Sally went twice per week for the physical therapy sessions, finishing up on 10/17/95. The exercises were provoking her pain problem, but the Dilaudid® injections helped her endure this very necessary part of her rehabilitation.

She next saw Dr. Smith on 10/20/95. He removed the knee splint and noted mild atrophy of the leg. Her knee was stiff from being in the splint for 7 weeks. He sent her to physical therapy, including warm pool therapy, with a note directing her therapist to work on the range of motion and strength of the right hip, knee, and ankle. Dr. Smith told Sally she could begin bearing as much weight as possible on the right leg while using the crutches.

During the period of recovery, Sally told Dr. Smith that because of the pain severity, her energy level had gone down, her sleep was disrupted, she was putting on weight again, and she felt depressed. None of the above-indicated medications had helped.

He therefore increased her prescription for 10-mg time-release Dexedrine® capsules. She was to take one to four of these capsules each morning as needed to bring her energy level up. Additionally, he told her to raise the dose of bedtime methadone to two to four tablets at bedtime for better nighttime pain control. The idea with the use of the Dexedrine® was to enhance her energy during the day, promote weight loss through energy enhancement, and tire her out enough to rest better at night. He also reminded her to take up to one to three Soma 350® tablets per night if needed to help her sleep.

The Dexedrine® combined with the other medications was working well until 11/3/95. For reasons unknown, Sally ran out of her methadone, Dilaudid® tablets, and Dilaudid® injection. About 5 hours after her last dose of Dilaudid® tablets and Dilaudid® injection, her pain began to intensify. The severity of the pain was unbelievably intense. By the sixth hour, the pain was so severe that her arms and legs began to tremble. All she could do was lie on the bed and cry and tremble. (One might think this was a case of drug withdrawal [or abstinence syndrome] in a person "addicted" to the type of medications Sally was on. It was my opinion, based on dealing with hundreds of patients of this type, that this reaction was not drug withdrawal. Sally depended on these medications to be independent and active. The two types of Dilaudid® she was using are powerful and can block much pain. When she ran out of her pain medications, including her methadone, she felt what the Dilaudid® had been blocking, and it was very severe. When pain of her type escalates this high and quickly in a chronic pain patient, it is not unusual to tremble and/or sweat because of the intensity of the pain that becomes prominent.)

Richard put in a call to Dr. Smith and explained the situation. Dr. Smith said the pharmacist would probably be available to fill a prescription on a semi-emergency basis such as this. Dr. Smith called the pharmacist and explained the situation to him. Dr. Smith issued prescriptions to cover all the medications Sally had used up, and Richard went to pick them up.

Dr. Smith told Richard that since Sally's body had used up a great deal of the Dilaudid® stored in her tissues (her system had become virtually "dry" of all opioids), he would have to start her with three of the 4-mg tablets and 8 mg of the Dilaudid® injection. The next injection would be 6 mg 2 hours later, and then she could go back to her previous dosing. By 30 minutes after the 8-mg shot Sally could tell that the pain severity was lessening noticeably. By an hour after the first shot, she had 40% pain control and the trembling had stopped. By Monday, 11/6/95, Sally was feeling much better.

When circumstances appeared to stabilize, Dr. Smith told Sally it was time to begin working on the troublesome myofascial trigger points that had been set up during her fall of 9/3/95.

On her visit of 11/16/95, he began by drawing a pain chart for her that reflected her most problematic pain area. She pointed to the areas of pain, numbness, and burning on her body, and he drew them on the chart using a different color for each symptom.

Her worst area of problem was pain on the sides of both buttocks and hip areas. She also indicated pain at the sacroiliac joint and mid buttock area on the right. He had her lie on the exam table on her left side, right arm over her head and right knee bent, with knee and leg as flat as possible. Dr. Smith could get three fingers between the lower rib margin and the top of the pelvis on her right side. When he repeated this on the left side, he could get four fingers into the same area. Sally was premedicated with 6 mg of Dilaudid® injection. Twenty minutes later, Dr. Smith began injecting the quadratus lumborum in its superficial and deep fibers, first on the right and next on the left. When he was finished, he could get four fingers in the interval between the bottom of the ribs and the top of the pelvis. When she got up, he checked the alignment of the pelvis and found it to be of equal height on both sides. This meant she would not have to use the shoe lift anymore.

A week later, on 11/23/95, 20% of the severe pain in her back was gone. Overall, Sally said she was doing a lot better. Dr. Smith referred Sally to Amy Williams, a certified myotherapist. He spoke to Amy and asked that she work only with the comprehensive program of stretching at this point and hold back on the deep tissue work for a while. He spoke to Sally and warned her that the stretching exercises would be problematic to her chronic pain problem in that they might cause pain flare-ups. These were to be expected. He told her to use a little extra Dilaudid® going into the sessions. The frequency of therapy was to be once per week. If she encountered a significant flare-up, he told her to use the injection to bring the pain under control. One of the purposes of the stretch program was to flush out and further identify more of the problematic myofascial trigger points.

At her visit of 12/7/95, Sally stated that with the use of the medications, stretch program, myofascial trigger point injection, and other factors, she felt well enough to return to work. She felt she could not return to the hectic schedule she had been on before, but perhaps her schedule could be modified to get her back to the company slowly. Her old job was available. She discussed her return to work with her old supervisor, Gladys Washington, who was more than glad to see her again. Sally told Gladys about her pain problem and the need to take medication to function. Gladys told Sally that she, Tom Packard (the managing supervisor), and Dr. Smith should get together to discuss the practicalities about Sally coming back to work and how to go about it.

At her visit of 12/17/95, Sally reported that the stretching program was helping. She told Dr. Smith that pain and resistance to full range of motion was becoming a problem in the right shoulder. When he tested the strength of the right shoulder, she was graded as follows (5/5 is normal; see Appendix 4 for muscle grading definitions):

Muscle (right side)	Grade
Biceps	4/5
Triceps	4/5
Brachialis	3+/5
Shoulder extension	4/5
Shoulder forward flexion	3+/5
Shoulder abduction	3+/5
Grip strength (JAMAR)	12 kg (normal for Sally should have been about 36 kg)
Wrist extension	3+/5

Before the myofascial trigger point injection, she was premedicated. The premedication consisted of two injections. One contained 4 mg of Dilaudid® plus 1 cc of 2% Xylocaine®. The other shot contained 35 mg of Phenergan® plus ½ cc of 2% Xylocaine®. The first set of myofascial trigger point injections was to the brachialis, coracobrachialis, and triceps 1, 2, and 3 trigger points. By the end of the injections, the Dilaudid® was wearing off and the myofascial trigger point injections were becoming too painful for her to tolerate.

Sally had arranged a conference with Dick, Gladys, Tom, and Dr. Smith. Tom and Gladys told Dr. Smith that Sally was a valuable employee and they would do all they could to get her back to work. Dr. Smith explained the nature of Sally's pain problem and the use of strong analgesics to give her enough ongoing pain relief to return to work. He told them that she would not be on the strong analgesics forever, but might need to use them for another year. He suggested they start her at 20 hours per week and add an additional 5 hours a week or as Sally could tolerate the increase in work schedule. Everyone agreed that only those at the meeting would be aware of her medications.

Sally returned to work the following week, on 1/2/96. She was glad to be back, and many of her colleagues who missed her when she left because of her pain problem were glad to see her. Sally immediately got in contact with the shops and stores she had dealt with in the past. Just getting back to work was a real emotional boost for her.

Throughout January 1996 to April 1996, the following myofascial trigger points were evaluated and injected by Dr. Smith (each time the same premedication was used): right brachioradalis; right gastrocnemius 1, 2, 3, and 4; right gluteus maximus 1, 2, and 3;

iliocostalis lumborum L1, 2, and 3; and iliopsoas 1, 2, and 3. All the myofascial trigger point injections from that group helped her in the following ways. The last three got rid of her hip flexion contractor. Some of the others either decreased her remaining shoulder and arm pain and/or relieved a great deal of her back pain.

By April 1996, she was working 40 hours a week and had lost all the weight she had gained. Her medication consumption was down to 1–2 cc of injectable Dilaudid® (mostly in the morning when painful stiffness was a problem), 4-mg time-contingent Dilaudid® tablets at one every 4 hours, and 10 mg of methadone at bedtime. The amount of premedication needed for myofascial trigger point injection had dropped to half of what she used to need.

From 5/8/96 to 6/5/96, the following additional myofascial trigger point injections were carried out: right levator scapula; longissimus thoracis at T3, 4, 6, and 11; right sacral multifidus; right pectoralis major and minor; and right scalene medius and posterior.

Her shoulder muscle strengths were repeated. It was also noted that she had 90% return to normal of the range of motion of the right shoulder.

Muscle	Grade
Biceps	5/5
Triceps	5/5
Brachialis	4+/5
Shoulder extension	4+/5
Shoulder forward flexion	4+/5
Shoulder abduction	4+/5
Grip strength (JAMAR)	25 kg (normal for Sally should have been about 36 kg)
Wrist extension	4+/5

From 7/11/96 to 8/15/96, she had the final series of myofascial trigger point injections: right peroneus longus, right and left piriformis 1 and 2, right rhomboid major, right serratus anterior, right serratus posterior superior, right supraspinatus, and right vastus lateralis 4.

By the time of her visit to Dr. Smith on 9/17/96, she was taking three to six Vicodin® per day and no more. She looked forward to the day when she would be off all pain medications, but realized that she may have to be on small doses of a medication like Vicodin® for the rest of her life. Dr. Smith told her to stay on all the oral vitamins, minerals, and hormones that she had been told to take for the rest of her life. He tapered her to a half-strength vitamin shot program with one day between injections and planned to keep her on those an additional 2 years. He would then taper her to quarter-dose shots for an additional year, and then she would go off the vitamin shots. However, he told her she might have to be on the vitamin shots for the rest of her life.

SUMMARY OF SIGNIFICANT POINTS IN THIS CHAPTER

One of the main points in this case study is to demonstrate that as patients with severe and/ or progressive fibromyalgia syndrome/MPS/posttraumatic hyperirritability syndrome recover, the dose of medication needed for recovery may escalate as physical recovery occurs (or it needs to escalate to help them recover). This does not mean the person has become tolerant or addicted to the medication.

This issue addressed in this chapter is that as increasing physical demands are placed on a painful body (i.e., as rehabilitation is undertaken, either at a physical therapist's office or elsewhere), the need for analgesic medication may be increased. The reliance on opioids usually decreases or ceases as rehabilitation is completed.

BIBLIOGRAPHY

Burnette, J. and Ayoub, M. (1989). Cumulative trauma disorders. I. The problem, *Pain Management,* 2, 196–209.

Elson, I. (1990). The jolt syndrome. Muscle dysfunction following low-velocity impact, *Pain Management,* 3, 317–326.

Kendall, F. and Kendall, E. (1963). *Muscle Testing and Function,* 3rd ed., p. 12.

Margoles, M. (1983). Stress neuromyelopathic pain syndrome (SNPS): report of 333 patients, *Journal of Neurological and Orthopedic Surgery,* 4, 317–322.

Simons, D.G. (1996). Clinical and etiological update of myofascial pain from trigger points, *Journal of Musculoskeletal Pain,* 4, 93–121.

Travell, G. and Simons, D.G. (1992). Post-traumatic hyperirritability syndrome (PTHS), in *Myofascial Pain and Dysfunction: The Trigger Point Manual,* Vol. 2, Williams and Wilkins, Baltimore, p. 545.

Vecchiet, L., Dragnai, L., de Gigontina, P., Obletter, G., and Giamberardino, M. (1993). Experimental referred pain and hyperalgesia from muscles in humans, in *New Trends in Referred Pain and Hyperalgesia,* No. 27, Series in Pain Research and Clinical Management, Vecchiet, L., Able-Fessard, D., Lindblom, U., and Giamberardino, M.A. (Eds.), Elsevier Science Publishers, Amsterdam, pp. 239–249.

APPENDIX 1: VITAMIN INJECTION PROGRAM INSTRUCTIONS

The general approach to using vitamin injections for chronic pain patients with MPS is as follows. The patient is taught the quarter dose of syringe #1. After a week or two at that dose, the quarter dose of syringe #2 is taught. Injections are given in an alternating fashion: #1 injection, then skip a day, #2 injection, skip a day, #1 injection, skip a day, etc. This is called the primary program. If nerve regeneration pain flare-ups occur at that dosing, the injections are stopped for a week and then started at 4-day intervals between the shots. When the quarter-dose shots can be done with the primary program for a month, the patient is progressed to the primary program using the half-strength doses.

Full-strength doses are used daily (#1 one day, #2 the next, #1 the next, etc.) for 10–14 days each time the patient is injured, reinjured, has an accident, or suffers trauma.

Separate syringes are used for different components because combining all ingredients would cause some to bind to each other and become inactivated (of no medical benefit).

None of the vitamin injections should be self-administered until the patient has been shown and told how to proceed. No harm will result from accidentally injecting one of these vitamin products into a vein. Fidgeting about small mounts of air in the syringe (up to as much as $1/2$ cc) is unnecessary and if injected will cause no harm.

1. Remove the bottle(s) from storage. Protection from light and temperatures above 110 degrees is recommended. Storage in the refrigerator is not necessary.
2. Open one of the alcohol skin swabs (tear it at the middle, not at the end).
3. Thoroughly coat the top of each bottle to be used.
   a. Be certain to eliminate any contamination of the rubber before inserting the needle into the top of the bottle.
4. Remove the syringe from its package.
   a. Use a new syringe with attached needle, swab, and separate needle for injection for each injection session.
   b. Peel apart the wrapper and pull the syringe with attached needle out of the wrapper.
   c. You will be using a 3-cc syringe, with any of a number of needles that commonly come attached to it.

    d. Make sure the needle is screwed securely onto the syringe by twisting the protected needle until it locks into place.

    e. Remove the plastic protector from the end of the needle so that you will be able to pressurize the bottle(s) as indicated in #5 below.

5. Each bottle must now be pressurized by injecting air into it with the syringe. Put air into the syringe by pulling back the plunger by the amount of air needed, which may be $2/_{10}$, $5/_{10}$, or 1 cc. Insert the needle into the middle of the top of each vitamin bottle, and inject the air into the bottle. Continue to do this with each bottle until pressurized as indicated below. Bottles are pressurized at each session. The needle pressurizing the bottle penetrates the rubber on the bottle by only $1/_4$ inch. Hold the bottle on a flat, secure surface while pressurizing it.

    Pressurize the bottles in the following order:

Syringe #1	Riboflavin
	B-complex (B-Plex 100)
	Xylocaine® (lidocaine) or Novocain® (procaine)
	Dexpanthenol
Syringe #2	Hydroxocobalamin
	Folic acid or Folvite
	Riboflavin
	Dexpanthenol

6. Then draw up the amounts of vitamin solution indicated for the specific syringe number. Draw up from the bottles in the reverse order that they were pressurized.

    a. Take the bottle to be used and turn it upside down.

    b. With the bottle upside down, insert the needle $1/_4$ inch through the rubber and draw up the recommended amount of solution.

    c. Do this until all the components of the injection have been drawn into the syringe.

7. Take the small injection needle out of its container. Change needles by unscrewing the needle attached to the syringe. Then screw the small-gauge injection needle onto the syringe until it locks into place.

8. Swab the injection site with the alcohol swab and inject.

9. After the injection is complete, pull the needle out and, using the swab, put pressure on the injection site for a minute to decrease bruising.

APPENDIX 2: WHERE TO GET INJECTABLE VITAMINS

Because of FDA intervention and changes in demand, the B-complex injection products listed below are not always available from the distributor listed. You may have to contact a number of those listed in order to obtain the desired product.

Product	Brand name	Distributor
Riboflavin (B2), 50 mg/ml	Riboflavin	Santa Clara Drug (6)
Dexpanthenol (B5)	Dexpanthenol, 250 mg/ml	Merit (1)
		Family Pharmacy (9)
		Monterey Bay Pharmacy (10)
		Schein (3)
		McGuff (7)
Folic acid injection (Bc)	Folvite, 5 mg/ml	Any pharmacy
		IDE (2)

Product	Brand name	Distributor
Hydroxocobalamin (B12)	1000 µg/ml	Santa Clara Drug (6)
B-Plex 100 (30 cc) Contents per cc:	B-complex-100 and others	Merit (1) McGuff (7) Schein (3)
Thiamine (B1)	100 mg	
Riboflavin (B2)	2 mg	
Pyridoxine (B6)	2 mg	Family Pharmacy (9)
Panthenol (B5)	2 mg	
Niacinamide (B3)	100 mg	Monterey Bay Pharmacy (10)
27-gauge 1-inch needles		Family Pharmacy (9) Smith (5) Monterey Bay Pharmacy (10)
30-gauge 1-inch needles	In brand name from BD	Family Pharmacy (9) Smith (5) Monterey Bay Pharmacy (10)

(1) Merit Pharmaceuticals
2611 San Fernando Road
Los Angeles, CA 90065
213-227-4831

(2) Interstate Drug Exchange, Inc.
1500 New Horizons Blvd.
Amityville, NY 11701
1-800-626-DRUG

(3) Henry Schein, Inc.
5 Harbor Park Drive
Port Ishington, NY 11050
1-800-772-4346

(4) Obtain through local drugstore

(5) Smith + Nephew MPL
(orders of 1000 or more)
1820 West Roscoe St.
Chicago, IL 60657
312-248-3810

(6) Santa Clara Drug
2453 Forest Ave.
Santa Clara, CA 95128
408-296-5015

(7) McGuff Pharmaceuticals
3617 McArthur Blvd.
Suite 507
Santa Ana, CA 92704
714-545-2491

(8) Acuderm Inc.
(will fill orders of 100 or more)
5370 N.W. 35 Terrace Blvd.
Ft. Lauderdale, FL 33309
1-800-327-0015

(9) Family Pharmacy
2053 Lincoln Ave.
San Jose, CA 95125
800-939-DRUG

(10) Monterey Bay Pharmacy
798 Cass Street
Monterey, CA 93940
408-373-8888

APPENDIX 3: POSTTRAUMATIC HYPERIRRITABILITY SYNDROME

The term "post-traumatic hyperirritability syndrome" (Travell and Simons, 1992, p. 545) was introduced to identify a limited number of patients with myofascial pain who exhibit marked hyperirritability of the sensory nervous system and of existing trigger points (myofascial trigger points). This syndrome follows a major trauma, such as an automobile accident, a fall, or a severe blow to the body, that is apparently sufficient to injure the sensory modulation mechanisms of the spinal cord or brain stem. The patients have constant pain, which may be exacerbated by the vibration of a moving vehicle, the slamming of a door, a loud noise (such as a firecracker at close range), jarring (bumping into something or being jostled), mild thumps (a pat on the back), severe pain (a trigger point injection), prolonged physical activity, and emotional stress (such as anger). Recovery from such stimulation is slow. Even with mild exacerbations, it may take the patient many minutes or hours to return to the baseline pain level. Severe exacerbation of pain may require days, weeks, or longer to return to baseline.

These patients almost always give a history of having coped well in life prior to their injury, having paid no more attention to pain than did their friends and family. They were no more sensitive to these stimuli than other persons. From the moment of the initial trauma, however, pain suddenly became the focus of life. They must pay close attention to the avoidance of strong sensory stimuli and must limit activity, because even mild to moderate muscular stress or fatigue intensifies the pain. Efforts to increase exercise tolerance may be self-defeating. Such patients, who suffer greatly, are poorly understood and, through no fault of their own, are difficult to help.

In these patients, the sensory nervous system behaves much as the motor system does when the spinal cord has lost supraspinal inhibition. In the latter, a strong sensory input of almost any kind can activate nonspecific motor activity for an extended period of time. Similarly, in these patients, a strong sensory input can increase the excitability of the nociceptive system for long periods. In addition, these patients may show lability of the autonomic nervous system with skin temperature changes and swelling that resolve with inactivation of regional trigger points. Since routine medical examination of these suffering patients fails to show any organic cause for their symptoms, they are often relegated to "crock" status.

Any additional fall or motor vehicle accident that would ordinarily be considered minor can severely exacerbate the hyperirritability syndrome for years. Unfortunately, with successive traumas, the individual may become increasingly vulnerable to subsequent trauma. A frequent finding is a series of motor vehicle accidents over a period of several years.

Similar phenomena have been described as the cumulative trauma disorder (Burnett and Ayoub, 1989), the stress neuromyelopathic pain syndrome (Margoles, 1983), and the jolt syndrome (Elson, 199) .

APPENDIX 4: TABLE OF MUSCLE GRADING (KENDALL AND KENDALL, 1963)

Test performance	Percent	Word and letter		Numeral
The ability to hold the test position against gravity and maximum pressure, or the ability to move the part into test position and hold against gravity and maximum pressure	100	Normal	N	5
	95	Normal–	N–	5–
Same as above except holding against moderate pressure	90	Good+	G+	4+
	80	Good	G	4
Same as above except holding against minimum pressure	70	Good–	G–	4–
	60	Fair+	F+	3+
The ability to hold the test position against gravity, or the ability to move the part into test position and hold against gravity	50	Fair	F	3
The gradual release from test position against gravity, or the ability to move the part toward test position against gravity almost to completion or to completion with slight assistance, or the ability to complete the arc of motion with gravity lessened	40	Fair–	F–	3–

Test performance	Percent	Word and letter		Numeral
The ability to move the part through partial arc of motion with gravity lessened: moderate arc, 30% or poor+; small arc, 20% or poor	30	Poor+	P+	2+
To avoid moving a patient into gravity-lessened position, these grades may be estimated on the basis of the amount of assistance given during antigravity test movements: a 30% or poor+ muscle requires moderate assistance, a 20% or poor muscle requires more assistance	20	Poor	P	2
In muscles that can be seen or palpated, a feeble contraction may be felt in the muscle or the tendon may become prominent during the muscle contraction, but there is no visible movement of the part	10	Poor−	P−	2−
	5	Trace	T	1
No contraction felt in the muscle	0	Zero	0	0

GLOSSARY OF TERMS FOR MYOFASCIAL PAIN SYNDROME*

The diagnosis of myofascial trigger points (TrPs) depends on the history and on its confirmation by physical examination. There is poor agreement among authors as to the most appropriate diagnostic criteria. Numerous clinical features have been associated with myofascial TrPs, but only recently have interrater reliability studies been reported that give some guidelines. No satisfactory laboratory or imaging test is currently available for making the diagnosis of myofascial TrPs.

Clinical features.   Several clinical features are commonly associated with the diagnosis of myofascial TrPs. These include a confusing mixture of sensory and motor phenomena:

- *History of spontaneous localized pain associated with acute overload or chronic overuse of the muscle.* The mildest symptoms are caused by latent TrPs that cause no pain but cause some degree of functional disability. More severe involvement results in pain related to position of the muscle or muscular activity. The most severe level involves intermittent or continuous pain at rest.

   The precise pattern of pain described by the patient is THE most valuable clue for finding where the TrP is located. Recognizing the pattern of pain as characteristic of a particular muscle tells the clinician where to look for the TrP or TrPs that are responsible for at least part of the patient's pain.
- *Palpable band.* A cord-like band of fibers is palpable in the involved muscle. This band helps to locate spot tenderness, but it may be inaccessible because of overlying muscles or thick [or tense] subcutaneous tissue. Its tendon attachment may evidence the spot tenderness of enthesopathy.
- *Spot tenderness.* This involves a VERY tender and VERY small spot which is found in a palpable band when the band is accessible to palpation. The sensitivity of this spot [the TrP] is increased by increasing the tension on the muscle fibers of the taut band.
- *Jump sign.* Pressure on the spot of tenderness causes the patient to physically react to the pain with a spontaneous exclamation or movement. This finding gives an

---

* This material is quoted from Simons' (1996) diagnostic criteria for MPS.

indication of the degree of spot tenderness, but the results are strongly dependent on the amount of pressure exerted by the examiner

- *Pain recognition.* Digital pressure on a tender spot [the TrP] or needle injection of an active locus induces at least some of the pain of which the patient complains, and the patient recognizes it as his or her pain. This finding by definition identifies an active TrP.

- *Twitch response.* The local twitch response is a transient contraction of the fibers of the taut band associated with a TrP. It can be elicited by vigorous snapping palpation of the taut band [when accessible] at the TrP or by needle penetration of an active locus in the TrP. The latter is an important phenomenon for assuring effective injection of a TrP. Snapping palpation is effective only in a taut band that is in a sufficiently superficial and accessible muscle. It also requires much skill.

- *Elicited referred pain and tenderness.* An active TrP refers pain in a pattern characteristic of that muscle. The pain is often not located in the immediate vicinity of the TrP, but is referred to a distant site. On initial examination, the patient is often surprised at the location and tenderness of the TrP. Eighty-five percent of the reported pain patterns project distally The deep tissue nature of the referred pain that is described by patients is substantiated by Vecchiet et al. (1993), whose study demonstrated the persistence of deep tenderness in the reference zone for a day or more after injection of hypertonic saline into a proximal limb muscle. Subcutaneous tissue is found to be more tender than the skin over both TrPs and FM tender points.

  Unfortunately, when the referred pain is elicited by the application of pressure to a tender location it is a non-specific finding. Whether one elicits only local pain, referred pain, or reaches pain tolerance depends upon the amount of pressure applied. Elicited referred pain did not clearly distinguish latent TrPs from active TrPs. Latent TrPs simply require more pressure.

- *Restricted range of motion.* Full-stretch range of motion of the affected muscle is restricted by pain. This restriction is relieved by the release of the palpable taut bands through inactivation of associated TrPs.

  The importance of this finding is relatively muscle-specific because it varies considerably from muscle to muscle; therefore, it is more useful as a diagnostic criterion in some muscles than in others. When movement is markedly restricted, measurement of increase in range of motion becomes a useful objective measure of progress. Relatively inexpensive, accurate, and convenient electronic inclinometers are now available for measuring range of motion. The restricted range of motion of patients with active TrPs provides an objective diagnostic distinction from patients with FM who characteristically show joint hypermobility (emphasis by the author).

- *Muscle weakness.* Clinically, the patient is unable to develop normal strength on static testing, as compared to testing of a contralateral uninvolved muscle. Static strength is measurable using a force meter. Dynamic testing of muscles with active TrPs is just beginning to be explored using surface electromyographic [EMG] techniques. The involved muscle may initially evidence fatigue, which is indicated by increased average amplitude of integrated EMG. Reduced mean spectral frequency and reduced forcefulness of movement look promising as additional measures of "initial fatigue" in pilot studies.

24 Louise's Story: Misunderstandings About Postoperative Analgesic Dosing

Louise T.

I am a 54-year-old housewife. As a result of several automobile accidents and falls while horseback riding during my childhood, I have lived with a lot of pain most of my life. For the past 22 years, as the result of another accident, I have lived with constant, severe intractable pain with nearly total body involvement. During this time, I have also had to undergo four surgeries. During the postoperative period of the last three surgeries, I have had a terrible experience because the doctors would not prescribe adequate pain medication for me. As a result of this, my postoperative recovery was traumatic and slow each time.

The first surgery involved three surgical sites, including each foot and one wrist. I had already been in excruciating and constant pain in most of my body for 9 years when I entered the hospital for the surgery. During all of those years, I had never had a prescription for pain medication that provided me any relief and in fact had taken very little pain medication at all during the previous 9 years. I was not taking any pain medication prior to the surgery. Before I entered the hospital, this was discussed with the surgeon and the anesthesiologist. I also explained to them that even although I was a small woman (5 feet tall and 103 pounds), I had a high tolerance to drugs. They assured me they would make sure that I was kept comfortable after the surgery.

During the postoperative time that I was in the recovery room, I was well medicated, but after that I was in trouble. About 3 hours after I left the recovery room, I began asking for more medication for the pain. I was given an injection but experienced little relief. I waited several hours, trying to be positive and suffer in silence, a behavior I had learned early in my life. I was given more injections throughout the night, but they were not strong enough to relieve the pain, even slightly. I could not sleep and had to concentrate very hard on my deep breathing and progressive relaxation techniques to maintain mentally and emotionally. I had been doing self-hypnosis and other relaxation techniques for many years to help me live with the constant, unrelenting, intractable pain. At that time (1984), it had been 9 years since I had slept any longer than a few minutes. I suffered from serious sleep deprivation, and that was another factor of my complicated pain problems.

The day after the surgery, I found out my doctor had left town after my surgery and had not left an order for an increase in the pain medication. By then, I was emotionally and physically drained because of the pain from the surgery and the flare-up of the preexisting pain was so severe. I was so traumatized and exhausted I felt like I would totally lose control and have a breakdown and not be able to come out of it. It was just beyond my comprehension that I could be so neglected and abused postoperatively. Finally, a nurse made the effort to call the doctor at his hotel, and he gave an order for a different, stronger medication. It gave me a little relief, but not a significant amount. Later that night, they began giving me oral medication instead of injections. The oral medication gave me no relief.

It was not only the lack of enough pain and sleep medication that traumatized me, but also the lack of caring from the doctor, nurses, and other staff. No one seemed capable of grasping the severity of my pain problem, and it seemed to me that they did not take me seriously. I had been dealing with the problem of trying to verbalize how much pain I was enduring for most of my life (by this time I was 42 years old). I grew up in an environment where people did not complain about things and just dealt with their difficulties without making an issue of them. There was never much verbal communication. For me, it seemed that if I was strong and stoic, people did not think I was hurting a lot. If I broke down and cried or got angry and spoke out, people acted like I was just a complainer and then disregarded me. It was very degrading to be in such excruciating, constant pain and not be believed about it.

My stay in the hospital was for 4 days, even though people with similar surgeries often stay fewer days. By the time I left, I was completely exhausted, humiliated, and an emotional wreck. I never did sleep while there and had only a slight amount of pain relief once I left the recovery room.

My recovery from the surgery was long and slow. For the next 10 years, I could not stand on my feet without having shoes on, with thick, soft insoles and soles. I could never go barefoot. I think if I had been given enough pain medication postoperatively so I could have slept and relaxed, perhaps my healing would have been sooner and I would not have been so traumatized. My body could not heal well after the surgery with the sleep deprivation and the physical and mental stress.

In 1989, I had to face the fact that I needed to undergo another spinal surgery. After seeing the CAT scan pictures and the results of the nerve conduction studies, and consulting with several specialists, I knew surgery was definitely necessary. I had been seeing Dr. S., a chronic pain specialist, for almost a year, and since he was an orthopedic surgeon, he was going to assist the neurosurgeon doing the surgery. He assured me he would make sure I had adequate pain medication after the surgery. After the terrible experience after previous surgeries, I was very reluctant to consent to this surgery but was convinced it was medically necessary.

The neurosurgeon, Dr. G., and Dr. S. practiced in the New Jersey area, and I lived in northern New Jersey, so I had to have the surgery in a hospital in New Jersey. It meant that I would again be in the hospital alone, with my husband miles away at work in northern New Jersey. After much conversation, both doctors told me that I would be given adequate pain medication postoperatively and that I would be listened to and believed if I expressed a need for more medication than was usual for other patients. They said the preexisting pain situation would be considered. At that time, it had been 14 years that I had lived with the constant, unrelenting pain in most of my body. The only way I could try to describe it was to say that it felt like a migraine or a giant toothache in all of my body, the kind of toothache you have when nerves are affected. The only problem with that was if the person hearing about it had never experienced severe nerve pain or a migraine, they had no frame of reference for understanding. This often was the problem when I was dealing with doctors and nurses.

Prior to entering the hospital, I had been taking some pain medication, but it really did not provide me with a measurable amount of relief. I kept taking it, hoping it would help, but to no avail.

The day before the surgery, I checked into the hospital. The next morning, I went into surgery, and when I woke up I was in my room. My usual pain flared up to an unbelievable level, along with the added pain from the surgery. I began asking for more medication. Guess what? Again, they refused to give me adequate medication.

I suffered that day and night, unable to have even the edge taken off the pain, and therefore, I could not even doze, let alone sleep. The next day, Dr. G. came into my room. I told him I was in intolerable pain. His reply was that he had a "standard medication order" for "all" of his surgical patients and it worked for "most" of them. I explained that it was definitely not adequate for me. He said that was too bad, he was not going to change it, and he was on his way out of town to spend the weekend at his beach house. Then he left. Later, I asked several nurses about his method of prescribing medication for his patients, and they all told me the same thing. He had a standard medication order, the same for all of his surgical patients. Of course, that is not what he told me before the surgery or I would have gone to a different surgeon. I suppose I had reason for a lawsuit against him, but I am not the type of person to do that. Perhaps in retrospect, I should have.

After Dr. G. left my room, I telephoned Dr. S. He told me that he was also leaving town for several days. I told him I was in trouble and really needed help with my pain medication. He ignored my comments, said my voice sounded great, and hung up. I was devastated. Here I was again, postoperatively, in such intolerable pain. I thought I would die, and not one person was willing to do a thing to help me. I tried to keep myself calm and rest, even though I couldn't sleep. I asked repeatedly to see a doctor, but my requests were refused. The second night after the surgery, in the middle of the night, my medication was decreased again, from injections to one pill. The dosage was less than I had been taking daily before the surgery.

I telephoned my husband at four in the morning and told him to come and get me out of the hospital. I might as well be at home where at least I had a supportive husband. He arrived at the hospital early and stayed with me until I was released. My requests to see a doctor still were not accommodated, and they released me from the hospital without letting me ever see a doctor. I had never been released after surgery without an examination by a doctor.

By this time, I was very nearly out of my mind. I was totally exhausted, due to never sleeping since the surgery, and emotionally destroyed. I could not stop crying. I am sure all of the stress postoperatively again interfered with the healing of my body and caused the long, slow recovery. Because of the lack of medical care and the emotional abuse, I probably did not improve as much after the surgery as I might have.

After we got home from the hospital (a long, difficult journey in my condition), my husband called Dr. S.'s wife and found out he was there and had never gone out of town. After hearing of the condition I was in, he wrote a prescription for injections of morphine for me. My husband had to then drive all the way back up to New Jersey, get the prescription, drive to the hospital to get it filled, and then drive all the way back home. It took him 5 hours to do that, and I was home alone while he did it. All of this could have been avoided if Dr. S. had notified the hospital that he had not left town after all. He should have examined me and been aware of the condition I really was in at the time before I left the hospital.

After I began to use the morphine injections, I was able to relax enough to sleep. Within a week, I was sleeping from 8 to 14 hours a night, the first normal sleep I had in the past 14 years.

In 1994, I unfortunately had to face the necessity of another surgery. Since I had been doing an aggressive physical therapy program in the swimming pool the past several years, I had been able to rehabilitate my body and was in better condition overall than I had been in for many years. The strong pain medication Dr. S. prescribed for me daily helped to facilitate the physical therapy regime and kept the constant, intractable pain to a more tolerable level. Because I was stronger, I hoped the surgery would go well for me.

As before with the previous surgeries, I discussed at length with the surgeon and anesthesiologist my long history of pain problems. I asked them to talk to Dr. S. to help them understand the complexity of my situation. They agreed and said they would get input from him to help with my postoperative pain management. It was decided that after the surgery I would be using a machine that dispenses pain medication as needed by the patient and is operated by the patient. I spent a great deal of time talking with them. I asked them repeatedly if I would really be able to use enough medication to keep me comfortable, even if it was a lot more than other patients used. They said that I would be in control of the quantity and could use it whenever I needed. When I felt the doctors did understand my special needs, and I understood what the surgery would entail, I agreed to proceed with it.

I awoke from the surgery in my room and, of course, feeling terrible. A few hours later, they connected the pain medication machine to me so I could self-administer the medication. I used it throughout the night and was able to sleep a few hours. The next day, the nurses said they would be getting me up out of bed to walk. When I tried to get up, I had excruciating pain and complete instability in my hips, groin, lumbar-sacroiliac joint, and low back. Those areas could not bear my weight and enable me to stand up. I had experienced this problem for many of the past 19 years, and it had kept me from being able to stand, sit, or walk for much of that time. I knew after talking to the surgeon that the position I had been placed in during the surgery had reinjured those areas of my body. That gave me another major problem and added pain that other women who have similar surgery do not encounter. Several of the nurses attending to me also were shocked to see how much more swollen and bruised my body was from the surgery than anyone they had seen before.

I began to need more pain medication than the machine would dispense. I observed that the strength of the medication was less than the medicine I had been using at home before the surgery. I was supposed to be able to get what I needed from the machine, but it was not programmed to give me enough. Here I was again, in more pain than other patients and more disability because of the surgery. And again the doctors and nurses did not understand the severity of my problems. They kept telling me that I was already using more pain medication than other people use and that it should certainly be enough for me. The doctor told me one of his nurses had used the machine after her surgery and had been so drugged that she slept all day and night for 3 days and "didn't feel a thing." I could not understand why he still refused to give me as much as I needed. I was still in so much pain that I could not sleep, and the sleep deprivation was damaging to me. I was exhausted and an emotional wreck, and I am a very strong person.

I requested an examination by an orthopedic surgeon I had consulted previously. He gave me a thorough physical examination and concurred with me. The position I had been placed in for the surgery had, in fact, reinjured those weak areas of my body. He prescribed total bed rest until those injuries were calmed down. It was 2 months after the surgery before I could finally stand and walk a few steps. It took longer than that for me to be able to sit.

Throughout my hospital stay, I struggled with the constant, acute pain and not enough pain medication. I had been using more on my analgesic dose at home before the surgery than they were giving me in the hospital. I was also suffering from intense headaches because my neck was also reinjured from the position I was in during the surgery.

The doctor and nurses did not seem to be able to grasp the complexity and severity of my physical problems. They were so used to their routine with patients who were only dealing with postoperative pain — patients who were feeling fine when they entered the hospital, had their surgery, got up and walked that day or the next, sat in a chair to eat, and then went home in a day or two after the surgery and resumed their usual life. The surgeon who did my surgery told me about his wife having surgery and then going home and mowing the lawn 2 days later. This is the type of patient he and the nurses were familiar with, but I did not fit that profile. Instead of being understanding and compassionate, it seemed to me that they were just inconvenienced by me because I had special needs. I was in so much more pain than other patients and unable to take care of myself. Since I could only lie in bed, I needed more help. I could not fend for myself at all. I could not even be propped up to eat. I could not even reach the tray to get the food, and no one would assist me. Fortunately, I was in the hospital in northern New Jersey where we lived, and my husband was able to be with me for several hours during the day.

Again, I could not understand why I was being misunderstood and neglected by the staff. I was in the hospital and obviously very miserable. It seemed that everyone's usual "routine" was more important than "the care of individual patients."

Most women who have similar surgery leave the hospital in 2 or 3 days. After 8 days, even though I still had a catheter in my bladder through an abdominal hole and I was nonambulatory and physically not ready to leave the hospital, I was released. It was because the insurance company refused to allow any more hospital time.

My husband was nervous about taking care of me in this condition, but it was good to be home in my own bed, and I was able to go back to my usual pain medication, with Dr. S. supervising the dosage. I was finally able to get more pain relief, and I started sleeping better.

The surgeon came to my home the next week to remove the catheter and examine me. After that, I had a portable commode placed up against my bed, and my husband would help me get off the bed and onto it. I used that until I was able to stand up and walk, 2 months after the surgery.

After this surgery, as with the others, my postoperative time was painful, traumatic, and physically and emotionally exhausting. My healing was slow and recovery time was extremely long. It was impossible for my body to begin healing after surgery with the level of trauma I suffered and inadequate pain medication and sleep deprivation. Some of it could have been avoided if the surgeons and anesthesiologists had been more responsible and understanding of my entire physical situation. They were always treating me as though the surgery performed was the only thing to consider. It was not. I have been living with complex, painful physical abnormalities for most of my life. These have all been aggravated, and they all flare up and become even more painful after the surgeries. To not consider this and realize the existence of the added pain I suffer with has been beyond my ability to comprehend.

Editors' note. The problem that Louise shares addresses patient individuality. Had her various surgeons listened to her reasons for additional postoperative analgesic medication, her recovery after each surgical procedure would have been reduced by one-half her usual recovery time.

25 Nina: The Use of Potent Opioids in a Complex Chronic Pain Patient

Michael S. Margoles, M.D., Ph.D.

HIGHLIGHTS OF THE CASE

- 1986: Rear-end auto collision
- 1994: Worked 60+ hours per week and aggravated the residual pain from the 1986 auto accident
  11/94: Enters Selogram program
- 3/13/95: Garage door strikes her between shoulder blades
- 9/11/95: Dr. Bojeff performs radiofrequency rhizotomy at right C3, 4, 5, and 6
- 2/2/96: Progressive neurodegeneration noted
- 3/7/96: Rear-end auto collision
- 5/9/96: Marital stress due to pain problem

The following is background information that occurred before this patient's readmission to my pain program on 11/18/94.

This patient had been originally seen by me in 1986 for residuals of an automobile accident. Her old chart material had unfortunately been disposed of because of the length of time between 1986 and her readmission to my program in 1994.

The patient reconstructed her 1986 injury. She was stopped at a stoplight in a right turn lane. She was alone and had her seat belt on in a 1984 Pontiac Firebird. Another car going an estimated 20–25 miles per hour struck her car from behind. After the impact, she banged her head against the headrest; she had her head turned left to watch for oncoming traffic. The patient reported that there was no damage to her car. Five hours after the injury, she began to experience pain in the right occipital area. The date of the injury was 1/7/86. The accident occurred on Wednesday, and she saw a physician at a walk-in clinic in Cupertino, California, on Friday. He prescribed 6 weeks of physical therapy, which provided her with no help. She was also sent to an orthopedic surgeon who provided her with no help. She then began to see Budd Fordyce, D.C. He was able to provide her with some relief.

1-57444-103-5/99/$0.00+$.50
© 1999 by CRC Press LLC

The patient stated that as of April of 1986, she was able to perform no work at all. She began in my pain program in July of 1986. She had pain in the neck area extending to T5 on the right side and numbness in the right arm. After the initial history and physical, the patient was diagnosed as having a posttraumatic myofascial pain syndrome. Routine therapy for this type of problem was administered according to the textbook material from Janet G. Travell and David G. Simons (Travell and Simons, 1983). This consisted of treating the perpetuating factors, replacing vitamin factors, stretch and spray, and myofascial trigger point injections to the neck. Medication treatment consisted of Vicodin® and Soma® at no more than one of each tablet every 4 hours. The patient stated that other medications had been tried before, but the combination of Vicodin® and Soma® provided her with best relief. The Vicodin® and Soma® were stopped in May of 1988.

The patient stated that she was off work for several months and took a year to get back to full-time work after treatment began in my program. She stated that in August of 1988, she was able to return to work. She stated that she was discharged from therapy in my program as of August of 1988. The patient stated that following discharge from the program, she still had pain every day. She would take Tylenol® to medicate for the residual pain. She was able to get back to full-time work and regular activities but was never able to return to hard aerobic workouts, which she had been doing frequently before the automobile accident. In early 1994, she was able to return to weight training. This patient stated that she kept getting better every year following the combined therapy of Dr. Hondiman and myself.

CHIEF COMPLAINT

The patient stated that in 1993, she obtained a job that made her work so hard and so many hours that she eventually began to experience a flare-up of her old pain problem and burnout in the months prior to seeing me in November of 1994. When she was seen on 11/18/94, her chief complaint was pain in the neck, back, and right arm for 1 month.

HISTORY OF PRESENT ILLNESS

The patient was 40 years old at that time, and she stated that her job had ridiculous hours. She stated that every calendar quarter she had a project that went to 60 hours a week and that the overtime was flaring up her pain. She had seen a local medical doctor who gave her Naprosyn®, which helped with mobility but gave no significant pain relief. She stated that she had recurrent pain since the auto accident in 1986. "Neck, back, and right arm pain 'went bonkers' 1 month ago." She stated that 3–4 weeks prior to November of 1994, she began to lose mobility in the right arm and neck. She had to stop her usual workouts for 1 month before seeing me. Her present vitamin program consisted of calcium and a B stress vitamin. She appeared to be in moderate distress.

REVIEW OF SYSTEMS

In the Global Activity Assessment Test (a copy is provided as part of the sample intake packet at the end of this chapter), she indicated that of all the activities she was performing, she had a 50% reduction in sports activities. Otherwise, she was performing up to the 80–100% mark in most of the other 13 activities evaluated. She said that her pain woke her up from sleep at night once; she found that her sleep was restless and that she had to take Benadryl® on occasion because she had difficulty falling asleep. In the Physiologic Dysfunction Question-naire (also part of the sample intake packet at the end of this chapter), she indicated significant problems with energy, such as decreased energy, tires easily, wakes up tired, gets tired by afternoon, does not tolerate stress well, cannot work as hard as she used to, and cannot work as much as she used to. She indicated weakness in the right arm and weakness of the back muscles. She also noted pain up and down the spinal area. In the Work and Employment Status part of the form, she stated she was doing her regular work full time and was working 40+ hours per week. She had been employed in her present position for 2 years, for a total of 9 years with the company. The reason she had to cut back on some of the work was pain in the neck, although she had not lost any time from work. She listed her occupation as a marketing communications manager. In the Provocative Activity Test, she checked off sometimes when she is not doing anything, rainy weather, exposure to cold, sitting, driving a car, lying on her back or belly, bending forward to brush her teeth, bending down to pick up something, bending her head from front to back, going down stairs, taking a deep breath, fatigue, and emotional stress or anxiety.

Under surgeries, she indicated tonsils in 1960, wisdom teeth in 1971, and a radical hysterectomy in 1988 with removal of uterus and both ovaries. The radical hysterectomy was performed because of a cancerous lesion in the cervix.

She stated that her skin was dry constantly and that she had occasional problems with sweating excessively. She had an allergy to sulfa and Motrin®. Problems with the neck consisted of stiffness, limited or restricted motion, and pain. She further indicated occasional orthostatic hypertension, occasional cold hands and cold feet, and occasionally nocturia times one or two. In the emotional checklist, she listed that she felt frustrated and angry. In the mental status check, she stated that she felt that her life was too demanding and she stated that she worried about her job. Under alcohol and tobacco, she denied smoking but stated that she used alcohol less than once per week. She stated that her marriage was very satisfactory. She stated that occasionally she could find no comfortable sleeping position. There was a family history of pernicious anemia, with a number of deaths from that disease.

Evaluation of the symptom chart revealed that she rated her pain at about 75% of the worst ever; intensity was moderate, which means it caused a marked handicap in the performance of activities of daily living, and the frequency of pain symptoms was constant. There was pain noted in the posterior neck on the right side extending anteriorly and from C1 to T1 on the right and from C6 to T1 on the left. There was paraspinal pain noted from T4 to L4 on the right and T5 to L3 on the left. There was pain down the ulnar aspect of the upper and lower parts of the upper right extremity and numbness indicated in the medial aspect of the right forearm and medial aspect of the right hand, both dorsally and on the volar surface.

PHYSICAL EXAMINATION

The patient was noted to be well developed, well nourished, well hydrated, and in moderate distress. As she disrobed, it was noted that she was able to take off her shoes standing up with no loss of balance and had no difficulty removing her tight-fitting jeans. Passive hyperextension of the left index metacarpophalangeal joint was carried out as a relative gauge for this patient's overall flexibility. On range of motion of the neck, she missed touching her chin to her chest by four finger breadths. She could extend to 15 degrees. She missed touching her shoulder with her ears by four finger breadths on each side. Rotation of the neck was 55 degrees to the right and 46 degrees to the left. A plastic goniometer was used to determine all ranges of motion numerically reported.

On range of motion of the shoulders, she had forward flexion to 140 degrees bilaterally, extension to 67 degrees on the right and 64 degrees on the left, and abduction of 167 degrees on the right and 185 degrees on the left. On maximum forward flexion of the arms, she stated that if she went further than 140 degrees, she felt tightness in the upper back musculature. On maximum abduction of the right arm, she felt tightness in the paraspinal muscles in the thoracic region and a taut band could be seen in the posterior paraspinal thoracic muscles with her in the sitting position. She also felt tightness in the upper right trapezius muscle. Grip strength testing was carried out, and she was found to be two-thirds of normal for each hand. The hand-to-shoulder blade test (Travell and Simons, 1983) revealed that she missed touching her right fingertips to the top of her shoulder blade by 7 cm on the right and 0 cm on the left. On the mouth wraparound test (Travell and Simons, 1983), she missed by 10 cm with the right hand and 11 cm with the left. Deep tendon reflex testing revealed (right/left): triceps 1+/1, biceps 1/±, brachioradialis 1+/2, patellae 2+/2+, and Achilles 1/1 (normal = 2/2).

Pinprick sensation testing was carried out using a pinwheel and standardizing at C4 on both sides. She had hypesthesia to pinprick in the right upper extremity at C5, C6, C7, C8, and T1. Pinprick sensation testing in the left upper extremity was normal from C5 to T1. In the lower extremities, on the right side there was hypesthesia to pinprick in L4, L5, and S1. On the left side, L4 and L5 were normal and there was pinprick hypesthesia at S1. The patient was then placed in the prone position and the following muscles were palpated for the presence of taut bands, tenderness, and jump signs. On both sides, there were taut bands, tenderness, and jump signs in the trapezius, sternocleidomastoids, pectoralis major, and latissimus dorsi bilaterally, with the only exception being a negative jump sign in the right pectoralis major muscle. (Note: Tenderness is reported by the patient. A taut band is found by the examiner. The jump sign is observed by the examiner and can sometimes be felt by the patient.) The jump sign is defined as an involuntary withdrawal response of the patient to a painful stimulus which comes on suddenly and is significantly painful (can be caused by physical examination or myofascial trigger point injections). Straight leg raising was 75 degrees on the right and 85 degrees on the left. On the right side, she felt tightness and pain in the posterior thigh. The rectus femoris muscle was checked for taut bands, tenderness, and jump signs bilaterally. Taut bands, tenderness, and jump signs were positive on the right side and just taut band and tenderness were present on the left side. The right knee could be passively flexed to 120 degrees and the left knee could be passively flexed to 115 degrees with the patient's leg hanging over the edge of the table. Manual muscle testing was carried out to some muscles of the lower extremities (right/left): EHL 4/4+, ankle dorsiflexion 4+ to 5−/5−.

The patient was then placed in the prone position and the paraspinal muscles were palpated for taut bands, tenderness, and jump signs. The taut bands, tenderness, and jump signs were noted from T4 to T12 on the right and T5 to T12 on the left. The jump signs were noticeably more pronounced in these muscles than in the previous muscles about the neck and shoulder tested. Range of motion of the lumbar spine revealed that she missed touching her toes by 1 inch, could extend 6 degrees, and could laterally bend 30 degrees to the right and 35 degrees to the left. When she performed a deep knee bend, the range of motion was 98% of normal, strength was 95%, balance was 95%, smoothness of movement was 95%, and there was no change in her pain intensity.

At the end of the physical examination, the following diagnoses were made:

1. Painful polyneuropathy: 356.4
2. Myofascial pain syndrome, multifocal, moderately severe: 729.1
3. Fibromyalgia: 729.0

A comprehensive panel of blood testing was ordered on 11/19/94 to assess for the presence of metabolic perpetuating factors (Travell and Simons, 1983) and any other metabolic dysfunction that might be noted. Blood count, liver function tests, cholesterol, triglycerides, and urinalysis were within normal limits. The patient had a less than optimal potassium level of 3.9 meq/ml (normal range = 3.5–5.4 meq/ml) and a deficiency of B12. Her B12 level was 79 pg/ml (normal range = 200–1240 pg/ml). The patient reminded me that there was a history of pernicious anemia in the family, and numerous relatives had died before the use of intrinsic factor and B12 injectable was initiated. The patient's serum folic acid level was found to be 15.5 ng/ml on a normal range of 2.0–17.0.

On the blood testing it was also noted that her free thyroxin was at 1.2 (normal range = 0.8–2.5) and would be consistent with less than optimal according to the criteria of Travell and Simons (1983). Therefore, treatment was initiated with the use of low-dose L-thyroxine at 0.025 mg/day and K-Tab® at two twice per day. The patient was placed on Vicodin® tablets at one-half to one tablet every 3–4 hours as needed for pain following the conclusion of the evaluation.

When she returned on 11/30/94, the blood tests (which were received on 11/28/94) were discussed with the patient. With respect to the thyroid problem, the patient indicated that she had a thyroid problem in the seventh or eighth grade. She stated her resting pulse had been 140, the gland was enlarged, and she had to be at home with a teacher. She was put on thyroid supplementation at that time. She reported that the pain medication helped most of the time.

The patient was placed on initial dosing with B-complex injections using a two-syringe formulation. (Note: This would be the quarter-strength dose and can be seen on the form at the end of this chapter.) Broad-spectrum B complex is used in any of these patients who have one or more of the B vitamins found to be deficient or below normal as defined by the criteria of Travell and Simons. On the initial injections, the riboflavin and dexpanthenol were not put in the #2 shot and the dexpanthenol was not put in the #1 shot. Review of the symptom chart of 11/30/94 showed that about 30% of her presenting symptoms were being relieved by her pain medication.

She was next seen on 12/21/94. The patient had been treated for an upper respiratory infection, and on 11/30/94 she had been instructed to add dexpanthenol injection (3 cc) twice a day for 2 days and then daily for 5 days as adjunctive treatment to the antibiotics that her local medical doctor was prescribing for her. The patient was told to buy Mineral Insurance Formula from Bronson and take three tablets per day. She had been on a generic B-complex tablet from a local drugstore and was told to discontinue that and begin nontime-release B complex with C and E by Bronson at two tablets twice per day. At that visit, her L-thyroxine was increased to 0.05 mg/day. Her B-complex injection was upgraded to the components of a half-strength shot, still minus the components indicated previously.

She was noted to be in mild distress and had a discharge from her nose, plus erythema of the nares on both sides. She was alert, coherent, demonstrated no slurred speech, thinking was clear, no evidence of drug toxicity, and her ability to hear and understand what I was saying was within normal limits. The symptom chart analysis revealed that about 15% of her initial symptoms remained. (Note: All references to trigger point injections are classic Travell and Simons myofascial trigger point injections as outlined in their two textbooks on the subject [Travell and Simons, 1983, 1992]).

At that visit, a classic latissimus dorsi trigger point (refer to Chapter 10 for location of myofascial trigger points) injection was carried out to a very large taut band in her right latissimus dorsi muscle. Injection of the muscle demonstrated a large, visible local twitch response and a total body jump sign on the patient's part. She noted that she had this same problem with trigger point injections in the years during which she had been in my program previously. This was a situation that was beyond her ability to tolerate because of the severe pain flare-up that was generated by the huge local twitch response and marked jump sign, which then aggravated pain in numerous other areas of the body.

The patient did not return until 1/4/95 and expressed that she was very apprehensive about considering further trigger point injections because of the marked pain flare-up due to the large jump sign from the latissimus dorsi myofascial trigger point injection. She was then spoken to about the use of opioid premedication for trigger point injections and assured that this would probably increase her ability to tolerate this very necessary procedure. At that visit, I told her that I could demonstrate to her that use of proper premedication could reduce the amount of pain generated by a trigger point shot. The patient was then told to palpate the most painful area that she could find. This was at the eighth thoracic paraspinal level. The patient's vital signs were then taken on automated equipment. After the second set of readings, the patient had 6 mg of morphine sulfate injected into the right upper quadrant of her buttock. Fourteen minutes postinjection, she sensed a feeling of heaviness but no loss of consciousness. By 15 minutes postinjection, the patient's tenderness rating had gone from an 8 to a 6 (the rating would be 0 for no tenderness at all and 10 would be the maximum tenderness possible). By 21 minutes postinjection, the patient's sensation of heaviness was gone and palpable tenderness was at a rated level of 4. By the time 24 minutes had passed, the patient indicated that the palpatory pain that she could obtain at T8 in the paraspinal muscles was a 2.

The patient was impressed that premedication could significantly reduce the amount of pain produced by her palpation, and I assured her that this would also have a positive effect on trigger point injections. At that visit, she stated that there was no problem with her sleep. Also at that visit, her problem was rated, as far as medical decision making was concerned, as follows: The number of diagnoses or management options was extensive. The amount and/or complexity of the data to be reviewed was extensive. The risks, complications, and/or morbidity was between high and moderate, and the type of decision making was moderate to highly complex.

At her visit of 1/11/95, she indicated that she was doing "fair." She stated that she was having trouble getting to sleep because of the pain. I recommended that she add Soma® and perhaps some Vicodin® at bedtime to improve her sleep. Palpation was carried out in the trapezius no. 2 and trapezius no. 3 areas on the right side. There was a trigger point with a jump sign associated with it on trapezius no. 3. At that visit, I drew a pain chart for the patient, and she stated that she had constant pain in the classic trapezius no. 2 distribution, in the paraspinal muscles from T2 to T11 on the right, and in the ulnar nerve distribution in the right upper extremity. At that visit, she was premedicated with 8 mg of morphine sulfate, and 20 minutes later the trapezius no. 3 on the right side was injected. The patient indicated that the 8 mg of morphine sulfate was minimally effective with respect to subduing the unpleasant symptoms of the trigger point injection. She was referred to Bonnie Pruden, a certified myotherapist, for adjunctive therapy to my program. At that visit, she was moved up to a full half-strength B-complex injection as delineated on the attached forms.

She was next seen on 1/25/95. She stated that the trigger point injection of her previous visit had helped the right arm and the medial right scapular pain. She stated that her insurance company would not pay for the treatment from the myotherapist and therefore she could not afford that therapy. She stated that her neck pain felt like "a vise" and was very problematic. She had problems with tiredness and fatigue due to irregular sleep. She stated that she had hunger problems associated with missing meals, and therefore I recommended she use Ensure to bridge the gap between meals. Palpation revealed problems in the scalene muscles on both sides. Therefore, it was recommended that 3 to 3.5 inches of telephone books be placed under the head of the bed (Travell and Simons, 1983). She stated that she was not sleeping well. She stated that she was waking up more and the problem had been most noticeable for the four nights preceding her visit. She was given 0.5-mg tablets of Ativan® at one to two tablets at bedtime as needed for sleep. The patient reported on her subsequent visit that she felt too hung over when using this medication for sleep. She then stated, comparatively, that the 350-mg Soma® tablets were better for sleep.

Evaluation of her symptom chart revealed that about 15–20% of her original symptoms remained on the chart. At that visit, the patient was premedicated with morphine sulfate (10 mg), and 15 minutes later the following muscles were injected: left trapezius no. 3, three times and right trapezius no. 3, four times. At that visit, the patient had hydrocortisone acetate prescribed and was told to take 5–7.5 mg daily to attempt relief of her fatigue. She indicated that the 10 mg of morphine that had been used for the trigger point injection produced satisfactory results.

Based on what the patient stated, it was felt that one-half to one Vicodin® tablet at 3–4 hours as needed for pain was not sufficient for what she was experiencing; therefore, on 1/28/95, she was switched to Lorcet® 10/650 at one tablet every 4–6 as needed for pain. A scan of her intake of Lorcet® 10 between January 1995 and October 1995 revealed that the patient averaged three to four tablets per day.

She was next seen on 1/31/95. A partial drug history was taken, and the patient indicated no problems with morphine sulfate. She stated that the Lorcet® helped, but was not very effective in the evening when her pain problem flared up. The use of Percodan® was considered at that time, but the patient stated she had an aspirin allergy. Therefore, she was given a prescription for morphine sulfate (15-mg tablets) with instructions of one to three tablets every 3 hours as needed for control of neuropathic or myofascial pain. In my clinic note, I indicated that she looked better than usual at that visit. She was alert and coherent, with no slurred speech, good cognition, no evidence of drug toxicity, and her ability to understand what I was saying was within normal limits. Symptom chart evaluation revealed that about 15% of her original problem was still present. At that visit, the patient was given a number of upper extremity stretching exercise sheets titled "Torso Stretching Instruction" and "Neck, Head, and Upper Back Stretching Instructions" and was told to perform a number of these exercises. (Copies of these sheets appear at the end of this chapter.)

I filled out a doctor-drawn pain chart and identified the levator scapulae as the most likely contributor to the pain pattern described. The patient was given premedication of 10 mg of morphine sulfate, and 21 minutes later five trigger point injections were placed into the levator scapulae muscles on both sides. The patient tolerated the procedure well.

The patient was questioned about the use of Ativan® for her sleep, and she stated that the medication caused her to be too hung over. She was therefore continued on Soma® for sleep. She was then questioned about her use of hydrocortisone acetate injectable. She stated that the 7.5-mg shot on Wednesdays and Fridays help with her energy. At about that time, she was switched to 5-mg tablets of Cortef (hydrocortisone acetate tablets), with a direction to take them at one-half tablet twice per day.

She was next seen on 2/22/95. She stated that for the 2 days preceding the visit, her pain that was worse toward the end of the day became very problematic, causing her sleep to be disrupted. She had trouble getting to sleep and staying asleep. She stated that two Soma® tablets at bedtime was of some help. She stated that the morphine sulfate tablets caused swelling, itching, and allergy and indicated that hives may become a real problem with that particular medication. The overall areas of pain involvement were noted to be decreasing with about 10% of her presenting symptoms still present. It was decided to do a number of trigger points relating to her residual upper pain problem, and she was premedicated with an equianalgesic dose of Dilaudid® injection (equal to the dose of morphine that had been given previously). Twenty minutes after the Dilaudid® injection was given, the patient had injection of one trigger point in the left trapezius no. 2 and two trigger point injections into the right trapezius no. 2.

Because of her sleep disruption, it was decided to place her on 10-mg tablets of Elavil®, at one to five tablets 2–3 hours before bedtime. In addition to the other adverse problems with morphine sulfate, the patient indicated itching and swelling from the medication as of 2/22/95, and she stopped the medication. On 2/23/95, she was issued a prescription for a small dose of Levo-Dromoran® (2-mg tablets) at one-half to one tablet every 4–6 hours as needed for pain.

During the time that she was on Levo-Dromoran®, she also took small doses of three to four tablets of Lorcet® 10/650 per day. About 4 days after initiating the Levo-Dromoran®, the patient stated that it helped for her pain and also stated it was also good for her evening pain.

She was next seen on 2/27/95, and it was noted that about 5–8% of her original symptom chart symptoms remained. By way of a doctor-drawn symptom chart, she indicated pain in the middle of the right trapezius no. 2 trigger point and some tightness in the sternocleidomastoid muscle at its distal end on the right side. She was given a 1-mg Dilaudid® injection for premedication, and about 20 minutes later two trigger point injections were carried out to the right trapezius no. 2 trigger point and one to the right levator scapulae muscle. It was on that visit that the patient indicated that the Levo-Dromoran® was good to help for her evening pain. I made a notation in the physician's treatment plan of 2/27/95 that if the patient's pain was gone, we were to taper her analgesics and perform muscle testing with a referral for physical therapy.

The next visit was 3/7/95. She stated that the Friday before the visit, she was able to sit through two movies, whereas before she could barely sit through one movie. It was noted that the turnaround time from the pain flare-ups was markedly improved. The patient continued on the previously indicated oral and injectable vitamin program. At that visit, the patient indicated by way of symptom chart a small amount of pain at the angle where the upper shoulder intersects the base of the neck on both sides, more prevalent on the right than the left, and about 5–10% of what had been previously recorded on her initial pain charts. On the doctor-drawn pain chart, she indicated a paraspinal muscle pain on the right side from T2 to T7, which was aggravated by standing a lot. At the visit of 3/7/95, the patient also indicated that the 1-mg Dilaudid® injection had made her slightly spacey after the trigger point shots were over.

At this visit, she was premedicated with 1 mg of Dilaudid® injection and the right scalene medius muscle was injected. During the procedure, the muscle demonstrated two local twitch responses and the patient demonstrated a large jump sign. She stated immediately after the injection procedure that the 1 mg of Dilaudid® injection was not enough to block the shock response to her body caused by the trigger point injection. (Note: It is not unusual for patients to be tolerant to small doses of premedications with opioids in certain areas of the body, but to require larger doses of opioids for premedication when more active trigger points are injected in other parts of the body.)

Her next visit was on 3/13/95. The patient indicated that the injection of 3/7/95 had cut her overall pain medication consumption (for Lorcet®) approximately in half; however, it had no effect on her consumption of Levo-Dromoran®. Because of increased pain due to stress at work, the patient was progressed to full-strength B-complex shots and told to alternate these injections for 10 days and then return to the half-dose program that was given to her on 1/25/95.

At that visit, she reported an accident that had occurred the day before. The garage door to her house was waterlogged. She bent forward to pick up something from her car and the waterlogged garage door hit her between the shoulder blades. At that visit, the patient was noted to be in moderately severe distress. The pain was back to about 15% on her original pain chart and there was also the appearance of a midline component from T5 to T8. The patient was premedicated with 0.6 cc of Dilaudid® injection (2 mg/ml) plus 25 mg of hydrocortisone acetate in the right upper quadrant. (Note: Hydrocortisone acetate injection is given via a systemic injection to persons who may become inordinately or abnormally stressed by a trigger point injection or series of trigger point injections. When the patient has a large jump sign during these trigger point injections, it taxes the adrenal gland, sometimes to the extent that the patient is tired and worn out for 2–3 days after the trigger point injection. The shot of hydrocortisone acetate solves that problem in approximately 90% of patients who have it.)

At this visit, the right scalene anterior, scalene medius, and scalene posterior were injected. The patient was also told to administer the following schedule of hydrocortisone acetate injections at home: On 3/14/96, 7.5 mg every 8 hours; on 3/15/95, 5 mg every 8 hours; on 3/16/95, 2.5 mg every 8 hours; and on 3/17/95, she was told to resume her previous intake of Cortef tablets.

She was next seen on 4/4/95. Review of her pain chart revealed that about 50% of the symptomatology had returned as compared to her original visit, and there was a definite concentration of pain in the paravertebral muscles on the right side from T1 to T8. She had constant pain in the trapezius no. 2 area and positional pain in the paraspinal muscles. There was pain in the musculature of the posterior right upper part of the right upper extremity and posterolateral part of the upper right lower extremity. At that visit, the patient was informed that within the next few months she would have to have her medication consumption reviewed by an independent medical consultant as specified by California state law.   ·

Because of incomplete coverage by her previous premedication, she was given 0.7 cc (1.4 mg) of Dilaudid® plus 25 mg of hydrocortisone acetate as a premedication to trigger point injections. The trigger points were injected in the trapezius no. 5 and right serratus posterior superior muscles. Following the injections, it was noted that she had improved lateral bending and lateral rotation of her neck compared to her original examination of 11/18/94. It was noted that her consumption of Lorcet® 10/650 and Levo-Dromoran® showed no increase compared to previous weeks. By calculation in the medication sheet, it was deemed that her use of Soma® went from an average of 1.3 tablets per day to 2.3 tablets per day.

Because of difficulties that she was having in the use of the right upper extremity, at that time consideration was given to, and discussed with the patient, sending her to a soft tissue chiropractor for adjunctive therapy to my program and also a physical therapy referral for a few weeks to increase her pinch strength, opponens strength in the right hand, grip strength, range of motion of the shoulder and neck, and strength of the right arm and shoulder.

She was seen on 4/12/95 and reported that she was working out with weights progressively. She was noted to be in moderate distress. She was alert and coherent, with no slurred speech, good cognition, no evidence of drug toxicity, and her ability to hear and relate to what I was saying was within normal limits. She noted at that visit that the paraspinal muscle pain on the right side was better and gave no indication of it on the pain chart. On the pain chart, she indicated that her pain was about 70% of the worst it had ever been, the intensity was moderate, and the frequency was constant. She still had difficulties at the base of the neck on both sides. It was felt that the splenius cervicis was a big contributor to the residual pain at the base of the neck. At that visit, I documented that she had lost range of motion with respect to lateral bending and rotation of the neck..

In order to enhance the effect of the premedication of the trigger point shots, the patient was given 12.5 mg of Phenergan® in addition to the 1.4 mg of Dilaudid® as premedication.

She also received 25 mg of hydrocortisone acetate. At that visit, three trigger points were injected in the right splenius cervicis muscle. (Note: Phenergan® had to be given in a separate syringe because it does not mix with injectable Dilaudid®.)

The next visit occurred on 4/19/95. The patient stated that she obtained 2–3 days of help and then all of the pain came back. She stated that overall she was doing well and continued with progressive weight training. On her pain chart, she indicated a minor flare in the thoracic paraspinal muscles on the right side and the usual pain at the base of the neck on both sides. On the doctor-drawn pain chart, the patient outlined pain in the angle of her jaw, pain throughout the entire right sternocleidomastoid muscle, and classic pain from a trigger point in the trapezius no. 2 on the right side. At that visit, the patient was premedicated with 1.8 mg of Dilaudid® injection, 12.5 mg of Phenergan®, and 25 mg of hydrocortisone acetate. The right trapezius no. 1, the right scalene posterior, and another two trigger points in the right trapezius no. 1 were injected. (Note: The reason for increasing this patient's premedication related to my desire to suppress unnecessary muscle jerking [jump sign] that this patient demonstrated. This type of patient is rare with respect to these extreme body jumps on trigger point injection. This is a clinical situation that the clinician has to deal with in order to successfully inject the myofascial trigger points that contribute to the patient's ongoing disability. The goal here is not to totally anesthetize the patient with medication before the procedure, but instead to be able to suppress as much jump-sign-related activity as possible while the very active myofascial trigger points are being injected. The patient will usually let the physician know when enough medication has been utilized to produce this quieting-type response in the irritable muscles. Also, once the procedure has been started, I never add additional premedication to help the situation; I merely stop injecting when the patient appears to be demonstrating too much bothersome jump sign activity. The next injection session is when I take the premedication up a few more milligrams, if needed.)

Her next visit was 5/11/95. This patient indicated that the flare-up of pain which was occurring subsequent to her garage door injury was up to about 80–85% of her original presenting pain complaints. The patient stated that she was frustrated. A big flare-up of pain caused loss of work activity in the preceding week. Whereas pain had been spilling over onto her left side from the right side of the trigger points, there was no more of this happening and it was reflected on her pain chart. She stated that the Levo-Dromoran® might not be strong enough for her pain spikes. She had returned to using Elavil® in an attempt to help her sleep, but reported that it caused too much hangover, and therefore she discontinued the Elavil® and continued with the Soma®.

At that visit, she was referred to the physical therapy department of a local hospital and a specific therapist whom I felt performed well with patients who have chronic pain syndrome. She was referred for two visits per week for 12 weeks. The reason for two visits per week instead of three visits per week is that this type of patient sometimes obtains too much muscle soreness from closely timed physical therapy workouts and is not given enough time to rest and recover between physical therapy sessions. The main area of problem at that visit was the paraspinal muscles from T4 to T12 on the right side. Therefore, the patient was premedicated with 2 mg of Dilaudid®, 12.5 mg of Phenergan®, and 25 mg of hydrocortisone acetate. Myofascial trigger point injections were carried out to the right iliocostalis thoracis T11 times two, the left iliocostalis thoracis T11, and the right iliocostalis thoracis T8. The observation was made that the jump signs generated by the trigger point injections were usually big, causing spontaneous contraction of muscles in the area injected and for a distance away from it, and this had been the case on all previous injection sessions.

As of 5/2/95, the patient stated she was on two 5-mg Cortef tablets per day. She was having some problems with constipation at that time, a problem unusual for her, and she was directed to take one to two senna tablets three times a day as treatment for that problem. She continued on her half-strength B-vitamin shots, containing all the components indicated on the sheet at the end of this chapter, and she was on an odd/even-day schedule (#1 injection was given on even-numbered days and #2 injection was given on odd-numbered days).

Her next visit was on 5/19/95. The patient was noted to be alert and coherent, with no slurred speech, good cognition, no evidence of drug toxicity, and comprehended what I was saying. Her pain was rated at about 75% of the worst she ever had. She indicated that she could sit for 30 minutes, stand for 30 minutes, and walk for 90 minutes. The intensity of the pain was moderate and the frequency was constant. The pain was depicted on both sides in the lower neck, paraspinally from T5 to T8 on the right side with noticeable intensity, and from T10 to L2 bilaterally with minimal intensity. At that visit, the patient was premedicated with 4 mg of Dilaudid® and 12.5 mg of Phenergan®. She was also premedicated with 25 mg of hydrocortisone acetate. Trigger point injections were carried out to the right T7, T8, and T9 multifidus. Before the third trigger point was carried out, the patient had a classic osteopathic release procedure performed from T2 to T7. She then had a trigger point injection into the right-sided multifidus at T10. The patient was noted to be conversant but somewhat light-headed, and therefore 0.13 cc (0.4 mg/ml) of Narcan® was administered subcutaneously. Immediately after that, the patient was noted to be conversant, had a mild flush on her face and low back, and was noted to be alert. The patient inquired about using larger dose B-complex shots at that time, and I told her it was okay to be on the 3-cc shots, and when she felt she was doing better, she could put one day between the shots.

Her next visit was on 6/1/95. The patient stated that she was having difficulty with sexual dysfunction. Her sex drive was down and her ability to reach an orgasm was down. She stated that the pain medications played a role in interfering; however, she stated that if she did not take enough pain medication, she would be in too much pain to be interested in sexual activity. She stated that at that time she was not able to control her pain. This was despite the fact that she might use Levo-Dromoran® all day long. She was depressed, grieving, and anxious. When I asked her about psychotherapy, she stated that she could not afford it. An official diagnosis of "depression related to anxiety and grieving reaction" was placed on the physician's treatment plan.

The patient stated that she could call the therapist she had seen previously after her 1986 accident. She stated that if she took three Soma® tablets, it helped her to get to sleep, but she had difficulty getting up in the morning. Therefore, the use of Halcion® for purposes of facilitating sleep was discussed in detail, and the patient was given a prescription for 0.125-mg tablets of Halcion® and instructed to take up to four of these tablets at bedtime to help induce sleep. Calculation of the patient's consumption of this medication over the next 2 months revealed that the medication successfully helped her initiate sleep at two tablets per night.

The patient had had a routine comprehensive panel of blood testing on 5/18/95. These were reviewed with the patient. Her free thyroxine level was below midline and the T3 total was in the upper quartile of the normal range. The TSH was high at 6.0 (normal range = 0.34 to 5.0 mIU/ml). The patient was on 0.05 mg of Synthroid® at that time. As of the end of June, she was told to progress to three tablets per day. The laboratory testing showed no abnormalities of blood counts, the sedimentation rate was normal, routine chemistries were within normal limits except for a low serum iron level, and there were no abnormalities of the liver function tests. The urinalysis was unremarkable.

The next visit was 6/13/95. Her pain chart looked as though it had about 10–15% of her original pain pattern; however, on the doctor-drawn pain chart she stated that she had new symptomatology for the preceding 30 days. This consisted of pain in both cheeks and malar areas, pain in both sides of the low back extending from T7 to the lumbosacral junction and out to the posterior axillary line, and pain on the dorsum of both hands. There was also a problematic area indicated in the right paraspinal thoracic musculature at T5. Notes on a trigger point adjunct sheet indicated that she had gotten her best response for trigger point injections with the combination of 4 mg Dilaudid® plus 12.5 mg Phenergan®. (Note: Phenergan® will not mix in the same syringe with Dilaudid®, and therefore these two medications have to be given in separate syringes.)

The patient was given 4 mg of Dilaudid® plus 12.5 mg of Phenergan® intramuscularly plus hydrocortisone acetate (25 mg by injection). About 30 minutes following the premedication, injection was carried out to the right sternocleidomastoid; sternal division in its mid length; right scalene anterior, just behind the sternocleidomastoid and close to the sternal area; and into the right scalene anterior about 1 cm away from the procedure mentioned above. On the last two trigger point injections, the patient had significant jump signs, either indicating that the premedication was not sufficient or that the patient's trigger points were extremely irritable. Nine minutes after the last trigger point injection was given, the patient was given 0.1 cc (0.4 mg/ml) of Narcan® to counteract some slight dizziness that she was having from the Dilaudid® injection.

At that visit, the patient asked for Valium® to use for daytime muscle tension. A small prescription of 2-mg tablets was issued. Up to this time, it was noted that the patient's intake of Levo-Dromoran® was steady at two to three tablets per day, with no dosage escalation.

Her next visit was on 6/29/95. The patient was asked about the efficacy of daytime Valium® and stated that the Soma® worked better. She stated that she had gone back to her massage therapist and three treatments had provided improvement. It was noted that she looked a lot brighter at that visit but was still in moderate distress. When asked about the Halcion®, she stated that it worked "great" and her sleep was more normal with that medication. The pain distribution as indicated by her was about 15–30% of what she had on her initial pain chart. The pain intensity was rated at about 65% of the worst she ever had. The intensity was moderate and the frequency was constant.

On the doctor-drawn pain chart, the patient indicated bilateral pain in the posterior paracervical musculature on head forward posture. At a previous visit, the patient had been given a review document which made an assessment of about 60% of the questions in the original questionnaire filled out for admission. She was still having problems with energy and stamina and there was weakness in the right upper extremity. She had pain up and down her back. She stated that she had problems with memory and verbalizing at her place of employment, but that had been getting better. She stated that reading and writing with the head tilted forward were very difficult because of pain. The global activity assessment test showed readings that were similar to her first visit; however, she rated her overall strength and endurance as being slightly less. Sleep was restless and she had difficulty staying asleep and falling asleep. She was able to work 40 hours a week, and the reason she could not do more was pain and fatigue.

In her review of systems, she stated that she generally found her life too demanding. She indicated that she felt cold most of the time. She felt her marriage was satisfactory. She stated she could find no comfortable sleeping position. At that visit, she was premedicated with 4 mg of Dilaudid® and 12.5 mg of Phenergan®. About 16 minutes later, she had trigger point injections to the right T6 rotator, T6 right semispinalis, right T6 multifidus, and right trapezius no. 3. A number of these muscles caused significantly large jump signs. Twenty-two minutes after the last trigger point injection, the patient stated that she was feeling slightly light-headed and therefore was given 0.11 cc (0.4 mg/ml) of Narcan® subcutaneously.

In June and July of 1995, the patient had an evaluation at the El Camino Center for Osteoporosis. The referral was made by her local medical doctors. Bone density was evaluated in the left spine and hip. The risk factors were "some physical characteristics," "obligatory protracted use of thyroid," "early oophorectomy, age 34," "potential hereditary predisposition," "the use of thyroid and steroids," and "limited antigravity exercises." The findings indicated that the lumbar spine bone mineral density was significantly greater than her age-matched group. There was a fracture risk in the right hip that was greater for a matched group and was noted to be mild, and the reason for this could not be immediately determined.

Her next visit was 6/30/95. She stated that she had a pain flare-up since the day before and stated that it felt like the flare-up when the garage door hit her back. She noted pain with motion and stabbing pain which occurred that morning. She was noted to be in moderate distress. She was alert and coherent, with no slurred speech, good cognition, no evidence of drug toxicity, and her ability to process what I was saying appeared to be within normal limits. Pain chart depiction of her pain problem showed that it demonstrated about 25% of the pain on her original pain chart. On the doctor-drawn pain chart, I indicated, at her direction, that there was pain at about T8 in the paraspinal muscles radiating distally and laterally. She was premedicated with 4 mg of Dilaudid® and 12.5 mg and Phenergan®, and 20 minutes later she was injected in the right T5 multifidus and right T4 multifidus in the paraspinal area. She was also noted to have tenderness with a jump sign in the right serratus anterior muscle.

As of 6/29/95, she was progressed to 0.05 mg of Synthroid® per day. She remained on her time-release potassium tablets at two tablets twice a day.

She was next seen on 7/13/95. She stated her depression was better and that her sleep was "pretty good." She was walking 5 miles three times per week. On her pain chart, she indicated the pain was 70% of what it was at its worst, she could sit for 30 minutes, stand for 30 minutes, and walk for 1 hour. The intensity of the pain was moderate and the frequency was constant. Compared to her original pain chart of 11/18/94, she had about 65% of the symptomatology depicted; however, the distribution was different in a number of areas. The distribution was the same in the posterior cervical region and localized in the right paraspinal muscles from T5 to T7. She had a band of pain going across her back from the left posterior axillary line to the right posterior axillary line from T9 to T11. She stated that this band was intermittent but was the most bothersome problem when it occurred. She said it was one of her most disabling pains, and the intensity was equal on both sides. She stated that area of pain began in May of 1995, and the origin was unknown. She stated that she might wake up with the pain and have it all day. She stated the frequency of this bothersome pain was less now than previously. It occurred 3–4 days a week and was not related to activity.

The pain distribution was compared to the Travell and Simons figures from the wall charts that were produced in 1993. The pain distribution most closely resembled that produced by the upper rectus abdominis muscle trigger point. The patient had previously indicated that she could have benefited from a bit more premedication prior to her trigger point shots; therefore, on her visit of 7/13/95, she was premedicated with 5 mg of Dilaudid® plus 12.5 mg of Phenergan®. She was also given an injection of 25 mg of hydrocortisone acetate. The right and left upper rectus abdominis trigger points were injected beginning 26 minutes after the injection of the Dilaudid®. Each side demonstrated one local twitch response and three jump signs. The last injection was given at 5:21 p.m. Six minutes later, the patient was given 0.12 cc (0.4 mg/ml) of Narcan® because she stated that she felt light-headed. At 5:35 p.m., the patient was alert, conversant, and had no more light-headedness.

Her next visit was 7/20/95. She stated that she had obtained good results from the last trigger point injections and was feeling better overall. She stated that her sleep was good and she still needed two Halcion® tablets to initiate sleep. She stated that with even using a down pillow, there was tenderness up and down the neck, and pressure on the neck was painful. Comparing the pain charts of 7/20/95 and 11/18/95, there was significant reduction of the pain across her back from the T8 to T11 level, and the patient stated that the trigger point injections had significantly improved that area of pain. She still had residual areas of pain in the neck, most prominent on the right paracervical musculature and in the right paravertebral muscles from T4 to T6 on the right.

She was premedicated with 5 mg of Dilaudid® plus a 12.5-mg Phenergan® injection and 25 mg of hydrocortisone acetate. Approximately 32 minutes after the premedication was given, injection was carried out to the right C3, C4, and C5 deep paraspinal muscles. Nine minutes after the last trigger point injection, the patient was given 0.1 cc (0.4 mg/ml) of Narcan®. By this time, the records reflect that the patient was no longer using Valium® (2-mg tablets). Her consumption of Soma® 350 was averaging approximately three tablets per day. She was taking approximately three tablets per day of Lorcet® 10. Consumption of Levo-Dromoran® tablets was averaging approximately 6 mg/day.

Her next visit was 7/27/95. The patient stated that her recovery from minor reinjuries was becoming faster and more complete. She said the areas of pain involvement were decreasing, but the intensity was not. With respect to the state of her psyche, she was more frustrated than depressed because of the remaining areas of pain. She stated that 4 days after the last trigger point shots, her sleep was very disrupted. She stated that three Halcion® tablets at bedtime corrected the sleep disruption. The most problematic pain areas were at the angle of the neck and the shoulder and were especially problematic on the right side. At this visit, the patient was premedicated with 4 mg of Dilaudid® and 25 mg of Benadryl®. (Note: It was noted that Benadryl® and Dilaudid® can be mixed in the same syringe without any precipitation problems.) She was also given an injection of 12.5 mg of hydrocortisone acetate. Sixteen minutes after the Dilaudid® was injected, trigger point injections were carried out to the right scalene anterior, scalene medius, and scalene posterior. A second injection was also given to another trigger point in the right scalene anterior. The patient tolerated the procedure well and did not need any Narcan® after the trigger points were finished.

She was next seen on 8/2/95. My note reads: "Overall, continues to improve." She was somewhere in between mild to moderate distress, alert, coherent, no slurred speech, good cognition, no evidence of drug toxicity, and had no problems understanding what I was saying. Once again, it was noted that some of her main problem areas were in the muscles at the neck/shoulder junction, with most problems on the right side. There were also areas of pain indicated in the right sternocleidomastoid muscle.

The patient was having some problems of an ergonomic nature with respect to her chair at work. She was referred to an occupational therapist to remedy the problem by obtaining a more appropriate chair for her. At that visit, she was premedicated with a 4 mg of Dilaudid® and 25 mg of Benadryl® injection. About 20 minutes later, an injection was carried out to the right T4 iliocostalis thoracis and two injections to the lower right splenius cervicis. The next two injections were carried out to the undersurface of the splenius cervicis taut band.

The patient had demonstrated a number of jump signs during the visit of 8/2/95, but it is my belief that the use of the injectable Dilaudid® and Benadryl® combination helped keep the number of trigger point injection-related jumps to a minimum.

Her next visit was 8/10/95. The patient stated that the pain caused by the garage door incident was mostly gone. She stated that overall she was doing well. She said that the week preceding the visit was the best that she had had since starting my pain program. She stated that the pain usually worsened in the evening. Medication consisted of three doses of Lorcet® 10 during the day for pain control and then the use of two Levo-Dromoran® tablets in the evening. She was noted to be in moderate distress and was alert and coherent, with no slurred speech, good cognition, no evidence of drug toxicity, and her ability to understand what I said was within normal limits. She stated that she had begun to use a yoga exercise tape to increase her range of motion.

At that visit, a physical examination update was performed. The neurologic part of the examination revealed the following (right/left): deep tendon reflexes — biceps 1/0, triceps ±/0, brachioradialis 1/0, patellae 2/2, Achilles 1/1. All of her abdominal reflexes were noted to be absent. Pinprick sensation testing in the upper and lower extremities revealed no deficits from C5 to T1 and from L4 to S1 bilaterally. Range of motion of the neck revealed that she missed touching her chin to her chest by one finger breadth and could extend to 30 degrees. She missed touching her ear to her shoulder on the right side by four finger breadths and on the left side by four and one-half finger breadths. Rotation of the cervical spine was to 70 degrees bilaterally. All ranges of motion of the cervical spine were accompanied by pain. Range of motion of the shoulders revealed 155 degrees of forward flexion on the right side and 150 degrees on the left. External rotation was to 65 degrees on the right and 58 degrees on the left. Abduction was carried out to 155 degrees bilaterally. All ranges of motion of the shoulders were accompanied by pain. In the recumbent position, palpation of the trapezius, sternocleidomastoid, pectoralis major, and latissimus dorsi revealed taut bands and tenderness in all of these muscles. On the right side, the trapezius demonstrated a jump sign and likewise for the latissimus dorsi. The jump sign elicited on the right sternocleidomastoid was greater than expected. On the left side, jump signs were found in the sternocleidomastoid muscle and latissimus dorsi. Straight leg raising could be carried out to 81 degrees on the right with problematic tight hamstrings and 82 degrees on the left with problematic tight hamstrings.

The patient was told to move to the edge of the table, still in the recumbent position, and allow her leg to slowly drop over the side of the exam table. The degree of extension to the right hip was 0 degrees and on the left side was 12 degrees. In the prone position, she had taut bands, tenderness, and marked jump signs from T5 to T12 on the right and T3 to T12 on the left. On range of motion of the lumbar spine, she could touch her toes in flexion, extend to 10 degrees, and lateral bend to 27 degrees to the right and 45 degrees to the left. When asked to do a deep knee bend, she had 100% for range of motion, 100% for strength, 100% for balance, 100% for smoothness of movement, and no change in her pain level.

Manual muscle testing revealed the following (right/left): Hip flexion 4+/4–/5–, hip extension 4+/4 (prone), hip abduction 4+/5-, knee extension 4+/4+, knee flexion 4+/5–, ankle dorsiflexors 5/5. Grip strength testing showed 20 kg and 16 kg on the right side and 22 kg and 21 kg on the left side. At the end of the examination, the patient was given an injection of 4 mg of Dilaudid® and 25 mg of Benadryl®, followed by three trigger point injections into the right scalene posterior. The jump signs elicited by these trigger point shots were unremarkable. Seven minutes after the last injection, the patient was given 0.1 cc of Narcan®.

On 8/1/95, the patient had been referred to Jeffrey Bojeff, M.D., for an independent medication review as required by state law. At the time of that review, I indicated to him that she was taking 0.125-mg Halcion® tablets at up to three at bedtime and had been on the medication since 6/1/95. I indicated she was on 2-mg Levo-Dromoran® tablets at two to three per day since 2/3/95. I also indicated that she was on Lorcet® 10/650 at three to four per day since 1/28/95. The diagnoses given to the reviewer were (1) polyneuropathy: 356.4, (2) myofascial pain syndrome, multifocal: 729.1, (3) fibromyalgia: 729.0, and (4) depression related to anxiety. A copy of the form utilized for these reviews is provided at the end of this chapter.

Dr. Bojeff felt that the patient had intractable pain, no evidence of drug-dependent syndrome, no indication that medications were used to obtain euphoria, and no indication of abstinence syndrome, and he felt that the medications were being used to facilitate pain control. He did not detect any drug-seeking behavior. He did not observe any evidence of toxicity to the medication. He felt that the medications were being used to accomplish goals of household work and chores, enhanced overall independence in physical functioning, and improved ability to interact with friends or family members. He also felt the medication was appropriate for the patient's needs. His suggestion was to use the Levo-Dromoran® only on a daily basis and Lorcet® for the "bad days." He felt that she had a C6 radiculopathy that might be helped with a cervical plexus block. He felt that magnetic resonance imaging (MRI) might be useful.

The MRI was performed on 8/23/95 and the radiologist's conclusion was, "There is very mild cervical spondylosis with possibly some foraminal narrowing at the C3-4 level on the right side. Otherwise, unremarkable MR of cervical spine with no evidence of disc herniation or cord compression."

The patient was next seen on 8/17/95. She stated that she had seen Dr. Bojeff and that he gave her an eight-pack sample of Ultram® tablets. She stated that the Ultram® tablets were taking the edge off of her pain and that she obtained more energy with the combination of the Ultram®, Levo-Dromoran®, and Lorcet®. The use of the Ultram® also allowed her to decrease the intake of Lorcet® and Levo-Dromoran®. She stated that the Soma® might be sedating her too much. With respect to sleep, she stated that even with up to three Halcion® tablets at bedtime, she might have "bad nights" and not be able to sleep through the night. On her pain chart, she had about 15–20% of her previous symptomatology, with the problem areas being at the neck/shoulder junction, more prominent on the right than the left, and also along the ulnar border of the left upper extremity, extending from the axilla to the little finger.

With the use of no premedication, the patient had skin trigger points injected with benzyl alcohol preservative to areas of the skin above the right scalene medius, right and left trapezius, right scalene posterior, right trapezius no. 1, and right scalene medius. There were some minor jump signs noted, but nothing of significance. (Note: The use of stretch and spray had been attempted on many of her visits, but to no avail. Most of the time stretch and spray was used, it appeared to aggravate her muscle pain problem.)

Because of her continued difficulty sleeping, the patient was given a prescription for Thorazine® (10-mg tablets) and told to take one to five tablets 2–3 hours before bedtime.

Her next visit occurred on 8/24/95. The patient stated that her pain was still "real bad in the evenings." She stated the Levo-Dromoran® did not help significantly in the evenings and noted that the evening pain flare-ups started at about 6 p.m. She stated that the Ultram® helped her feel psychologically better. She was noted to be alert and coherent, with no slurred speech, good cognition, no evidence of drug toxicity, and her ability to understand what I was saying was within normal limits. She was premedicated with 4 mg Dilaudid® and a 20-mg Benadryl® injection. Following that, the right sternocleidomastoid was injected twice near the manubrium. A third trigger point was injected in the T8 deep paraspinal muscle on the right side.

Her next visit was 8/31/95. She commented that the injections of 8/24/95 had caused better results with respect to postinjection soreness. She indicated that one of the problems that she had was inability to wear a necklace.

The patient stated that she had seen Dr. Bojeff on the same day and that some nerve conduction studies were done. The patient was of the opinion there was a 50% conduction deficit on the right compared to the left in the upper trapezius muscle. Dr. Bojeff also said that she had a problematic C3 and C4 on the right side. He proposed injecting C3 and C4 on the right side and 2–3 weeks later the cervical plexus. This procedure was to be scheduled by the patient.

The patient and I discussed the procedure, and it was my opinion that it might be of some value for her remaining areas of problem in the right posterior paracervical musculature. The patient stated that she felt that Ultram® took the place of Soma® during the day but was not of help at bedtime. She was still using Soma® at bedtime. She felt that her use of the Ultram® helped her to sleep better at night. When I reviewed her use of Thorazine® at bedtime, she stated that she was taking 20 mg at bedtime and still not sleeping well. She was waking up two to three times per night. I told her that it was okay to go up on the Thorazine® or use one Soma® plus Thorazine®.

The patient stated she had no soreness after the previous injections and was using a grip strength device to strengthen her grip. The pain distribution was similar to previously in the posterior paracervical musculature and had a very faint remnant of pain in the right paraspinal musculature from T4 to T8. There was still some numbness in the right upper extremity in the ulnar nerve distribution.

Throughout the entire time of her treatment at my pain management facility, and up to and including 8/31/95, this patient was gainfully employed. She was also given a prescription for an occupational therapy evaluation at her place of employment, with the message to the therapist indicating the patient had myofascial pain syndrome and fibromyalgia and needed a proper ergonomic chair and keyboard for her computer work. At that visit, she was premedicated with 4 mg of Dilaudid® and 25 mg of Benadryl®, and 20 minutes later three myofascial trigger points were injected in the right sternocleidomastoid muscle and three myofascial trigger points were injected in the right pectoralis minor muscle.

About 7 minutes after the procedure, the patient was put through a range of motion of the upper extremities (right/left): forward flexion 180/170, external rotation 72/62, abduction 173/173. When compared to her original evaluation of 11/18/94, it was deemed that the patient had shown improvement on both sides for forward flexion, essentially no change in the external rotation on either side, slight improvement for right-sided abduction, and slight decrease in the range of motion for abduction of the left side.

The patient's next visit was 9/5/95. She stated that overall her pain problem was not as bad as previously. She was able to drive a van the preceding weekend with less of the usual pain from performing that activity. She stated that she was going to go ahead and schedule the nerve block with Dr. Bojeff. Grip strength was briefly tested and found to be slightly higher than the values of 11/18/94 on the right side, with an average of 1 kg gain. Grip strength testing on the left side, however, revealed an average of 6 kg gain. The patient was alert and coherent, with no slurred speech, good cognition, no evidence of drug toxicity, and no difficulty understanding what I was saying.

The patient stated at that time that she was having problems with Thorazine® in that it was causing too much of a hangover in the morning. I recommended that she use Restoril® or Valium® at one to two tablets at bedtime to attempt to normalize her sleep. Pain chart depiction showed some decrease in the posterior paracervical pain pattern on the right and left, and also the right parathoracic pain area had decreased some more. On the doctor-drawn pain chart, I diagnosed the subclavius trigger point as being problematic. After premedicating the patient with 4 mg of Dilaudid® and 25 mg of Benadryl®, the right subclavius muscle was injected, with three big jump signs generated during that trigger point injection. The patient stated that she obtained major pain relief from the subclavius trigger point injection, which allowed her to cut back on her pain medication.

As of 9/5/95, the patient was still continuing on her K-Tabs® at two twice a day and remained on her L-thyroxine at 0.15 mg/day. Her consumption of Soma® was averaging two to three tablets per day. She had tapered off the Halcion® as of 8/17/95. She was continuing the Halcion® at about eight tablets per day. Her consumption of Levo-Dromoran® averaged 6–8 mg/day.

On 9/11/95, this patient had a procedure performed by Dr. Bojeff. The patient stated, and I always found her to be reliable, that she was under the impression that she was going to undergo a nerve block in the cervical spine and possibly the cervical plexus. There was no signature given for performing any lesioning procedure in the cervical spine area. The following is a quote from the operative note of that date. The note was dictated by Dr. Bojeff:

> The patient was positioned on the x-ray table, an intravenous axis line was placed. IV Versed was given for preop sedation. Monitors were placed and vital signs were obtained and recorded. Then landmarks were checked and the appropriate levels were marked.
>
> After adequate anesthesia was obtained, the block was then performed with a 22 gauge SMK block needle advanced to the lateral border of the lateral body of the vertebrae. Position confirmed by A/A-P and lateral views. The nerve was stimulated at 2 Hz and again at 50 Hz and was checked for sensory distribution and lack of motor function. Then aspirated to confirm that it was not in a vascular space before injection. Blocked the nerve with 1 cc 0.5% Marcaine under fluoroscopic guidance. Then the nerve was lesioned with RF to produce a lesion at 80 degrees centigrade for 90 seconds at each site in the C3, C4, C5 and C6. Discharged home in good condition, pain free.

There is no time indicated on the report as to when the procedure was done. On the same date in the afternoon, the patient called my office and stated that she "had C3–4 spinal nerve block done by Dr. Bojeff. Was in excruciating pain. What should she do? Grin and bear it or come in?" I returned the patient's call the next day, and I told her that if the pain flare continued, we would get her into the office on 9/13/95.

The next office visit was on 9/13/95. The patient was seen at 6 p.m. She stated that the treatment from Dr. Bojeff on the preceding Monday had consisted of a lesion of C3–6, lateral end of lateral body–medial communication branch. She stated that the doctor told her it would take 90 days to get the full results from the procedure and 10 days for the burning to calm down. The patient stated that she had been off work for 3 days because of pain from the procedure done by Dr. Bojeff. She was experiencing dizziness and exhaustion. Pain control was poor. She was noted to be in moderate to severe distress. She was alert and coherent, with no slurred speech, good cognition, no evidence of drug toxicity, and her ability to understand what I was discussing with her was within normal limits.

Review of her pain chart showed that there were new areas of problems in the paraspinal musculature of the thoracic region bilaterally from T7 to T11. The patient rated her pain at about 85% of the worst that she experienced; the intensity of pain was severe and the frequency constant. She could sit for 15 minutes, stand for 15 minutes, and walk for 30 minutes. She also stated that the pain at the angle of her neck and shoulder junction on the right side had been made worse by the procedure that Dr. Bojeff had carried out. The area on the right was also made worse by bending or twisting the neck to the left.

At that visit, the patient was told to stop her Levo-Dromoran® and was begun on Dilaudid® oral solution (1 mg/ml). About that time, the patient was switched to 5-mg Valium® tablets to be used at bedtime instead of the 2-mg tablets that had been ordered previously. On the date of that visit, the patient was premedicated with 4 mg of Dilaudid® and 25 mg of

Benadryl®, and about 40 minutes later myofascial trigger point injections were carried out to the right trapezius no. 2, the right longissimus thoracis at T8, iliocostalis thoracis on the right at T8, right iliocostalis thoracis at T7, right iliocostalis thoracis at T5, and right iliocostalis thoracis at T6. The patient was also put on a tapering hydrocortisone acetate injection schedule, in addition to her oral Cortef, starting at 20 mg on 9/14/95 and tapering down to none of the injectable on 9/18/95.

She was next seen on 9/18/95. She said her neck was very tender on the right side where the lesions were put into her neck during the radiofrequency procedure. She stated that even the liquid Dilaudid® did not give symptomatic relief, and the same was true for the two Levo-Dromoran® tablets every 3 hours. When I asked her what the net gain from the procedure performed by Dr. Bojeff was, she said that she was able to put a pillow in back of her neck for the first time in 1½ years. She stated that she was currently using two tablets of Valium® at bedtime instead of Soma®.

On her symptom chart, the pain was rated at 90% of the worst ever, intensity was severe, and frequency was constant. There was right paracervical pain from C2 to C7 that had not been present previously and also some of her usual shoulder/neck angle pain on the right side. She stated that the paraspinal thoracic pain described on her pain chart of 9/13/95 was spreading laterally on both sides and becoming very painful in the morning. She stated that when those pain attacks occurred, she could hardly breathe. At that visit, the patient was premedicated with 5 mg of Dilaudid® and 25 mg of Benadryl®. Twenty minutes later, the upper rectus abdominus muscles on the right and left side were injected in the exact same area that they had been injected previously on 7/13/95. (Note: The following is a point of information. When myofascial trigger point injections are carried out appropriately, it is very unlikely that the same myofascial trigger point will occur in a previously injected site.)

Ninety minutes after the procedure, the bowel sounds were checked and found to be active. Seventeen minutes after the procedure, the patient was given 0.1 cc (0.4 mg/ml) of Narcan®. On the subsequent visit (9/28/95), the patient stated that the relief from these trigger points (relating to the pain in the lower parathoracic spine) lasted for about 4–5 days.

She was next seen on 9/21/95. She stated that the neck had flared up from the lesions placed by Dr. Bojeff. The area of problem describing the posterior cervical spine on 9/18/95 was slightly widened laterally. The flare-up was causing her noticeable distress. She was noted to be in marked distress. The skin on the back of the right side of the neck was so sensitive that she could not wash it. I recommended that she wait on the brachial plexus block until the 3-month mark after the lesioning in the neck. My note on the physician's treatment plan for 9/18/95 indicated that the patient needed more abduction of the right shoulder. Therefore, the patient was premedicated with 4 mg of Dilaudid® and 25 mg of Benadryl®, and the right infraspinatus was injected. When that muscle was injected, there were four local twitch responses and one jump sign. One week later, a note was made that the range of motion of the right shoulder was better.

The patient was next seen on 9/28/95. She stated that Dr. Bojeff had put her on Neurontin®. She stated that even a low dose the medication made her feel "rotten." The medication was stopped and nothing was substituted for it. She stated that the preceding Monday she had gotten a prescription from Dr. Bojeff for Catapres® patches. We discussed her work situation for a while. She stated that the competition was high at work. With respect to hours of work per week, she stated, "I'm trying to keep it at 40 hours" per week. She was also trying to stay away from 60-hour work weeks. She was noted to be in moderate distress. She stated that she was sleeping much better since the block to her neck.

The patient had been instructed to put the Catapres® patch over her posterior cervical pain on the right side. By way of a doctor-drawn pain chart, the patient stated there was a band in the trapezius no. 3 area on the right side "that wouldn't let go." The patient was medicated with 4 mg of Dilaudid® and 25 mg of Benadryl®. Myofascial trigger point injections were carried out to the right T6 deep paraspinal, right T7 deep paraspinal, left T6 deep paraspinal, iliocostalis thoracis T6 on the right, right trapezius no. 3, right T9 iliocostalis thoracis, right T11 iliocostalis thoracis, and right T11 longissimus thoracis.

Throughout the entire preceding period of time, the patient continued to take the B-complex injections as indicated. She was taking the half-strength shots on alternating days. On even-numbered days, she would take injection #1, and on odd-numbered days, she would take injection #2.

Her next visit was on 10/5/95. I detected that she was showing signs of stress and recommended psychotherapy. When asked what her stresses were, the patient said her husband, work, Dr. Bojeff, and myself. In order to cut her stress level down, she decided to change her work so that she could work 2 days a week at home. The patient stated that her husband had a big problem with psychotherapy based on events related to psychotherapy following her 1986 accident. At that visit, the patient was referred to David Bevone, Ph.D., clinical psychologist and board certified in pain management.

When asked about her sleep, she stated that she woke up stiff and painful. She was noted to be in moderately severe distress. A pain chart filled out by the patient showed about 15% of her original symptoms and then the lower thoracic paraspinal involvement from T8 to T11 extending bilaterally to the posterior axillary line. Trigger points were palpated at T10 bilaterally, and there was tenderness in the T10 iliocostalis thoracis muscle. The patient was premedicated with 4 mg of Dilaudid® and 25 mg of Benadryl®, and then the T11 deep paraspinal muscles were injected on the right and left side. It was noted that her consumption of Soma® remained constant at that time, averaging about three tablets per day. Her consumption of oral Dilaudid® solution was 17 mg/day. Her use of Soma® at bedtime continued. Her use of Lorcet® continued at about three tablets per day.

Her next visit was 10/12/95. She stated that she was very pleased with the work that Dr. Loquila (a chiropractor) was performing for her. She stated that after one of the treatments, she was plagued by low back pain, nausea, and vomiting. She was told to take 25-mg Phenergan® suppositories every 3–5 hours as needed to combat the nausea and vomiting. Her pain chart following the chiropractic treatment showed paraspinal pain extending from the base of the occiput to just above the lumbosacral junction. She had pain in all of the paraspinal soft tissues out to the medial scapular border and in the lower thoracic and upper lumbar spine out to the posterior axillary line.

The patient was premedicated with 35 mg of Phenergan® plus 0.75 cc of 2% Xylocaine® and then in a separate syringe 4 mg of Dilaudid®. Trigger point injections were carried out to the right and left rectus abdominis muscles just below the umbilicus. She had been complaining of a great deal of belching after the chiropractic treatment and therefore the "belch button" trigger point was injected on the right and left sides.

Her next visit was on 10/26/95. The patient said she had been doing very well with the therapy from Dr. Loquila and that beginning his therapy had had a marked effect on improving her sleep. She was noted to be in moderately severe distress. She stated that she used the Dilaudid® liquid in the morning to control the stiffness and pain that is so characteristic of this type of patient. She stated that 4 hours later, she used Lorcet® 10/650. On that date, the patient was told to discontinue the use of Lorcet® in favor of the Dilaudid®. This was done for better overall control of her pain severity. She continued on the Valium®. Also on that date, the patient was told to discontinue the use of Ultram®. It was felt that this medication was giving her insignificant control of her pain level at that time. In retrospect, her use of Levo-Dromoran® continued through October of 1995 and then ceased.

Continuing with the visit of 10/26/95, on her pain chart she rated her pain about 85% of the worst that she has ever felt; intensity was severe, and frequency was constant. She could sit for 30 minutes, stand for 30 minutes, and walk for 30 minutes. Pain distribution on the charts was posterior paracervical from C3 to C7 bilaterally, thoracic paraspinal musculature extending out about 2 inches from the midline bilaterally from T3 to T5 and then T11 to L2, a band of about 2 inches in width, extending to the posterior axillary line bilaterally.

On that visit, she related that the most bothersome area of pain was in the thoracic spine area from approximately T4 to T6 bilaterally, and it was pain that was related to the old car accident of 1986 and the area where the garage door had hit her in the back. At that visit, she was premedicated with 4 mg of Dilaudid® and 25 mg of Benadryl®. Following that, myofascial trigger point injections were carried out on the right at the T10 deep paraspinal muscles, with one local twitch response and one jump sign. The right T8 deep paraspinal muscle was injected, the right T8 iliocostalis thoracis and longissimus thoracis were injected with two jump signs, and the right T7 iliocostalis thoracis and longissimus thoracis were injected with three jump signs. The injection solution for these trigger points was 0.25% Marcaine without epinephrine.

On 10/31/95, the patient left a note on my answering machine stating that she needed a medical leave of absence because of pain and dysfunction related to pain. The initial request was for a 2-month leave of absence.

On 11/1/95, I spoke with her over the phone, and she indicated she was going to start her leave of absence that Friday. The plan was to keep her off for a couple of months. I asked if she had seen Dr. Bevone; she said "not yet," but she said she would go soon.

The next visit is dated 11/9/95. The patient stated, "Ever since the nerve block I have been on a downward spiral." (This refers to the radiofrequency lesioning that she had in September.) She was noted to be in moderately severe distress and stated that she was going to be starting her sessions with the clinical psychologist the following Monday. Symptom charting at that visit revealed that she rated her pain at 90% of the worst that she has ever had; sitting could be accomplished for 15 minutes, standing for 15 minutes, and walking for 1 hour. The intensity of the pain was severe and the frequency constant. The area of pain chart involvement now surpassed that of her original chart of a year earlier. There was cervical pain on the right side, both anteriorly and posteriorly, interscapular pain from T4 to T7 bilaterally, lower thoracic and lumbar pain from T11 to L4 with extension to the posterior axillary line bilaterally, pain in the right buttock, and pain down the lateral side of the right thigh and leg. There was also the previously mentioned ulnar pain on the right upper extremity, both above and below the elbow.

On that date, the patient was premedicated with 4 mg of Dilaudid® and 25 mg of Benadryl®. The right gluteus minimis was injected in two areas. The solution used was 0.25% Marcaine. Between the two shots, the patient had five jump signs and additionally ten local twitch responses.

In a telephone note of 11/13/95, the patient indicated that she met with Dr. Bevone and was thankful for the referral. A recommendation was made for the patient to be put on an antidepressant. I started her on low-dose Norpramin® (10-mg tablets), to be taken at one to five tablets before retiring.

She indicated that with the help of the chiropractic work, her sleep continued to improve and she was tapering her use of Valium®.

She was next seen on 11/22/95. The patient was emotionally distraught, the reason being that pain restricted her ability to work. Her sexual life was very adversely affected by the lack of pain control. She stated that the injections of Dilaudid® that she had obtained at the office as premedication for her trigger point injections were more effective than the oral liquid

Dilaudid®. She stated that her yoga classes were progressing well and that she had better control of her sciatic pain. She was noted to be alert and coherent, with no slurred speech, good cognition, no evidence of toxicity, and her ability to hear and understand were within normal limits.

Review of her symptom chart showed that the symptoms were an additional 10% worse in terms of geographic distribution compared to 11/9/95. She stated that the interscapular pain that she had at that time and the sciatic pain down the right leg were new since the radiofrequency procedure had been carried out.

(Note: Making the decision to put an intractable pain patient on injectable opioids, such as Dilaudid®, is a very difficult decision since the inappropriate use of the medication can be accompanied by unnecessary complications of addiction, overutilization, and use of the medication for psychologic purposes instead of physical pain abatement purposes. I had known this patient for essentially 8 years at the time of her request for the use of injectable Dilaudid®. I had observed that she was a sincere individual, had a stable marital relationship of 19 years, and a stable husband. I had gotten to know her husband following her 1986 injury. She was a goal-oriented person who was very accurate in her reporting and very sensitive to requests to use medications in accord with my directions. She was being seen very frequently at the office. She had no excuses about losing her medications or other indicators of being a poor candidate for the use of injectable analgesics.)

Therefore, on her visit of 11/22/95, dosing, and the direction of eventually considering the injectable Dilaudid®, was started with the use of 4-mg Dilaudid® tablets. She was given a prescription for 400 tablets with directions for one to three tablets every 4 hours as needed for neuropathic or myofascial pain. It was also obvious, from observation of this woman's progress, emotional status, and general response to the pain she was feeling, that her pain level had moved into the range of being severe. At the same time that the Dilaudid® tablets were issued, the patient was given a prescription for 80 cc of Dilaudid® (2 mg/ml injectable) with directions for 0.5–2 cc every 3 hours as needed for severe pain. The idea here was to use the Dilaudid® injectable for breakthrough pain that could not be treated with the use of Dilaudid® tablets.

At the visit of 11/22/95, the patient was premedicated with 4 mg of Dilaudid® and 25 mg of Benadryl®. A left-sided upper rectus abdominis trigger point injection was carried out as related to the horizontal band of pain across the lower thoracic and upper lumbar region. She reported on her visit of 12/12/95 that the relief of pain in that band lasted 1 day. (Note: The interpretation here was that one of the myofascial trigger points contributing to the band of pain had been relieved, but others contributing to that same pain site needed to be located and properly injected.)

In a telephone note of 11/29/95, she left a message stating that the Norpramin® was not helping her significantly with respect to sleep. This was noted at the three- to four-tablet dose. She stated that she would elevate the dose to 50 mg at bedtime and see if the quality of her sleep improved. She stated that the sleep seemed to be worse with Norpramin® and had been better with Soma®.

On 11/23/95, this patient was referred for an MRI of the cervical spine because of her progressive right-sided pain. I felt at that time that because the problem had progressed to not only involve her entire right upper extremity but also the lower extremity, there was a need to rule out cord damage that might have occurred from the radiofrequency lesioning. The procedure was done on 12/1/95 and compared with the previous cervical spine study. Essentially, the study of 12/1/95 failed to reveal any significant change from the previous study.

Her next visit was 12/12/95. She was alert and coherent, with no slurred speech, good cognition, no evidence of drug toxicity, and her ability to understand what I was saying was within normal limits. When inquiring about the results of the Norpramin® for purposes of mood elevation, she stated that she was not as teary and did not feel "up." When I inquired about her employer, she stated they wanted her to have as much time off work as needed. With respect to her activity level, she stated that she could do many activities, but sitting, such as the type she did at work, was most provocative to her pain problem. She stated that up to 4 mg of intramuscular Dilaudid® did not help the pain that occurred when she sat. (Note: This patient had initially been taught to administer her vitamin shots drawing up the injections with a 3-cc syringe plus 20-gauge 1½-inch needle. When the proper amounts were drawn up, the needle was exchanged for a 30-gauge 1-inch needle. This needle is extremely well tolerated by chronic pain patients who frequently have sensitive muscle, skin, and subcutaneous tissue. Therefore, when it came to having this patient draw up Dilaudid® shots for herself, there was no need to repeat the instructions which I had given her when she first began her vitamin injections.)

Her sleep had been irregular since being off work. She stated that the Norpramin® was not much help for sleep and that it caused night sweats, which were bothersome. She stated that, in general, her morning pain was better. I recommended that she return to the use of Thorazine® at bedtime. Review of her symptom charting showed that the pain was severe and constant and rated about 80–85% of the worst she ever had. It was obvious that the chiropractic work had helped relieve some of her interscapular pain and also had cut back on the pain that was radiating into her right upper and lower extremity. There was numbness noted in the lateral border of the right lower extremity from the hip to the lateral border of the foot and the medial surface of the right upper extremity in the distribution previously described for pain.

The patient had been given a 3-day pain diary which covered 11/24 to 11/27/95. On a scale of 10 being the worst pain severity and 0 being none, over those days her pain ranged from a low of 5 to a high of 8. The activity level during those days ranged from resting or sleeping to doing half of all the usual work inside the home. The predominant mode during the hours of 4 a.m. to 6 p.m. each day was activity in which she was doing half of all of her usual work inside the home and related activities.

At the visit of 12/12/95, she was premedicated with 4 mg of Dilaudid® and 25 mg of Benadryl®. Following that, the deep paraspinal muscles on the right side were injected at the C3, C4, C5, and C4–5 level. During the procedure, she had a jump sign averaging about two per procedure and a local twitch response on each of the four injections.

On her visit of 12/15/95, she indicated that at times up to 15 mg of oral Dilaudid® solution by mouth did not provide much pain control. At that period of time, she continued on the thyroid medication at 0.15 mg/day. She also continued on the potassium tablets at two twice per day. At that visit, the possible use of Duragesic® patches was discussed in a preliminary fashion. She stated that when she slept on her left side, both her right and left arm went to sleep, and this consisted of a tingling sensation in the upper extremities. She was alert and coherent, with no slurred speech, good cognition, no evidence of toxicity, and her ability to hear and understand what I was saying was within normal limits.

On her visit of 12/19/95, she reported localized relief only at the previous areas of myofascial trigger point injections. At that visit, two pain diary sheets were reviewed, spanning the time from 12/13/95 to 12/19/95. Her overall energy level was rated at 40–50% of what she had before the pain problem started. The pain severity ranged between a level of 5 and 9 throughout. Her overall activity level was graded at about 50% of what she had prior to the onset of her pain problem. Medications that she was using during that time period consisted of Dilaudid® tablets, Dilaudid® injectable, Soma® 350, Norpramin® 10, 10-mg Thorazine® tablets, and oral Dilaudid® liquid. Using the Dilaudid® solution, her intake between 9/13/95 and 9/15/95 averaged 17–30 mg/day. Some of the comments that the patient made regarding the Dilaudid® oral solution were as follows: The solution gave her much better control of her pain and faster onset of pain relief than Levo-Dromoran® or Lorcet® 10. During attacks of acute pain, she used 1 teaspoon every 2 hours for best pain control. She stated that 1 teaspoon every 2 hours gave her 30% pain relief and that if she used too much of the oral solution, she had problematic itching.

At the visit of 12/19/95, the patient was given a prescription for 50-μg/hour Duragesic® patches and told to leave the patches on for 3 days. Each new patch would be applied at the 2½-day mark and the old patch removed at the 3-day mark. She was told that 4 hours after the patch had been put on, she was to cut her usual Dilaudid® dose in half and wait for the Duragesic® patch to begin working at the 8- to 12-hour period from the time of application. After the Duragesic® went to work, she was to supplement with Dilaudid® injectable for her pain spikes, as needed.

Review of her pain chart of 12/19/95 revealed bilateral posterior cervical pain from the occiput to C7 and including from the midline to the lateral-most aspect of the neck on both sides. There was anterior pain in the sternocleidomastoid muscles on both sides and in the trapezius no. 2 on the right side. Tingling in the ulnar nerve distribution and down the lateral aspect of the right leg was indicated by the patient to be "minimal." She was premedicated with 4 mg of Dilaudid® and 25 mg of Benadryl®. Following that, the right L1–2 longissimus thoracis was injected, with four jump signs, the right L4 iliocostalis lumborum was injected, with three jump signs and one local twitch response; and the right T11 longissimus thoracis was injected with 0.25% Marcaine, with two local twitch responses and two jump signs.

Her next visit was 12/28/95. The patient stated that the Duragesic® patches were helping. She was using the injectable Dilaudid® to supplement the patches. Neurologic reevaluation was carried out and compared to her values of 8/10/95. There was no hypesthesia or hyperesthesia in the upper or lower extremities. She stated that the use of the Duragesic® patches had made a difference in respect to controlling the pain that was making her feel "nuts." The patient had stopped the Norpramin®; it did not seem to help that much with the sleep or mood elevation. Also, the Norpramin® had been responsible for troublesome night sweats. When asked how she was doing with her psychologist, she said she was making progress. When asked about her sleep, she stated that one 10-mg Thorazine® tablet was okay but one and one-half tablets a day gave too much of a hangover. I recommended that she use one Soma® and one Thorazine® at bedtime to improve her sleep.

On the pain chart, she had 10–15% of her original symptomatology on her pain chart of 11/19/94 and a thin stripe of pain extending from the mid buttock to the posterior mid lateral thigh into the lateral aspect of the calf and ending at the ankle. There was numbness in the ulnar nerve distribution in the right upper extremity. She stated that the frequency of the pain radiating down her right leg was becoming less. She stated that the worst part of the area in her bilateral neck pain region was gone since the last trigger point injection procedure.

The patient submitted a pain diary that covered 12/22/95 to 12/25/95. The pain intensity ranged between 7.5 and 5.5. Her energy level was still about 40–50% of normal. The frequency of the pain was constant. The pain intensity ranged between moderate to severe, and activity level was about 50% of her usual prepain level.

The patient was premedicated with 4 mg of Dilaudid® and 25 mg of Benadryl® plus 0.5 cc of 2% Xylocaine®. Following that, myofascial trigger point injections were carried out to the right iliocostalis thoracics T11, with three jump signs; the right iliocostalis thoracis T9, with one local twitch response and two jump signs; the right iliocostalis thoracis T6, with three big jump signs and one local twitch response; and the right iliocostalis thoracis T3, with one local twitch response and three big jump signs.

At her visit on 12/28/95, the patient was placed on 100-mg Serzone® tablets.

On 1/6/96, I received a call from her psychotherapist. He stated that the patient had called him to discontinue the treatments. He stated that she had had about five sessions by that time and had gained insight. She stated that she had financial problems. He stated this patient said she would follow up before return to work in a few months. He felt that she had resolved a number of major issues. He stated that he had performed surface electromyography on the patient and that she had excess muscle tension in the upper right trapezius. He stated that she continued with cold hands and sympathetic overactivity. He also stated that he had enjoyed working with her.

Her next visit was on 1/11/96. The patient had had a radical hysterectomy because of some cervical carcinoma on reviews previously. She stated that she was presently on "high dosage" of birth control pills. She was getting an interview form for hypothyroidism and adrenal insufficiency, and it was noted that she had quite a number of positives on both of the tests. She was continued at 0.075 mg of thyroid supplementation and was told to increase the dose to 0.1 mg/day. The patient was questioned about the thyroid problem, and she stated that it was problematic in high school. She had 2 years of home teaching during this problem and was treated with thyroid medication. She stated that the medication helped. She was kept out of physical education in high school. The patient stated that the response to the thyroid treatment was that her pulse rate went from 140 bpm down to 120 and she stopped losing weight. On her visit of 1/11/96, her pulse rate was 100 bpm and regular, her blood pressure was 90/80, and her temperature was 99.1. She was alert and coherent, with no slurred speech, good cognition, no evidence of drug toxicity, and her ability to understand what I was saying to her appeared to be within normal limits. Review of the pain chart showed that the radicular component in the right upper extremity was gone. The posterior paracervical pain pattern remained less prominent, but geographically was still the same. There was pain noted radiating from the sternoclavicular joint on the right side down to the anterior axillary line in about a 2- to 3-inch-wide pattern. There was approximately 35% of the pain in the lower thoracic distribution left, about 50% of the right paraspinal thoracic pain from T4 to T6, and presence of the radicular pain from the mid buttock area on the right side down the lateral aspect of the leg and foot.

The patient returned a form that was used to repeat some of the initial review of systems (see Update of Progress in Program at the end of this chapter). On that form, she indicated problems with energy and stamina, which included decreased energy, tires easily, gets tired by afternoon, does not tolerate stress well, cannot work as hard as she used to, cannot work as much as she used to, and has to rest more now than before her pain problems started. There was weakness of the right arm and left leg, as well as the back muscles. The Global Activity Assessment Test (see form labeled Update of Progress in Program) was compared with her original version, and it was noted that overall she was abut 40% down as far as physical functioning was concerned. Sleep was a bigger problem in January of 1996 than originally. Whereas she had originally rated her overall strength and endurance at 8 (on a scale of 0 to 10), she rated herself at a level of 5 in January 1996. In the Provocative Activity Test, there were many physical activities that provoked her pain. She noted that she had been out of work for 2 months at that time. She stated that she felt life was satisfactory, but had worries about money and her job. She stated that she felt cold most of the time. She felt that her marriage was very satisfactory.

Her next visit was 1/17/96. Inquiry was made about the effectiveness of the Duragesic® patches. She stated that the pain relief was better than that obtained with the Dilaudid® injection alone, and she supplemented the patches with Dilaudid® injection. She stated that the 75-μg/hour patch did not provide enough pain relief. As of that date, she was switched to the 100-µg/hour patches. My note on that date read, "Patch or no patch, she feels she is getting better. Flare-ups are not as bad as before." She stated that the pain still became worse as the day went on. She was noted to be in moderately severe distress, but I observed, "Overall looks bright and positive." She was alert and coherent, with no slurred speech, good cognition, no evidence of drug toxicity, and her ability to understand what I was saying was within normal limits. She stated sleep was a problem in general, but the Thorazine® was helping. On the pain chart that I drew for the patient that day, she indicated a tightness in the upper one-third of the trapezius muscle. At that visit, a skin trigger point injection was carried out to the trapezius no. 2 trigger point, which she indicated at a subsequent visit was of no help.

Her next visit was 1/25/96. She stated that she had had a bout with the flu since the early part of the month and this caused her energy to go down. At that time, she was on 0.125 mg of Synthroid® and indicated no problems. The patient was told to elevate her intake of Synthroid®, going up by 0.025 mg weekly until she got to a maximum of 0.175 mg/day. She stated that her activity level had not improved since December. She stated that compared to the first visit to the office, overall she was worse. She stated that her sleep was better and she did not have to use Thorazine® at that time. She was continuing the use of Soma® at the rate of two to three tablets per day. She was on Cortef at one-half tablet twice per day. Her intake of Dilaudid® injectable was averaging about 12 mg/day. Her consumption of Serzone® was 100 mg twice per day. A comprehensive panel of laboratory testing was order and showed no problems for the complete blood count. The chemistries were essentially unremarkable. Electrolytes showed that her potassium was 4.3 (normal range = 3.4–5.5) on four K-Dur® tablets per day. Liver function tests showed no abnormalities. There was a very slight elevation of her triglycerides. Sedimentation rate was unremarkable. Her free thyroxin level was 0.9 ng/dl (normal range = 0.6–1.5) on 0.1 mg of Synthroid® intake per day. Urinalysis was within normal limits. At that visit, the patient was premedicated with 4 mg of Dilaudid® plus 25 mg of Benadryl® and 0.5 cc of 2% Xylocaine®. The left and right trapezius no. 2 muscles were injected. There were two local twitch responses and four jump signs in each muscle that was injected.

On 1/30/96, Dr. Bevone was contacted about the patient. He stated that the patient had stopped coming, but then had come back on the Monday before I called him. She was more depressed and there was a recommendation to increase the Serzone®. I expressed to him a concern about this patient's neediness and that others feel sorry for her. Some guidelines were asked for. He stated that the patient was scared. He stated that she needed to be encouraged to develop a support system. She needed encouragement to continue her appointments with Dr. Bevone. He reiterated my position that the patient's visits needed to be structured and time limits needed to be adhered to.

The next visit was 2/2/96. The patient stated that she had gotten some impressive relief from the trigger points that had been previously injected and that the overall result was that they had helped.

On 2/2/96, a repeat of her physical examination had been scheduled. In preparation for this repeat examination, and to further evaluate the role of the analgesic medication in her case, the patient was told to drop from the 100-µg/hour Duragesic® patches to the 75-µg/hour patches 3 days before the examination. She was also told to take no Dilaudid® injections after 5:00 p.m. the night before the evaluation. The office visit began at 11:20 a.m. that day. The patient was noted to be alert and coherent, with no slurred speech, good cognition, no evidence of drug toxicity, and was processing what I was saying within normal limits. It was noted on her symptom charting that she indicated that her pain was 95% of the worst that she had ever had. Sitting tolerance was 10 minutes, standing tolerance 10 minutes, and walking tolerance 15 minutes. Intensity of the pain was severe and frequency was constant. Compared to some of her previous checks, there was marked pain in the right paracervical musculature, interscapular pain from T4–T6 was marked, pain was radiating down the ulnar aspect of the entire right upper extremity, pain was noted from T12 to the lumbosacral junction and extended to the posterior axillary line, there was pain in the left buttock, and there was pain in the right buttock extending down the lateral side of the thigh and leg. Because the colored pencils that patients use to fill in the chart can be used in a heavy shading or light shading fashion, it was easy to see that the intensity of her pain in all the areas mentioned was much more significant than previously. She was noted to be well developed, well nourished, well hydrated, and in moderately severe distress. When she got up from the examining chair, she was noted to be stiff; she had to use the exam room chair armrest to push herself up. It was noted that as she disrobed, she could take her sweater up to about 7 level, but no higher. She had to remove one arm at a time, then push the garment up over her head. She was in noticeable distress while doing this; the same was true for a turtleneck sweater which she slipped her arms out of first and then slipped over her head slowly. It was noted that as she removed her shoes, she lifted her right leg up with her right hand and then took the shoe off with the opposite hand. She also had to assist her left leg with her left hand to get her shoe off. (Note: This is an indicator of extensive hip weakness.) There was no problem with removal of her sweatpants. Although the room temperature was essentially normal, the patient felt cold and had goose bumps on her upper extremities. With the hands outstretched, there was no tremor noted. The neurological examination was repeated, and this time there was found to be hypesthesia to pinprick in the upper extremity in the right C5 and C7. Findings were negative for any pinprick pathology on the left side. In the right lower extremity, there was pinprick hypesthesia in the L5 dermatome; otherwise, for all the dermatomes in the lower extremities on the left and right side, there were no abnormalities found. Range of motion of the cervical spine was compared to her original exam of 11/18/84. There was mild improvement with respect to flexion and extension. Lateral bending had stayed the same on both sides, and there was approximately a 10-degree increase in rotation on both sides. Range of motion of the shoulders was essentially the same as it had been initially, except for a 30-degree decrease in abduction of the left shoulder on the exam of 2/2/96. More extensive manual muscle testing was carried out at the visit of 2/2/96 than previously. Manual muscle testing revealed (right/left): shoulder forward flexors 4+/4+ with breakaway weakness on both sides, shoulder abduction 4+/4+, wrist extension 4+/5–, hip abduction 4/5– with pain in the hip on the right and pain in the anterior thigh on the left, hip adduction 4/4 with pain in the back of the hip on the right and pain in the back of the leg on the left, knee extension 4/4+ with pain in the back of the leg on the right and pain in the back of the leg on the left, ankle dorsiflexion 5/5–, and EHL 4+/4+. Grip strength testing was carried out using a Jamar Grip Strength Tester. The net result was approximately two-thirds of normal anticipated strength on both sides for a female her age. It was noted that on resisted abduction, the patient had a tremor on both sides when resistance was attempted in the shoulders. Straight leg raising was 45 degrees on the right with pain in the back of the leg and 40 degrees on the left with pain in the back of the leg. This represented a 30- to 40-degree difference when compared to the original testing which had showed 75 and 85 degrees, respectively. Range of motion of the lumbar spine was essentially similar to the previous test, except she lacked 10 degrees of lateral bending to the right. In the sitting position, rotation of the lumbar spine was carried out and was found to be 0 degrees to the right and 24 degrees to the left, with both of these tests causing pain in the neck and back. The deep knee bending maneuver showed that overall her score was worse this time by about 20–30% in all categories measured. This maneuver caused pain on the evaluation of 2/2/96 and had not caused any discomfort on the prior examination. It was noted that in the recumbent position, she was most comfortable with her hips and knees bent almost maximum. (Note: This usually indicates a trigger point in the area of the iliopsoas muscle on the side on which the flexion occurs.) The patient was noted to be in marked distress and was instructed to give herself an injection of 4 mg of Dilaudid®. In the recumbent position, she was checked for taut band signs and jump signs in the trapezius, sternocleidomastoid, pectoralis major, and latissimus dorsi muscles. All muscles had taut bands, tenderness, and jump signs. The jump signs were most noticeable in the right sternocleidomastoid muscle, left trapezius, left sternocleidomastoid muscle, and the left latissimus dorsi. Palpation was also carried out in the posterior right triceps, right brachioradialis, mid upper forearm, lower chest on both sides, and both tibialis anterior muscles. Tenderness with accompanying jump signs was found in all areas tested. At the same visit, the patient was given a verbal evaluation for signs of symptoms of estrogen deficiency (a copy of that form is appears at the end of this chapter). She had a lot of positives on the examination. She stated that she was taking high-dose Ovral® every day. (Note: It was decided to put her on an additional 0.3 mg of Premarin® because of the numerous positives in that test, such as anxiety, cold hands and feet, depression, painful sexual activity, fatigue, forgetfulness, headaches, inability to concentrate, inability to cope, insomnia, loss of creativity, loss of libido, nervousness, night sweats, palpitations, paresthesias, and weakness, with the presence of a severe myofascial pain syndrome and thinning of the genital skin area, plus osteoporosis.)

On 2/6/96, I spoke to Dr. Bevone about her progress. He stated that the patient would be coming in with her husband the following week. He stated that she was more depressed. I indicated to wait a week to see the effect the extra estrogen would produce; if it had no significant benefit, then the psychiatrist should be called in. A decision was made to refer her to a psychiatrist for therapy and administration of additional antidepressant medication.

The patient was next seen on 2/7/96. She stated that she was not feeling good. She stated that her energy was better, but the night sweats still woke her up. A checklist hyperthyroid test was carried out verbally, and the patient was found to have many positives. She was noted to be in moderately severe to marked distress. She stated that her sleep was not good. Palpation of the right scalene medius muscle revealed a taut band with a noticeable jump sign.

The patient's next visit was on 2/15/96. She stated that the estrogen had helped her mood and pain a little. She had, therefore, seen Dr. Ralston (a psychiatrist), who was taking over the management of her psychologic medication. She stated that her evening pain was still problematic. There was no problem with the thyroid dose. She was noted to be somewhat between moderate distress to moderate severe distress. She seemed slightly better emotionally. The patient had gone back to use of the 100-μg Duragesic® patches and injectable Dilaudid®, and the pain symptomatology intensity was noticeable reduced between the charts of 2/15/96 and 2/2/96. Posterior paracervical musculature on both sides was involved, the interscapular musculature from T3 to T6, on the arm from the axilla to the ulnar two fingers, and buttock from the mid buttock down the lateral aspect of the thigh and leg. The patient was premedicated with 4 mg of Dilaudid® and 25 mg of Benadryl®, plus 0.5 cc of 2% Xylocaine®. About 40 minutes later, the right scalene medius was injected with 0.4% procaine. There were two local twitch responses and one jump sign. She was referred to myofascial physical therapy, a special type of therapy with resistive exercises, massage, and ischemic compression plus range-of-motion restoration two to three times a week for 3 months. She was continuing her therapy with Dr. Loquila. On 2/15/96, she was told to take one and a half of the 0.3-mg Premarin® tablets. In follow-up about a week later, she indicated that the sweating problem was less. She was told to go to two of the 5-mg Cortef tablets each morning. She remained off of the Levo-Dromoran® tablets and the Valium® tablets. She continued to use small amounts of Benadryl® with each of her Dilaudid® injections. She had been back on the 100-µg Duragesic® patches since 1/17/96. Her consumption of Dilaudid injection averaged 10–20 mg/day.

Her next visit was 2/22/96. I informed her of the need for Independent Medication Review. Dr. Ralston had put her on Paxil®. The patient felt that Dr. Ralston could help her. I made some increase in her intake of Dilaudid® injectable, and the patient stated that this was because some of the flare-up symptoms remained subsequent to the physical reexamination of 2/22/96. She was in mild distress at that visit and looked more composed. She was much less teary. (Note: From the time of her having to leave work because of the pain flare-up due to the radiofrequency procedure on her neck, through 2/2/96, the patient had been noticeably emotionally labile. She would cry easily during our sessions, and this became a fairly constant occurrence. This was based on a number of factors, one of which was her loss of stature in the world of employment. It also turned out that a great deal of that emotional lability was due to her low estrogen level, which will be further explored as this synopsis continues.) The symptom chart showed about 15% of the symptomatology that was demonstrated on her pain chart of 11/22/95. The patient was premedicated with 4 mg of Dilaudid® plus 25 mg of Benadryl® plus 0.5 cc of 2% Xylocaine®, and myofascial trigger points were injected in the right posterior latissimus dorsi two times and the right iliocostalis thoracis. The patient had one big jump sign (which shook her whole body) and two smaller jump signs during the latissimus muscle injections and one jump sign with the iliocostalis thoracis injection.

The next visit was 3/1/96. She stated that she was doing better and her pain level was down. She stated that when Dr. Loquila treated her muscles, they were less tender. She stated that the physical therapy program was helping. She stated that she and her husband had seen Dr. Bevone on the preceding Monday. Clinically, there was no weeping or crying during the visit. She was alert and coherent, with no slurred speech, good cognition, no evidence of drug toxicity, and her ability to understand what I was saying was within normal limits. She was premedicated with 4 mg of Dilaudid® plus 25 mg of Benadryl® plus 0.5 cc of 2% Xylocaine®, and myofascial trigger points were carried out into the left deep quadratus lumborum two times, the right superficial quadratus lumborum, and the right iliocostalis lumborum L2. She demonstrated a number of jump signs, and this was especially noticeable when the superficial quadratus lumborum was injected. The patient stated that Premarin® was elevated to 0.6 mg/day. The plan was to keep her at that dose for a couple of weeks and then taper her down.

Her next visit was on 3/6/96. She stated that she had been bruising and bleeding from vitamin shots for a few weeks preceding that visit. Inspection of her injection sites revealed some mild superficial bruising about 1.5 cm in diameter in two areas of injection. She mentioned that the use of the estrogen had reduced some of her problems with night sweats. She stated that she was having more good days and having them more often. She continued on Paxil® and was using it at bedtime. When asked how things were going with Dr. Bevone, she stated that he was nice, but that she didn't feel that he understood some of the important intricacies of her problems. The pain chart showed about 20% of the symptomatology that was on her symptom chart of 2/22/95. At that visit, she was premedicated with 4 mg of Dilaudid® plus 1 cc of 2% Xylocaine®. In a separate syringe, an injection of 25 mg of Phenergan® plus 0.5 cc of 2% Xylocaine® was given. Four myofascial trigger points were injected in her gluteus minimus anterior muscle. During these injections, she had a limited number of jump signs, but had three of them when trigger point no. 4 of the vastus lateralis was injected. She had injection of gluteus maximus no. 1 on the right side with three local twitch responses and five jump signs. Lastly, the piriformis no. 2 trigger point was injected on the right, with three local twitch responses and five jump signs.

Her next visit was two days later, on 3/8/96, and was the result of being rear-ended in an automobile accident on 3/7/96. The patient stated that she was stopped at a light and was hit from behind at low speed. She stated that her car lurched forward and her head went back onto the headrest. She stated that her neck felt "a little funny" at the time and pain continued to worsen through that evening. She stated that as of 3/8/96, the neck pain was a lot worse. With my permission, she had increased her dose of injectable Dilaudid® to compensate for the pain flare-up. She was told to increase her intake of Cortef to 35 mg/day for 1 week and then return to her dose of two tablets per day (10 mg). She was noted to be in moderate distress. When asked about her sleep, she stated that she had taken extra Soma® and extra Thorazine® the evening of 3/7/96 to compensate for the increased pain. Compared to one of her recent symptom charts, the pain intensity had gone from about 70% to 85% on visual analogue scale (i.e., 85% of the worst pain she has ever had). Her walking tolerance had gone down, and the same was true for her sitting tolerance. Standing tolerance remained the same. Pain distribution was bilateral posterior cervical involving the entire posterior neck. The pain extended to the sternocleidomastoid muscle on the right and the neck/shoulder junction of the trapezius muscle on the left. The interscapular pain had become more intense, but the geographic distribution was the same. There was pain from T11 to L1 and extending out to the posterior axillary line on both sides. The only leg pain that was seen on her chart of 3/8/96 was distal to the tibialis anterior and the medial lower leg in its lower half on the right side down to the ankle, but not any further. Repeat physical examination was carried out. The patient stated that she had her last injection of 1.5 cc (2 mg/ml) of Dilaudid® at 8:00 that morning. The physical examination started at 10:09 a.m. From the disrobing maneuver, it was noted that as she went to remove her shoes, she used her right hand to assist the right leg and left hand to assist the left leg. She removed her slacks standing up against the examining table and used the right hand to assist the right leg out of the pant leg, but did not use the left hand to assist the left leg in getting out of the slacks. Neurologic testing was carried out for deep tendon reflexes. This was compared to the three sets that had previously been generated on 8/10/95, 12/28/95, and 2/2/96. Deep tendon reflex testing revealed (right/left): triceps 1+/1, biceps 1/±, brachioradialis 1/±, patellars 3/3, and Achilles 2+/2. This testing revealed that her right and left triceps reflexes were coming back and that her patella reflexes were becoming more hyperactive. The findings on the 3/8/96 examination were compared to 2/2/96. Range of motion of the neck with respect to forward flexion and extension had improved by about 20%. Lateral bending was the same on the right side and lacked about 20% of range of motion on the left side. Lateral rotation of the neck was approximately the same as the previous exam. There was pain in her neck on all range of motion. Range of motion of the shoulders revealed a 30-degree increase on both sides with forward flexion, essentially no change with external rotation, and a 15-degree increase of abduction on the left side. There was no pain on any range of motion of the shoulder. She assumed the recumbent position with no problem. Taut bands, tenderness, and jump signs were found bilaterally in the trapezius, cervical and mastoid, pectoralis major, and latissimus dorsi muscles. Straight leg raising could be carried out to 65 degrees on the right side and 81 degrees on the left side. This represented a 20-degree increase on the right and a 41-degree increase on the left. Hip extension was 25 degrees on the right and 15 degrees on the left. There was pain in the low back on the right side, but no pain on the left. This particular test had to be compared to the findings of 8/10/95. There was a 25-degree increase in hip extension on the right side and a 3-degree increase in hip extension on the left side. Range of motion of the lumbar spine revealed that she could touch her thumbs to the floor. Extension was the same as previously at 10 degrees. Lateral bending was 25 degrees to the right and 45 degrees to the left. This represented a 5-degree increase on both sides. Rotation of the lumbar spine revealed 37 degrees of rotation on both sides. This represented a 37-degree increase on the right and a 13-degree increase on the left. Having to do a deep knee bend, her overall rating was 100% for range of motion, 85% for strength and balance, and 90% for smoothness in movement, and it was noted that this maneuver did make her pain worse. This represented a 40% gain in range of motion, a 15% gain in strength, a 15% gain in balance, and a 20% gain in smoothness of movement. In the prone position, palpation of the paraspinal muscles from T3 to T12 on the right and T4 to T12 on the left revealed taut bands, tenderness, and jump sign. There was one point in the left thoracic paraspinal muscles of the longissimus thoracis at the T8 level which when palpated and snapped caused a large jump sign and was the most tender area of her paraspinal muscles. The patient was told to go to full-strength vitamin shots daily for 10 days (series #1 on even-numbered days and series #2 on odd-numbered days).

The next visit was 3/14/96. On that visit, she mentioned that she had problems with urinary retention on Paxil®, and therefore Dr. Ralston switched her to Zoloft®. She stated that since her recent auto accident, her pain level had gone way up. She stated that her need for injectable pain medication had increased to 3 cc (2 mg/ml) of Dilaudid® every 2 hours for increased pain relief. The patient's symptom chart on that date indicated that her pain level was up to the 85% mark, but the medication that she was on was giving good control of her pain symptomatology. The pain was still rated at severe and constant, but only showed 35% of the symptomatology noted on her worst recent pain chart of 2/2/96. The patient was premedicated with 4 mg of Dilaudid® and 25 mg of Benadryl® plus 0.5 cc of 2% Xylocaine®, and injection was carried out to the problematic taut bands in the paraspinal muscles on the left that were noted at the T8 and T11 during the examination of 3/8/96. The patient was sent for laboratory testing for assessment of her testosterone, FSH level, and estradiol levels. The testing showed that she was deficient in testosterone and that her estradiol level was at 87. Although this estradiol level was in the range for postmenopausal women, I felt it was too low for a woman her age.

The next visit was 3/21/96. She was noted to be alert and coherent, with no slurred speech, good cognition, no evidence of drug toxicity, and her ability to hear and understand what I was saying was within normal limits. Her overall pain level was stable as compared to the previous visit, and the pain was reported to be severe and constant. Because her sleep was disturbed, it was decided to add methadone at bedtime. The patient stayed on this medication for about a month. She commented that it produced better pain relief than Dilaudid® tablets. The medication helped her get to sleep, but she could not get up in the morning because of a problem with hangover from the methadone. Therefore, it was discontinued in May of 1996. Because of the inability of Premarin® to significantly raise this woman's estrogen level, she was put on Estratest® (1.25 mg esterified estrogen, 2.25 mg methyltestosterone). The patient was complaining of nocturnal myoclonus clonus. Her husband had commented that at times the problem became very severe. She was, therefore, put on 0.5-mg tablets of Klonopin®, one to six tablets at bedtime, for control of the myoclonus. She was told to begin at one tablet at bedtime and progress slowly until her sleep was restful. Unfortunately, the net effect of the Klonopin® over the next 2 weeks was that the dose that produced the proper therapeutic effects also caused too much morning hangover. Therefore, that medication was discontinued. She was continuing to use Benadryl® with her injectable Dilaudid® at home. The records showed that she did not use any Thorazine® after February of 1996. Her use of 350-mg Soma® tablets continued at about one to three tablets per day. At her visit of 3/21/96, she indicated that main problem was still the posterior paracervical musculature on both sides. She indicated that the pain area causing the most need for analgesic medication was at about the T5–T7 level, paraspinal muscles, and deep paraspinal muscles. She stated that at times this pain area compromised her breathing. She was premedicated with 4 mg of Dilaudid® and

25 mg of Benadryl® plus 0.5 cc of 2% Xylocaine®. Myofascial trigger point injections were carried out to the T6 right longissimus thoracis and left T7 iliocostalis thoracis, the left T5 and T6 multifidus, and the right T5 and T6 multifidus. There were numerous significant jump sides generated at each level that was injected.

On 3/1/96, she had been sent for medication review to an internist specializing in myofascial pain syndrome and chemical dependency (a copy of the referral form is provided in Chapter 22). At the time of her visit to the specialist, her diagnoses were (1) myofascial pain syndrome, progressive, multifocal, severe: 729.1; (2) fibromyalgia: 729.0; (3) power neuropathy: 356.4; and (4) depression. Medications listed were 100-µg/hour Duragesic® patches at three per day with a starting date of 2/19/95; 2-mg/ml Dilaudid® injections at 10–20 mg/day since 11/22/95; and 10 mg methadone three times per day since 3/20/96. He thought the patient did have intractable pain, no evidence of drug-dependent syndrome, no limitations of using drugs through euphoria, no evidence of abstinence syndrome, no evidence of drug-seeking behavior, and no evidence of toxicity to the medications. He felt the medications were used for obtaining appropriate goals of normal daily living, felt the medications were appropriate for the patient's needs and goals, and felt there was no additional diagnosis. He did recommend ruling out a levator scapula syndrome, and if present, injecting it.

Her next visit was on 3/27/96. At this visit, the patient stated that she was doing much better. She was told to stop her Ovral® and continue with the Estratest®. She also stated that the female hormone regimen had not produced any increase in her sex drive. She was noted to be in moderate distress and much brighter and less stressed than on numerous recent visits. Pain symptomatology was similar to previous visits as listed on the pain chart; pain level on the visual analogue scale was down to 60% of the worst it had ever been. Sitting tolerance was 30 minutes, standing tolerance was 30 minutes, and walking tolerance was 1 hour. Pain was still rated at severe and constant. One additional area of pain had been added to the pain chart and that was in the paraspinal muscles on the right side from T8 to T12, in the area of the longissimus thoracis. On the back of the doctor-drawn pain chart, this last area mentioned was highlighted and had a radiating component down to the lateral aspect of her right buttock. The patient was premedicated with 4 mg of Dilaudid® plus 25 mg of Benadryl® and 0.5 cc of 2% Xylocaine®. Myofascial trigger points were injected in the right T4 iliocostalis thoracis and longissimus thoracis, left T4 iliocostalis thoracis, and left T4 longissimus thoracis. There was a minimum of local twitch responses and a minimum of jump signs associated with this procedure. She had been changed to the 50-µg/hour Duragesic® patches on 3/11/96. However, because of the subsequent intensity of her pains once she attempted that dosing, she remained at the 100-µg/hour intake through the end of April 1996.

Her next visit was 4/3/96. At that visit, she was switched from Estratest® to Estrace (a natural estrogen derived from soybean). She had been retested on a number of her hormonal levels on 3/28/96. The T4 total was at 12.0 (normal range = 4.5–12.3), testosterone remained in the deficient part of the range, FSH was satisfactory, and the estradiol was 94 pg/ml. On her visit of 4/3/96, I inquired about her psychotherapy. She indicated that she wanted some work with boundary issues, and a number of resources were mentioned to her. She stated that Dr. Raghavn had her on 100 mg of Zoloft® per day. On the symptom chart, there were numerous problem areas which amounted to 40% geographically compared to the chart of 2/2/96. She had to drive a long distance to see Dr. Light, the consultant who performed her Independent Medication Review. She stated that since that time, she had a flare-up of the pain in the interscapular area from T4 to T6. She was premedicated with 3 mg of Dilaudid® plus 0.5 cc of Benadryl® and 0.5 cc of 2% Xylocaine®, and myofascial trigger point injections were carried out in the right scalene medius and the left scalene posterior muscle using 0.4% procaine. There was a minimum of jump signs and a minimum of local twitch responses. For purposes of improving her sleep and improvement of the myoclonus, the patient was put on one to two Ambien® tablets at bedtime.

Her next visit was on 4/10/96. She continued with the Cortef tablets at two each morning. She stated that in the week prior to the visit, she had noted some increased depression and increased urinary retention. She felt that this was most likely due to the use of methadone. She stated that her night sweats were less since her estrogen intake was going up. She continued on Dilaudid® injections at about 20–30 mg/day. Soma® intake was about one tablet per day. She was taking no Valium®. A note had been placed in the chart that as of the visit of 4/10/96, her auto accident of 3/7/96 was closed out. She was noted to be between moderate distress and moderately severe distress. She was alert and coherent, with no slurred speech, good cognition, no evidence of drug toxicity, and her ability to understand what I was saying was within normal limits. The symptom chart revealed some new findings, and this was compared to the pain chart of 2/2/96. Pain severity was about 85%, with a sitting tolerance of 20 minutes, standing tolerance of 30 minutes, and walking tolerance of 45 minutes. Pain was still rated at severe and constant. Posterior paracervical pain was present on both sides, but more prominent on the right than the left. The interscapular area mentioned previously, extending from T4–T7 and out about 2 inches from the midline, was more dense than she had noted previously. Parascapular pain on the right side extending from T4 to T8 and the T10–L1 bilateral pain extending out to the posterior axillary line was noted, and the radicular pains on the right leg were less prominent than previously. She had an area of pain in the anterolateral inferior chest wall on the left side and pain in the right sternocleidomastoid muscle. I drew the most problematic area of pain on a doctor-drawn pain chart, and this was the midline pain from T8 to T9, which extended about an inch and one-half out laterally on both sides. The patient was premedicated with 3 mg of Dilaudid® plus 25 mg of Benadryl® and 0.5 cc of 2% Xylocaine®, and the right serratus anterior was injected in two different locations, demonstrating a total of one local twitch response and four jump signs during that procedure. The injection solution was 0.25% Marcaine. She was given a sleep abnormalities interview form that I had developed (provided at the end of this chapter), and it was noted that myoclonus was still a problem, but there was no problem with nightmares, no sleeping in the tense attitude, and no abnormal breathing while sleeping. She stated that she felt beat up when she awoke in the morning and also woke up tired.

The next visit was on 4/17/96. She was having problems with boundary issues, both at home and at her place of employment. She indicated that the right scapula felt "sticky" on most days. Range of motion of the scapula was checked on both sides and was found to be within normal limits. The symptom chart was similar to what was described in the previous visit. The patient was premedicated with 3 mg of Dilaudid® plus 25 mg of Benadryl® plus 0.5 cc of 2% Xylocaine®, and the following myofascial trigger points were injected: right triceps no. 1 two times, right T6 and T5 paraspinal, and left T6 and T5-6 paraspinal (paraspinal means deep paraspinal). Injection solution was 0.25% Marcaine, and each muscle demonstrated two to five large jump sign reactions. In that visit, the patient was referred to Jesse Forde, MFCC.

Looking back (on 10/3/96) over the numerous myofascial trigger point injections that were performed on this patient, it is my opinion that all the trigger point injections helped this woman; some gave temporary relief, and some gave more permanent type relief. It was the totality of the myofascial trigger point injections, over time, that gave the best overall improvement in physical performance and functioning.

The next visit was on 4/24/96. She stated that her visits with Jesse Forde, MFCC, had good initial results. She had begun to experience pain in her left heel of a week's duration, and this pain was worse when she was up on the foot. She stated that the Estrace was helping her overall pain and energy, and she stated, "I feel like me again." She said that her sexual activity was better. She stated that the Klonopin® helped her get to sleep and that her sleep was fair, but she had difficulty getting up in the morning. She stated that she could sit for longer periods of time with less distress. On her symptom chart, she indicated that pain symptoms were about 65% of the worst pain she ever felt. She could sit for 30 minutes, stand for 30 minutes, and walk for an hour, and the pain was severe and constant. Other than the heel pain on the left, her symptom chart showed a pain distribution that was about 15% of what it had been at its worst (on the pain chart of 2/2/96). The most problematic area on the doctor-drawn pain chart was the superior medial border of the right scapula. Therefore, the patient was premedicated with 3 mg of Dilaudid® plus 25 mg of Benadryl® plus 0.5 cc of 2% Xylocaine®, and myofascial trigger points were injected with 0.4% procaine in the right scalene anterior, generating a big jump sign; right scalene posterior; and right trapezius no. 3 (the right trapezius no. 3 was injected about 2 inches superior to that depicted in the 1983 Travell and Simons textbook on the subject).

Her next visit was on 5/2/96. She stated that she was doing fine with her licensed marriage and family counselor. She stated that the counselor was helpful, and she was working on boundary issues for return to work. She felt that Jesse Forde was able to work with her on areas of concern and need that Dr. Bevone had not been able to address. The patient stated that she was physically overdoing and the increased activity had pushed the need for pain medications up. It was noted that in late April and early May of 1996, her intake of injectable Dilaudid® went to about 40–60 mg/day. She stated that 1–2 months previously, she could do no evening work, and at the time of the visit she could do errands in the evening. She was noted to be in moderate distress. She was alert and coherent, with no slurred speech, good cognition, no evidence of drug toxicity, and her ability to hear and understand what I was saying was within normal limits. She stated that the Ambien® was helping with respect to her sleep. The patient was given an attention deficit disorder screening test, since I felt that problem might be part of her pain syndrome. She was also given a Copeland Symptom Checklist for Adult Attention Deficit Disorders. Both tests pointed out that she probably had attention deficit disorder. The patient also stated that she could benefit from enhancement of her overall energy level. Therefore, she was started on Dexedrine® 10-mg spansules at one capsule per day. Her symptom chart showed that the medial scapular border pain on the right side had been eradicated. Posterior paracervical pain remained in the cervical occipital junction to C7 bilaterally, and the interscapular pain remained with a dominance on the right side from T4 to T8. She had persistence of the left heel pain and also indicated early involvement of pain in the plantar aspect of the right heel. She was premedicated with 3 mg of Dilaudid® plus 25 mg of Benadryl® and 0.5 cc of 2% Xylocaine®, and then myofascial trigger point injections were carried out to the right scalene posterior three times and the left scalene posterior. All these injections demonstrated at least one jump sign in addition to a local twitch response, and the last trigger point injection demonstrated three jump signs. The patient had repeated testosterone and estradiol levels, and the testosterone was deficient, but the estradiol read 1027 pg/ml. Therefore, the patient was taken off of the Estrace tablets. (Note: I believe that this relatively high level of estradiol was due to laboratory error.) Because of the patient's deficiency of testosterone, she was placed on 5 mg of oral methyltestosterone daily.

Her next visit was on 5/7/96. She indicated that her pain was worse when she was sitting. She stated that overall she was much better. She was able to stretch the intervals between the pain medication doses. Hip muscle strength testing was carried out, and she was found to have 5/5 strength on the right (on 2/2/96, she had 4/4 strength), and on the left she had 4+ with breakaway weakness (on 2/2/96, she had a 4/5 rating of the left hip). She stated that the posterior paracervical pain was a lot better. The interscapular pain was clearing up. The heel pain was essentially the same. Problem areas remained in the posterior paraspinal cervical musculature and the trapezius no. 2 trigger point area. She was checked for iliac crest height and found to be within normal limits. She was checked for a short hemipelvis and found to be short on the right side, needing 0.5 cm of correction, using a magazine or similar material, under the right ischial tuberosity to the level of the pelvis when she was sitting. She was premedicated with 3 mg of Dilaudid® plus 25 mg of Benadryl® plus 0.5 cc of 2% Xylocaine®. Then the following myofascial trigger points were injected: left gluteus minimus anterior, with one local twitch response and six big jump signs; left gluteus minimus anterior and posterior, with three local twitch responses and ten big jump signs; and right iliocostalis thoracis T4, with two local twitch responses and six jump signs. (Note: The weight-bearing muscle at the hip was injected with 0.4% procaine since I did not wish to incapacitate her for ambulation. The iliocostalis thoracis was injected with 0.25% Marcaine because it is not a weight-bearing muscle. Recent studies by Hubbard [1993] have revealed the presence of sympathetic nerve supply in the center of the trigger point. The reason for using Marcaine for injection purposes was to perform a sympathetic nerve block with the Marcaine as an adjunct to mechanically breaking up the trigger point with the needle that was being used for injection.)

Her next visit was 5/15/96. She stated that during the preceding week she had a few days of encouraging pain relief and restoration of function. Her comment about the butt lift was that it may have been helping, but she noted that the results of using it were not significant as far as pain relief was concerned. Her work with her therapist was progressing very nicely. The patient was working through a great deal of anger that had been associated with what she felt was an inappropriate procedure that had been performed by Dr. Bojeff. She felt the therapy was proceeding well and that Mrs. Forde was helping her to obtain additional insights and help from where her previous therapy had left off. Previously, I had asked the patient's husband to monitor her for nocturnal myoclonus, and the report was that there was none present as of that visit. She had had some pain flare-up for the 2 days preceding her office visit. She stated that her sleep was good and that the Ambien® was giving her a normal sleep. Her dreams were good and the dream patterns were good. She stated that the day before, she had had a marked pain flare-up in the medial location in her back and in a 2-hour period she had taken two Levo-Dromoran®, two Soma®, and 2 cc of Dilaudid® injectable plus one Lorcet®, which did not provide adequate relief from that particular pain. She stated that her evening pain was still the most problematic. She was noted to be alert and coherent, with no slurred speech, good cognition, no evidence of drug toxicity, and her ability to hear and understand what I was saying was within normal limits. On her symptom chart, I noted the appearance of a new pain. There was a right parascapular thick, intense band at about the T5 level that extended down to just below the mid section of the right buttock. She was premedicated with 3 mg of Dilaudid® plus 25 mg of Benadryl® plus 0.5 cc of 2% Xylocaine®. The following myofascial trigger points were injected: right iliocostalis thoracis, T8–T9; right iliocostalis thoracis and longissimus thoracis at T7; right T7 longissimus thoracis; left iliocostalis thoracis T7; and left longissimus thoracis at T7. All of these were injected with 0.25% Marcaine. All muscular injections demonstrated at least two local twitch responses and one to two jump signs, with the last muscle demonstrating two referred jump signs. (Note: When I indicate that the jump sign was big, it means that the patient's whole body twitched or jerked noticeably in response to the needle going through the muscle. This type of response during a myofascial trigger point injection can be very counterproductive in that it can activate and/or aggravate other myofascial trigger points in local or distant regions from the trigger point being injected. The best approach in cases of this type is to administer enough premedication to minimize the number and intensity of jump signs, and yet not administer so much premedication that the patient is excessively sedated. The idea in premedication for myofascial trigger point injections is to help the patient endure this procedure which can, at times, be from mildly to extremely painful. Also, in patients who are less than optimally premedicated, there is an "aftershock" that the patient can feel throughout the whole body for days after the trigger point injection has been carried out.).

The patient was next seen on 5/24/96. Based on the pain distribution that she had, including the cervical problem, it was felt that there may be an irritated-disc-related problem that was causing complications. I gave her a lengthy explanation about the use of intravenous colchicine in such patients and gave her a study that had been published on administering this type of therapy to 3000 patients. (Note: Colchicine is a strong anti-inflammatory drug that is derived from the autumn crocus plant. When taken by mouth, it is as potent as Motrin®, Naprosyn®, aspirin, and other such drugs. However, when given intravenously, it is a very powerful anti-inflammatory that is capable of shrinking inflamed and swollen spinal discs and can shrink down the inflammation of swollen nerve roots. In some patients, I use it intravenously for its very strong anti-inflammatory capabilities. In this patient's case, I considered that she might have a disc problem.) An intravenous butterfly needle was inserted into the patient's antecubital vein, and infusion was started with normal saline. Next the injection was switched to 2 cc of colchicine (1 mg) and injected over a period of 4 minutes. The line was then flushed with normal saline and the butterfly needle removed. Seven minutes following the injection, the patient was able to bend forward and touch her proximal interphalangeal joints to the floor on both sides. This would be considered a good initial response with a colchicine injection. The patient indicated that her evening pain was still a problem. When I inquired about the Dexedrine®, she stated that it was a big help; it helped decrease her pain in the evening and increased her energy. She actually went off the medication for a few days to assess its overall effectiveness in her recovery. In the 10 days before her visit of 5/24/96, the patient went on and off the medication a number of times to assess its efficacy in her overall rehabilitation. She stated that if she took the medication in the evening, it would help her get through the evening better. As of the visit of 5/24/96, directions were written for her to take one to three capsules each morning as needed. She had gone back to using Levo-Dromoran® for additional pain control as of 5/9/96. Her usage of the medication averaged about 10 to 12 tablets per day (20–24 mg/day). She was noted to be in moderate distress, was more alert, and was more animated than usual. She was alert and coherent, with no slurred speech, good cognition, no evidence of drug toxicity, and her ability to hear and understand what I was saying was within normal limits. A review of her opiate intake was carried out. The patient was using the 50-μg Duragesic® patches and had been doing so since 3/27/96. She was taking Levo-Dromoran® at the dosage indicated above and injectable Dilaudid® at 7–20 mg/day. It was planned that at the time of her next Duragesic® renewal, she would be converted to the 75-μg/hour patches to cut down on her need for some of the other opiates. On this visit, she was given 2 cc of colchicine intravenously. Two hours after her first colchicine injection, the patient indicated she had 50% pain relief. Also, the colchicine injection got rid of her heel pain problem.

Her next visit was on 5/29/96. At that visit, she stated that the results from the colchicine shot gave marked increase in flexibility and converted the heel pain to intermittent. She stated that the pain in general was 20% better until her night pain set in. The patient had experienced a pain flare-up from dancing at a wedding she had attended, and the flare-up itself was removed by the colchicine injection. She continued to see Dr. Ralston and continued on Zoloft®. Range of motion of the lumbar spine was checked, and it was noted that she could get her palms to the floor. She rated her sleep at "fair." Symptoms on the symptom chart distribution were limited to the posterior paracervical musculature and the sternocleidomastoid on the right side, with some involvement of the trapezius. Paraspinal muscles showed involvement on the right side from T4 to T10 and on the left side from T4 to T6. At that visit, the patient was given a 2.5-cc colchicine injection intravenously into the right antecubital vein. The patient was asked to do a repeat symptom chart 17 minutes after the colchicine shot had been administered. The pain level went from 75% to 50% and the pain distribution was decreased overall by 40%. Five minutes after the patient filled out her follow-up symptom chart, myofascial trigger points were injected in the right levator scapula three times and the left levator scapula three times. No premedication other than intravenous colchicine was used. The patient had the usual number of jump signs for muscular injection, but indicated that the procedure was overall too painful without the use of premedication with Dilaudid®.

It was in May of 1996 that this patient's 20-year marriage became very stressful and difficult. The patient planned to return to work on 6/3/96.

Her next visit was 6/4/96. Her injectable Dilaudid® intake ranged from 12 to 20 mg/day. This patient's use of oral hydrocortisone ceased in approximately June of 1996. The patient had been off of Soma® between March of 1996 and the middle of May of 1996. When she went back on the medication, her dosing between May and June averaged one to two tablets per day. Her chiropractor had ordered a cervical pillow and cervical traction. She was referred to Dr. Bondo, a dentist with expertise in treating myofascial pain syndrome. The intent here was to have her evaluated to see if any component of her cervical problem was related to malocclusion or dental imbalances. (If present, these problems can be very problematic perpetuating factors in patients with myofascial pain syndrome.) The patient said that, over-all, she was doing much better. When the subject of return to work was brought up, the patient informed me that both her employer and the disability insurance company were "playing games." She stated that her sleep was not too good over the preceding $1^{1}/_{2}$ weeks. She felt that Ambien® may have been affecting her memory and she was, therefore, switched back to Soma®. On her symptom chart, pain was rated at about 70% of the worst she had ever had. She could sit for 30 minutes, stand for 30 minutes, and walk for 1 hour. Pain was rated at severe and constant. The pain patterns depicted on her chart were the usual posterior cervical musculature bilaterally, with emphasis on the right side. The sternocleidomastoid muscle on the right was involved, as was the upper trapezius near the neck/shoulder angle. Previously noted thoracic paraspinal pain extending from T4 to T8 was noticed. There was radicular pain down the right arm in an ulnar nerve distribution. There was radicular pain down the right leg extending from the iliac crest through the middle of the buttock and then down the lateral aspect of the thigh and lower leg. The heel pain was about one-quarter of what it had been previously. At that visit, she was given a 3-cc intravenous colchicine injection, and 26 minutes later the left soleus no. 3 trigger point was injected with 0.25% Marcaine. The patient experienced three intense jump signs when the injection of the muscle was carried out.

The patient's next visit was on 6/11/96. A short time before coming to the office, the patient had an estradiol level drawn. At that visit, she was put back on the Estrace at 1 mg/day. I discussed her return to work status with her. She stated that she had discussed the return to work with her work supervisor, and the disability insurance company was willing to have her return to any type of work. She stated that she was merely waiting for a call from her supervisor. Dr. Ralston had her on 150 mg of Zoloft® at that time. The patient was noted to be in between moderate distress and moderately severe distress. She was alert, cooperative, and oriented, with no slurred speech, good cognition, no evidence of drug toxicity, and her understanding of what I was saying was within normal limits. Pain chart distribution was similar to previously, although there was more pain noted in the distal two-thirds of the left calf posteriorly. At the time of that visit, she had been switched to 100-µg/hour Duragesic® patches. Sleep was still a problem, and therefore she was given a prescription for 10-mg Mellaril tablets and told to take between one-half to five tablets 2 hours before bedtime. The Dilaudid® injection remained constant at about 20 mg/day. She was premedicated with 4 mg of Dilaudid® plus 25 mg of Benadryl® and 0.5 cc of 2% Xylocaine®, and then palpation was carried out to the right iliocostalis thoracis muscles from T1 to T6, with no tenderness, taut band, or jump sign elicited. She was injected into the left gastrocnemius no. 1 with 0.4% procaine, the right iliocostalis thoracis T10, iliocostalis thoracis on the right at T8, and iliocostalis thoracis on the right at T9. Multiple intense jump signs were elicited at each level injected.

Her next visit was on 6/18/96. At that visit, I inquired about the results of the 3-cc colchicine shot which was given on 6/4/96. The patient stated that 24 hours after the injection, she felt remarkable relief which lasted an additional 24 hours, and then her pain reverted to its usual. She stated that she had been walking 3–4 miles a day for a number of months before that visit. She stated at the visit that she could not walk more than half a mile "without screaming" pain since a month prior to the visit. The repeat estradiol testing had shown a malabsorption problem and an observation that the patient got some results from the oral supplementation, but nothing of significance. She was, therefore, referred to Phillip Renraw, M.D., because of his expertise in female hormone balancing. With respect to return to work, she indicated that she was getting the runaround from her supervisor. It was her impression that if she did return to work, she would have to do quite a bit of her work in an upright standing position because of her back pain problem. She was, therefore, referred to another patient from my practice who had worked with success with that problem for a number of years. When asked about the quality of her sleep, she said it was "not too bad." She stated that she used Soma® when she needed it. On her symptom chart, the areas of involvement were down to about 15% of what they had been at their worst on 2/2/96. The visual analogue pain scale rating was at 70%. She could sit for 20 minutes, stand for 20 minutes, and walk for 20 minutes. The pain was rated at severe intensity, and the frequency was constant. She still had problematic pain in the left calf, and at this time the pain involved the entire calf from the popliteal fossa to the heel. Pain was also into the arch of both feet, more prominent on the right than the left. She was premedicated with 4 mg of Dilaudid®, 25 mg of Benadryl®, and 0.5 cc of 2% Xylocaine®. Trigger point injections with 0.25% Marcaine were carried out to the left L1–2 longissimus thoracis, left L2–3 longissimus thoracis, and four injections into the left piriformis muscle. The longissimus thoracis injections demonstrated one significant jump sign per muscle. The piriformis muscle, when it was injected, demonstrated eight significant jump signs.

She was given an endocrine testing follow-up form which I had put together for my patients (a copy is provided at the end of this chapter). With respect to the low thyroid function, she clinically had numerous problems checked off. Her low estrogen symptom checklist showed about 70% of the items were checked off. In the low adrenal gland function, approximately 60% of the items were checked off. It is noteworthy that as of her visit of 7/3/96, after having had the estrogen and testosterone implants put in by Dr. Renraw, she had less problem with fluid retention, better ability to cope and concentrate, and all areas checked off in the low adrenal gland functions were improving on the systemic estrogen.

Into the month of June, the patient was seen by Dr. Bondo for evaluation of possible myofascial pain dysfunction syndrome) of the jaw and fascial muscles.

She was also referred to an occupational therapist to obtain proper ergonomic seating and helpful devices for her return to work. She was told to discontinue her use of Levo-Dromoran® and continue with Duragesic® patches and Dilaudid® injection. A small protocol was developed in mid-June for the left leg pain problem. It was felt that the piriformis muscle and medial hamstrings were the most likely problematic muscles contributing to dysfunction in that leg. Other muscles considered for that problem were the gluteus medius, gluteus minimus, vastus lateralis, and gastrocnemius no. 1. It is noteworthy that a number of times during the entire treatment plan, I performed stretch and spray in the classic textbook patterns of the books by Travell and Simons. The patient never demonstrated anything more than a slight response to this modality of therapy. It has been my experience that patients with multitudes of myofascial trigger points that affect one extremity or in one geographic area will not respond to stretch and spray as well as patients with a single-muscle myofascial pain syndrome. Another contributing muscle was felt to be the splenius cervicis muscle on the right side. During early June, I noted in my physician's treatment plan that consideration was being given to use of 10 mg/ml of Dilaudid-HP®, depending on her overall response to the program that was being utilized at that time.

Her next visit was on 6/25/96. She stated that she was getting better and doing more activity around the house. She was back to work and was working on Monday, Wednesday, and Friday for 3 hours a day. She stated that she had to increase her Dilaudid® intake to go on with her work at home and at the office. She stated that she was working with Yale Jons, a disability specialist. She appeared to be in moderate to moderately severe distress. She was alert and coherent, with no slurred speech, good cognition, no evidence of drug toxicity, and her ability to hear and understand what I was saying was within normal limits. On the symptom chart, she rated her pain on the visual analogue scale at 65%. Sitting tolerance was 20 minutes, standing tolerance was 20 minutes, and walking tolerance was 20 minutes. The intensity of the pain was moderate and the frequency of the pain was constant. Distribution of pain was posterior paracervical on both sides and less intense than on previous charts. The same is true for the thoracic paraspinal pain from T4 to T7. The pain in the left calf and heel was also less intense, but it was also noted that there was involvement of the dorsum of her right foot. The patient was premedicated with 4 mg of Dilaudid®, 25 mg of Benadryl®, and 0.5 cc of 2% Xylocaine®. Following that, two separate trigger point areas were injected in the splenius services on the right side, and two separate trigger points were injected in the levator scapula on the right side. All injections were carried out with 0.4% procaine, and all muscles demonstrated at least two local twitch responses and two jump signs, with one of the levator scapula injections demonstrating a large jump sign.

At my request, the patient submitted a copy of one of her paychecks covering the pay period from 6/16 to 6/30/96.

The next visit was on 7/3/96. She stated that she had seen Dr. Renraw for the consultation. After reviewing my laboratory testing, it was decided that the patient did not absorb estrogen well via the oral route, and therefore he implanted pellets of estrogen and testosterone subcutaneously. A week prior to implantation of the pellets, the patient had received an injection of estrogen from him, and she experienced a marked increase in her overall energy. At about this time, her need for Dexedrine® oral spansules ceased. Her recent 100-μg/hour Duragesic® patches were continuing at one patch every 3 days. Her recent Dilaudid® injection was averaging about 20 mg/day. She was still having marked problems with pain in her right foot. The symptom chart findings were essentially the same as her previous visit. Extensive examination of this patient with palpation in the lower extremities and the use of a pressure threshold meter (a device for testing the patient's threshold to pain) revealed that in general as the testing went from T9 to the calves, the readings went down (indicating a lower pain threshold to mechanical stimulus). There was significant palpable tenderness in both lower extremities, which was most marked on the lateral aspect of the left leg from the distal thigh to the dorsum of the left foot. On the dorsum of the left foot, palpation produced a bent jump sign. Based on that evaluation, an additional protocol was developed for the approach to the pain in the lower part of the body. These trigger point injections were to follow in the order left iliocostalis thoracis T8, left longissimus thoracis T8, left gluteus medius, piriformis on both sides, left gluteus minimus, left tibialis anterior, and left extensor digitorum brevis. Laboratory testing on 7/13/96 showed that her free thyroxin was 0.9 and the TSH was 0.04 (normal range = 0.34–5.50). Her estradiol level was 471 and her testosterone level was 301 ng/dl (normal range = 12–90).

She was next seen on 7/16/96. She stated that she had noted easy bruising at her vitamin and Dilaudid® injection sites from the previous 2 months. Inspection of those areas revealed some minimal areas of bruising in three to four areas, about 1–1.5 cm in diameter. (Note: Her allowable dosage of injectable Dilaudid® had been increased to 1–4 cc every 2–3 hours as needed for severe pain.) At that visit, she indicated that she was taking 6–10 mg of injectable Dilaudid® per injection. At that visit, 10 mg/ml of Dilaudid-HP® (high potency) was added to her treatment program, and the patient was shown how to draw up an injection from an ampule. She was also continuing her 100-μg/hour Duragesic® patches. She was continuing at work, working Monday, Wednesday, and Friday for 5 hours a day. The following week she planned to progress to Monday, Tuesday, Thursday, and Friday for 5 hours a day. I issued a slip to her employer indicating the need for her work schedule to increase in hours and indicating that she could increase by 1–3 hours per week. She stated that since Dr. Renraw had implanted estrogen pellets, her overall well-being was much improved, as was her sex drive. With respect to sleep, she was using three to four Soma® tablets at bedtime. On the pain symptom chart, she had the usual posterior paracervical musculature involvement bilaterally, the previously mentioned paraspinal thoracic involvement, and involvement of both calves, the dorsum of the left foot, the left heel, and the arch of the left foot. She was premedicated with 4 mg of Dilaudid®, 25 mg of Benadryl®, and 0.5 cc of 2% Xylocaine®. She was also given an additional injection of Vistaril® plus 0.5 cc of 2% Xylocaine® (Vistaril® and Dilaudid® do not mix in the same syringe). Myofascial trigger point injections were carried out at the left T8 and T9 iliocostalis thoracis, left T9 and T10 iliocostalis thoracis, left longissimus thoracis at T8, and left T8–9 longissimus thoracis. At every level, at least two big jump signs were elicited, and it was my observation that the jump signs were too strong at every level, posing a risk of activating secondary and tertiary trigger points that may have been detrimental to her overall pain syndrome and progress. Therefore, a decision was made to use more Dilaudid® on the future injection sessions. At this time, the patient was getting into complex emotional issues with her therapist, Mrs. Forde. At some of her visits, she was noted to be emotionally labile, but not as much as in the past, and I could tell by talking to her that strong emotions were related to the issues she was working on with her therapist. Her total injectable Dilaudid® intake went to a range of between 50 and 80 mg/day. Her intake of thyroid was increased to one of the 0.2-mg tablets per day plus two of the 0.025-mg tablets per day.

Her next visit was 7/24/96. She stated that 2–3 weeks after the estrogen and testosterone pellets had been implanted, she went off of her Zoloft® and had experienced no depression. However, with respect to the complex issues that she was dealing with, the patient had lost 8 pounds in a week. She stated that she had not slept well for the preceding 1½ weeks. She stated that she was having problems with hyperventilation and overreacting. She stated that Valium® was a help, and therefore she was given a prescription for 50 5-mg Valium® tablets with one refill. After that prescription was given, the patient was not in need of Valium®. Review of the symptom chart revealed that the geographic distribution of pain was approximately similar to the previously dictated chart, and the visual analogue scale; sitting, standing, and walking times; plus intensity and frequency of pain were the same. She filled out another endocrine testing and follow-up sheet. This time, 40% of the low thyroid function symptoms were gone, 40% of the previously indicated low estrogen dysfunction symptoms were gone, and 90% of the low adrenal function symptoms were gone. A low testosterone function in the female scale had been added to the test, and the patient checked off no areas of problem. The free thyroxin blood test showed 1.5 ng/dl (normal range = 0.6–1.5). The T3 total was 172 ng/dl (normal range = 60–181). Both Dr. Renraw and I were following the patient with respect to blood testing. The patient was continued on her oral vitamins and minerals and her prescription of potassium as previously indicated. She was also continued on her Cortef tablets at two per day. Because of the noticeable stress that was evident in her life at that time, the patient was told to go to full-strength B-complex injections daily (#1 shot on one day, #2 shot next day, #1 the next day, etc.) for 2 weeks and then return to the half-strength shots, with 1 day between each of the B-complex injections after that.

On 7/31/96, I spoke to the patient's therapist, and we agreed that a number of stress-related emotional issues were aggravating the organic aspects of her pain problem.

The patient turned in a pay stub for 7/16 to 7/31/96. (Note: This proof of employment was not required of the patient regularly, but only at monthly intervals.)

Her next visit was 8/7/96. Injectable Dilaudid® intake was in the range of about 40–60 mg at that time. The patient reiterated the extensive anxiety with her husband at that time, but stated that they were working with the licensed marriage and family counselor to resolve their issues. She was off Zoloft® for 3 weeks at that time. A review of her symptom chart revealed a rating of 90% on the visual analogue scale and her ability to sit was 15 minutes, stand 15 minutes, and walk 15 minutes. The pain was rated at severe and constant. Geographic distribution of the pain was bilateral paracervical posterior, bilateral thoracic paraspinal from T4 to T7, bilateral paraspinal from T8 to L2 and extending out to the posterior axillary line bilaterally, bilateral calves, and in the arch and dorsum of the left foot. It was my estimate that about 30% of the pain representation was augmentation of her underlying myofascial pain syndrome due to severe emotional stress. She was alert and coherent, with no slurred speech, good cognition, no evidence of drug toxicity, and was able to correctly process complex issues that we discussed. She was premedicated with 6 mg of Dilaudid® plus 25 mg of Benadryl® and 1 cc of 2% Xylocaine®. A second syringe containing 35 mg of Vistaril® plus 0.5 cc of 2% Xylocaine® was administered. Trigger points were injected in the iliocostalis thoracis T10 muscles bilaterally, with two local twitch responses per injection and three jump signs on each side.

The next visit was on 8/14/96. She said that as of 9/1/96, her employer would switch her to the status of being a subcontractor. She was working 20 hours a week at that time. She stated that the stress and tension in her marital relationship at home was mounting. Comments on the symptom chart were essentially the same as the previous visit. In addition to the previously read geographic distribution of pain, the patient had mild markings of pain in both buttocks, with radiation down the posterior lateral aspect of both thighs to the popliteal fossa on the right and to the mid calf on the left. She was premedicated with 6 mg of Dilaudid® and 25 mg of Benadryl®, plus 2% Xylocaine®. She was injected in the left gluteus medius number one trigger point with 0.4% procaine; there was one local twitch response and two jump signs. The left gluteus medius no. 2 and no. 3 myofascial trigger points were palpated and found to be negative for the presence of tenderness or trigger points.

Her next visit was on 8/21/96. When I inquired about her work, she said that her employer was terminating her at the end of the month, but would hire her back as a consultant. At that visit and subsequent visits through 9/10/96, a questionnaire/physical examination form that I had developed for evaluating arachnoiditis was gone over with the patient. After reviewing the form, it appeared as though the patient had a component of arachnoiditis as part of her ongoing pain syndrome. On 8/21/96, she was premedicated with 6 mg of Dilaudid® plus 25 mg of Benadryl® and 2 cc of 1% Xylocaine®. She was also premedicated with 25 mg of Vistaril® plus 0.5 cc of 2% Xylocaine®. Following that, the left piriformis was injected four times in the areas of trigger points no. 1 and 2. There were at least one to three local twitch responses and two to four jump signs per injection site. The myofascial trigger points were injected with 0.4% procaine.

Her next visit was on 8/27/96. At that visit, the patient related that she had moved out of her home, leaving her husband behind, and into the home of a friend. She was sleeping on a mattress that was not comfortable and there was a flaring of her pain problem. Some of the emotional stressors that were high at the time were the fact that she felt that her husband did not understand her pain problem and also the change in status at her place of employment. She was alert and coherent, with no slurred speech, good cognition, no evidence of drug toxicity, and her ability to hear and understand what I was saying was within normal limits. She appeared very stressed at that visit. She was premedicated with 10 mg of Dilaudid-HP® plus 25 mg of Benadryl® and 0.5 cc of 2% Xylocaine®. She was given additional injections of 25 mg of Vistaril® plus 0.5 cc of 2% Xylocaine® and a separate injection of 40 mg of Depo-Medrol plus 0.5 cc of 2% Xylocaine®. Four trigger points were injected in her piriformis muscle on the right to trigger points no. 1 and 2. There was an average of two local twitch responses per injection site and two jump signs per injection sign. The patient submitted a payment document from her employer indicating employment from 8/16 to 8/31/96. Her intake of Dilaudid® injectable at that point was averaging approximately 90 mg/day. At that visit, the patient and I agreed to a maximum of 10 mg of Dilaudid® every 3 hours as needed for her pain control.

The next visit was on 9/3/96. She stated that she had flown in a small plane recently and had flared up the band of pain in the lower thoracic–upper lumbar region. She said that her pain problem had become extremely intense for the 2 days before the visit. She pointed out that she had continuing stressors with her employer and with her husband. This had also been adversely affecting her sleep because of the anxiety and pain flare-up. She was noted to be in moderate distress, but was sedated because of taking Soma® before coming to the office. She was alert and coherent, but her speech seemed to be slightly slurred; she had good cognition and mild evidence of drug toxicity, but was able to hear and understand what I was saying within normal limits. The band of pain that she had indicated on her pain chart actually extended from the inferior aspect of the shoulder blade on both sides to the top of the pelvic brim on both sides and extending laterally out to the posterior axillary line. The patient was premedicated with 10 mg Dilaudid®, 25 mg Benadryl®, and 0.55 cc of 2% Xylocaine®. In a separate syringe, she was given 25 mg Vistaril® plus 0.5 cc of 2% Xylocaine®. Twenty minutes later, she had three trigger point injections into the right rectus femoris muscle 2 inches lateral to the midline, on the right side. One was 2 inches above the umbilicus, one was at the same level as the umbilicus, and the other was 2 inches below the umbilicus. There was an average of one local twitch response per injection. There were seven jump signs generated from the upper injection, and two jump signs accompanied the lower injections. During the procedure, the patient had vital sign monitoring approximately every 10 minutes. Her vital signs remained stable. It was felt that she was a bit too sedated at the end of the procedure, and therefore she was given 0.15 cc (0.4 mg/ml) of Narcan® right after the last trigger point injection, and 20 minutes later 0.1 cc of additional Narcan® was administered.

On 9/5/96, the patient called in early for her refill of Dilaudid-HP®. I called the patient to inform her that early renewal at that time would reflect that her usage of the medication was escalating too fast. Therefore, I reminded her that we had agreed to a maximum of 80 mg/day of the injectable Dilaudid®, and the patient was fully cooperative when I pointed out the problem and our agreement. The patient did not use Dilaudid-HP® after this date.

Her next visit was on 9/10/96. She stated that she was down to 3 cc (2 mg/ml) of Dilaudid® every 3 hours for pain control. She stated that she had been dropped from her place of employment and was bothered by this. Her overall attitude seemed to be good. She stated that the pain in the calves was better. She was alert and coherent, with no slurred speech, good cognition, no evidence of drug toxicity, and her ability to comprehend and understand what I was saying was good. Review of the system chart showed a rating of 85% on the visual analogue scale. She could sit for 30 minutes, stand for 30 minutes, and walk for 30 minutes. Intensity of her pain was rated at moderate and frequency at constant. Pain distribution showed posterior paracervical involvement on the right side only from the suboccipital area to C7. The paraspinal thoracic area was evolved from T2 to T8 and filled up most of the area between the spine and the medial border of the right scapula. The pain in the lower thoracic area occurred from T10 to L2 and went out to the posterior axillary line in a band-like shape. There was radicular pain going down the right leg, the mid buttock, lateral right thigh, and lateral calf. On the left side, the pain was going down the middle of the calf to the heel, with a thin stripe of pain in the left heel. She was premedicated with 10 mg Dilaudid-HP® plus 25 mg Benadryl® and 0.5 cc of 2% Xylocaine®. A second injection of 25 mg Vistaril® plus 0.5 cc of 2% Xylocaine® was given. Four trigger point injections were carried out to the left piriformis in the no. 1 and no. 2 trigger point areas. There was an average of two local twitch responses per injection and an average of three jump signs per muscle.

At her next visit on 9/18/96, she stated that morning stiffness (due to onset of cold weather) had become a problem. She was noted to be in moderate severe distress. On the symptom chart, all the patterns mentioned on 9/10/96 were present, plus there was radicular pain and paresthesias into the right upper extremity. She was premedicated with 8 mg of Dilaudid®, 40 mg of Benadryl®, and 0.5 cc of 2% Xylocaine®. The upper rectus abdominis trigger points were injected on both sides using 0.25% Marcaine. There was one local twitch response per muscle and three jump signs accompanying each injection. The patient was sent for a comprehensive panel of laboratory testing which revealed the following results: Complete blood count was within normal limits. The sedimentation rate was at 44 (normal range = 1–20). The chemistry showed no abnormalities of glucose, urea nitrogen, iron, calcium, phosphatase, and uric acid. The electrolyte panel revealed that the patient's potassium was at 3.6 (normal range = 3.5–5.5). She stated that she had had some upper respiratory symptoms at the time on that drawing, and she had been vomiting secondary to the upper respiratory infection. Liver function tests were within normal limits. Free thyroxin was 1.3 (normal range = 0.75–2.0 ng/dl). Urinalysis was within normal limits. The estradiol (now under the care of Dr. Renraw) was 469 pg/ml.

Her next visit was on 9/23/96. The patient was noted to be in moderate distress and had taken her last dose of 3 cc of Dilaudid® (6 mg) at 10:05 that morning. The physical examination repeat was conducted at noon that day. The results were compared to her testing of 3/8/96. There was less range of motion of the cervical spine for flexion and extension, but better range of motion for lateral bending. Lateral rotation was approximately the same. Range of motion of the shoulders was essentially the same as previously. The trapezius, sternocleidomastoid, pectoralis major, and latissimus dorsi muscles all had taut bands, tenderness, and jump signs, and this was the same as what was found on 3/8/96. Straight leg raising was approximately the same as previously. The ability to extend her hip over the side of the table had improved by 7 degrees on the right side and 11 degrees on the left side. The paraspinal muscles from T1 to T12 demonstrated taut bands, tenderness, and jump signs. With respect to range of motion of the lumbar spine, previously she had been able to touch her thumb to the floor; at this visit, all fingers and thumbs touched the floor. Extension was at 22 degrees; it had previously been at 10 degrees. Lateral bending was approximately the same as previously. She had lost about 10 degrees in respect to rotation of the lumbar spine. Her ability to do a deep knee bend had improved from the previous examination and at the visit of 9/23/96; there was no pain provoked by the deep knee bend. Pinprick sensation testing revealed that there was now a hypesthesia to pinprick in the upper extremities at C5, C7, and C8. This was the most extensive hypesthesia that she had had since coming back into the program. There was no hypesthesia in the left upper extremity. In the lower extremity, there was hypesthesia on the right at L5 and S1, which represented one more dermatome of involvement as compared to previously. There was no hypesthesia in the left lower extremity. Her intake of injectable Dilaudid® from 9/15/96 to 10/3/96 averaged 15–40 mg/day.

Her most recent visit occurred on 10/3/96. I think she may have again mentioned the problem with respect to vomiting. She was noted to be in moderately severe distress. She was alert and coherent, with no slurred speech, good cognition, no evidence of drug toxicity, and her ability to hear and understand what I was saying was within normal limits. It was noted that her pain distribution had reverted very closely to the distribution that she had upon first entering the program on 11/1894. However, the symptom chart of 10/3/96 showed the radicular pain down the lateral right thigh and lateral right calf. On her visual analogue scale, the rating was exactly the same as 1994. Her ability to sit, stand, and walk was increasing, and she could sit 20 minutes, stand 30 minutes, and walk 45 minutes. She was premedicated with 8 mg of Dilaudid®, 40 mg of Benadryl®, and 0.8 cc of 2% Xylocaine®. Approximately 20 minutes later, trigger point injections were carried out to three areas in the right trapezius no. 3 and to the longissimus thoracis T5 on the right. (Note: On this visit, as on all previous visits where trigger points were injected, the specific trigger point was sought out in its respective taut band and then injected.) These muscles each demonstrated two local twitch responses and an average of one jump site.

HIGHLIGHTS

In conclusion, this case of a chronic pain patient with four major insults to her body has demonstrated:

1. In the responsible chronic pain patient, potent opioids can be used to keep the patient physically functional
2. Potent opioids can be used to facilitate injection of hyperirritable myofascial trigger point
3. Some of the multisystem abnormalities in this type of patient
4. Some of the problems associated with the use of potent opioids in the treatment of chronic pain patients
5. Physiological problems related to less than optimal levels of estrogen and testosterone
6. Problem of nocturnal myoclonus that may be problematic in some chronic pain patients
7. Some of the physical examination procedures that I believe are useful in the evaluation of chronic pain patients with soft tissue pain problems

Items referenced to Bronson Pharmaceutical, 1945 Craig Road, P.O. Box 46903, St. Louis, MO 63146 (phone 1-800-610-4848).

GLOSSARY

See Chapter 10 on myofascial pain syndrome for definition of terms.

BIBLIOGRAPHY

Rask, M.R. (1980). Colchicine use in five hundred patients with disk disease, *The Journal of Neurological and Orthopedic Surgery,* 1(5).

Travell, J.G. and Simons, D.G. (1983). *Myofascial Pain and Dysfunction, The Trigger Point Manual,* Williams and Wilkins, Baltimore.

Travell, J.G. and Simons, D.G. (1992). *Myofascial Pain and Dysfunction, The Trigger Point Manual,* Vol. 2, Williams and Wilkins, Baltimore.

Name _____

Date _____

ENDOCRINE TESTING AND FOLLOW-UP

Code to be used: check mark = I have the condition
question mark = I don't understand the term
leave blank = I don't have the condition

Low Thyroid Function

Some of the symptoms and signs of hypometabolism that you may experience are

_____ Apathy
_____ Balding
_____ Bloating
_____ Cold intolerance
_____ Constipation
_____ Decreased memory
_____ Depression
_____ Difficulty sleeping
_____ Dry hair
_____ Dry skin
_____ Dryness of eyes
_____ Dryness of other mucous membranes
_____ Dyslexia
_____ Early morning stiffness
_____ Excessive use of clothing or blankets
_____ Fatigue
_____ Fluid retention
_____ Hoarseness
_____ Impotence
_____ Infertility
_____ Joint pains
_____ Lack of attention span
_____ Lethargy
_____ Loss of sex drive
_____ Menstrual irregularities
_____ Muscle cramps
_____ Muscular aches and pains
_____ Nasal congestion
_____ Peeling or cracking fingernails
_____ Puffy eyelids
_____ Tingling, numb, and burning sensations
_____ Tiredness
_____ Weight gain: # lbs in last 12 months ____

_____ Cold skin
_____ Diffuse muscle tenderness may be present
_____ Eyelids may be puffy
_____ Facial swelling
_____ Hair dull, may be thin
_____ Heart rate may be slow
_____ Loss of hair
_____ Lowered basal temperature
_____ Muscles stiff, tender; occas. weak
_____ Often overweight
_____ Skin dry, sallow, rough occas. carotinemic
_____ Swelling of the eyelids
_____ Swelling of the feet
_____ Trigger points are frequent
_____ Voice may be hoarse
_____ Weakness of the shoulder girdle

Low Estrogen Function

Some of the symptoms and signs of estrogen insufficiency you may experience are

_____ Anxiety
_____ Cold hands and feet
_____ Burning sensation
_____ Depression
_____ Fatigue
_____ Forgetfulness
_____ Genital skin becomes thin and pale with decrease in the size of the labia minora, clitoris, and uterus
_____ Headaches
_____ Hot flushes
_____ Inability to concentrate

_____ Inability to cope
_____ Insomnia
_____ Irregular menses
_____ Joint pain
_____ Loss of creativity
_____ Loss of libido
_____ Muscle pain
_____ Myofascial pain
_____ Nervousness
_____ Night sweats
_____ Osteoporosis
_____ Painful sexual intercourse
_____ Can feel heart pounding in chest
_____ Numbness or tingling
_____ Trigger points
_____ Variable absence of periods
_____ Vertigo
_____ Weakness
_____ Weight gain

Low Adrenal Function

Some of the symptoms and signs of adrenal insufficiency you may experience are

_____ Apathy
_____ Decreased bodily energy
_____ Decreased mental energy
_____ Dehydration
_____ Depression
_____ Diarrhea is not uncommon
_____ Dizziness when standing up
_____ Fatigue

_____ Headache is a frequent symptom
_____ Irritability of the stomach
_____ Loss of appetite
_____ Low blood pressure
_____ Mucous membrane pigmentation
_____ Muscle cramps
_____ Muscle pain
_____ Muscle spasm
_____ Nausea
_____ Negativism
_____ Nervous symptoms may occur
_____ Psychosis
_____ Salt craving
_____ Skin pigmentation
_____ Vague abdominal pain
_____ Vomiting
_____ Weakness
_____ Weight loss

Low Testosterone Function in Women

Some of the symptoms and signs of testosterone insufficiency women may experience are

_____ Low energy
_____ Loss of sex drive
_____ Slowed down
_____ Mildly depressed mood
_____ Fewer dreams
_____ Thin, fine hair
_____ Dry, thin skin

MICHAEL S. MARGOLES, M.D.
177 San Ramon Drive
San Jose, California 95111-3615
(408) 226-0318

To:_____

Please help us by filling out these information sheets as accurately as you can. If there is a question that you do not understand, go on to the next section. We will help you fill in the unanswered parts when you come to the office for your first visit.

When you come, **BRING WITH YOU**
    (1) THESE COMPLETED FORMS
    (2) A COMPLETED INSURANCE FORM
    (3) ALL YOUR MEDICATION AND VITAMIN BOTTLES
    (4) FINANCIAL PAYMENT _____
Work-injured patients please ignore (2) and (4).

ASSIGNMENT OF BENEFITS: I hereby assign all medical and/or surgical benefits, to include major medical benefits to which I am entitled, including Medicare, private insurance, and other health plans, to MICHAEL S. MARGOLES, M.D.

_____   _____
         Signature of patient   Signature of witness

A photocopy of this assignment is to be considered as valid as an original. This assignment will remain in effect until revoked by me in writing. I understand that I am financially responsible for all charges whether or not paid by said insurance. I hereby authorize said assignee to release all information necessary to secure the payment.

RELEASE OF MEDICAL INFORMATION:
I hereby authorize _____ to release to MICHAEL S. MARGOLES, M.D., any desired medical/surgical records regarding my medical history, including consults, X-rays, reports, progress notes, diagnostic evaluations, laboratory reports, and diagnoses. A photocopy of this form shall be considered as valid as the original.

_____   _____
         Signature of patient   Signature of witness

EDUCATIONAL RELEASE: I give Michael S. Margoles, M.D., permission to use photographs, videotape, and/or records related to my case, but not my name or face, for professional communication with other members of the medical profession.

_____   _____
         Signature of patient   Signature of witness

Name _____

Date _____

PERSONAL IDENTIFICATION DATA

Name:_____
                          Last   First   Initial

Address:_____
                     Street   City   State   Zip Code

_____   _____   _____
     Date of birth   Age   The hand you write with (left or right)

Telephone number (Home): (   )_____

Telephone number (Work): (   )_____

Name of nearest relative or friend for us to contact in case of emergency or to get a message
to you:

_____
                          Name

_____
                          Address   Phone Number

Marital status:
___ Single (never married)
___ Married   Number of years_____
___ Divorced   Number of years _____

Family doctor:_____
                               Name   Phone Number

Your employer:_____
                               Name   Phone Number

Your occupation:_____

Employer of spouse:_____
                               Name   Address

                     _____
                               Occupation   Phone Number
Your:
    Social security number:_____

    Driver's license number:_____

    Car license plate number:_____

Name _____

Date _____

FINANCIAL POLICY TO PATIENTS

FEES FOR SERVICE: are to be paid in full at each visit. We accept cash, cashier's check, money order, and a number of credit cards.

INSURANCE: We ask you to file with your insurance company. We will give you copies of your office visit charges, which you can staple to your form. If the company denies charges, you may bring in the explanation. If necessary, we will submit a letter of explanation, which may be of help. There may be a charge for this service.

More and more, insurance companies are asking for copies of your medical records. If this occurs, and your records are only 10 pages or less, we will do the copy work for $0.25 per page. If the chart is larger, we will ask you or your insurance company to take care of the copy work. Medical charts are not released from the office under any circumstance.

AUTOMOBILE INSURANCE: We ask that you pay the doctor directly for his services. You may take the billing to your agent and ask for payment. We will cooperate and complete forms for your company as they request, but only with your written authorization. There will be a charge for this service. The fee will vary with the complexity of the material requested.

MISCELLANEOUS FORMS: such as disability, life insurance, social security, etc. will also be completed with your written authorization for release of the requested medical information. There may be a charge for this service. The charge will vary with the complexity of the material requested.

MISSED APPOINTMENTS: Patients having scheduled visits and not giving 24 hours advance notice for cancellations will be charged the full amount of the missed visit. Exceptions will be made for emergencies.

I AGREE THAT I AM FINANCIALLY RESPONSIBLE TO PAY FOR MEDICAL AND/OR SURGICAL FEES TO DR. MARGOLES, REGARDLESS OF MY INSURANCE COMPANY RESPONSE TO PAYMENT. IF I AM SEEING THE DOCTOR FOR A WORK-RELATED INJURY, I AGREE TO PAY FEES FOR MISCELLANEOUS FORMS, SUPPLIES, AND OFFICE VISITS NOT COVERED BY THE INSURANCE COMPANY.

_____   _____
Patient signature   Date

PHYSICIAN–PATIENT ARBITRATION AGREEMENT

In consideration of the agreement of Dr._____

herein called Doctor, to serve as physician for _____

herein called Patient, Doctor and Patient do hereby agree as follows:

(1) It is understood that any dispute as to medical malpractice, that is as to whether any medical services rendered under this contract were unnecessary or unauthorized or were improperly, negligently, or incompetently rendered, will be determined by submission to arbitration as provided by California law, and not by a lawsuit or resort to court process except as California law provides for judicial review of arbitration proceedings. Both parties to this contract, by entering into it, are giving up their constitutional right to have any such dispute decided in a court of law before a jury, and instead are accepting the use of arbitration.

(2) Any such arbitration proceeding shall be administered by the AMERICAN ARBITRATION ASSOCIATION, through its appropriate medical panel as designated by the said AMERICAN ARBITRATION ASSOCIATION.

(3) Any such arbitration proceedings shall be governed by California Code of Civil Procedure, sections 1280, *et seq.*

(4) If any court action is undertaken to set aside or otherwise attack the arbitration award, the losing party in the court action shall bear all costs of such action, including reasonable attorney's fees for the prevailing party.

Entered into this _____day of_____, 19____.

NOTICE: BY SIGNING THIS CONTRACT YOU ARE AGREEING TO HAVE ANY ISSUE OF MEDICAL MALPRACTICE DECIDED BY NEUTRAL ARBITRATION AND YOU ARE GIVING UP YOUR RIGHT TO A JURY OR COURT TRIAL. SEE ARTICLE 1 OF THIS CONTRACT.

Signed: (Patient)_____

Signed: (Physician)_____

Witness:_____

Name _____

Date _____

NARRATIVE SUMMARY SECTION

You can help us with the assessment of your pain and disability problem by writing a summary of your medical history as it relates to the problems you will be asking us to treat. You can write this out or type it up. For the narrative, tell us about your problem:

- When did it begin?
- How has it affected you?
- Who did you see?
- What did they say?
- What did they do?
- What did you do?

Write this on a separate sheet of paper, as though you were writing an article for the *Reader's Digest*. You may use the fill-in-the blank questions on the following pages to give you some ideas about what to cover in your summary. If you do not care to do the narrative, just fill in the blanks below.

MULTIPLE QUESTION SECTION

Complete the answers to the following questions. Describe, circle, or check off an appropriate answer to the following:

Date pain problem began: _____

The onset of original pain problem was: ☐ Sudden ☐ Gradual

The cause of original pain problem was: ☐ Injury ☐ Accident ☐ Assault ☐ Unknown

Other (explain):_____
_____

Location where it happened: ☐ Home ☐ Work ☐ Car ☐ Other: _____

What were you doing at the time? ☐ Bending ☐ Sitting ☐ Lifting ☐ Twisting
☐ Falling ☐ Driving Other:_____

How much time went by between your injury and the beginning of your pain problem?
____immediate ____hours ____days ____weeks ____months ____not applicable

How much time went by between the start of your pain problem and your first visit to a health care professional? ____immediate ____hours ____days ____weeks ____months ____years ____not applicable

Did your pain problem go away or get better and then return? If it returned, explain.
_____
_____

Total number of doctors seen for your problem _____

Please list the doctors that you have seen for your pain problem, beginning with the first doctor you saw. Include the following information (if these items were performed):

Testing: Myelogram, EMG, MRI scan, evoked potential test, X-rays, referral to consultant, CT scan, CAT scan, bone scan

Diagnosis: The clinical term(s) used, or in your own words

Treatment: Medications, physical therapy, appliances (brace, corset), surgery, rehabilitation, hospitalization, and others

Your response: Did the treatment help you?

FIRST DOCTOR SEEN: _____

Testing:_____

Diagnosis:_____

Treatment:_____

Response:_____

SECOND DOCTOR SEEN: _____

Testing:_____

Diagnosis:_____

Treatment:_____

Response:_____

THIRD DOCTOR SEEN: _____

Testing:_____

Diagnosis:_____

Treatment:_____

Response:_____

You may list other doctors on the back of these sheets or on a separate sheet of paper.

Please indicate which one of the following treatments you have tried for your pain problem and the results of each (leave blank if not tried).

Write: A if tried and major relief
         B if tried and some relief
         C if tried and no relief
         D if tried and the pain got worse
         If not tried, please leave blank.

_____ Acupuncture	_____ Nerve blocks	_____ Traction
_____ Biofeedback	_____ Other counseling	_____ Tranquilizers
_____ Braces or cast(s)	_____ Pain relievers	Transcutaneous
_____ Chiropractic	_____ Physical therapy	electrical nerve
_____ Exercise program	_____ Psychotherapy	stimulation (TENS)
_____ Homeopathy	_____ Relaxation training	_____ Trigger point
_____ Hypnosis	_____ Spinal injection	injections
_____ Massage	_____ Surgery	_____ Other_____

How has the intensity of the pain changed throughout the time you have had it?
☐ increased   ☐ decreased   ☐ stayed the same

If you have pain-free periods, how long do they last? ____minutes   ____hours   ____days
____weeks   ____months

For the next question put an "X" on the line that shows where you are at:

Effect on my mood since my pain problem began. How have you felt during the last two weeks?

No effect |_____| Overwhelmingly depressed
                                                                    and suicidal

What is your worst fear associated with your pain problem?

_____

_____

What is the most aggravating thing about your pain problem?

_____

_____

IN THE CHART BELOW PUT DOWN ALL THE MEDICATION
YOU ARE PRESENTLY TAKING; INCLUDE VITAMINS

Medication	Strength	Number/day	Reason you take it	For how long?

MEDICATIONS PREVIOUSLY TAKEN

Please list all of the medications that have been used to treat you for your pain and problems related to your pain, and code the results as follows:

0 = excellent results (100% relief)   4 = made things worse
1 = good results (50% relief)   5 = nausea
2 = fair results (25% relief)   6 = vomiting
3 = poor results (none)   7 = upset stomach

For 8 and 9, put in your own definitions

8 = _____

9 = _____

If you don't know why the medication was given, put unknown on the line for "reason it was given." You can put more than one number in the lines under "results."

Medication	Reason it was given	Results

GLOBAL ACTIVITY ASSESSMENT TEST

For each category of activity listed below, put a number (from 10 to 0 or "—") on the line indicating what your present capability is compared to before the pain problem began (prepain status).

Scoring to Use

10 = doing everything without problem in that group
9 = 90% of prepain status
8 = 80% of prepain status
7 = 70% of prepain status
6 = 60% of prepain status
5 = 50% of prepain status
4 = 40% of prepain status
3 = 30% of prepain status
2 = 20% of prepain status
1 = 10% of prepain status
0 = can't do any more
— = normally never do this

1. Your usual job   _____
2. Work around the home   _____
3. Socialization activities   _____
4. Getting up or down out of a chair   _____
5. Sports   _____
6. Hobbies   _____

7. Sexual activity   _____
8. Sleep   _____
   Number of times the pain wakes you up per night? _____
   How many hours of sleep do you usually get per night? _____
   Is sleep restful or restless? _____
   Take medications for sleep? _____
   If yes, which ones? _____
   Check any of these that apply:
        ___ Have trouble falling asleep
        ___ Have trouble staying asleep
9. Hygiene (shower, grooming, shampooing, toilet, etc.)   _____
10. Eating and feeding   _____
11. Chewing (food, etc.)   _____
12. Dressing and undressing   _____
13. Driving a vehicle   _____
14. The overall strength and endurance   _____

PHYSIOLOGIC DYSFUNCTION QUESTIONNAIRE

Directions for Taking This Test

In the sections listed below, put a check mark in front of any statement that relates to current problems that you have had for more than one month.

1. Energy and stamina (check all applicable items)
   ___ (a) Decreased energy
   ___ (b) Tire easily
   ___ (c) Wake up tired
   ___ (d) Get tired by lunch time
   ___ (e) Get tired by afternoon (by 4–5 p.m.)
   ___ (f) Do not tolerate stress well
   ___ (g) Cannot work as hard as I used to
   ___ (h) Cannot work as much as I used to
   ___ (i) Have to rest more now than before my pain problem started
2. Muscular problems (check all that apply)
   ___ (a) Weakness of the arm
        ___ (1) Right
        ___ (2) Left
   ___ (b) Dropping things with hand
        ___ (1) Right
        ___ (2) Left
   ___ (c) Weakness of the leg
        ___ (1) Right
        ___ (2) Left
   ___ (d) Weakness of abdominal (stomach) muscles
   ___ (e) Weakness of back muscles
   ___ (f) Buckling of leg or leg gives out without warning
        ___ (1) Right
        ___ (2) Left
   ___ (g) Loss of urine when coughing or sneezing

___ (h) Have to use a cane to walk
___ (i) Need a wheelchair
    ___ (1) All of the time
    ___ (2) Most of the time
    ___ (3) Some of the time
___ (j) Pain up and down the spinal area (from neck to low back)
___ (k) Bending the head forward causes:
    ___ (1) Increased spinal pain that shoots into tailbone area
    ___ (2) Electric shock-like sensations that shoot into arm(s) and/or leg(s)
___ (l) Tendency to lose my balance and fall when I am standing up with my eyes closed
___ (m) Needs crutches to walk

3. Thinking problems (check all that apply)
___ (a) Memory does not function as well as it used to
___ (b) Get confused more now than before
___ (c) Make thinking errors
___ (d) Behavior has changed; it is worse now than before
___ (e) Sometimes thinking gets "fuzzy"
___ (f) Not as smart as I used to be
___ (g) Have lost interest in social activities such as parties, going out to dinner, or being with friends
___ (h) Feel depressed
___ (i) Problems with dizziness
___ (j) Vision is blurred (answer only one)
    ___ (1) All the time
    ___ (2) Some of the time
___ (k) Hand(s) tremble
___ (l) I feel weak all over

4. PCS (check all that apply)
___ (a) Have difficulty following directions
___ (b) Have difficulty with reading
___ (c) Have difficulty with understanding
___ (d) Have difficulty understanding what people are saying to me
___ (e) Had loss of consciousness after an accident
___ (f) Have ongoing blackouts

WORK AND EMPLOYMENT STATUS

Please check the category or categories that relate to your current work or employment status.

___ (a) I am a housewife and do not work outside the home for gainful employment
___ (b) I am doing my regular work full time
___ (c) I am doing my regular work part time
___ (d) I am doing modified regular work full time
___ (e) I am doing modified regular work part time
___ (f) I am doing light work part time
___ (g) I am going to school full time
___ (h) I am going to school part time
___ (i) I am disabled from working because of an injury that occurred while I was at work (work-related injury). (Employed but not working)

___ (j) I am unemployed and not working
___ (k) I am presently retraining for another type of work
___ (l) I am presently going on job interviews
___ (m) I am legally retired because of a work-related injury
___ (n) I am not working because I have reached retirement age and ceased working
___ (o) I do volunteer work only
___ (p) I am receiving workman's compensation benefits
___ (q) I am receiving state disability benefits
___ (r) I am receiving social security disability benefits
___ (s) I am receiving disability benefits from insurance that I purchased on my own or
         through the company I work for

Number of hours presently working per week: _____

How long working at the present job?_____

Reason not able to do all of usual work_____
_____

Number of work days missed per month because of the pain problem_____

If not presently working, write in the number of months off work_____

What was the date last worked? _____

PROVOCATIVE ACTIVITY LIST

The following aggravate my pain problem (put a check mark in front of all those that apply):

___ Sometimes when not doing anything
___ Rainy weather
___ Exposure to cold
___ Hot climate
___ Noise
___ Vibration
___ Alcoholic drinks
___ Caffeinated drinks (coffee, tea, cola)
___ Sitting
___ Driving a car
___ Lying on back
___ Lying on belly
___ Lying on right side
___ Lying on left side
___ Bending forward to brush teeth
___ Bending down to pick up something
    from the floor
___ Bending from side to side at the waist
___ Bending head from front to back
___ Crossing legs: right over left
___ Crossing legs: left over right

___ Going up stairs
___ Going down stairs
___ Walking
___ Running
___ Sexual relations
___ Other movements (explain)

_____

___ Standing
___ Coughing
___ Sneezing
___ Taking a deep breath
___ Bowel movements
___ Menstrual periods
___ Certain clothes worn
    Which?_____
___ Fatigue
___ Emotional stress or anxiety
___ Bending backward at the waist
___ Going to work or coming home from
    work
___ Spouse (wife or husband)

GOALS

If your pain was reduced to an acceptable level, list the activities that you would engage in that your current pain level prevents you from doing. Be specific.

1. _____

2. _____

3. _____

4. _____

5. _____

6. _____

PREVIOUS PAIN PROBLEMS

If you have had any pain problems in the past, please list them:

Area	Cause	Date	Length
Example: low back	Work injury	8/19/79	Six months

INJURIES/ACCIDENTS

List all injuries, broken bones, and auto accidents:	Date of injury

SURGERIES

List all surgeries and dates.

Area operated	Date	Surgeon

FAMILY HISTORY

Put an appropriate letter(s) in front of any disease that is (was) present in your mother (m), father (f), sister (s), brother (b), children (c), aunt (a), uncle (u), grandmother (gm), or grandfather (gf).

___ Alcoholism	___ Emotional problems	___ Liver disease
___ Allergies	___ Epilepsy	___ Mental retardation
___ Anemia	___ Foot pains	___ Muscle pain
___ Arthritis	___ Glaucoma	___ Neck pain
___ Asthma	___ Gout	___ Seizures
___ Back pain	___ Growing pains	___ Spinal cord disease
___ Brain disease	___ Headaches	___ Stroke
___ Bursitis	___ Heart disease	___ Suicide
___ Cancer	___ High blood pressure	___ Tendonitis
___ Depression	___ Joint pains	___ Thyroid disease
___ Diabetes	___ Knee pains	___ Tuberculosis
___ Disc problems	___ Leg cramps	___ Weak legs
		___ Weakness

REVIEW OF SYSTEMS

In the sections that follow, unless told to do otherwise, put a letter in front of any of the items that relate to you. Use the following letters:

O = Occasionally
C = Constantly
P = In the past, but not now
SP = Since the pain problem began
SA = Since the accident or injury (problems that have only begun since the time of your accident or injury)

IS = Intensified since the time of your accident or injury (problems that you had before your accident or injury, but they have intensified since that time)

Skin

___ Dry skin
___ Itching
___ I get "gooseflesh"
___ Sweat excessively
___ Brittle fingernails
___ Skin rash
___ Canker sores
___ Warm intermittent (off and on) flushed sensations in skin of face and other body areas

Lymph nodes

___ Enlargement
___ Tender

Blood system

___ Bruise easily
___ Bleeding tendency
___ Frequent nosebleeds
___ Anemia

Allergy

Please list all foods and drugs that you are allergic to.
Item   Reaction
_____ _____
_____ _____
_____ _____
_____ _____
_____ _____

Head

___ Loss of hair
___ Dandruff
___ Headaches

Eyes

___ Difficulty driving at night
___ Loss of vision
___ Blurred vision
___ Double vision
___ Eyes water
___ Eyelid twitches
___ Pain in the eye
___ Reddening of the eye

___ Bright sunlight hurts eyes
___ Drooping eyelid
___ Eyeglasses
___ Contact lenses
___ Feeling of pressure in the eye or eye socket

Ears

___ Decreased hearing
___ Ringing in ear(s)
___ Hissing sound
___ Roaring sound
___ Clogged ear
___ Crackling sound
___ Vertigo
___ Drainage from ears
___ Wear hearing aid
___ Pain inside the ear without infection

Nose

___ Sinus trouble
___ Stuffy nose
___ Runny nose

Mouth

___ Burning tongue
___ Sore tongue
___ Pain in tongue
___ Discomfort in the mouth
___ Pain in cheek muscles
___ Pain in roof of mouth
___ Burning of the lips
___ Difficulty chewing
___ Pain in tooth or teeth
___ Gums bleed when brushing teeth
___ Clicking or popping of jaw joints
___ I get pain in my mouth when I yawn
___ Difficulty with speaking or speech
___ Limited opening between the teeth
___ I wear dentures

Throat

___ Difficulty swallowing
___ Tightness of the throat area
___ Sore throat without infection
___ Voice fluctuations
___ Persistent hoarseness

Neck

___ Swelling of any glands
___ Stiffness
___ Limited or restricted motion
___ Pain

Breasts

___ Pain
___ Discharge from nipple
___ Enlargement
___ Breast lump
___ Cancer of the breast
___ Tender nipples

Respiratory system

___ Shortness of breath
___ Chest pain or pressure attacks
___ Frequent coughs
___ Cough up blood
___ Trouble breathing
___ Tight chest
___ Asthma
___ Pick up colds, flu, and bronchitis easily
___ Hayfever

Heart and circulation

___ Cold hands
___ Cold feet
___ Low blood pressure
___ Heart problems
___ High blood pressure
___ Circulation problems
___ Swelling of feet
___ Irregular heartbeat
___ Wear a pacemaker
___ Fast heartbeat
___ Get dizzy when stand up

Gastrointestinal system

___ My bowels are regular
___ I have to use laxatives
___ Constipation
___ Diarrhea
___ Heartburn
___ Indigestion
___ Vomiting
___ Hernia
___ Liver trouble
___ Disease of the pancreas
___ Abdominal pain
___ Bloating
___ Anal itching
___ Weight gain
___ Weight loss
___ Nausea
___ Jaundice
___ Hemorrhoids
___ Stomach ulcer
___ Loss of bowel control
___ Blood in stool
___ Change in bowel habits
___ Gall bladder disease
___ Colitis
___ Bowel is irritable
___ Gas
___ Anal pain
___ Loss of appetite
___ Diverticulitis
___ Spastic colon
___ Hiatus hernia
___ Have to use antacids

Urinary system

___ Loss of bladder control
___ Kidney stones
___ I have blood in my urine
___ Kidney trouble
___ Irritation of the bladder

___ Frequent urination
___ Infection of the bladder
___ Burning with urination
___ Difficulty passing urine
___ When I cough I lose urine
___ I have to get up ____ times per night to urinate
___ Interstitial cystitis of the bladder

Male reproductive system

___ Discharge from penis
___ Prostate trouble
___ Pain in testicle
___ Sore penis
___ Difficulty having an erection
___ Lump in testicle

Infectious diseases

___ Recurrent pneumonia
___ Frequent colds or flu
___ Recurrent sinus infections
___ Mononucleosis
___ Venereal disease

Nervous system

___ Difficulty with smell
___ Blackout spells or fainting
___ Stroke
___ Seizures
___ Convulsions
___ Difficulty walking in a dark room
___ I bump into doorways as I go through them
___ I walk into walls
___ Difficulty walking on uneven ground
___ Burning in foot
___ Difficulty with taste
___ Pinched nerve in neck

___ Incoordination
___ Pinched nerve in low back
___ Numbness in face
___ Paralysis
___ Wasting of muscles
___ Tingling in my hand(s) and/or finger(s)

Misc.

___ Night sweats
___ Inappropriate sweating
___ Sweaty palms
___ Lack of ambition and desire
___ Writer's cramp
___ Problems with charley horses
___ I have to pick leg up with hand to get it into the car

I get electric shock-like sensations in my:

___ Neck
___ Right arm
___ Left arm
___ Back
___ Right leg
___ Left leg

I feel:

___ Depressed
___ Frustrated
___ Helpless
___ Withdrawn
___ Discouraged
___ Angry
___ Nervous
___ I have many fears
___ Anxious
___ Agoraphobic
___ Hopeless
___ Worried
___ Bitter
___ Fearful
___ Irritable
___ Apathy
___ Drowsiness

Mental status

___ I'm a nervous wreck
___ I'm very emotional
___ I have extreme highs and lows
___ I'm not having any fun anymore
___ Even when I'm with people, I feel as though I'm not there
___ It feels as though I'm acting
___ I'm hostile
___ I'm angry
___ Feel like going into a rage
Do you find your life (check):
___ Generally unsatisfactory
___ Too demanding
___ Boring
___ Satisfactory
Do you worry about (check):
___ Money
___ Job
___ Marriage
___ Home life
___ Children
Do you (check):
___ Cry easily
___ Feel inferior to others
___ Feel shy
___ Feel things often go wrong
___ Often feel depressed
___ Have unnecessary or irrational fears
___ Feel anxious or upset
Have you (check):
___ Seriously considered suicide
___ Attempted suicide

Endocrine (glands)

___ Thyroid problem
___ Adrenal problem
___ Hypoglycemia

___ Thirsty all the time
___ Cold most of the time
___ Too warm most of the time
___ Unusually jumpy and nervous
___ Diabetes

Use of alcohol and tobacco

How often do you usually drink alcoholic beverages (beer, wine, brandy, whisky, cocktails, etc.)?
___ Never drink alcohol
___ Less than once per week
___ Once per week
___ 2–3 times per week
___ 3–6 times per week
___ Every day
Do you smoke?____ If you answered yes, which of the following:
___ Cigarettes ___ Pipe
___ Cigars ___Other
How many per day? ____
For how many years? ____

Marriage

If you are married, how would you describe your marital relationship?
___ Very satisfactory
___ Satisfactory
___ Tolerable
___ Intolerable
___ Minor but persistent conflicts
___ Major and persistent problems and conflicts

The following is for men

Check all that apply to you. If any of the coding (SA, C, etc.) applies, use it.

___ Poor sexual performance
___ Enlargement of the breasts
___ Loss of sex drive
___ Loss of interest in sexual intercourse
___ Consistent inability to achieve or maintain penile erection that is adequate for completion of sexual intercourse
___ Hot flushes
___ Have become passive
___ Lack motivation
___ I'm irritable

Sleeping

Number of pillows I usually sleep with _____
___ The bed sheets hurt my feet
___ I have nightmares
___ I'm being chased in my dreams
___ I'm exhausted when I wake up
___ I can find no comfortable sleeping position

Other

___ My shoes hurt my feet

The following is for women (female reproductive system)

Menstrual problems: Premenstrual syndrome (PMS or PMT). Symptoms usually begin 10 days before the onset of the menstrual flow and consist of swelling, fluid retention, tiredness, stress, anger, anxiety, nervousness, hostility, emotional ups and downs, mental confusion,

weakness, and others. If you have this problem, check the severity.
___ Mild (occasionally)
___ Moderate (every month + tolerable)
___ Severe (every month + very distressing)
In the last few months is your PMS getting (check):
___ Better
___ No change
___ Worse
Pain with menstrual periods (cramps and low back and leg pain):
___ Mild
___ Moderate (requires medication for relief)
___ Severe (medication + bed rest + miss work)
Other problem areas (use coding)
___ Bleeding between periods
___ Excessive menstrual flow
___ Clots
___ Endometriosis
___ Irregular menstrual periods
___ Vaginal discharge
___ Vaginal yeast infection
___ Other vaginal infection
___ Vaginal irritation
___ Hot flashes
___ Possibly pregnant

Pregnancies

Number of pregnancies
_____
Number of live births
_____
Number of c-sections
_____
Were any of your births (labors) difficult?
_____ yes ___ no

How many were difficult?

_____

Were there complications during your pregnancies?

_____ yes _____ no

Were there complications during the birthing of your children?

_____ yes _____ no

Undergarments

Please answer the following about wearing a brassiere. Check all that apply to you. If any of the coding (SA, C, etc.) applies, use it.

___ No problems

___ I never have worn one

___ I used to wear a brassiere but don't at present because of pain or discomfort

___ I wear a brassiere that buckles in the front because the buckle in the back hurts my back

___ I wear a brassiere that buckles in the front because buckling in back hurts my shoulders or other anatomy

___ I use a brassiere that buckles in the back, but begin by buckling in the front and twisting it to the back

___ I wear strap pads

___ Underwires bother me (pain or soreness)

Comments

_____

_____

_____

_____

_____

Religious preference

_____

_____

Name _____

Date _____

UPDATE OF PROGRESS IN PROGRAM

Directions: Fill in/answer all the questions below and either hand in at the front desk or mail back to the office.

PHYSIOLOGIC DYSFUNCTION QUESTIONNAIRE

Directions for Taking This Test

In the sections listed below, put a check mark in front of any statement that relates to current problems that you have had for more than one month.

1. Energy and stamina (check all applicable items)
   ___ (a) Decreased energy
   ___ (b) Tire easily
   ___ (c) Wake up tired
   ___ (d) Get tired by lunch time
   ___ (e) Get tired by afternoon (by 4–5 p.m.)
   ___ (f) Do not tolerate stress well
   ___ (g) Cannot work as hard as I used to
   ___ (h) Cannot work as much as I used to
   ___ (i) Have to rest more now than before my pain problem started
2. Muscular problems (check all that apply)
   ___ (a) Weakness of the arm
       ___ (1) Right
       ___ (2) Left
   ___ (b) Dropping things with hand
       ___ (1) Right
       ___ (2) Left
   ___ (c) Weakness of the leg
       ___ (1) Right
       ___ (2) Left
   ___ (d) Weakness of abdominal (stomach) muscles
   ___ (e) Weakness of back muscles
   ___ (f) Buckling of leg or leg gives out without warning
       ___ (1) Right
       ___ (2) Left
   ___ (g) Loss of urine when coughing or sneezing
   ___ (h) Have to use a cane to walk
   ___ (i) Need a wheelchair
       ___ (1) All of the time
       ___ (2) Most of the time
       ___ (3) Some of the time
   ___ (j) Pain up and down the spinal area (from neck to low back)
   ___ (k) Bending the head forward causes:
       ___ (1) Increased spinal pain that shoots into tailbone area
       ___ (2) Electric shock-like sensations that shoot into arm(s) and/or leg(s)

___ (l) Tendency to lose my balance and fall when I am standing up with my eyes closed
___ (m) Needs crutches to walk

3. Thinking problems (check all that apply)
   ___ (a) Memory does not function as well as it used to
   ___ (b) Get confused more now than before
   ___ (c) Make thinking errors
   ___ (d) Behavior has changed; it is worse now than before
   ___ (e) Sometimes thinking gets "fuzzy"
   ___ (f) Not as smart as I used to be
   ___ (g) Have lost interest in social activities such as parties, going out to dinner, or being
            with friends
   ___ (h) Feel depressed
   ___ (i) Problems with dizziness
   ___ (j) Vision is blurred (answer only one)
            ___ (1) All the time
            ___ (2) Some of the time
   ___ (k) Hand(s) tremble
   ___ (l) I feel weak all over

4. PCS (check all that apply)
   ___ (a) Have difficulty following directions
   ___ (b) Have difficulty with reading
   ___ (c) Have difficulty with understanding
   ___ (d) Have difficulty understanding what people are saying to me
   ___ (e) Had loss of consciousness after an accident
   ___ (f) Have ongoing blackouts

GLOBAL ACTIVITY ASSESSMENT TEST

For each category of activity listed below, put a number (from 10 to 0 or "—") on the line indicating what your present capability is compared to before the pain problem began (prepain status).

Scoring to Use

10 = doing everything without problem in that group
9 = 90% of prepain status
8 = 80% of prepain status
7 = 70% of prepain status
6 = 60% of prepain status
5 = 50% of prepain status
4 = 40% of prepain status
3 = 30% of prepain status
2 = 20% of prepain status
1 = 10% of prepain status
0 = can't do any more
— = normally never do this

1. Your usual job   _____
2. Work around the home   _____
3. Socialization activities   _____

4. Getting up or down out of a chair   _____
5. Sports   _____
6. Hobbies   _____
7. Sexual activity   _____
8. Sleep   _____

    Number of times the pain wakes you up per night? _____

    How many hours of sleep do you usually get per night? _____

    Is sleep restful or restless? _____

    Take medications for sleep? _____

    If yes, which ones? _____

    Check any of these that apply:

        ___ Have trouble falling asleep

        ___ Have trouble staying asleep

9. Hygiene (shower, grooming, shampooing, toilet, etc.)   _____
10. Eating and feeding   _____
11. Chewing (food, etc.)   _____
12. Dressing and undressing   _____
13. Driving a vehicle   _____
14. The overall strength and endurance   _____

IN THE CHART BELOW PUT DOWN ALL THE MEDICATION YOU ARE PRESENTLY TAKING; INCLUDE VITAMINS

Medication	Strength	Number/day	Reason you take it	For how long?

WORK AND EMPLOYMENT STATUS

Please check the category or categories that relate to your current work or employment status.

___ (a) I am a housewife and do not work outside the home for gainful employment

___ (b) I am doing my regular work full time

___ (c) I am doing my regular work part time

___ (d) I am doing modified regular work full time

___ (e) I am doing modified regular work part time

___ (f) I am doing light work part time

___ (g) I am going to school full time

___ (h) I am going to school part time

___ (i) I am disabled from working because of an injury that occurred while I was at work (work-related injury). (Employed but not working)

___ (j) I am unemployed and not working

___ (k) I am presently retraining for another type of work

___ (l) I am presently going on job interviews

___ (m) I am legally retired because of a work-related injury

___ (n) I am not working because I have reached retirement age and ceased working

___ (o) I do volunteer work only

___ (p) I am receiving workman's compensation benefits

___ (q) I am receiving state disability benefits

___ (r) I am receiving social security disability benefits

___ (s) I am receiving disability benefits from insurance that I purchased on my own or through the company I work for

Number of hours presently working per week: _____

How long working at the present job?_____

Reason not able to do all of usual work_____
_____

Number of work days missed per month because of the pain problem_____

If not presently working, write in the number of months off work_____

What was the date last worked? _____

PROVOCATIVE ACTIVITY LIST

The following aggravate my pain problem (put a check mark in front of all those that apply):

___ Sometimes when not doing anything	___ Going up stairs
___ Rainy weather	___ Going down stairs
___ Exposure to cold	___ Walking
___ Hot climate	___ Running
___ Noise	___ Sexual relations
___ Vibration	___ Other movements (explain)
___ Alcoholic drinks	_____
___ Caffeinated drinks (coffee, tea, cola)	___ Standing
___ Sitting	___ Coughing
___ Driving a car	___ Sneezing
___ Lying on back	___ Taking a deep breath
___ Lying on belly	___ Bowel movements
___ Lying on right side	___ Menstrual periods
___ Lying on left side	___ Certain clothes worn
___ Bending forward to brush teeth	Which?_____
___ Bending down to pick up something from the floor	___ Fatigue
	___ Emotional stress or anxiety
___ Bending from side to side at the waist	___ Bending backward at the waist
___ Bending head from front to back	___ Going to work or coming home from work
___ Crossing legs: right over left	
___ Crossing legs: left over right	___ Spouse (wife or husband)

REVIEW OF SYSTEMS

In the sections that follow, unless told to do otherwise, put a letter in front of any of the items that relate to you. Use the following letters:

O = Occasionally
C = Constantly
P = In the past, but not now
SP = Since the pain problem began
SA = Since the accident or injury (problems that have only be-

gun since the time of your accident or injury)

IS = Intensified since the time of your accident or injury (problems that you had before your accident or injury, but they have intensified since that time)

Skin

___ Dry skin
___ Itching
___ I get "gooseflesh"
___ Sweat excessively
___ Brittle fingernails
___ Skin rash
___ Canker sores
___ Warm intermittent (off and on) flushed sensations in skin of face and other body areas

Lymph nodes

___ Enlargement
___ Tender

Blood system

___ Bruise easily
___ Bleeding tendency
___ Frequent nosebleeds
___ Anemia

Allergy

Please list all foods and drugs that you are allergic to.
Item   Reaction
_____   _____
_____   _____
_____   _____
_____   _____
_____   _____
_____   _____

Head

___ Loss of hair
___ Dandruff
___ Headaches

Eyes

___ Difficulty driving at night
___ Loss of vision
___ Blurred vision
___ Double vision
___ Eyes water
___ Eyelid twitches
___ Pain in the eye
___ Reddening of the eye
___ Bright sunlight hurts eyes
___ Drooping eyelid
___ Eyeglasses
___ Contact lenses
___ Feeling of pressure in the eye or eye socket

Ears

___ Decreased hearing
___ Ringing in ear(s)
___ Hissing sound
___ Roaring sound
___ Clogged ear
___ Crackling sound
___ Vertigo
___ Drainage from ears
___ Wear hearing aid
___ Pain inside the ear without infection

Nose

___ Sinus trouble
___ Stuffy nose
___ Runny nose

Mouth

___ Burning tongue
___ Sore tongue
___ Pain in tongue
___ Discomfort in the mouth
___ Pain in cheek muscles
___ Pain in roof of mouth
___ Burning of the lips
___ Difficulty chewing
___ Pain in tooth or teeth
___ Gums bleed when brushing teeth
___ Clicking or popping of jaw joints
___ I get pain in my mouth when I yawn
___ Difficulty with speaking or speech
___ Limited opening between the teeth
___ I wear dentures

Throat

___ Difficulty swallowing
___ Tightness of throat area
___ Sore throat without infection
___ Voice fluctuations
___ Persistent hoarseness

Neck

___ Swelling of any glands
___ Stiffness
___ Limited or restricted motion
___ Pain

Breasts

___ Pain
___ Discharge from nipple
___ Enlargement
___ Breast lump
___ Cancer of the breast
___ Tender nipples

Respiratory system

___ Shortness of breath
___ Chest pain or pressure attacks
___ Frequent coughs
___ Cough up blood
___ Trouble breathing
___ Tight chest
___ Asthma
___ Pick up colds, flu, and bronchitis easily
___ Hayfever

Heart and circulation

___ Cold hands
___ Cold feet
___ Low blood pressure
___ Heart problems
___ High blood pressure
___ Circulation problems
___ Swelling of feet
___ Irregular heartbeat
___ Wear a pacemaker
___ Fast heartbeat
___ Get dizzy when stand up

Gastrointestinal system

___ My bowels are regular
___ I have to use laxatives
___ Constipation

___ Diarrhea
___ Heartburn
___ Indigestion
___ Vomiting
___ Hernia
___ Liver trouble
___ Disease of the pancreas
___ Abdominal pain
___ Bloating
___ Anal itching
___ Weight gain
___ Weight loss
___ Nausea
___ Jaundice
___ Hemorrhoids
___ Stomach ulcer
___ Loss of bowel control
___ Blood in stool
___ Change in bowel habits
___ Gall bladder disease
___ Colitis
___ Bowel is irritable
___ Gas
___ Anal pain
___ Loss of appetite
___ Diverticulitis
___ Spastic colon
___ Hiatus hernia
___ Have to use antacids

Urinary system

___ Loss of bladder control
___ Kidney stones
___ I have blood in my urine
___ Kidney trouble
___ Irritation of the bladder
___ Frequent urination
___ Infection of the bladder
___ Burning with urination
___ Difficulty passing urine
___ When I cough I lose urine
___ I have to get up ___ times per night to urinate
___ Interstitial cystitis of the bladder

Male reproductive system

___ Discharge from penis
___ Prostate trouble
___ Pain in testicle
___ Sore penis
___ Difficulty having an erection
___ Lump in testicle

Infectious diseases

___ Recurrent pneumonia
___ Frequent colds or flu
___ Recurrent sinus infections
___ Mononucleosis
___ Venereal disease

Nervous system

___ Difficulty with smell
___ Blackout spells or fainting
___ Stroke
___ Seizures
___ Convulsions
___ Difficulty walking in a dark room
___ I bump into doorways as I go through them
___ I walk into walls
___ Difficulty walking on uneven ground
___ Burning in foot
___ Difficulty with taste
___ Pinched nerve in neck
___ Incoordination
___ Pinched nerve in low back
___ Numbness in face
___ Paralysis
___ Wasting of muscles
___ Tingling in my hand(s) and/or finger(s)

Misc.

___ Night sweats
___ Inappropriate sweating
___ Sweaty palms

___ Lack of ambition and desire
___ Writer's cramp
___ Problems with charley horses
___ I have to pick leg up with hand to get it into the car

I get electric shock-like sensations in my:

___ Neck
___ Right arm
___ Left arm
___ Back
___ Right leg
___ Left leg

I feel:

___ Depressed
___ Frustrated
___ Helpless
___ Withdrawn
___ Discouraged
___ Angry
___ Nervous
___ I have many fears
___ Anxious
___ Agoraphobic
___ Hopeless
___ Worried
___ Bitter
___ Fearful
___ Irritable
___ Apathy
___ Drowsiness

Mental status

___ I'm a nervous wreck
___ I'm very emotional
___ I have extreme highs and lows
___ I'm not having any fun anymore
___ Even when I'm with people, I feel as though I'm not there
___ It feels as though I'm acting

___ I'm hostile
___ I'm angry
___ Feel like going into a rage

Do you find your life (check):
___ Generally unsatisfactory
___ Too demanding
___ Boring
___ Satisfactory

Do you worry about (check):
___ Money
___ Job
___ Marriage
___ Home life
___ Children

Do you (check):
___ Cry easily
___ Feel inferior to others
___ Feel shy
___ Feel things often go wrong
___ Often feel depressed
___ Have unnecessary or irrational fears
___ Feel anxious or upset

Have you (check):
___ Seriously considered suicide
___ Attempted suicide

Endocrine (glands)

___ Thyroid problem
___ Adrenal problem
___ Hypoglycemia
___ Thirsty all the time
___ Cold most of the time
___ Too warm most of the time
___ Unusually jumpy and nervous
___ Diabetes

Use of alcohol and tobacco

How often do you usually drink alcoholic beverages

(beer, wine, brandy, whisky, cocktails, etc.)?
___ Never drink alcohol
___ Less than once per week
___ Once per week
___ 2–3 times per week
___ 3–6 times per week
___ Every day

Do you smoke?____ If you answered yes, which of the following:
___ Cigarettes   ___ Pipe
___ Cigars   ___ Other

How many per day? ____
For how many years? ____

Marriage

If you are married, how would you describe your marital relationship?
___ Very satisfactory
___ Satisfactory
___ Tolerable
___ Intolerable
___ Minor but persistent conflicts
___ Major and persistent problems and conflicts

The following is for men

Check all that apply to you. If any of the coding (SA, C, etc.) applies, use it.
___ Poor sexual performance
___ Enlargement of the breasts
___ Loss of sex drive
___ Loss of interest in sexual intercourse
___ Consistent inability to achieve or maintain penile erection that is adequate for completion of sexual intercourse

___ Hot flushes
___ Have become passive
___ Lack motivation
___ I'm irritable

Sleeping

Number of pillows I usually sleep with _____
___ The bed sheets hurt my feet
___ I have nightmares
___ I'm being chased in my dreams
___ I'm exhausted when I wake up
___ I can find no comfortable sleeping position

Other

___ My shoes hurt my feet

The following is for women (female reproductive system)

Menstrual problems: Premenstrual syndrome (PMS or PMT). Symptoms usually begin 10 days before the onset of the menstrual flow and consist of swelling, fluid retention, tiredness, stress, anger, anxiety, nervousness, hostility, emotional ups and downs, mental confusion, weakness, and others. If you have this problem, check the severity.
___ Mild (occasionally)

___ Moderate (every month + tolerable)
___ Severe (every month + very distressing)
In the last few months is your PMS getting (check):
___ Better
___ No change
___ Worse
Pain with menstrual periods (cramps and low back and leg pain):
___ Mild
___ Moderate (requires medication for relief)
___ Severe (medication + bed rest + miss work)
Other problem areas (use coding)
___ Bleeding between periods
___ Excessive menstrual flow
___ Clots
___ Endometriosis
___ Irregular menstrual periods
___ Vaginal discharge
___ Vaginal yeast infection
___ Other vaginal infection
___ Vaginal irritation
___ Hot flashes
___ Possibly pregnant

Pregnancies

Number of pregnancies
_____
Number of live births
_____
Number of c-sections
_____

Were any of your births (labors) difficult?
_____ yes _____ no
How many were difficult?
_____
Were there complications during your pregnancies?
_____ yes _____ no
Were there complications during the birthing of your children?
_____ yes _____ no

Undergarments

Please answer the following about wearing a brassiere. Check all that apply to you. If any of the coding (SA, C, etc.) applies, use it.
___ No problems
___ I never have worn one
___ I used to wear a brassiere but don't at present because of pain or discomfort
___ I wear a brassiere that buckles in the front because the buckle in the back hurts my back
___ I wear a brassiere that buckles in the front because buckling in back hurts my shoulders or other anatomy
___ I use a brassiere that buckles in the back, but begin by buckling in the front and twisting it to the back
___ I wear strap pads
___ Underwires bother me (pain or soreness)

Comments

_____

_____

_____

Religious preference _____

Name _____

Date _____

A copy of this direction sheet is given to the patient.

B-complex injection #1	**Full**	**Half**	**Quarter**
Dexpanthenol, 250 mg/ml (B5)	1 cc	$\frac{1}{2}$ cc	$\frac{2}{10}$ cc
2% lidocaine (Xylocaine®)	$\frac{1}{2}$ cc	$\frac{1}{2}$ cc	$\frac{2}{10}$ cc
B-complex 100 (mixed B complex)	1 cc	$\frac{1}{2}$ cc	$\frac{2}{10}$ cc
Riboflavin, 50 mg/ml (B2)	$\frac{1}{2}$ cc	$\frac{1}{2}$ cc	$\frac{2}{10}$ cc

Frequency: _____

B-complex injection #2	**Full**	**Half**	**Quarter**
Dexpanthenol, 250 mg/ml (B5)	$1\frac{1}{2}$ cc	$\frac{1}{2}$ cc	$\frac{2}{10}$ cc
Folic acid, 5 or 10 mg/ml (Bc)	$\frac{1}{2}$ cc	$\frac{1}{2}$ cc	$\frac{2}{10}$ cc
Hydroxycobalamin, 1000 μg/ml (B12)	$\frac{1}{2}$ cc	$\frac{1}{2}$ cc	$\frac{2}{10}$ cc

Frequency: _____

General approach to using these vitamin injections. The patient is taught the quarter dose of syringe #1. After a week or two at that dose, the quarter dose of syringe #2 is taught. Injections are given in an alternative fashion: injection #1, then skip a day, injection #2, skip a day, injection #1, skip a day, etc. This is called the **primary program**. If nerve regeneration flare-up occurs at that dosing, the injections are stopped for a week and then started at 4-day intervals between the shots. When the quarter-dose shots can be done with the primary program for a month, the patient is progressed to the primary program using the half-strength doses.

Full-strength-doses are used daily (#1 one day, #2 the next, #1 the next, etc.) for 10–14 days each time the patient is injured, reinjured, has an accident, or suffers trauma.

_____ Use alternate injection program: Inject a #1, skip a day, inject a #2, skip a day, inject a #1, skip a day, inject a #2, etc.

_____ Inject _____ cc of dexpanthenol, 250 mg/ml, daily for _____ days.

Injection Procedure Instructions

Please do not self-administer any of the vitamin injectables until you have been shown and told how to proceed. No harm will result from accidentally injecting one of these vitamin products into a vein. Fidgeting about small amounts of air in the syringe (up to as much as $\frac{1}{2}$ cc is unnecessary) and if injected will cause no harm.

1. Remove the bottle(s) from the storage place. Protection from light and temperatures above 110° is recommended. Storage in the refrigerator is not necessary.
2. Open one of the alcohol skin swabs (tear if at the middle, not at the end).
3. Thoroughly coat the top of each bottle to be used.
   a. You want to be certain to eliminate any contamination of the rubber before inserting the needle into the top of the bottle.

4. Remove the syringe from its package.
   a. Use a new syringe with attached needle, swab, and separate needle for injection for each injection session.
   b. Peel apart the wrapper and pull the syringe with attached needle out of the wrapper.
   c. You will be using a 3-cc syringe with any of a number of needles that commonly come attached to them.
   d. Make sure the needle is screwed securely onto the syringe by twisting protected needle until it locks into place.
   e. Remove the plastic protector from the end of the needle so that you will be able to pressurize the bottle(s) as indicated in #5 below.
5. Each bottle must now be pressurized, except riboflavin, by injecting air into it with the syringe you have. Put air into the syringe by pulling back the plunger by the amount of air needed, which may be $2/10$, $5/10$, or 1 cc. Insert the needle into the middle of the top of each vitamin bottle, and inject the air into the bottle. Continue to do this with each bottle until pressurized as indicated below. Bottles are pressurized at each session.
   The needle pressurizing the bottle penetrates the rubber on the bottle by only $1/4$ inch. Hold the bottle on a flat, secure surface while pressurizing it.
   Pressurize the bottles in the following order:
   Syringe #1
      Riboflavin
      B complex (B-Plex 100)
      Xylocaine® (lidocaine) or Novocain® (procaine)
      Dexpanthenol
   Syringe #2
      Hydroxocobalamin
      Folic acid or folvite
      Riboflavin
      Dexpanthenol
6. Then draw up the amounts of vitamin solution indicated for the specific syringe number. Draw up from the bottles in the reverse order that you pressurized them.
   a. Take the bottle to be used and turn it upside down.
   b. With the bottle upside down, insert the needle $1/4$ inch through the rubber and draw up the recommended amount of solution.
   c. Do this until all the components of the injection have been drawn into the syringe.
7. Take the small injection needle out of its container. Change needles by unscrewing the needle attached to the syringe. Then screw the small-gauge injection needle on the syringe until it locks into place.
8. Swab your injection site with the alcohol swab and inject.
9. After the injection is complete, pull the needle out and, using the swab, put pressure on the injection site for a minute to decrease bruising.

Name _____

Date _____

SYMPTOM CHARTING

On the figures that appear on the front and/or back of this page, use the indicated colors to show me where you have the indicated problem or symptom. If you do not have any of the symptoms called for on a set of figures, skip it and go on to the next. New patients, please give me what symptoms you have had for the last two months; established patients, please give me the symptoms you have had for the past week. If a symptom is more intense in certain areas, shade heavier in that area. If you are color blind, please go according to the number at the top of the pencil.

Rate your overall pain intensity by putting an "x" on the line:_____

How long/far can you: sit _____;   stand _____;   walk _____ (in hours)

Intensity of pain symptoms (check the one that best applies to you)
_____ Minimal — an annoyance. Causes no handicap in the performance of activities of daily living (ADL) or job duties
_____ Slight — causes some handicap in the performance of ADL and duties that bring the pain on
_____ Moderate — causes marked handicap in the performance of ADL and duties that bring the pain on
_____ Severe — precludes the performance of ADL and/or job duties that bring on the pain

Frequency of symptoms (check the one that best applies to you)
_____ Occasional (about 25% of the time)   _____ Intermittent (about 50% of the time)
_____ Frequent (about 75% of the time)   _____ Constant (100% of the time)

(Note: Numbers that appear after the name of a color refer to Berol prismacolor pencils.)

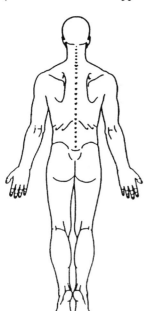

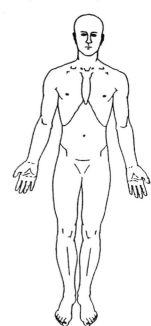

Indigo Blue #901
for dull or sharp, constant
or intermittent pain,
aching, or soreness

Canary Yellow #916
for numbness, tingling, or
dead areas

Crimson Red #924
for burning or hot areas

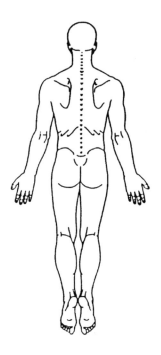

True Green #910
for cramping or
charley horses

Cold Gray Medium #966
for areas of twitching,
jumping, or jerking

Pink #929
for pressure, tension,
tightness, or twisting

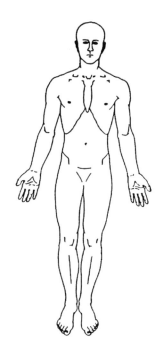

Orange #918
for sharp, shooting,
stabbing pains of
short duration (fleeting)

Brite Violet #988
for swelling or
sensation of swelling

Grass Green #909
for areas that feel well

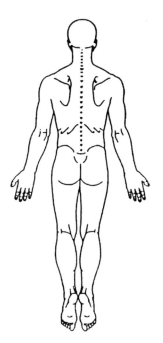

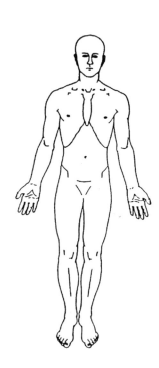

Name _____

Date _____

PAIN CHART DRAWN BY DR. MARGOLES

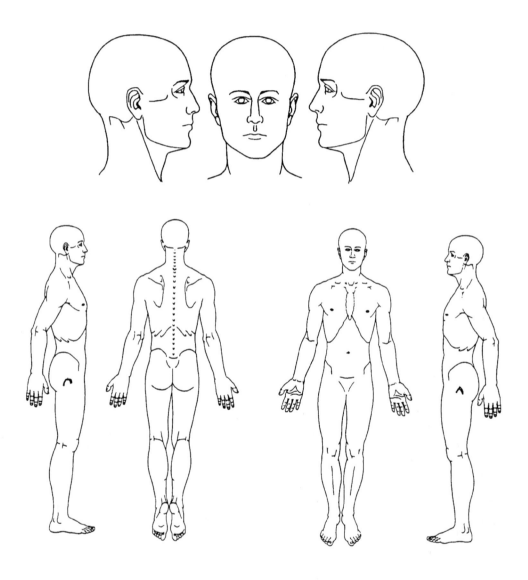

PHYSICIAN TREATMENT PLAN

Name_____

NOTE CODING TO BE USED

TO DO TODAY	

TO DO NEXT VISIT	

ONGOING	

WAITING FOR	

//// = Done   \\\\ = Deleted (not done)   ▦ = Carried forward

TB = taut band; TPI = trigger point injection; TrP = trigger point; ROM = range of motion

PHYSICIAN TREATMENT PLAN

Name_____

DIAGNOSES AND ICD- CM-9 NUMBERS
1
2
3
4
5

INFORMED CONSENT OF THE PATIENT: I understand and have been informed of the risks and benefits of the narcotic(s) (opioid(s)) medication that may be used in my treatment. I understand the addiction potential, the possibility of adverse reactions to the medication, and the possibility of developing dependency on the medication. I understand the risks and benefits of this (these) drug(s) compared with other treatment methods. I understand that if I fail to obtain medical and/or medication reviews, laboratory tests, or if I fail to keep up with return visits to Dr. Margoles' office, I may be tapered off my medication(s) and discharged from Dr. Margoles' practice with notice being given. I will disclose to Dr. Margoles all other sources of medication.   Patient signature_____ Date _____

TREATMENT PLAN OBJECTIVES (check all that apply)

Pain relief	Return to work	Correct sleep problem
Improved physical function	More work around the home	Improve endurance
Improved psychologic function	Behavior modification	Teach injury prevention
Improved social function	Teach coping skills	Teach pacing skills

PHYSICAL EXAM UPDATES DONE	SPOUSE INTERVIEW	PAYCHECK STUB	LABORATORY DATE ORDERED	UPDATES DATE RECEIVED

M.D. MEDICATION REVIEW			PHARM.D. REVIEW		
NAME	DATE SENT	DATE RECEIVED	NAME	DATE SENT	DATE RECEIVED

ABNORMALITIES OF SLEEP

Name: _____

Date: _____

Score: yes = 1   no = 0

Date → Symptom ↓				
Myoclonus?				
Nightmares?				
Tense?				
Abnormal breathing?				
Feel beat up when awake in AM?				
Wake up tired?				
Do muscle jumps wake you up?				
Medication Rx'd				
Total score				

PAIN DIARY HELPS

Pain Severity

A = Minimal. An annoyance. Causes no handicap in the performance of activities of daily living (ADL).

B = Slight. Causes some handicap in the performance of ADL and duties that bring on the pain.

C = Moderate. Causes marked handicap in the performance of ADL and duties that bring on the pain.

D = Severe. Precludes the performance of ADL and/or job duties that bring on the pain.

Pain Frequency

1 = Occasional — about 25% of the time

2 = Intermittent — about 50% of the time

3 = Frequent — about 75% of the time

4 = Constant — 100% of the time

Energy Level

The range here is from 10 = as much energy as ever to 0 = constantly fatigued and seriously tired all the time. Pick a number at or between those numbers that reflects your current energy level.

Quality of Sleep

S1: Poor. Many awakenings (greater than five awakenings). Nightmares. Need to take pain medicine during the night.

S2: Better than poor. Two to three awakenings. Need to take pain medication during the night.

S3: Restful. One to two awakenings. No need for pain medications during hours of sleep.

S4: Peaceful and restful. No awakenings.

Activity Level

0 = Resting or sleeping.

1 = Minimal. Doing one-fourth of all usual work inside the home and/or one-fourth of all duties of usual employment.

2 = Moderate. Doing one-half of all usual work inside the home and/or one-half all duties of usual employment.

3 = Normal. Doing all usual work inside the home and all duties of usual employment.

PAIN DIARY

Patient name _____

Dates		/	/	/	/	/	/	/	/	/	/	/	/	/	/	/
Item[1]		A P m m	A P m m	A P m m	A P m m	A P m m	A P m m	A P m m	A P m m	A P m m	A P m m	A P m m	A P m m	A P m m	A P m m	A P m m
Pain severity																
Worst ever	10															
	8															
Moderate	6															
	4															
Minimal	2															
	1															
None	0															
Pain frequency																
None 0%																
Occasional 25%																
Intermittent 50%																
Frequent 75%																
Constant 100%																
Pain intensity																
Minimal	A															
Slight	B															
Moderate	C															
Severe	D															
Energy level																
Worst ever	0															
	2															
	4															
	6															
	8															
Best Ever	10															
Sleep quality																
Poor	S1															
	S2															
	S3															
Good, restful	S4															
Activity level																
Resting or sleeping	0															
Minimal	1															
Moderate	2															
Normal	3															

OFFICE VISIT RECORD

Name _____ Date _____

___Office visit ___Tele. Call ___Private ___Pers. injury ___Industrial   Reason: ___Follow up evaluation
___New patient evaluation ___Consult ___Established patient with new injury / problem

Times[1]: E/M: _____ to _____   Injections: _____ to _____   Consult: _____ to _____

_____
_____
_____
_____
_____
_____
_____
_____
_____
_____
_____
_____
_____
_____
_____
_____
_____

EXAMINATION (there may be forms attached to this office visit record that give supplemental information)
Vital signs: PR:_____ B/P:_____ Wt.:_____ Temp:_____ Resp: _____

No distress	Mod. severe distress	
Mild distress	Marked distress	
Moderate distress	Severe distress	

ASSESSMENTS
PROGRESS

	Better	Worse	No change
Ambulation	____	____	____
Facial	____	____	____
Distress	____	____	____
Pain	____	____	____

MENTAL STATUS CHECK

Yes	No	
__	__	Alert
__	__	Coherent
__	__	Slurred speech
__	__	Good cognition
__	__	Evidence of drug toxicity
__	__	Hearing (listening) OK

OTHER
___ Medication usage
___ Amount of pain behavior
___ Memory
___ Assessment for presence of depression
___ Assessment for secondary gain factors
___ Detailed evaluation of symptom chart

Sleep: _____

Analgesic medication_____ Pain relief, etc., rating _____

OFFICE VISIT RECORD

Name _____ Date _____

Work status: Returned to work on (date) _____   Able to return to work on (date) _____   Work

restrictions: ___ No restrictions ___ Part time: specify hours per day _____ Modified work   Restrictions _____

_____ Duration _____

___Continues usual work status and duties.   ___ Total restriction; not a candidate for return to work.

_____

_____

_____

_____

_____

_____

_____

_____

_____

_____

Counseling:
__ Diagnostic results, impressions, and/or recommended diagnostic studies.   __ Patient and family education.
__ Importance of compliance with chosen management (treatment) option.   __ Prognosis.
__ Instructions for management (treatment) and/or follow-up.   __ Risk factor reduction.

Management and instruction given:

___ Medication management	___ B-complex injections	___ Injury prevention
Tablets or pills	___ Hydrocortisone or similar steroid	___ Pacing skills
___ Time-contingent pain med. dosing	___ Other:_____	___ Proprioceptive assessment
___ Flexible time-contingent dosing	___ Behavior modification	___ Review of x-rays
___ Single and multiple drug format	___ Cognitive skills	___ Stretching exercises
___ Muscle relaxer/tranquilizer	___ Coping skills	___ Therapeutic exercises
___ Other_____	___ Correction of sleep dysfunction	___ Work with patient's spouse
Injectable medication	___ Dietary related to the pain	
___Injection of medication for use at home	___ Home spray and stretch program	

Nature of presenting problem(s):

__ Minor - good prognosis with management/compliance.

__ Low severity - full recovery without functional impairment is expected.

__ Moderate severity - uncertain prognosis. Increased probability of prolonged functional impairment.

__ High severity - high probability of severe prolonged functional impairment.

Medical decision making: (circle 2 out of 3)

Number of diagnoses or management options	Amount and/or complexity of data to be reviewed	Risk of complications and/or morbidity	Type of decision making
minimal	minimal or none	minimal	straight- forward
limited	limited	low	low complexity
multiple	moderate	moderate	moderate complexity
extensive	extensive	high	high complexity

Diagnoses: (see billing sheet for this visit)

_____M.D.

Patient_____

Date → | | | | | | | |

TEST ↓

DEEP TENDON REFLEXES
(for grading see below)
  Triceps right
  Biceps right
  Brachioradalis right
  Patellar right
  Achilles right

  Triceps left
  Biceps left
  Brachioradalis left
  Patellar left
  Achilles left

CLONUS (see below)
  Right
  Left

BABINSKI
  + = present - = absent
  Right
  Left

ABDOMINAL REFLEXES
  + = present   - = absent
  Upper right
  Middle right
  Lower right

  Upper left
  Middle left
  Lower left

Patient_____

Date → | | | | | | | |

TUNING FORK TEST
n = normal   a = abnormal

Right

| Index MCPJ | Index MCPJ | Index MCPJ | Index MCPJ | Index MCPJ | Index MCPJ | Index MCPJ |
| Medial Malleolus | Medial Malleolus | Medial Malleolus | Medial Malleolus | Medial Malleolus | Medial Malleolus | Medial Malleolus |

Left

| Index MCPJ | Index MCPJ | Index MCPJ | Index MCPJ | Index MCPJ | Index MCPJ | Index MCPJ |
| Medial Malleolus | Medial Malleolus | Medial Malleolus | Medial Malleolus | Medial Malleolus | Medial Malleolus | Medial Malleolus |

Right

| Therapist | Therapist | Therapist | Therapist | Therapist | Therapist | Therapist |
| Patient | Patient | Patient | Patient | Patient | Patient | Patient |

Left

| Therapist | Therapist | Therapist | Therapist | Therapist | Therapist | Therapist |
| Patient | Patient | Patient | Patient | Patient | Patient | Patient |

RHOMBERG (see below) | | | | | | | |

PINPRICK TESTING
See below
Standardized at
  C5 right
  C6 right
  C7 right

C5 right						
C6 right						
C7 right						

Patient_____

Date →							
C8 right							
T1 right							
C5 left							
C6 left							
C7 left							
C8 left							
T1 left							
L4 right							
L5 right							
S1 right							
L4 left							
L5 left							
S1 left							

Deep tendon reflex grading
4 = Very hyperactive (++++)
3 = Hyperactive   (+++)
2 = WNL (Normal)   (++)
1 = Weak   (+)
± = Trace
0 = Absent   (Absent)

Clonus grading
0 = Absent
1 = Very slight (1 - 2 movements)
2 = Slight (3 - 4 movements)
3 = Moderate (short of sustained)
4 = Sustained

*Rhomberg test*_____   *Grade Meaning*
                            1   Steady
                            2   Sl. unsteady
                            3   Unsteady
                            4   Short of falling
                            5   Falls
                            6   Falls with eyes open (feet together and arms crossed)

Pinprick testing grades
///// = deficit   0 = within normal limits   X = hyper-response

MYOFASCIAL PAIN SYNDROME SCREENING TEST

RIGHT	*PAIN*	*SITTING*	*LEFT*	*PAIN*
		Hyperextension left index finger : degrees _____		

ROM Neck

		Forward (FB)...	_____	_____
		Extension...	_____	_____
_____	_____	Lat. bend (FB)	_____	_____
_____	_____	Rotation..	_____	_____
		3 Knuckle test	_____	_____

ROM Shoulder

_____	_____	Forward..	_____	_____
_____	_____	External rotation......................................	_____	_____
_____	_____	Abduction..	_____	_____
_____	_____	Adduction..	_____	_____
_____	_____	Hand to shoulder blade (cm)......................	_____	_____
_____	_____	Mouth wrap around test (cm)...................	_____	_____

Notes _____

_____

TB	TNDR	JS	DEGR	*RECUMBENT* [1]	TB	TNDR	JS	DEGR
				Trapezius taut band...................................				
				Sternocleidomastoid taut band				
				Pectoralis maj. taut band				
				Latissimus dorsi taut band**.....................				

---

[1] In columns for TB, TNDR and JS answer Y = yes or N = no. In DEGR give degrees of flexion or SLR obtained before pain.

	DEGR	*RECUMBENT*		DEGR
Pain at:		Straight leg raising test.............................	Pain at:	
Pain at		Hip extension	Pain at	

TB	TNDR	JS	Tx - Tx	*PRONE*	TB	TNDR	JS	Tx - Tx
				Thoracic paraspinals taut band				

RIGHT   *PAIN*   *STANDING*   *LEFT*   *PAIN*

ROM Lumbar Spine

Forward "/deg... _____ _____

Extension.. _____ _____

_____ _____ Lat. bend .... _____ _____

_____ _____ Rotation... _____ _____

SQUAT TEST (deep knee bend)

Range of motion (ROM)......... .... _____ _____

Strength .... _____ _____

Balance .... _____ _____

Smoothness of movement .... _____ _____

Need to grasp table or leg....... .... _____ _____

Pain intensity: 1 = better 2 =   no change   3 = worse............................. _____ _____

Definitions: Tenderness — patient states muscle is tender when palpated. Taut band (TB) — an involuntary sustained contraction of a small or large segment of a muscle. The band can be recognized by specific palpation. Jump sign (JS) — an involuntary withdrawal response that occurs when an abnormally tender trigger point is palpated or injected. The patient may wince or cry out. Local twitch response (LTR) — an involuntary contraction of taut band in a muscle that occurs when the trigger point in the taut band is snapped or pierced with a needle.

* Diagnostic therapy may be administered using Fluori-Methane to increase the ROM and/or decrease the pain in any area of abnormality indicated above. If this is done and a good response obtained, put an asterisk in the "normal" column to indicate a positive clinical response. ** Can also be tested in recumbent position.

CODING TO BE USED: T = tender, P = painful. Use the following with T or P: 1 = mild, 2 = moderate, 3 = severe, 4 = excruciating. Example: T3, P2. TB = taut band. JS = Jump sign LTR = local twitch response. Taut band grading: 1 = thin, up to ⅛ inch at its greatest diameter; 2 = moderate, up to ¼ inch at its greatest diameter; 3 = up to ½ inch or more at its greatest diameter. Grading of degree of restriction: 0 = within normal limits , 1 = mild (up to 90% of normal ROM), 2 = moderate (up to 60% of normal ROM), 3 = severe (up to 30% of normal ROM), 4 = no motion.

26 Stewart's Story: The Use of Injectable Analgesic for Maintenance of Gainful Employment

Michael S. Margoles, M.D., Ph.D.

Stewart I.* was 46 years old when he came for evaluation and treatment. He was a consulting engineer to three major software companies. His work was very tedious and technical. He related an 8-year history of progressive low back and sciatic leg pain. Sometimes the leg pain was on the right side and sometimes it occurred on the left. On rare occasions, when the pain got real bad, it might radiate down both legs. When a search was carried out for the most likely cause(s) for his pain problem, the history revealed that he had been involved in four automobile accidents over a number of years: one "fender bender," one rear-end whiplash, one in which the car was totaled by crashing into a heavy-duty pole, and the most recent, a major crash into another vehicle in 1987. After that, he came under the care of Dr. Piashonie (anesthesiologist and specialist in pain management). As of this writing, he had been in my pain management program for 3 years.

In the past history, Stewart related four high school soccer injuries and three college soccer injuries. Each injury kept him out of playing soccer for 2–3 weeks and necessitated that he see a doctor for evaluation and treatment. Once, while working after school one day, he slipped on liquid soap at the top of a flight of stairs. He slid and tumbled down the entire flight. The doctor diagnosed sprain of the wrist and ankle, plus contusion to the back.

The significance of the past history of numerous high school and college injuries is that they act like a cumulative trauma injury effect. They set the stage for subsequent injuries (which may occur years later) to have a more severe and adverse effect on the patient than would be expected. The pain and dysfunction produced by subsequent injures will produce more pain and more physical dysfunction compared to a patient who has a similar injury and no past history of injuries.

Stewart said:

---

* Name changed to protect the patient.

It wasn't until recently that the doctor informed me that I've had progressive, severe, multifocal myofascial pain syndrome for at least 10 years. The headaches that had begun at age 16 were probably myofascial in origin. I have tried many medications. Nonsteroidal anti-inflammatory drugs used to be helpful for the first 10–15 years, but then they began irritating my gut whether I took them with food or not. Tagamet®, Prilosek®, and Cytotec® were of help when I began using them, but have not been of much help in recent years

I've used Soma 350® over the last 8 years, at two to four tablets per day. It is a good muscle relaxer and also of help for going to sleep on those nights when my muscles are too tight or nights that I just can't settle down. I usually take no more than four Soma 350® per day. Occasionally, if needed, I am permitted to take up to six tablets per day of the Soma 350®.

All his medication treatment was combined with other therapies for chronic pain to enhance the effect of the other treatments used. These other therapies consisted of the following (note that only one or two of these therapies were administered conjointly with or without a specific analgesic medication): psychotherapy, behavior modification, cognitive restructuring, two lumbar epidurals, two lumbar MRIs, distraction therapy, group therapy, exercises, stretches, hypnosis, epidural spinal stimulator, walking up to 3 miles per day, and taking analgesic medication on a time-contingent basis and/or on an as-needed basis. The analgesic medications were most helpful when used in conjunction with physical therapy, exercises, stretches, and walking.

I've had some very severe attacks of pain, sometimes lasting months. Numerous myofascial trigger point injections have given good partial relief during the pain flare-ups. I understand that it may take a number of years to get rid of all the pain and other symptom-producing myofascial trigger points. Over the last 7 years, numerous pain medications, including Darvon®, Darvocet-N® 100, Vicodin®, Lorcet 10®, Percodan®, Percocet®, injectable Nubain®, injectable Buprenex®,* injectable Dalgan®, methadone, morphine sulfate tablets, MS Contin® (time-release morphine), and injectable morphine sulfate, have been tried. They were all used to obtain pain relief, but all produced troublesome side effects and no significant pain relief. All types of morphine sulfate used produced significant side effects of severe constipation, urinary hesitation, urine retention, nausea, occasional vomiting, and sedation that was very troublesome and interfered with my ability to work. Dilaudid® tablets at up to 6–8 mg every 4 hours were tried and minimal relief** was obtained. The Dilaudid® produced no bothersome side effects. The medications that gave satisfactory pain control were injectable Buprenex® (0.3 mg/ml), injectable Dilaudid® (2 mg/ml), and injectable Dilaudid-HP® (10 mg/ml). The most predictable pain relief came from Dilaudid-HP®.

As part of his medication management, a "pain cocktail"*** was used to taper him off all pain-relieving (Dilaudid-HP®) and related medications (Soma 350®, etc.) for 3 months to assess benefit of discontinuing pain medication. His pain got noticeably worse during the first

---

* This medication was first taken by the sublingual route, then later by injection.

** Means that lack of adequate pain relief made it impossible to run his business for more than 2–3 hours a day, instead of the usual 8–10 hours a day.

*** This is a combination of medications consisting of variable amounts of Elavil® and methadone. The patient does not know the contents.

2 months he was tapered off his usual pain-relieving medications, and the physical dysfunction secondary to being in more pain and discomfort became more pronounced. He was not able to perform enough physical activity to run his business and produce income. His business began to go downhill due to lack of finances. His credit rating began to suffer. He was refused a business improvement loan because of the recent risks associated with his declining income. In order to keep him gainfully employed, at week 8 of his medication taper, he was put back on the Dilaudid-HP® and Soma 350®. Immediately after going back on the medications, he was able to return to his usual work and activity level. His doctors seemed baffled by these events.

> I run a very successful business. About two to three times per week, I finish up at 7:00 to 9:00 p.m. At those times, I am stiff and sore and have painful muscles in the back, legs, buttock, and shoulders. On some days, cramping may occur in those same areas along with the pain. I also become so tired that I want to take a nap for an hour. In addition to the pain, cramping, and sore muscles, I become irritable.

It was then that an injection of 3.5–4.0 mg of Dilaudid-HP® resolved most of the stiffness, soreness, and diffuse muscle pain within 10–30 minutes. It was surprising that he noted that the tiredness and irritability left about as fast as the pain, soreness, and stiffness. If he added equal parts of 0.5% Marcaine with epinephrine to the Dilaudid-HP®, he could extend the relief by an extra 1–2 hours. After the pain relief set in, Stewart could finish up the day with good pain control (up to 60–80% pain relief) that carried him through until bedtime (at about midnight). All the members of the treatment team agreed to trust Stewart to administer the medication to himself, instead of having to go to their offices or the emergency room every time he needed a dose of potent injectable analgesic medication.

> When Dilaudid-HP® was the only analgesic I was using, I began to have mild withdrawal episodes during the night. That is because the Dilaudid® acts for a short period of time. The withdrawal was manifested by mild to moderate sweating that became very annoying. I awoke with the pillow drenched with perspiration. This was resolved by using 30 mg of methadone at bedtime. The methadone acts for a long period of time. Methadone had been a problem when I took it twice per day, causing bothersome sedation. However, taking it only once, at bedtime, kept side effects from it to a minimum.

The problem mentioned above was due to taking a short-acting medication, with a duration of action of 3–4 hours, and trying to make it last all night. By adding the methadone at bedtime (duration of action was 10–30 hours), the problem of nighttime withdrawal was eliminated.

> At times, Buprenex® injection has provided pain control similar to Dilaudid-HP®, but the overall quality of the pain control has not been as good as the Dilaudid-HP® injection. If the pain becomes great (grade 7 out of 10 or above), the Buprenex® does not seem to work at all compared to the Dilaudid-HP®.
>
> Most mornings, I wake up at 7:00 a.m., stiff as a board in the back, and also very painful in that area. A 4- to 5-mg injection of Dilaudid-HP® gets me up and prepared for the work day within 30 minutes instead of the usual 2 hours that it took prior to the use of Dilaudid-HP®. By the time lunch rolls around, at 12:30–1:00 p.m., the pain is back up to a 6–8 rating again. Usually 3.5 mg of Dilaudid-HP® helps me continue with most of the necessary activities for the rest of my work day.

In his use of the Dilaudid-HP®, Stewart discovered that there is a dose of medication that modifies and *blocks some of the pain,* and a higher dose that *reestablishes and/or returns him back toward the normal activity level that it takes to run his business.* The dose of Dilaudid-HP® that blocks some of the pain is 2 mg. The dose that modifies the pain level and gets him back to a normal activity level (and allows him to run his business) is 3.5–5.0 mg given every 3–6 hours, as needed.

In conclusion, this chapter presents an aggressive 46-year-old engineer who had chronic back and leg pain after numerous injuries spanning his teen years to adulthood. The therapeutic approach consisted of numerous treatments from each of the following categories: medication, psychiatry/psychology, physical, and invasive. A medication taper was also attempted, but almost caused a disaster with respect to loss of his business. The Dilaudid-HP® and Soma® were restarted and were instrumental in saving his consulting job. Use of Dilaudid-HP® as the primary analgesic caused a problem of withdrawal at night, during sleep. This problem was remedied using methadone at bedtime.

27 Glossary of Terms for Opioids and Opioid-Containing Analgesic Medication in the Management of Chronic Intractable Pain

Michael S. Margoles, M.D., Ph.D.

ABSTINENCE SYNDROME

The abstinence syndrome (withdrawal) is characteristic of the person with drug dependence syndrome and is characterized,* in the acute phase, by:**

- **Early:** Yawning, lacrimation, rhinorrhea, sweating
- **Intermediate:** Extreme dilation of the pupil(s), piloerection, flushing, tachycardia, twitching, tremor, restlessness, irritability, anxiety, anorexia
- **Late:** Muscle spasm, fever, nausea, diarrhea, vomiting, severe backache, abdominal and leg pains, abdominal and muscle cramps, hot and cold flashes, insomnia, intestinal spasm, coryza and repetitive sneezing, increase in body temperature, increase in blood pressure, increase in heart rate, increase in respiratory rate, spontaneous orgasm, chills, bone and muscle pain in back and extremities due to controlled substance withdrawal and not due to the underlying disease process

ADDICTION — SEE DRUG DEPENDENCE SYNDROME

COMMUNITY STANDARD

This is the body of prevailing medical knowledge and acceptable methods of medical practice. It is considered on a nationwide basis.

---

* The source for this is *Drug Facts and Comparisons*, J.B. Lippencott, Philadelphia, 1991, pp. 994–995.
** With short-acting narcotics maximizes at 36–72 hours and continues to 5–10 days.

COMPLIANCE

1. Taking medications according to directions
2. Calling to clarify questions about dosing of controlled substance
3. Reporting medication side effects promptly
4. Not sharing medications with others
5. Demonstrating no drug-seeking behavior
6. Demonstrating no unsanctioned use of medication
7. Demonstrating only situational dose escalation with return to steady-state levels after the situation has passed

CONTROLLED SUBSTANCE

A controlled substance is any medication or substance that is "scheduled" (rated), according to abuse liability, by the U.S. Department of Justice. These substances can only be prescribed by specialists who are licensed to practice in the fields of medicine, dentistry, and podiatry. Actual controlled substance prescribing privileges are granted by issuance of a special numbered certificate by the Department of Justice. Some examples of schedule III medications are Tylenol® and codeine, Fiorinal® with codeine, Valium®, and Vicodin®. Some examples of schedule II medications are morphine, Percodan®, Dilaudid®, and Demerol®.

INTRACTABLE PAIN

As used here, intractable pain means a pain state in which the cause of the pain cannot be removed or otherwise treated. In the generally accepted course of medical practice, no relief or cure of the cause of the pain is possible or none has been found after reasonable efforts to do so. "Reasonable efforts" include, but are not limited to, evaluation by the attending physician and one or more physicians specializing in the treatment of the area, system, or organ of the body perceived to be the source of pain.

OPIOID

Opioids include any of the synthetic or natural medications that are commonly used for the management of pain symptoms. These are also commonly called narcotics. The term refers to morphine, codeine, Dilaudid®, Levo-Dromoran®, methadone, Demerol®, Percodan®, Percocet®, Vicodin®, Lorcet 10®, and many other medications.

PHYSIOLOGICAL

Most chronic pain patients can stop taking a controlled substance abruptly and not suffer any consequence. However, a small number of chronic pain patients will, after being on a controlled substance for a number of weeks or months, develop physiological dependence.

In this condition, the medication or drug actually replaces (or alters) vital chemical substances and/or neurotransmitters that are normal to the body. Therefore, the medication becomes an integral part of the body's normal physiology (all the processes that are vital and normal to the body's day-to-day functioning) while the medication is being used. When this type of patient abruptly stops taking the medication, a mild form of the abstinence syndrome occurs. Whereas this event is common in persons with drug dependence syndrome, it is rare and very mild in chronic pain patients taking medications for therapeutic purposes.

This is also true for some chronic pain patients who may be taking a therapeutic dose of a medication such as 10–20 mg of Valium® per day or three to four Tylenol® and codeine tablets per day. After suddenly stopping the medication, they may experience mild chills, mild "shakes" and nervousness, and a flare-up of the pain that was suppressed by the narcotic and/or narcotic-containing analgesic they were taking. They do not experience the typical drug dependence syndrome abstinence symptoms of craving the drug, recidivism, convulsions, flushing, fast heart rate, fever, nausea, vomiting and retching, intestinal spasm, spontaneous orgasm, and other characteristic occurrences once the medication is stopped.

If mild abstinence symptoms occur in a chronic pain patient after stopping the use of an analgesic, tranquilizer, or muscle relaxer, this can be remedied by the use of a short tapering of the drug. The formula to use is take one-half the medication dosage for 4 days, half of that dose (one-fourth the original dose) for the next 4 days, half of that dose (one-eighth of the original dose) for 4 days, and then stop.

This problem does not signal that the chronic pain patient was a "drug addict," but merely that the patient had physiological dependence and because of that needed to be tapered off the medication instead of being acutely withdrawn from it.

TOLERANCE IN OPIOID-RELATED EUPHORIA

In narcotics, tolerance to the euphorigenic effects develops faster than any other type of tolerance and may result in progressive escalation of the amount consumed to obtain the same euphoric effect.

This should not be confused with the chronic pain patient's legitimate need for increased dosing of pain medication when a pain flare-up occurs or as the pain problem becomes progressively more severe with the passage of time.

28 Acetaminophen and Hydrocodone Levels in Chronic Pain Patients

Harvey Rose, M.D.

OBJECTIVE

The purpose of this report is to measure serum levels in patients with chronic nonmalignant pain requiring larger than the usual doses of a combination of acetaminophen and hydrocodone. Serum levels were measured in these patients from 1.5 to 2.5 hours following ingestion of the dose of acetaminophen and hydrocodone that they were taking for pain relief.

The setting was the office of a solo family practitioner, and bloods were drawn by that practitioner in the office. All patients had their blood drawn following ingestion of the medicine within 1.5–2.5 hours after ingestion, except patient #1, whose first two bloods were drawn at random without the patient being aware that it was being done. The other specimens were drawn after the determined time.

The main outcome showed that the serum levels of acetaminophen and hydrocodone do not necessarily follow the amount of medication ingested. Each patient is individual, and the pharmacokinetic/pharmacodynamic uniqueness of each person seems to determine the amount of medication that is actually in the serum following ingestion.

RESULTS

The data show that the amount of acetaminophen, even when large doses were taken, did not exceed the reference lab level; the amount of hydrocodone did exceed reference lab levels in a few patients.

CONCLUSIONS

In patients who require larger than usual doses of acetaminophen and hydrocodone, it is important to obtain serum levels to be sure that toxic levels of acetaminophen do not occur and also to make sure that the patient is taking the medicine and is achieving a serum level that may ensure some analgesic effect. Also, in the current regulatory climate, it is important

1-57444-103-5/99/$0.00+$.50
© 1999 by CRC Press LLC

to show that large doses do not produce dangerous serum levels in patients who require these medications over a long period of time.

Some patients who are given chronic opioid therapy for nonmalignant pain appear to require larger than the usual amounts of these medications to lessen pain and improve functioning. This situation often raises concern about tolerance and dependency or addiction and greatly increases the discomfort of the physician, who may fear charges of excessive prescribing when the amount or duration of therapy exceeds some ill-defined "norm" or "community standard."

In an effort to evaluate factors that may lead to this apparent need for relatively high doses, I recently measured serum drug concentrations in patients requiring higher than usual doses of a combination product containing 500 mg acetaminophen (A) and 5 mg hydrocodone (H). These patients have all been successfully managed for long periods (up to 20 years) without any physical or laboratory evidence of hepatic or renal toxicity.

My major concern in looking at these levels was related to the potential toxicity of A, for there is no long-term toxicity associated with H. All patients received consultations regarding their problems to comply with California's new Intractable Pain Treatment Act (1990).

Patient #1 in Table 28.1 is considered an index case. She was on five A-H tablets a day, in addition to large doses of nonsteroidal anti-inflammatory drugs and intermittent trigger point injections. She felt that the A-H gave only slight pain relief. Random blood levels showed no detection of H and low levels of A. Because she was taking generic A-H, she was given a brand name and the same results were found. With three A-H tablets taken at once, she had significant pain relief and was more mobile; nevertheless, her blood levels for A-H were in the very low reference range (blood was drawn 2.5 hours postingestion of A-H).

Patient #3 has a strong family history of migraine and has had cluster-type headaches for 30 years. Various alternative therapies have been tried unsuccessfully. Brain scans have been negative. She does achieve partial pain control with steady 20–25 A-H per day. She has occasional severe exacerbations which have been controlled with a combination of intravenous steroids, DHE 45, narcotic agonist/antagonist (despite chronic hydrocodone use), and prochlorperazine.

Patient #7 has a similar family history. She has occasional acute exacerbations that respond to increased A-H use and also intramuscular promazine, prochlorperazine, or methotrimeprazine.

Serum concentrations of A-H were measured 1.5–2.5 hours after ingestion in nine patients by a special commercial lab. Most patients were in a steady state, except for patient #1 who was given the three A-H tablets after no detection at lower doses. As seen in Table 28.1, the blood levels of A-H were lower than would be expected. The concentration of A never exceeded the reference lab range. The H levels did significantly exceed the reference levels in three cases, but considering the amounts taken by patient #5 and patient #7, it was less than would be expected.

Thus, a "standard" or "usual" dose of A-H does not guarantee an adequate serum concentration. Whether these reference lab levels correspond to therapeutic levels is not known at this time and requires further research. The cause of these individual variations is unknown, but could reflect intestinal malabsorption or abnormal liver metabolism. The latter has been described with codeine, which is less efficiently demethylated to morphine in about 10% of Caucasians (Mikus et al., 1991). These poor metabolizers would probably not attain pain relief from usual analgesic doses of codeine. Other opioids including hydrocodone have not been widely studied.

The potential value of therapeutic monitoring is well recognized for many medications, including anticonvulsants, amitriptyline, digoxin, lithium, and others. There has been limited use of this technique for opioids, however. A blood level of 150–600 ng/ml has been found

TABLE 28.1   Patient Data

Test date	Diagnosis	A-H dose	Tabs/day	Current years/ current/ dose	Total years on opiate	Drawn 1.5–2.5 hours postinjection A level[a] (5–30 µg/ml)	H level[a] (17–36 ng/ml)
Patient #1	Age 52/female						
04-19/91	Fibromyalgia	1	5	5	9	3	None det
05-22-91		1	5	5		3	None det
06-24-91		1	5			1	Note det
08-08-91		3	10–12	0.5		5	16
Patient #2	Age 74/female						
07-23-91	Fibromyalgia, degenerative discs	3	8–14	0.5	6	10	36
Patient #3	Age 48/female						
11-01-90	Chronic cluster	3	20–25	2	9	15	38
04-24-91	headaches	3	20–25			19	Not done
Patient #4	Age 58/female						
08-13-91	Old spine compression fracture with anterior fusion	3	14	2	7	14	41
Patient #5	Age 51/male						
09-08-91	Chronic cluster headaches, recent RA	7	15–20	1	20	12	74
Patient #6	Age 79/female						
09-15-91	Osteoarthritis and osteoporosis, prior disc surgery	3	12	1	13	9	64
Patient #7	Age 45/female						
11-09-91	Chronic mixed	4	20–25	4	15	12	58
11-17-91	headaches	4[a,b]				28	43
Patient #8	Age 66/female						
10-02-91	Multi neck fusions	3	10–12	0.5	10	9	17
Patient #9	Age 45/female						
10-28-91	Chronic mixed headaches, controlled paranoid schizophrenia	3	15	1/3	4	17	37

[a] Tests done by National Medical Services, Willow Grove, PA. Levels obtained were 1.5 hours after ingestion of 1000 mg acetaminophen and 10 mg hydrocodone.

[b] See patient #7. Also took, 3 hours prior to blood drawn, three tablets of a combination product containing butalbital (50 mg), acetaminophen (500 mg), and caffeine (40 mg).

necessary to prevent recidivism in methadone maintenance patients (Dole, 1988). A study of some chronic pain patients demonstrated that hydromorphone concentrations of more than 4 ng/ml were required for pain control (Reidenberg et al., 1988). The latter study identified some patients where hydromorphone concentrations were low even at high doses, and the authors concluded that the wide variation in pharmacokinetics probably adds to reports of poor analgesic control in chronic cancer pain using opioids. This observation has been made by others (Tennant et al., 1988). These findings are consistent with the large pharmacokinetic/pharmacodynamic variability observed in numerous studies of short-term opioid administration for acute painful conditions.

An interesting study done in Germany measured the response to various painful stimuli in patients with asymptomatic silent myocardial ischemia. By subjecting normal angina patients and silent ischemia patients to painful stimuli (i.e., electrical shocks, cold pressor tests, and tourniquet pain tests), they found that patients with silent ischemia tolerated these painful stimuli better than people with angina. They concluded that individual differences in sensibility to pain may partly explain lack of anginal pain in patients with silent ischemia (Droste and Roskamm, 1983).

This pharmacokinetic/pharmacodynamic variability observed in patients suggests that large doses of combination opioid and nonopioid analgesics may be both safe and necessary in some patients. It further contradicts the conclusion that patients are "addicted" merely by virtue of large doses or long duration. None of these patients described here has shown any desire for continued dose escalation or demonstrated any dysfunctional, addictive behavior or any harm in taking these medications. I prefer to call these patients "therapeutically dependent," for the medications have improved their quality of life (Rinaldi et al., 1988). Quality of life, not quantity of "pills," should be paramount in chronic pain management. Many physicians avoid such patients and such high doses, not so much for fear of addiction but rather for fear of the response by overzealous and misguided regulatory and licensing agencies.

It is my belief that this approach is appropriate as long as other reasonable and affordable methods of pain management have not succeeded and the patient shows pain relief and/or improved functioning without continued dose escalation or addictive behavior (Clark, 1988; Texas Intractable Pain Treatment Act, 1989; California Intractable Pain Treatment Act, 1990; Sacramento–El Dorado County Medical Society, 1990). In addition to close clinical monitoring of such patients, physicians may wish to consider the use of serum concentration measurements, which may provide reassuring information to all concerned: the patient, the physician, and the police.

BIBLIOGRAPHY

California Intractable Pain Treatment Act (1990). Business and Professions Code Section 2241.5.
Clark, H.W. (1988). Chronic pain and the chemical dependency specialist, *California Society for the Treatment of Alcoholism and Other Drug Dependencies News,* 15(1), 1–12.
Dole, V.P. (1988). Implications of methadone maintenance for theories of narcotic addiction, *Journal of the American Medical Association,* 260, 3025–3029.
Droste, C. and Roskamm, H. (1983). Experimental pain measurement in patients with asymptomatic myocardial ischemia, *Journal of the American College of Cardiology,* 1(3), 940–945.
Mikus, G., Somoqyi, A., Bochner, F., and Chen, Z.R. (1991). Polymorphic metabolism of opioid narcotic drugs: possible clinical implications, *Annals Academy of Medicine, Singapore,* 20, 9–12.
Reidenberg, M., Goodman H., Erle, H., et al. (1983). Hydromorphone levels and pain control in patients with severe chronic pain, *Clinical Pharmacology and Therapeutics,* 44, 376–382.
Rinaldi, R., Standler, E., Wilford, B., and Goodwin, D. (1988). Clarification and standardization of substance abuse terminology, *Journal of the American Medical Association,* 259, 555–557.
Sacramento–El Dorado County Medical Society (1990). The Painful Dilemma: The Use of Narcotics for the Treatment of Chronic Pain, November 1990.
Tennant, F., Robinson, D., Sagherian, A., and Seecof, R. (1988). Chronic opioid treatment of intractable non-malignant pain, *Pain Management,* 1(1), 18–26.
Texas Intractable Pain Treatment Act (1989).

Section VI

Miscellaneous

29 The Anesthesiologist's Role in a Pain Clinic

Joseph Lee, M.D.
Richard Weiner, Ph.D.

Chronic pain is often frustrating to patients, their families, and the therapists who attempt to treat them. Chronic pain is a big problem in the United States. It has become an epidemic. An estimated 35–40 million Americans have chronic pain problems, and this includes arthritics, patients with migraine headaches, and people with pain in the neck and low back.

These patients can be very demanding and often present problems that appear very complex and baffling to the physician. A young internist at a local hospital recently made the following statement: "I've been well trained and feel comfortable in diagnosing and treating acute health care problems. However, I have had no training in understanding chronic pain. No matter what I do they never seem to get better."

Although attitudes among the public and medical community are changing, it is still not uncommon to hear someone say that the most chronic pain patients are "crocks," "fakers," or "malingerers" trying to get out of work or make a fast buck. This attitude was expressed by a neurosurgeon who said: "I never accept those patients (chronic pain patients). When they call here I have my receptionist refer them elsewhere. The problem is, I never know when to believe them."

THE MULTIDISCIPLINARY PAIN CLINIC

Fortunately, new service delivery methods have been developed in the war against chronic pain. The multidisciplinary pain clinic (MPC) offers new hope to chronic pain patients and can be a community resource to the physicians who are trying to help them. The MPC utilizes a team concept that brings together numerous medical and clinical specialists who share a common goal of alleviating the chronic pain patient's pain, dysfunction, and suffering.

The anesthesiologist is an integral part of the MPC team. Many of the programs active in the treatment of chronic pain patients fall under the auspices of departments of anesthesia at major universities. Anesthesiologists are best known for their work in the operating room. They are the physicians who "put the patient to sleep" while the surgeon operates on them. Many anesthesiologists have training in the administration of spinal injections, nerve blocks (deadening nerves), injections into trigger points (painful areas in the muscles), and the intravenous (by vein) administration of numerous pain-relieving drugs. They may also be called upon to administer intravenous medications while another physician member of the team manipulates a stuck or painful joint. Their skills are employed by the MPC to evaluate the patient's need for medications ranging from local anesthetics to potent narcotic pain-relieving drugs.

SPINAL INJECTIONS

Spinal injections are administered by the anesthesiologist into the area of the spinal fluid (deep in the spinal area) or into the epidural space (a large space that surrounds the spinal cord from the base of the skull to the lower tip of the spine). He or she may inject one or more local anesthetics plus cortisone to relieve pain. Sometimes spinal injections are used to find out where the patient's pain is coming from. A therapeutic epidural block can be done in the neck, thoracic spine, low back, and/or sacral area, depending on the location of the pain.

EPIDURAL BLOCKS

Therapeutic lumbar epidural blocks are useful in the treatment of painful scarring that forms in the low back after surgery. Surgery on the back for disc disease, bony slippage, or spinal fusion sometimes leaves a scar around the epidural space which can irritate numerous spinal nerves as they travel through this space on their way out of the spine and down the leg. Sometimes the surgery leaves a severe inflammation called arachnoiditis (inflammation of the lining of the spinal cord) which is sometimes benefited by injection of cortisone into the epidural space. One of the newer techniques of epidural injection involves the use of morphine and cortisone in the epidural space for the relief of low back and leg pain.

ARM AND LEG PAIN

Arm and leg pain is sometimes caused by inadequate circulation to the extremities. Sometimes blocking the nerves that control circulation (sympathetic nerves) in the neck or low back with local anesthetic can open up the circulation to the arm and/or leg on the painful side.

CASE REPORTS

John P. was a 40-year-old Vietnam veteran who had injured his back while lifting a heavy object. He underwent two back surgeries with only transient relief. Because of his persisting pain and disability, he became progressively more depressed and gained 110 pounds. Family problems and suicide threats occurred as the problems worsened. He eventually had to be admitted to the psychiatric unit of a hospital. While in the hospital, he was seen by the pain clinic anesthesiologist, who felt that he had arachnoiditis. The anesthesiologist treated him with trigger point injections to the muscles of his low back, followed by a therapeutic lumbar epidural injection of local anesthetic and cortisone. His pain was dramatically improved by these injections, and with that stress decreased, he was better able to cooperate with his psychiatric rehabilitation. Since that time, it has also been possible for him to better manage his pain and depression problems. His family and social problems have improved, and he has been able to lose 50 pounds.

Karen F. was a 26-year-old woman who slipped at work and injured her back. When first seen at the pain clinic, she reported pain in the back which was also radiating down her leg.

After evaluation, it was felt that she had a slipped disc; however X-ray examination did not confirm that. She then had an examination of some of the deeper muscles in her buttock via a vaginal exam. An area of tenderness was located in her pyriformis muscle (in the middle of the buttock and deep inside). The tender muscle was injected by the anesthesiologist, using local anesthetic and cortisone, and her relief was immediate and permanent.

CONCLUSION

In order to reduce the intensity, frequency, duration, and frustration of pain experienced by many chronic pain patients, the MPC can be utilized as a readily available community medical resource for patients and physicians alike. The MPC may draw upon anesthesiology. There are certain problems which respond well to the kind of medication which is given by the anesthesiologist. You might ask your treating physician if he or she has considered a consultation with an anesthesiologist, or if not, why not.

30 My Story: Chronic Pain and How to Keep Your Friends

Ruth Fields

In November of 1976, while Jimmy Carter was being elected president, my husband and I were on vacation at Mikaha Beach, Oahu, Hawaii. We went there from the island of Kauai to see the world-championship board surfers. It was fun sitting on the beach watching those experts handle the waves.

The waves were unpredictable, constantly changing, and the force of the surf frightened me too much to go in myself. A couple of men were body surfing, and after a while my husband decided to join them. "Come on, honey, come on in," my husband kept calling. Reluctantly, I finally succumbed. What fun it was. Inexperienced as I was at body surfing, I tried to practice the little I knew to handle the waves. Before I knew it, a wave that looked as big as a mountain was coming at me. Frightened, I then ducked under the wave so low that I scraped my belly on the sand at the bottom. After the wave went over me, I stood up only to find a huge sister wave, just as mammoth and ferocious as the first one, coming toward me. I looked away toward the beach and saw that the first wave had not died down but instead had slammed into the beach with such force that it created an even bigger wave coming at me from the beach. There I was, caught between two enormous waves coming toward me from opposite directions. Not knowing which wave to duck under, I stood there and got hit by both waves at the same time. The force of the impact was so strong that I was thrown high up into the air in a somersault and landed hard on my back on the hard wet sand. I screamed, "My back, my back!"

Later the pain subsided and I thought I was alright. I was left with a "kink" in my back. There was pain only after bending forward for a few minutes.

When I returned home, my chiropractor checked me and told me no damage was done. He encouraged me to continue my very active lifestyle. I continued to manage my home, be a part-time chaplain at Juvenile Hall, play golf three times a week, swim 100 laps in the pool daily year round, and walk 40–60 minutes a day as rapidly as I could.

Ten months after the accident, after an extremely active weekend in Palm Springs, I awoke with horrible pain in my buttocks radiating down both legs to my heels. I thought, "Could this be happening to me?" My chiropractor tried to relieve my suffering to no avail. I could not sit, could not roll over on my side in bed, and could stand only for a few minutes. My buttocks felt like I was being gored by a bull, piercing me unrelentingly.

Thus began my sorrowful saga going from doctor to doctor, to chiropractor after chiropractor, and to physiotherapist after physiotherapist. I was in Stanford Hospital, U.C. Hospital, and also in emergency at Valley Medical Hospital. I even went to the Philippines to seek psychic healing, even though it was against my faith. Desperately, I even went to world-renowned doctors in Boston. My brother, who is also a doctor, could not help me. How helpless he felt, as did my family and friends. I was even required to seek psychological help with different therapists. I felt betrayed by God, as my total life was dedicated to him.

The night before my accident, my husband and I spoke before parishioners at the Lihuie Assembly of God Church in Kauai. We also had picked up a hitchhiker in Kauai a few days earlier, who was a Sephardic Jew, and had the joy of introducing him to our beloved Lord, Jesus Christ. We also had sent hundreds of dollars to feed the hungry just before leaving on our trip. How could my loving Lord leave me in such a destitute condition? My faith was being tested. I searched through the scriptures to find out how a loving God could allow me, his child, to suffer so much. Lots of friends came to see me and judged my walk with God while I was flat on my back in agony, which was and is to this day my only safe position. I am in intractable, severe, disabling cruel pain in most of my body from the waist down.

ABANDONMENT OF FRIENDS AND FAMILY

One by one, most of my friends either judged me (as a sinner) or abandoned me. The loneliness and despair caused much depression, and often I would entertain thoughts of suicide.

At the time of the accident, I was happily married and living with my husband, Bruce, and the youngest of my three children. Adam, age 8 years, was the only child remaining at home. In the beginning, Bruce would come home expecting a clean house, dinner, and a cheerful wife. Instead, he came home to me, a women on her back, desperately seeking help, compassion, understanding, and, above all, pain relief. After seeking help from a minister, in a few weeks my husband changed and understood my sorrowful plight with the tenderness, love, and understanding for which I had hoped. Adam had also begun to understand my position. Nevertheless, my suffering produced much suffering in both Bruce and Adam, and sometimes one or all three of us would end up sobbing.

At this time, I could not sit; I could only lay on my back. I could not stand or walk more than a minute or two at a time. During this time, several friends, who had previously professed to love me, accused me of either lack of faith, underlying emotional problems, or having deep-rooted marital problems which were the cause of my back pain. These were the people who were the first to abandon me, and good riddance! Other friends felt so helpless that they avoided me because my situation was so depressing. Even the neighbors that I was close to did not come to see me, except for one who once brought a casserole for our dinner. This abandonment often depressed me even more than the pain in my body; the hurt was horrible.

One friend did stick by me, primarily with phone calls only. She and her husband had their own travel agency. She was frequently traveling all over the world on gala holidays. Somehow it was easier to travel abroad than coming to visit or help me. She would call me and go on and on about the inconveniences she was "suffering" while traveling. These "inconveniences" were so petty to me and so inappropriate with all that I was going through that she was the only friend that I avoided. Her inappropriate conversation included agonizing over being stuck in New York with a tux and evening gown, and having to lug them to Europe or ship them back to California. In the meantime, I was agonizing over torturous pain, which doctor to go to, and friends and relatives disappearing out of my life. The whole thing was ludicrous and I felt like a victim. Eventually I forgave her and have since restored our relationship. This was several years later, after I got somewhat better.

My stepdaughter, Kyla, was the only one who cooked and helped us when she occasionally visited. My son and daughter-in-law at that time were busy with his chiropractic education, raising a family of three children, and making a living. However, a phone call from them gave me some needed emotional support.

At Adam's school, they had an extra little Christmas tree and Adam asked if he could have it for his Mom. He hauled it home, put it on a table in the corner of my bedroom, and proceeded to decorate it for me with all his heart. He wanted so much to make me happy, and he did.

An old Bible study leader, who was never a close friend before, helped me occasionally with errands or buying school clothes for Adam, which I really appreciated.

In spite of all the efforts of my doctors, I spiraled downward until I was completely bedridden, on my back only, in 1980. There I remained for the next 5 years until such time as I was taken to Denver, Colorado, for spinal implant surgery and then to a rehabilitation hospital. An ambulance took me to San Francisco and then I was put on a gurney on the plane, still on my belly. Another ambulance met me at the Denver airport and took me to Swedish Hospital, still an my stomach. What a trip!

I went to Denver one person and returned another person, due to the surgeries, teaching, and encouragement I received through the efforts of Dr. Jay Law, who did the spinal implant surgery, and Spalding Rehabilitation Hospital. To show you how bad my condition was, I was taken all the way to Denver on my stomach. I could tolerate no other position as I was on no pain medication. Dr. Law wanted me off all drugs in order to determine where to position the spinal implant according to my true pain pattern.

Needless to say, I was a sorry sight when I met Dr. Jay Law — I was a totally atrophied desperate woman, all skin and bones, weighing only 95 pounds. He had his psychologist examine me to be certain that my problem was strictly physical. She was very understanding. Dr. Law performed two surgeries.

My first surgery was performed while I was on my stomach. I was covered with heavy pads in an operating room while being fluoroscoped. It was necessary for Dr. Law to see where he was going in my spine. Lying on my stomach, I looked into a computer which was set up for me to punch as Dr. Law instructed during the surgery. Here he was putting needles into my spine with only local anesthetic, and some of those needles went where there was no anesthesia. I tried to be very brave and not react. I was so thankful that he opted to do the surgery, I didn't make a peep. Believe me, a few times I really could have yelled. Nevertheless, the surgery went well. After a severe accident in the hospital in which I sprained both hips severely, I worked with Dr. Law on the computerized spinal stimulator for 3 weeks. The second operation was performed successfully. Fully equipped with my new stimulator implant, I was sent to Spalding Rehabilitation Hospital for 3 more weeks.

HOW TO KEEP YOUR FRIENDS

For most of us, chronic pain is tough. All our lives, whenever we became sick we were treated or the body healed itself and we eventually got well. Now we find ourselves in chronic pain, often with intractable unrelenting severity, and after 1, 2, 10, or even 20 years we are still stuck with our suffering. Well, what about the rest of our lives, especially our friends and relatives? They bring the casseroles, flowers, get-well cards, and good wishes and then, when we don't get better, little by little, they disappear from our lives. The phone calls get farther and farther apart, as do the visits, and eventually we find ourselves desperately lonely, hurt, depressed, and abandoned. We lose our self-esteem, think we have done something wrong, and feel angry and depressed.

How can people be so uncaring? What is this world coming to? This abandonment coupled with our pain makes us often feel like giving up. Sometimes we wish we were dead. We "veg" out in front of the tube for company, but it isn't like a warm hug, a friendly smile, and someone caring.

We sink into self-pity. The whole thing is a downward spiral. Are you in this downward spiral, my suffering friend?

There is a way up and out of the pit. After 11 years of pain, 2 pain centers, and 63 doctors, physiotherapists, and chiropractors, I have learned how to live a joyful and victorious life, though in severe pain.

To begin with, the greatest strengthener of my life is the Lord Jesus Christ, and he is the greatest attitude changer, too. I have found in life that I cannot change others or the world, but I can change me. If you are willing to make these healthy changes, I can assure you that you will have all the friends you can handle.

1. First, commit to change.
2. You must make a decision to put all thoughts of pain on the back burner of your mind and leave them there as much as possible. "What?" you say, "This is impossible. She's crazy." No, just as an athlete must practice over and over to be perfect, we must discipline our minds to ignore the pain as much as possible to have a happy life. At first, it was like mental gymnastics, and I would time myself as to how long I could go without consciously thinking of pain. My first try lasted 5 minutes, then 15; it kept extending longer and longer. I had talked to an old man at a pain center and asked him how to do it. He simply said, "Just keep putting the pain thoughts on the back burner, and if they come forward, just put them back again and again." Ignore the pain message as best as you can. This is deliberate denial or, as I call it, selective perception. You select where you want your mind to go. You can do it. Others have done it. I have done it, and so can you. Tell friends and family not to discuss pain unless you bring it up and only briefly unless you need to work through a problem or decision with them.
3. Choose joy. Give up all the self-pity. Do not nurse thoughts of self-pity. Do not look for sympathy or discuss your last surgery or failure to get well. My past sufferings and present are my own "Vietnam." What joy is there in reliving any of it? Give it up! Who really cares or truly understands what you have gone through and are currently going through? Reliving your suffering is nonproductive for you and those around you. My favorite scripture from the Bible which helped me the most is Philippians 4:6-8: "Don't worry about anything, but in all your prayers ask God for what you need, always thanking him with a thankful heart. And God's peace, which is far beyond human understanding, will keep your hearts and minds safe in union with Christ Jesus. In conclusion, my brothers, fill your minds with those things that are good and that deserve praise: things that are true, noble, right, pure, lovely, and honorable." When in a fix, Philippians 4:6-8. You can train yourself to live Philippians 4:6-8. Write it on notes with a thick marking pen. Put it on your mirror, refrigerator, doors, and cabinets. Learn it and live it. The Bible says we shall be transformed by the renewing of our minds. As you keep giving your troubles back to God in prayer, mental and emotional relief will come. As you think of good things and talk of only good things, joy will begin to come. As we appreciate the good in our lives, we get happy. Good is there if you are willing to look. This

includes "Happy Talk" (from the musical "South Pacific"). Keep talking "Happy Talk."

4. Forgive family, friends, neighbors, doctors, and therapists who have hurt you mentally or physically, ignored you, shunned you, or misunderstood you. To err is human; to forgive, divine. Jesus on the cross (while uncaring men cast lots for his clothes) in agonizing torturous pain and dying said, "Forgive them Father, for they know not what they do." Not only forgive, but forget.

5. Assuming you have been through steps 1 to 4 and made a choice to implement these attitude changes, you are then ready to woo your friends and family back. When we are in severe pain, we tend to keep more to ourselves and not reach out to others. Our hope is that others will reach out to us. For most of us, this has not been the case. Even though you are still in severe pain, on your best of days I suggest you call your friends or relatives and find out how they are getting along. This assumes that you have already committed to putting your pain on the "back burner" of your mind. Listen to their hearts and hurts and give them your attention, affirmation, compassion, and understanding. Then, when your friends and relatives question you about your life, give them a brief report on how you are, minus self-pity. Remember to keep it brief. Now change the subject and get onto something else. Be sure to ask questions about your friends' and relatives' lives and circumstances and also to contribute anything newsy that you may have to offer. The point is, my fellow sufferers, to give your companion enough interest to keep their friendship and also to learn to consider others first and forget your pain by forgetting yourself. This may seem strange at first, because you probably would like to scream from the rooftop, "I hurt like hell. Doesn't anyone really care?" Yes, people care; however, they are helpless as to what to do or how to relate to you with your pain problem. Our society as a whole does not prepare people to deal with chronic illness or anything out of the ordinary. We cannot change our society, but we can change our own prison of loneliness and our own attitudes. For me personally, I needed the help of a loving God to achieve this.

Another thing to do to get your friends and relatives back is to extend invitations. If you are capable of getting out of the house, then perhaps you would like to invite a friend to lunch at a restaurant. If your friends are working, try to get together at night or on the weekends. Tell your friends how long you are capable of being up, sitting, etc. according to your individual condition. Otherwise they will wonder if you are still ill or if they might be causing you to overextend yourself. Try to be honest and up front and let them know your capabilities and limitations. Remember, you are doing this in a matter-of-fact, informative fashion without causing your companion discomfort or looking for sympathy. Let your friends know how special they are and how much they mean to you.

If you are shut in, ask a friend over for lunch. If you can put a lunch together, do it. If you cannot, then perhaps you could ask your friend to pick up a take-out lunch from a fast-food restaurant, Chinese food restaurant, health food store, or even the grocery store. This worked quite well for me once I got over the self-consciousness of asking. I learned to listen to my friends and ask questions to really get into what their activities were and what was going on in their lives. In all honesty, I was never this good a listener before my pain problem, and I can honestly thank my pain for teaching me how to really listen, to be happy, and much more. Like my husband says, "Out of the mud comes the lotus." In other words, out of my suffering came some beautiful growth. We either get bitter or better with suffering. I first got bitter toward God, my friends and relatives who let me down, doctors who caused me added horrendous pain and didn't get me better, and even the one doctor whose treatment made me much worse.

However, with God's help, I learned to turn it around, get rid of my hurts emotionally, forgive everyone, and make the most of every day. Every morning I would say, "This is the day the Lord hath made, I will rejoice and be glad in it." I learned to seize the day and make the best of it. This was not easy, especially being bedridden on my back for 5 years. The pain was so intolerable that I couldn't even walk down the hall to the kitchen to fix a sandwich. My husband fixed lunch for me before going to work and left it by my bed. A telephone, radio, and television kept me in contact with the outside world. Rarely did I go to the door during those years. The 62 doctors I had been to exhausted all their ideas to help me. I even needed to use a bedpan a third of the time. Sometimes it would spill or no one was home to empty it. After a long day all alone, I'd have a bedpan full of urine. I hated the stench of lying in my own urine or having to ask someone to empty it.

The loneliness and despair forced me to learn how to forget myself by helping others, and I tried to minister to the needs of my family, counseling them over the phone and praying for people as best I could. However, I still needed friends badly. Little by little, I learned that people couldn't handle my suffering. It made them feel helpless and depressed. Even though it was honestly the way I felt, people would call less and less or not at all. I had no one to counsel me on how to handle this. It was a cousin in Boston who suggested I call people for lunch and stop discussing my problem as much as possible. My husband really appreciated my effort to put away "pain talk" as much as possible. As you may have already discovered, chronic pain is a mystery, a bore, and a frustration to most people and most physicians.

Now on to the lighter side: How about asking people if they know any good jokes? The response will shift the conversation to the lighter side of life. Try to memorize one or two of these jokes; write them down and try them out on your spouse. You may want to use a little notebook to jot down your friends' or family's needs, interesting jokes, dates they are leaving town, etc. Our memory on pain medication can play tricks on us or fade, and you need to remember, so keep notes or a journal and review it every few days. Use a large calendar to write important appointments, events, and daily notes not only for yourself but concerning important dates reminding you of your friends' vacations, where they are going, operations, etc.

What I am going to tell you right now is very important and is the basis for your winning your friends back, making new friends, and keeping them all. "Whatsoever thou sowest also shalt thou reap." In other words, you "reap what you sow." If a farmer plants corn, what will he reap at harvest time? Corn, of course. If a farmer plants wheat, what will he reap at harvest time? That's right, wheat. If you give, or should I say plant, seeds of love, goodness, and generosity, what will you reap at harvest time? "Give and it shall be given unto you." Just keep giving and this great universal law will see to it that you receive in return. Don't worry about receiving. It will just happen. Remember that "inch by inch makes anything a cinch." It takes time.

When the farmer plants his seeds, he then has to water, fertilize, weed, and wait. God makes the increase. Then, eventually, the farmer sees a little sprout peeking through the soil. The sprout continues to get bigger and bigger and eventually there is a harvest. Your harvest is when your friends or relatives come back into your life and stay there. Since every seed does not sprout, every loved one will not respond. Some people refuse to be around sick people, period. Accept that and just enjoy the ones who return.

If you can find a good support group or at least one other person in pain who you can relate to, this would be ideal to fill your need to freely discuss your pain, sorrow, doctor, medication, or to just get your true feelings out in a climate of total acceptance, love, and understanding. After 10 years of pain, I have found such a friend. We talk every day. We are love therapy for one another and have developed a true friendship. This friendship came about by using the methods I have mentioned. In the beginning, I gave the love and compassion primarily and my seeds sprouted, and I have had a joyous relationship with this person since my harvest came in. She has returned all I gave and more. It can be done. Now, it's your turn. I challenge you to choose love instead of sorrow. Plant your seeds of love and goodness and have a great life starting today. Seize the day!

If you have needs that your friends and relatives could possibly be filling, you may want to use the following sample letter.

To my friends, relatives, and neighbors:

I know my illness has put a strain on some of you. You may have feelings of frustration, helplessness, compassion, sympathy, anger, or sorrow. I have all of those feelings, too. Presently, I am attempting to make a better life for my family and myself; if you would like to help me, here is a list of the help I can use:

1. A telephone call once a week (Please share your life with me, too.)
2. Sheets changed once a week
3. Shopping or errands once a week
4. Play scrabble, cards, backgammon, etc. once a month or occasionally
5. Hot dish or casserole once a month or occasionally
6. Take Johnnie shopping for school clothes
7. Cut toenails once a month or give me a home permanent
8. Tell me jokes and funny stories
9. Cards and letters are nice
10. Carpool help
11. Hair washing once a week
12. Straighten bedroom (I am in too much discomfort to keep things neat)
13. Transportation to doctors (very important)
14. Laundry once a month
15. Most important — please stay in my life

The items listed above are only suggestions of ways you can help me if you choose. This in no way obligates you to help me, and I want that clearly understood. I realize you have your own personal responsibilities and problems. Know that I love you and appreciate you either way. Just a phone call showing that you care can make my day.

Lovingly,

The above is a suggested list only. Make your own list tailored to your own needs. Use your own discretion to determine which friends should receive your letter and list. Don't be afraid. Go for it. Great challenges make great heroes. There will be days when you are so flared up and are suffering so much pain that it would be ridiculous to even try any of these suggestions. Just use what you can when you can and leave the rest in Gods' hands.

FRIENDS

The way to have a friend is to be a friend. Here are some suggestions:

1. Ask friends not to discuss your pain or how you are feeling. Ask them to talk about things like what's new, what's happening, etc.

2. Appreciate your friends. Thank them for calling. Tell them how much they mean to you. Thank them for their thoughtfulness.

3. Send thank-you cards and friendship cards, both funny and sentimental. Have a few on hand and send them out as you feel led. Remember birthday gifts.

4. Ask friends to pick up take-out food and join you for a meal; insist on paying.

5. Don't just be a "taker." Too many sick people forget to continue to give. I have given and given to sick people, and they usually keep taking and taking and do not make any effort on my behalf. I am in pain and have needs, too. Healthy people have needs too, especially for appreciation and someone to be interested in them.

6. Become a good listener. Get into your visitor's life. Listen and ask questions to show you really care. Don't take the conversation back to you and your life all the time. As you become an active listener, many people will keep coming back for your kindness and interest. People in our society are so busy that they usually do not have time to listen. Many people go to therapists just to have someone to listen. You can be that kind of person.

7. Become a joke teller. Everyone loves a good joke and everyone loves to laugh.

8. Hug, touch, and make eye contact. Do it sincerely.

9. Be sympathetic to your friends' ills.

10. Play games, cards, computer games, checkers, backgammon, scrabble, Chinese checkers, etc.

11. If you are home most of the time because of your illness, let your friends know that you are there for them if they just need to talk.

12. Ask friends to tell you all about their vacations; ask if they took pictures, and ask to see them. Ask questions. Most people are happy to share if you only ask. Take an interest in others and they will take an interest in you.

13. Be honest about your loneliness. Most people have no idea what you are going through.

14. Plan outings with friends within your limitations. Tell them you might not be able to make it but will try. Personally, I let them know I am only 70% reliable because of my pain. Then, if I have to cancel, they are somewhat prepared and are understanding.

Ask your doctor to put you in touch with another pain patient or two. They can make wonderful friends because they usually understand. Just don't get entrapped with too much "downer" conversation. Make a pact to try to encourage and cheer one another up. If in depression now, wait until you are leveled off with antidepressant, therapy, etc. before approaching friends. They feel so helpless when we feel helpless. They just run from us.

HOW TO PACE YOURSELF

Pacing your activity and rest time is truly an art. If you are one of the people in chronic pain who can be up all day, this message is not for you. However, if you are like me, and need to regulate your activities and your rest times, then the following is very important for you.

Measure your pain level from 0 to 10, with 0 being no pain at all and 10 being the worst pain you have ever had (intolerable pain.) When you awaken, observe your pain level. Let's say, for example, you awaken with a 3 or 4 pain level and begin your daily routine. When your pain reaches a 6, stop and rest until it goes down one or two points. Then resume activity again until your pain reaches a 6 again. It is recommended that you repeat this off and on all day. This can be very difficult because it is normal to get involved in a given activity and want to keep going until it is finished. However, by using your awareness and self-control, you will begin to develop the art of pacing and have more "up time" at the end of the day than if you kept going until your pain reached an 8 to 10 level.

As you may already have discovered, once your pain level reaches 8 to 10, it is almost impossible to get it back down unless you sleep through the night. At that level, the depression comes on strong. Self-pity sets in, and you often wish you had never been born. Also, you must consider what it must be like for your loved ones to come home and find you in the agony of "killer" pain. Wouldn't your family appreciate finding you smiling and reasonably comfortable? How terrible it was before I knew how to pace myself. My poor husband and son would return home after a hard day out in the world and find me agonizing in tortuous pain, crying, and needing them to hold my hand and comfort me. It was a bummer for them to come home to this day after day and also for me. We must not only consider ourselves but also consider the lives of those around us, so try to pace yourself. It is very important, so please give it the attention it deserves and try to become a really good pacer.

To begin, you may want to follow your usual daily routine for one day and keep a record of your pain levels throughout the day and evening and also keep a record of your activity level. Then, the next day, observe your pain level when you awaken, record it, and pace yourself through the day and evening. Add up your time and record your pain levels. Also observe how much better you feel by the evening when the family comes home. Most pain patients are in severe pain by evening. If you are such a patient, persevere and become a good "pacer," and you will greatly reduce those torturous evenings. Remember, "inch by inch anything's a cinch."

As you incorporate pacing and other modalities into your life, the quality of your life will eventually greatly improve. The happiest people I know are people in chronic pain who, like me, are determined to make every day the best day of their lives. You can start this right now. Because I am suffering, I have made a decision to choose joy instead of self-pity, limited productivity instead of inactivity, and you can, too. I have also found that we have to be our own "cheerleaders." Expecting others to applaud your efforts and bravery can be disappointing. Healthy people usually do not know or understand what you are going through unless they themselves have gone through something similar. Remember that if you can find another chronic pain patient for a friend, this can be the best therapy you can have. Of course, you will want this other person in pain to be encouraging and as positive as possible. Otherwise you can end up with a "pity party."

For me personally, I prefer to give and receive helpful ways to "make it." For those who need to discuss their pain over and over and get their feelings of frustration out, finding a good support group may be the answer.

Try to spend more time on good ideas and encouragement than on complaining. You will be happier in the end.

Ask your doctor, pain specialist, chiropractor, or principal therapist if he or she will introduce you to another pain patient or group. It may prove to be helpful. You may want to share this pacing information and compare notes on how it worked. You get out of something according to what you put into it, so do try.

In any event, do the best you can and leave the rest to God. He loves you and will get you through.

RELAXATION

1. For reducing pain
2. For general well-being
3. For relieving stress

When we are in pain, the alarm system of our mind and body turns on automatically. We become anxious, our adrenaline level goes up, and in general we are stressed. We then have the normal response of trying to protect our hurting area and also trying to get relief. In chronic pain, the relief does not come, and we have to live with our systems still in somewhat of a state of alarm. How, then, do we cope? When the family is in chaos and feelings are hurt, your pain level goes up to a 10 (the worst pain you have ever had), and you wish you could just die. What should you do?

There are many ways to relax. Sedentary ways to relax include card games, computer games, soaking in a hot tub, smoking a cigarette, drinking an alcoholic beverage, making a phone call to a good friend, watching a ball game or other sports on television, etc. Activity can also be relaxing, such as swimming, walking, tennis, table tennis, horseback riding, skiing, etc. These are all good in their own way and also serve as distractions and good recreation.

Formal relaxation techniques serve a different purpose and teach you how to deliberately relax your mind and every muscle in your body. The result will often reduce your pain level and also reduce or turn off your alarm system. The following is the most widely used technique I have experienced for pain therapy:

1. Sit or lie in your most comfortable position, using a pillow under the head and knees if lying on your back. Do this alone with no noise or disturbances, if possible.
2. Loosen any tight clothing or belts.
3. Close your eyes.
4. Take five very slow deep breaths. (When the breathing slows down, the entire body will in turn slow down also.) Extend every breath as long as you can.
5. Relax your body. Squeeze every body part as tight as you can; hold for 5 seconds and then relax. Then begin with one body part at a time. Starting with the eyes and working your way all the way down to the feet, hold each muscle contraction and count to 5 seconds. For example, squeeze the eyes tight, then tighter, hold, count to five, and then relax. Next squeeze your lips tight, then tighter, hold, count to five, and then relax. Drop your mouth open. Let it relax. Continue to breathe slowly. Do the shoulders next: shrug them tight, hold, count to five, and relax. Now the arms: tense your arms, tighten hard, hold, count to five, and relax. Clench your hands and fingers, make a tight fist, squeeze tighter, hold, count to five, and relax. Exhale and tighten your abdomen, tighten, count to five, relax, and breathe. Tense your thighs, tighten, count to five, and relax. Tighten your lower legs, hold to a count of five, and relax. Now let your entire body go limp and melt into the surface on which you are resting.
6. This is a good way to relax your mind: Perhaps you would like to envision some place in nature, possibly in the woods where you may have once had a lovely camping trip. Maybe you would prefer to be at the beach listening to the steady sound of the waves lapping over the wet sand. Some people might enjoy picturing themselves on a sailboat, sailing out on a calm bay. Some people may prefer an indoor scene such as a cozy room with a fire crackling in the fireplace. A warm spa with bubbling water might be your preference. Use your imagination and let your mind color this scene as if you were an artist. Put lovely details in your scene. Make it just right, perfectly comfortable, and perfectly beautiful.
7. Now mentally place yourself in this scene. Be sure to totally relax there. You may be basking in the warm sun in this scene. This is your time for you. If worries enter

your mind, let them go. Do not hold on to your thoughts; let them simply come and
go.

8. You have no worries, no fears, only pure relaxation and pleasure. Leave your
worries with God.

9. This is your sanctuary, your retreat. You deserve this special place — enjoy. Try
to visit this place once or twice a day. Enjoy your sanctuary and find peace and quiet
in it.

Some people will find that their pain level will go down. Others may fall asleep. Do not
worry about it if you napped. You truly relaxed. A little catnap can be very refreshing and
give you much needed respite from pain. Others will feel soft and content and maybe find
themselves smiling for no special reason.

A few may still feel restless. You may have a worry or concern that you are unable to put
aside. Do not think you have failed in any way. We all have good days and bad days, peaceful
days and fretful days. Simply try again tomorrow. It usually becomes easier and easier to
relax the more you try. Just take your little mind trips to your special sanctuary. This little
retreat can become your best time of day. You get out of something according to what you
put into it. So please try it; you'll love it.

RECREATION (TO RE-CREATE ONESELF)

When I was at Spalding Rehabilitation Hospital in Denver, Colorado, for 3 weeks in 1985,
I learned many new things about managing my life in chronic pain. One thing in particular,
which I am writing about in this chapter, is the importance of staying happy and scheduling
recreation as part of therapy on the road to good health.

Webster's Dictionary defines recreate as to create anew and to relax and divert oneself. The
definition of recreation is refreshment and relaxation of one's body or mind after work.

How we "recreate" depends on our own personal choices and also our own physical
limitations, but it is a very important therapy for us all. Some people enjoy crafts, oil painting,
embroidery, and other handiwork that can be done sitting down. Some people prefer card
games, scrabble, backgammon, pictionary, checkers, puzzles, etc. One friend in chronic pain
took up the keyboard 6 months ago and has been joyously happy singing and playing for her
own pleasure and occasionally at gatherings. I swim, do oil painting lying down, and have
occasional luncheons and shopping outings with friends. Listening to music is another
beautiful way of recreating. Since finding out what good therapy this is, I have discovered
all kinds of new music, which makes me feel good inside.

Physical activity is important. It gives us enjoyment and keeps our bodies in shape. "If you
don't use it, you lose it." This means if we neglect to use certain body parts, they become
atrophied, which means weak and flabby. Atrophy begins after 48 hours to a very minor
extent, but it is very important to realize that in time you will be out of shape. So we must
try our best to keep our hurting bodies moving, at least on our better days. You may only be
able to take a walk down your hallway, and someone else may be able to ride a bike or go
dancing, but do whatever you can to keep yourself going to whatever degree your pain level
allows you. When we are enjoying ourselves, our right brain secretes endorphins and healthy
substances which help us to heal and make us feel good. Feeling as good as you can, while
in chronic pain, is very important in keeping sadness and depression away.

The evening news can be so distressing as to cause one's pain level to go up. It is important
to surround ourselves with positive and happy people and circumstances as much as possible.

Complaining, critical, negative people can make us feel much worse and even depressed. It is best to avoid such people whenever possible. Every day, make a decision to make it the best day of your life. You will be surprised how fulfilled and happy your life will be even though you are suffering physically.

It is important to not only schedule your doctor appointments but also to schedule your recreation. Mark it down on your calendar and keep that appointment for your own pleasure therapy. You may have been brought up to believe that recreation is self-indulgent and irresponsible; however, you have a responsibility to yourself and those who love you to try to feel good and enjoy life. At first, I felt guilty scheduling my own recreation, but the payoff in emotional happiness has dissolved my guilt. So go for it, have a good time, and love life. Don't forget to bring your mate and healthy friends along for the fun. They will love it, and so will you. Our society is really quite busy and stressed on "overload." If you can find another pain patient as a friend, you can really enjoy your recreation together and understand each other's limitations. Maybe afterward, you can kick back in a hot tub together with a nice cool drink and tell each other some funny jokes.

This certainly does not mean that one cannot discuss problems and try to solve them. Of course this is necessary, but you may want to make a conscious decision not to allow discussion or worry about your problems to interfere with your recreation time. Sometimes during recreation, when a thought or concern worries me, I will either write it down in a notebook to deal with later or let those thoughts pass out of my mind so that I can continue my recreation therapy. Fun feels so good. Why ruin it?

Those of us in chronic pain have good days and bad days, or maybe I should say good days and "bite the bullet" days. For me, bad days are often spent flat on my back staring at the ceiling, listening to the radio or conducting our personal business from my bed. On those days, my recreation would only be listening to good music. It is impossible to have fun when in a flare-up and "biting the bullet." But on those better days, schedule your recreation as best you can. On bad days, don't fight it; try to rest and accept it as best you can. At those times, try to remember there will be better days around the corner.

You are a child of the universe. You have a right to be happy. Take charge of your life and make it a good one. You deserve it.

Finally, I would like to give thanks to my husband, Bruce, who has been there for me night and day all the way through. My illness has brought out nothing but the best in him. He is kinder, more compassionate, and more generous than ever, and he knows he has my heartfelt, undying appreciation. In this appreciation I include my beloved children, especially Adam and Steve, who have gone more than the extra mile for me time and time again. There are also a few friends and relatives who cared and let me know it. As for doctors, there were many who tried for me and helped, such as Dr. Jay D. Law and my brother, Dr. Bert Rettner, but the real star is Dr. Michael Margoles, who has done everything in his power to give me good conscientious treatment with a truly caring heart. As for chiropractors, my son Steven Davis has proven to be by far the best, with endless adjustments at all times of the day or night. My need for adjustments has gone down, as I am doing considerably better. With the help of these two great men, and I might add men of God, I am once again on my feet and happily leading a relatively active life. To my fellow sufferers, I would like to say: Hang in there. There is a light at the end of the tunnel. The best is yet to come, Seize the day. I am still in severe pain, and after 11 years of it, I *am still learning* every day how to make it. If it weren't for my medication, vitamin therapy, and chiropractic care, I'd be flat on my back again. Swimming and walking also help my back, and the spa often gives much needed relief. My pain is worse than most, but I am trying. Won't you, too?

Section VII

Appendix

The American Academy
of Pain Management

The American Academy of Pain Management is the largest society of multidisciplinary pain management professionals in North America. The academy is a nonprofit multidisciplinary society that provides a number of services that benefit the public. The services provided by the American Academy of Pain Management include:

- Multidisciplinary board certification
- Pain program accreditation
- Outcomes Measurement — National Pain Data Bank
- Continuing education

The academy holds full voting membership in the National Organization of Competency Assurance.

Certification by the American Academy of Pain Management is dependent upon criteria related to education and experience. Certified individuals must meet rigorous standards regarding certification. A psychometrically valid test is required. The written examination adheres to "Standards for Educational and Psychometric Testing" and the "Uniformed Guidelines on Employee Selection Procedures." An applicant must demonstrate and provide documentation of experience in pain management and meet other standards established by the American Academy of Pain Management to ascertain professional behavior in pain management.

Certified clinicians must abide by the Code of Professional Conduct and Patient Bill of Rights established by the academy. Continuing education is mandated.

Over 100 pain programs have been accredited by the American Academy of Pain Management. Over 7000 patients are listed in the National Pain Data Bank — Outcomes Measurement System. The National Pain Data Bank collects information on pain management at intake, discharge, and follow-up. The American Academy of Pain Management participates in the AMA Practice Parameter Forum.

HIGHLIGHTS OF ACADEMY ACHIEVEMENTS

- Authored *Innovations in Pain Management: A Practical Guide for Clinicians,* a multivolume textbook on pain management
- Produces the multidisciplinary journal *The American Journal of Pain Management*

1-57444-103-5/99/$0.00+$.50
© 1999 by CRC Press LLC

- Produces two quarterly newsletters, *The Pain Practitioner* and the *Pain Program Standard*
- Conducts an annual conference that attracts approximately 1000 multidisciplinary attendees yearly
- Conducted seven live international satellite teleconferences
- In conjunction with the University of the Pacific, co-sponsors the first accredited graduate program leading to a Certificate of Completion in Pain Studies
- Has a presence on the Internet (Internet address is http://www.aapainmanage.org)

For further information regarding board certification, pain program accreditation, outcomes measurement, or noncertified membership, contact the American Academy of Pain Management at 13947 Mono Way, #A, Sonora, CA 95370 (phone 209-533-9744, fax 209-533-9750, e-mail AAPM@AAPAINMANAGE.ORG).

Index

511